## Forthcoming Monographs in the Series

Bleck:    Orthopaedic Management of Cerebral Palsy

Burgess:    Amputations: Surgical Technique and Postoperative
            Management

Hughston, Walsh and Puddu:    Patellar Subluxation and Dislocation

Nelson and Nelson:    Orthopaedic Infections

Pappas and Akins:    The Child's Hip

Sarmiento and Latta:    Functional Bracing of Fractures

Southwick and Johnson:    Surgical Approaches to the Spine

# METABOLIC
# DISEASES
# OF
# BONE

*by*

## JENIFER JOWSEY, D.Phil.

Director, Orthopaedic Research,
Mayo Clinic and Mayo Foundation,
Rochester, Minnesota

*Volume I in the Series*
## SAUNDERS MONOGRAPHS
## IN CLINICAL ORTHOPAEDICS

*Consulting Editor*
CLEMENT B. SLEDGE, M.D.

1977    W. B. SAUNDERS COMPANY
Philadelphia • London • Toronto

W. B. Saunders Company:   West Washington Square
Philadelphia, PA    19105

1 St. Anne's Road
Eastbourne, East Sussex BN21 3UN, England

1 Goldthorne Avenue
Toronto, Ontario M8Z 5T9, Canada

Metabolic Diseases of Bone                                  ISBN 0-7216-5224-7

Last digit is the print number:    9    8    7    6    5    4    3    2    1

*In honor of*

C. JOWSEY ESQ., I.S.O., O.B.E.

# Foreword

This work by Dr. Jenifer Jowsey marks the beginning of a new series of Monographs in Clinical Orthopaedics. No series could wish for a more auspicious beginning than this scholarly work, *Metabolic Diseases of Bone*.

It is our purpose to present subjects of interest and importance in the field of musculoskeletal disease. The breadth of this field and the diverse sources of new information suggest that there is a need for timely and comprehensive coverage of current concepts, written by authorities who are encouraged to present the "whys" as well as the "hows" of disease and treatment.

It is especially fitting that the first work in this series concerns metabolic bone disease since the philosophy of the series was best expressed by the "Father of Metabolic Bone disease," Fuller Albright,* when he complained that he was "frequently asked in giving a talk to make it 'practical' and not too 'theoretical'. By 'practical' is usually meant 'therapeutic;' by 'theoretical' is usually meant 'fundamental.' The author has no patience with such a philosophy. One cannot possibly practice good medicine and not understand the fundamentals underlying therapy. Few if any rules for therapy are more than 90 per cent correct. If one does not understand the fundamentals, one does more harm in the 10 per cent of instances to which the rules do not apply than one does good in the 90 per cent to which they to apply."

If the sophistication of medicine in general, and of orthopaedics in particular, increases exponentially, it becomes even more difficult to keep abreast of current theories and practice. It is, therefore, our intention to select important broad areas of knowledge and recognized authorities in these areas and give them ample space to express the rationale of treatment as well as the techniques.

In keeping with this philosophy, Dr. Jowsey brings to her subject unique qualifications which have brought her wide recognition as a scientist with strong clinical interests. She received her undergraduate and graduate training at Oxford University, where she obtained her D. Phil. in 1955 under the tutelage of Dame Janet Vaughan. Dame Janet's laboratory in the mid-1950's was a center of exciting new work in bone kinetics and morphology. Armed with the new tool of radioactive isotopes for tracer studies, they developed to a high degree the new techniques of quantitative autoradiography. Dr. Jowsey's patience and keen eye led her to develop the methods of quantitative assessment of bone turnover by measurement of formation and resorption surfaces seen on microradiographs of bone. These techniques, of themselves, might have produced tables and figures of desiccated scientific interests but for Dr. Jowsey's keen insight into the real questions of human biology –

*Albright, Fuller, in Cecil, R. L., and Loeb, R. F.: *Textbook of Medicine* 8th ed. Philadelphia, W. B. Saunders Co., 1951, p. 1217.

the dynamics and pathophysiology of musculoskeletal disease. So, instead of dreary isolated facts, we see beautifully presented the "whys" and "hows" of metabolic bone disease, founding the theme for the series.

Fuller Albright would be pleased.

Clement B. Sledge, M.D.

# PREFACE

In spite of a detailed description of the symptoms of a bone disease with the associated biochemical data, one is unable to understand the disorder and accompanying disease until the bone tissue itself is examined. It is necessary to compare bone tissue from patients who have the same symptoms and the same biochemical abnormalities, indicating that they have the same diseases; the abnormality that is found to be similar in all tissue samples can then be regarded as the bone tissue abnormality in that disease. It must also be always kept in mind that the investigator who is searching for the truth must pay attention to all the details, even if the information is unexpected or vexing. Many of the most exciting developments in investigative medicine have originated from precisely this attitude.

Therefore, it is necessary to understand thoroughly bone as a tissue and bone cell behavior and response in normal bone and diseased bone. This permits a flexibility of thinking which is not otherwise possible. Such is the purpose of this book.

There are a number of books on various aspects of the material presented here which cover the ground in more detail, such as that on bone histology by Hancox,[1] on metabolic bone and stone disease by Nordin,[2] and on bone pathology by Collins.[3] The present volume describes the histology of normal bone, the pathology, the clinical picture, and the biochemical findings of bone disease. In addition, the methods of observing the skeleton are described, since without some knowledge of how the information is derived it is unreasonable to expect proper evaluation of the data.

The book is divided, therefore, into three parts. The first part deals with mineral metabolism and the structure of bone; the second part deals with the methods of examining bone and of quantitatively measuring certain parameters of bone and of hormones which affect bone; and the third section is concerned with bone disease.

The length of this book would be considerably increased if I were to write the names of all the people to whom I owe gratitude, not only for assisting in my career in research but also in the preparation of this book. However, there are some to whom I owe special thanks. For generosity in my education, my father and mother, and I cannot pass this point and not recall with great affection my sister. Without the encouragement of that generous person, Dame Janet Vaughan, my career may never have begun, and without the British–American Cancer Society and the help of Dr. Franklin C. McLean I would not have had the chance to come to the Land of Opportunity and continue my research. A significant amount of the work presented here was supported by a federal grant from the National Institutes of Health, AMO 8658. At the Mayo Clinic I have enjoyed the collaboration of many medical colleagues, in particular Dr P I Kelly and Dr. B. L. Riggs, and have found a pleasant sanctuary in the Orthopaedic Department with a special regard for Dr.

ix

M. B. Coventry. From day to day and week to week my job, and the writing of this book, have been made both possible and pleasant by the technical personnel of the Orthopaedic Research Department, perhaps the most loyal and helpful group I have ever had the pleasure to work with; special thanks in the preparation of this manuscript go to Mrs. Joan Toensing and Mrs. Randi Carlson. Finally, it would be remiss of me indeed not to mention my own family, Fen, Pamela, and John, who have regarded my book writing efforts with respect.

## *REFERENCES*

1. Hancox, N. M.: Biology of Bone. Cambridge, Cambridge University Press, 1972.
2. Nordin, B. E. C.: Metabolic Bone and Stone Disease. Baltimore, Williams and Wilkins Co., 1973.
3. Collins, D. H.: Pathology of Bone. London, Butterworth and Company, Ltd., 1966.

# Contents

**Part I**
**MINERAL METABOLISM AND BONE MORPHOLOGY**..........................................  1

*Chapter One*
MINERAL METABOLISM: CALCIUM  .......................................................  3

*Chapter Two*
MINERAL METABOLISM: PHOSPHORUS ...................................................  11

*Chapter Three*
MINERAL METABOLISM: ALKALINE PHOSPHATASE ............................  16

*Chapter Four*
MINERAL METABOLISM: MAGNESIUM....................................................  19

*Chapter Five*
MINERAL METABOLISM: PARATHYROID HORMONE............................  23

*Chapter Six*
MINERAL METABOLISM: VITAMIN D  ...................................................  31

*Chapter Seven*
MINERAL METABOLISM: CALCITONIN  ...................................................  35

*Chapter Eight*
BONE MORPHOLOGY: BONE STRUCTURE.................................................  41

*Chapter Nine*
BONE MORPHOLOGY: BONE TISSUE .......................................................  48

*Chapter Ten*

BONE MORPHOLOGY: BONE CELLS ............................................................ 58

*Chapter Eleven*

BONE MORPHOLOGY: TYPES OF BONE TISSUE ...................................... 78

**Part II**

**METHODS OF EVALUATION**.......................................................................... 85

*Chapter Twelve*

CALCIUM BALANCE ...................................................................................... 87

*Chapter Thirteen*

BONE DENSITY MEASUREMENTS ............................................................. 96

*Chapter Fourteen*

RADIOISOTOPE METHODS ......................................................................... 115

*Chapter Fifteen*

BONE GROWTH MARKERS ......................................................................... 124

*Chapter Sixteen*

AUTORADIOGRAPHY .................................................................................. 127

*Chapter Seventeen*

MORPHOLOGY .............................................................................................. 138

*Chapter Eighteen*

ORGAN AND TISSUE CULTURE ............................................................... 157

**Part III**

**METABOLIC BONE DISEASE**...................................................................... 161

*Chapter Nineteen*

PAGET'S DISEASE OF BONE ..................................................................... 163

*Chapter Twenty*

OSTEOPETROSIS............................................................................................ 172

*Chapter Twenty-One*
OSTEOGENESIS IMPERFECTA ..................................................................... 186

*Chapter Twenty-Two*
RICKETS AND OSTEOMALACIA ............................................................. 192

*Chapter Twenty-Three*
UNUSUAL FORMS OF OSTEOMALACIA ...................................................... 205

*Chapter Twenty-Four*
THYROID BONE DISEASE ......................................................................... 215

*Chapter Twenty-Five*
ACROMEGALY.......................................................................................... 219

*Chapter Twenty-Six*
HYPERCORTISONISM ............................................................................... 224

*Chapter Twenty-Seven*
HYPERPARATHYROIDISM.......................................................................... 229

*Chapter Twenty-Eight*
OSTEOPOROSIS: JUVENILE ...................................................................... 248

*Chapter Twenty-Nine*
OSTEOPOROSIS: IDIOPATHIC, POST-MENOPAUSAL, AND SENILE ......... 256

*Chapter Thirty*
THE TREATMENT OF OSTEOPOROSIS ....................................................... 296

**Index**.................................................................................................... 304

Part I

# Mineral Metabolism and Bone Morphology

# Chapter One

# MINERAL METABOLISM: CALCIUM

## GENERAL COMMENTS

The ion calcium is necessary for a number of essential physiologic processes. Calcium is abundant in sea water, where life is assumed to have originated.[1] However, the concentration of calcium in both marine animals and in man is less than that of sea water; this difference suggests that calcium had to be excreted or secreted by primitive marine animals, possibly in the form of a calcium-salt exoskeleton. Sodium parallels calcium in these respects and is also a physiologically important ion. However, calcium is not as abundant as sodium in the extramarine environment, and so, once out of the sea, animals evolved mechanisms to conserve calcium and devised the endoskeleton, which doubled as a supporting structure and a store of calcium (Table 1–1). Just as the exoskeleton may have originated primarily as a calcium excretion pool and secondarily (and fairly inefficiently) as a protective device, the vertebrate skeleton serves primarily as a supply of calcium should external sources fail, and secondarily as a means of support that became necessary when animals left the buoyant ocean for an existence on land and in air.

**Table 1–1**  CALCIUM CONCENTRATIONS IN WATER, FISH, AND MAN

|  |  | mg/dl |
| --- | --- | --- |
| Pacific Ocean water | = | 40 |
| Brackish water | = | 8–20 |
| Fresh water | = | 3.6 |
| Shark serum | = | 18 |
| Marine teleost serum | = | 15.4 |
| Freshwater teleost serum | = | 10.6 |
| Human serum | = | 9.28 |

From Love[2] and Copp.[3]

## THE ROLE OF THE SKELETON

In addition to acquiring a store of calcium, terrestrial animals had to develop a means of controlling this store and making it available when necessary. This led to the development of calcitonin, vitamin D, and, eventually, parathyroid hormone control of mineral metabolism, involving the gut, skeleton, and renal control of the movement of calcium ions into and out of the body and from bone to serum.

Calcium, with phosphate, accounts for the hardness of bone tissue and its ability to remain rigid. However, the extraskeletal role of calcium is more vital; calcium plays an essential role in blood coagulation as a cofactor in the conversion of prothrombin to thrombin. However, levels of calcium have to fall very low before impairment of the coagulation process becomes significant.

At less depressed calcium levels, neuromuscular excitability is affected; the myoneural function is exquisitely sensitive to small changes in ionized calcium concentrations, and depletion of calcium rapidly results in muscular weakness, tetany, and eventually convulsions, if the calcium is low enough to permit depolarization and central nervous system malfunction. Calcium is also an essential element in membrane transport and enzyme regulation and most peptide hormones are regulated by the adenyl cyclase system, which depends on calcium for stimulation.

The overwhelming majority (99.0 per cent) of the body calcium is in the skeleton. Of the remaining 1 per cent, 5g is in the extracellular fluid and is in equilibrium with the bone mineral by rapid or slow exchange processes. Although calcium enters the body through the gastrointestinal system and leaves by the kidney, the major source of calcium in the event that intake is inadvertently restricted, is bone. It is the goal of the elaborate mechanisms that have evolved and that affect bone metabolism to maintain a constant serum calcium level for the maintenance of proper physiologic function. This is achieved by a sensitive system that tends to prevent the development of high serum calcium levels when the serum phosphorus is elevated as well as preventing hypocalcemia. It is of interest that practically all hormones in the body are involved in calcium metabolism in some way; because of this, most abnormalities of hormone function result in bone disease or abnormalities in bone structure. This is to be expected of hormones such as parathyroid hormone and vitamin D, which have a specific function in calcium homeostasis, but it is also true of others, such as estrogens, thyroxine, and adrenal hormones.

## CALCIUM HOMEOSTASIS

All calcium that enters the body does so normally via the gastrointestinal system, and the amount is controlled by dietary intake and absorption. Dietary intake varies a great deal, mainly in relation to milk consumption. In the United States, the average intake is 650 mg per day. Of this, approximately 30 per cent is absorbed (250 mg) and 400 mg remains in the gut. Although maximum calcium absorption occurs in the stomach and duodenum, there is also significant absorption in the ileum. In the small intestine there is a continuous influx (endsorption) and efflux (exsorption) of calcium so that exchange of endogenous and exogenous calcium does occur beyond the stomach. However, the net amount of calcium absorbed depends mainly on the amount ingested in the diet and is proportional to that amount. The proportion absorbed depends on a number of factors; the most important one is vitamin D, which is specifically responsible for absorption of this ion. However, even under optimal conditions, calcium absorption rarely exceeds 40 per cent. The presence of steatorrhea, sprue, high levels of complexing substances such as phytates, or absence of part of the gut will diminish calcium absorption.

The kidney has perhaps a greater control normally, over calcium influx and efflux. Approximately 10 g of calcium is filtered by the kidney every day in a normal adult man, and the majority can be secreted by the kidney under certain conditions. However, in a physiologically normal situation 97 to 99 per cent is reabsorbed and only 1 to 3 per cent, or 100 to 300 mg, finds its way into the urine every day. If the serum calcium is raised, for example by a high calcium and vitamin D intake, the filtered load increases and the daily urinary calcium level increases. On the other hand, serum parathyroid hormone acts on the kidney to increase the amount of reabsorbed calcium and to decrease urinary calcium.

Although direct measurements are impossible, indirect techniques, notably radioisotope kinetic studies, have indicated that about 350 mg of calcium per day is added to or removed from bone by the mechanisms of exchange and bone remodelling. This is about twice the urinary excretion, which, in turn, is greater than the amount of calcium absorbed from a normal dietary intake. Thus the blood-to-bone flux is greater than the input and output of calcium from the body; this allows fluctuations in the latter to be balanced by alterations in the blood-to-bone flux. For example, during a period of starvation, the level of calcium intake will be zero and acidosis will increase urinary calcium excretion. In spite of these two factors, which will tend to lower serum calcium, precise homeostatic control is achieved by decreasing the calcium leaving the blood and going to the skeleton; after a short time bone resorption will also increase the amount of calcium leaving the skeleton for the blood.

In an adult man, urinary calcium excretion generally exceeds absorption by approximately 50 to 100 mg of calcium per day. If 10 per cent of body weight is bone and about 25 per cent of the weight of bone is calcium, the average person's skeleton contains 1500 g of calcium. If this rate of loss occurs over a thirty-year period, approximately one-half to two-thirds of the skeleton may be expected to be lost. In osteopenic bone disease, the rate of loss would be expected to be greater.

The minimal daily requirement of calcium has been stated as being 800 mg per day; however, more than 1.1g of dietary calcium is needed by the average person to maintain a zero or slightly positive calcium balance producing a physiologic situation where loss of calcium would not be occurring.

## SERUM CALCIUM

In man, the calcium in the serum is found in the following three forms: 3.5 mg is bound to protein; 1.5 mg is complexed with ions, mainly citrate; and 5.5 mg is in an ionized form. Summation of these values gives a total serum calcium of 10.5 mg, which is somewhat high and represents postprandial values. Fasting morning measurements would be slightly lower in all three categories (Table 1–2). The protein-bound form is an obligatory association, and this calcium is not available for physiologic functions, for which the ionic free calcium is responsible; this is also true for complexed calcium. The free, ionized calcium is the physiologically active ion and is responsible for muscle contraction, blood clotting, mineralization of ma-

**Table 1–2**   THE PARTITION OF CALCIUM IN THE SERUM
(values are mg/dl)

| | | | |
|---|---|---|---|
| | Globulin, 0.64 ⎱<br>Albumin, 2.44 ⎰ | Nondiffusible, 3.08 ⎱ | |
| | Ionized calcium, 5.0 ⎱ | | Total calcium, 9.2 |
| Bicarbonate, 0.6 ⎱<br>Phosphorus, 0.2 ⎰<br>Citrate, 0.3<br>Other ? | Complexes, 1.13 | Diffusible, 6.13 ⎰ | |

trix, and so on. This was shown by early experiments, using the frog heart method, in which the amplitude of the contraction was found to be related to the ionized calcium concentration, which demonstrated that calcium bound to protein or citrate did not alter the muscle response.[4] It is therefore physiologically most relevant to measure ionized calcium levels, since it is the ionized calcium that stimulates or suppresses the secretion of parathyroid hormone, thus producing a feedback system by which serum calcium levels are maintained at the expense of parathyroid hormone-induced bone resorption. However, ionized calcium is difficult to measure, and total serum calcium is therefore the value most often reported and is meaningful because the proportion of ionized to bound calcium is relatively constant. Therefore, by and large, changes in total serum calcium will reflect changes in ionized calcium; the two most common exceptions occur when there are fluctuations in serum phosphorus or in serum albumin. Serum phosphorus will rise or fall largely as a result of oral ingestion of this element, although it may also, of course, vary with renal or hormonal aberrations; ionized calcium will vary inversely with the serum phosphorus. Dehydration is probably the most frequent cause of abnormal levels of serum proteins; when the protein concentration is high, total calcium is high, but ionized calcium may be normal or decrease. Postural changes and venous occlusion during serum sampling may also cause changes in the protein-bound calcium fraction.[5] Since serum phosphate can be measured and the protein concentration can be evaluated simply by measuring the specific gravity using copper sulfate solutions,[5] a correction can be made, and even in these circumstances total serum calcium is physiologically meaningful.

## METHODS OF MEASUREMENT OF SERUM CALCIUM

Early methods developed to measure total serum calcium involved the precipitation of calcium as the oxalate by adding oxalic acid to the serum sample.[6] Hydrochloric acid is mixed with a recrystallized precipitate and excess acid titrated against sodium hydroxide in the presence of an indicator such as methyl red. The method is valid in the presence of large amounts of magnesium and phosphorus, and it is accurate. However, it is also cumbersome and has been succeeded by methods that involve binding of the calcium by strong complexing agents.

Ethylenediamine tetra-acetic acid (EDTA) will complex calcium from serum, and in an alkaline solution the indicator Eriochrome blue SE can be used and the end point read by a spectrophotometer. The procedure is automatic in that the speed of delivery of the titrating reagent (EDTA) is determined by a motor, and the color change is recorded photoelectrically on a moving chart; the only manual procedure is the measurement of the intercept of the curve, which is related to the amount of calcium in the solution.[7] As in the early oxalate method, magnesium and phosphorus are not important interfering elements in methods using complexing agents.

As orginally described, the method used relatively large volumes of serum, generally 1 ml. However, 0.1 or 0.2 ml volumes have been used with less than 1 per cent variance reported.[8, 9] More recently, GBHA has been used as the complexing agent. Glyoxal bis (2–hydroxyanil) (GBHA) complexes with calcium in an alkali solution to give a chloroform-extractable deep pink color that can be measured on a spectrophotometer.[10] Protein apparently does not interfere, and magnesium will only influence the results at high concentrations — some six times that of the calcium concentration. Amounts of calcium less than 0.2 $\mu$gm will give a positive recordable value with this method.

Atomic absorption spectrophotometry is probably the most commonly used method at this time, largely because it is rapid and can be accurate if care is taken. The major problem is with contamination of the sample by calcium in the tubes and stoppers; this difficulty is not unique to atomic absorption methods but becomes significant in all techniques utilizing small samples.[11] Atomic absorption spectrophotometry will measure all the calcium in the sample because the procedure of burning the element in a flame results in dissociation of any complex. This is in contrast to the EDTA methods, in which calcium, already complexed to a chelate as strong as or stronger than EDTA, will be "invisible." Occasionally, EDTA infusions have been used in an attempt to evaluate the ability of the body to respond to calcium deprivation. In such instances, an EDTA titration method would reflect the calcium remaining over and above that complexed with the infused EDTA, and the results will be different from those measured by means of atomic absorption spectrophotometry.

The first successful approach to the measurement of ionized calcium was the frog heart method of McLean and Hastings.[4] Ultrafilterable calcium is probably somewhat more reliable, but it measures complexed calcium in addition to ionized calcium.[12] Since the complexed calcium represents a relatively small proportion and is reasonably constant except when citrate levels vary, ultrafilterable calcium is a good measure of ionized, or physiologically available, calcium.[13] The proteins are filtered off with their associated calcium, and the remaining calcium is measured in a neutral solution with murexide as an indicator.

The flow-through ion-specific electrodes are now the preferred instruments, although it cannot be assumed that they are free from problems. Since pH is a major factor influencing the fraction of calcium which is ionized, the major concern is to prevent $CO_2$ loss (Table 1–3). The blood is drawn anaerobically by vacucontainer and spun down immediately after clotting. The serum is then drawn into an insulin syringe and mounted on the gear-driven pump; then the determination is made. In some investigators' experience, storage of the specimen in insulin syringes with no attempt at re-equilibration produces the most repeatable results.[14]

Leaving the specimens at room temperature results in a fall in ionized calcium, and in some laboratories keeping the specimens in ice cold saline or even frozen is considered unreliable. Recently a solid-state, specific dip electrode for calcium ion has been reported and appears to be reliable.[15]

**Table 1–3   VARIATION IN IONIZED CALCIUM RESULTING FROM DIFFERENT STORAGE PROCEDURES**

| Sample | Storage | Equilibrated | $Ca^{2+}$ mg./dl. | pH |
|---|---|---|---|---|
| 1 | None | — | 4.37 | 7.43 |
| 2 | None | — | 4.64 | 7.38 |
| 2 | Frozen in oil | None | 4.36 | 7.55 |
| 3 | None | — | 4.94 | 7.41 |
| 3 | Frozen (no oil) | Yes | 5.30 | 7.43 |
| 4 | None | — | 4.95 | 7.44 |
| 4 | Frozen (no oil) 1 day | None | 4.92 | 7.46 |
| 5 | Frozen (no oil) 3 days | — | 4.80 | 7.43 |
| 5 | None | None | 4.80 | 7.45 |

From Subryan et al.[14]

It is important to remember to draw blood without stasis; constriction of tissue around the vein causes false serum calcium values. Serum or plasma calcium values vary from one laboratory to another, depending largely on the technique. Any value quoted should be accompanied by the normal range for the laboratory in which the measurement was made. For example, at the Mayo Clinic the normal range is 8.9 to 10.1 mg/dl, which is similar to the figures of 9.0 to 10.2 mg/dl from the University College Hospital, London;[16] but in the Walter Reed Army Hospital the normal range is 8.2 to 10.1 mg/dl.[17] Variations also exist for ionized calcium measurements; at the Mayo Clinic the normal range is 3.35 to 5.05 mg/dl, while at Walter Reed it is 4.5 to 5.2 mg/dl. The variation in the normal range has significance only in what is considered abnormal; in addition, it is obvious that there would be grounds for believing that some individuals at the extremes of the normal range are not normal.

The last point raises the question of the meaning of the variation within the normal range. The average physician will frequently report values as within normal levels (WNL), regarding a value of 8.9 mg/dl as normal as one of 9.8 mg/dl. Although there is little data to convince anyone to the contrary, it is conceivable that

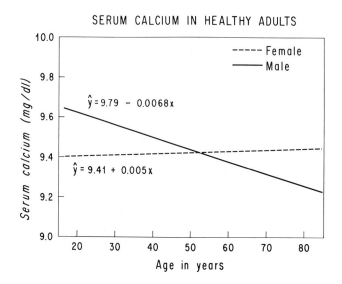

**SERUM CALCIUM IN HEALTHY ADULTS**

$\hat{y} = 9.79 - 0.0068x$

$\hat{y} = 9.41 + 0.005x$

Serum calcium (mg/dl)

Age in years

**Figure 1–1**   The serum calcium in males decreases with age increase in contrast to the slight rise in females. (Redrawn from Keating et al.[15])

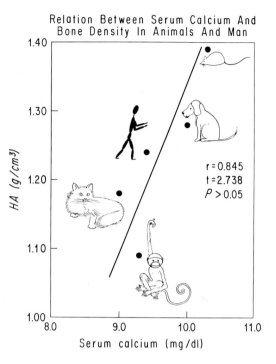

Relation Between Serum Calcium And Bone Density In Animals And Man

r = 0.845
t = 2.738
P > 0.05

HA (g/cm³)

Serum calcium (mg/dl)

**Figure 1–2** The relationship between the density of hydroxyapatite (HA) and the serum calcium level in man and different animals. The positive correlation suggests that the higher serum calcium and perhaps phosphorus are producing a more complete apatite crystal or possibly a higher density of crystals at the expense of non-mineral material.

values within normal levels have significance if they are far from the mean. For example, a study of serum calcium and phosphorus in normal men and women showed that the serum calcium remains constant with age in women but decreases in men[18] (Fig. 1–1). Later studies revealed a relationship between estrogens, parathyroid hormone, and bone resorption which explained the data.

In children the total serum calcium values have been reported as being high or normal compared with adults. The high values were from United States citizens, who can be expected to be consuming significant volumes of vitamin D-enriched milk[19] while the normal values were from London children,[16] where vitamin D is not added to the milk. There are also significant differences in normal calcium values in different animals; for example, the average normal serum calcium of an adult rabbit is 16 mg/dl., a larger percent being bound to citrate than in man. The serum calcium appears to influence the mineral density of bone; in any event there is a correlation between serum calcium and the average mineral density of the bone (Fig. 1–2).

## NON-SERUM CALCIUM

There is considerable interest in the movement of calcium into and out of cells, and it is tempting to speculate that the Aequorin luminescent reaction with calcium could be useful.[20] The problem is to get sufficient material through the hard cell membrane of cells such as osteoclasts and osteoblasts, and there is always the initial difficulty of obtaining preparations of any type of bone cell for study that is behaving like an osteoclast or osteoblast and has not reverted to a fibroblast.

## REFERENCES

1. Neuman, W. F., and Neuman, M. W.: In the beginning there was apatite. In Zipkin, I. (Ed.): Biological Mineralization. New York, John Wiley & Sons, 1973, pp. 3–19.
2. Love, R. M.: The Chemical Biology of Fishes. London, Academic Press, 1970, p. 114.
3. Copp, D. H.: The Ultimobranchial Glands and Calcium Regulation. In Fish Physiology. W. S. Hoar, and D. S. Randall (Eds.). New York, Academic Press, 1969, Vol. 2, pp. 377–398.

*Serum Calcium*
4. McLean, F. C., and Hastings, A. B.: The state of calcium in the fluids of the body. I. The conditions affecting the ionization of calcium. J. Biol. Chem., *108*:285–322, 1935.
5. Phillips, R. A., van Slyke, D. D., Hamilton, P. B., Dole, V. P., Emerson, K., Jr., and Archibald, R. M.: Measurements of specific gravities of whole blood and plasma by standard copper sulphate solutions. J. Biol. Chem., *183*:305–330, 1950.
6. Fiske, C. H., and Logan, M. A.: The determination of calcium by alkalimetric titration II. The precipitation of calcium in the presence of magnesium, phosphate, and sulfate with applications to the analysis of urine. J. Biol. Chem., *93*:211–226, 1931.
7. Jones, J. D., and McGuckin, W. F.: Complexometric titration of calcium and magnesium by a semi-automated procedure. Clin. Chem., *10*:767–780, 1964.
8. Copp, D. H.: Simple and precise micromethod for EDTA titration of calcium. J. Lab. Clin. Med., *61*:1029–1037, 1963.
9. Hargis, G. K., Sidwell, C. G., Jackson, B. L., and Williams, G. A.: An ultramicromethod for serum calcium determination. Am. J. Clin. Pathol., *52*:773–775, 1969.
10. Kuczerpa, A. V.: A rapid ultramicro method with an enhanced stability and range for the photometric determination of calcium using glyoxal bis (2-hydroxyanil). Anal. Chem., *40*:581–585, 1968.
11. Parsons, J. A., Dawson, B., Callahan, E., and Potts, J. T.: A method for the analysis of phosphate and calcium in small samples of plasma by atomic absorption spectrophotometry. Biochem. J., *119*:791–793, 1970.
12. Rose, G. A.: Determination of the ionized and ultrafilterable calcium of normal human plasma. Clin. Chim. Acta., *2*:227–236, 1957.
13. Terepka, A. R., Toribara, T. Y., and Dewey, P. A.: The ultrafilterable calcium of human sera. II. Variations in disease states and under experimental conditions. J. Clin. Invest., *37*:87–98, 1958.
14. Subryan, V. L., Popovtzer, M. M., Parks, S. D., and Reeve, E. B.: Measurement of serum ionized calcium with the ion-exchange. Clin. Chem., *18*:1459–1462, 1972.
15. Schwartz, H. D.: Serum ionized calcium by electrodes; new technology and methodology. Clin. Chim. Acta., *64*:227–239, 1975.
16. Round, J. M.: Plasma calcium, magnesium, phosphorus and alkaline phosphatase levels in normal British schoolchildren. Brit. Med. J., *3*:137–140, 1973.
17. Heath, H., III, Earll, J. M., Schaaf, M., Piechocki, J. T., and Li, T. K.: Serum ionized calcium during bed rest in fracture patients and normal men. Metabolism, *21*:633–640, 1972.
18. Keating, F. R., Jr., Jones, J. D., Elveback, I. R., and Randall, R. V.: The relation of age and sex to distribution of values in healthy adults of serum calcium, inorganic phosphorus, magnesium, alkaline phosphatase, total proteins, albumin and blood urea. J. Lab. Clin. Med., *73*:825–834, 1969.
19. Arnaud, S. B., Goldsmith, R. S., Stickler, G. B., McCall, J. T., and Arnaud, C. D.: Serum parathyroid hormone and blood minerals: interrelations in normal children. Pediatr. Res., *7*:485–493, 1973.
20. Johnson, F. H., and Shimomura, O.: Preparation and use of aequorin for rapid microdetermination of $Ca^{2+}$ in biological systems. Nature (New Biol.), *237*:287–288, 1972.

# Chapter Two

# MINERAL METABOLISM: PHOSPHORUS

## GENERAL COMMENTS

Phosphorus is the fuel supply of the body as well as an intimate part of its structure. It is abundant, and large fluctuations in serum phosphorus are physiologically tolerable; perhaps for this reason there is little control of the phosphorus level in the blood and little control of the amount absorbed from the diet. In contrast to calcium, in which ingestion of this ion results in only a small postprandial rise in serum calcium, large oral loads of phosphorus may result in postprandial rises in serum phosphorus of up to two-fold and beyond. Since blood passes through the kidney at a rate equal to twice the complete blood volume per day, there is adequate opportunity to remove the excess. Excess is that amount causing the serum phosphorus to be greater than normal, and having the added complication of combining with normal levels of calcium in the serum; if the calcium times phosphorus product is exceeded, there will be precipitation of calcium phosphate in the soft tissues.

## CONTROL OF PHOSPHORUS

Parathyroid hormone and calcitonin both lower the serum phosphorus, parathyroid hormone more effectively, by increasing the renal excretion of this ion. Since this hormone also causes release of bone mineral from the skeleton, the serum phosphorus reflects the sum of phosphorus coming from the skeleton and the effect on increased renal excretion. The renal excretion of phosphorus also reflects the filtered load, which will reflect oral intake; individuals receiving phosphate supplements, therefore, can be expected to show a urinary phosphorus level which closely resembles the dietary level. However, on a normal dietary intake of phosphorus the tubular reabsorption of phosphorus (%TRP) is generally over 80 per cent in normal individuals; abnormal parathyroid function is reflected in a decrease in %TRP below this level or by an absolute decrease in the TmP/GFR, the ratio of the tubular maximum for phosphorus (TmP) divided by the glomerular filtration rate (GFR).

## SERUM PHOSPHORUS

The level of phosphorus in the serum probably has a far greater impact on mineral metabolism than the serum calcium level. Although it is the ionized calcium that influences serum parathyroid hormone secretion, numerically quite small changes in serum phosphorus result in large fluctuations in ionized calcium. It is therefore not surprising, perhaps, to find that the most severe bone disease can develop rapidly when hyperphosphatemia occurs, such as in renal failure. Despite the importance of serum phosphate levels, these are often not measured in investigational studies of mineral metabolism, and yet, if there are no measurements of ionized calcium, the total serum calcium is relatively meaningless physiologically without an accompanying serum phosphorus, if this is abnormal.

By comparison with calcium, phosphorus is relatively simply distributed in the serum. There is almost no phosphorus bound to protein ( <10 per cent), and the majority is all ionized and filterable. Inorganic phosphate exists as $H_2PO_4^-$, $HPO_4^=$ and $PO_4^=$, the majority, (80 per cent) being $HPO_4^=$, with negligible amounts as $PO_4$ (Table 2-1).[1]

Two other features contrast phosphate with calcium and have practical implications. Serum calcium values vary comparatively little in normal individuals, probably because of the efficient feed-back system of the parathyroid. The total variation in normal man, including infants, is about 15 per cent. In contrast, the serum phosphorus may be as low as 2.5 mg/dl in an infant, a variation of 61 per cent. The same is true of the variations in different animal species; phosphorus values have a clearly larger range, again perhaps because there is no closely controlling feed-back system, as there is for calcium (Table 2-2). Of more technical importance is the low soft-tissue content of calcium in comparison with the high phosphorus content. The phosphorus content in most tissues is relatively high, since this element is a constituent of cells, membranes, cell enzymes, and so forth. It follows therefore that a sample of serum left in contact with the clot will gradually increase in phosphorus content with time; serum or plasma should be drawn off the cells as soon as the blood sample is spun down in the centrifuge.

In children both serum calcium and, particularly, phosphorus tend to be higher than in adults; perhaps this represents a physiologic adaptation to the greater demands for both calcium and phosphorus in the rapidly metabolizing and minera-

**Table 2-1**   THE DISTRIBUTION OF PHOSPHORUS IN WHOLE BLOOD
AND SERUM (range expressed in mg/dl × 10)

|  | Whole blood | Plasma or serum |
|---|---|---|
| Total | 28–48 | 10–14 |
| Inorganic | 2.1–3.1 | 2.2–4.4 |
| Organic | 19–29 | 0–4.0 |
| Lipid | 8–18 | 6.1–9.9 |
| Adenosine triphosphate | 5.1–10.4 | — |
| Diphosphoglycerate | 8.1–16.7 | — |
| Nucleotide | 2.2–3.4 | — |
| Hexose phosphate | 1.4–5 | — |

From Marshall and Nordin.[1]

**Table 2–2** SERUM CALCIUM AND PHOSPHORUS IN MAN AND DIFFERENT ANIMALS

|        | Ca mg/dl | | $P_i$ mg/dl | |
|--------|------|-----|------|-----|
|        | mean | SD  | mean | SD  |
| Man    | 9.4  | 0.4 | 3.4  | 0.4 |
| Monkey | 9.3  | 0.6 | 4.2  | 1.1 |
| Dog    | 10.0 | 0.8 | 4.5  | 0.9 |
| Cat    | 9.0  | 0.6 | 6.1  | 1.4 |
| Rabbit | 14.7 | 1.1 | 5.5  | 1.2 |
| Rat    | 10.3 | 0.5 | 10.2 | 0.9 |

lizing skeleton of the child, who is increasing bone mass. Perhaps as a corollary to this or perhaps merely as a result of the high serum calcium and phosphorus values, the osteoid border widths in children are lower than in adults. In the adult both serum calcium and phosphorus values are lower. By comparison with the elevations that are seen in renal failure or other bone diseases, the changes are small, but they are nevertheless significant clinically. For instance, an adult with a serum phosphorus of 5.2 mg/dl must be considered as hyperphosphatemic, while such a value in a child is normal (Table 2–3).

Above the age of 20 variations also exist with age and sex. In males the values fall steadily from a mean of 3.5 mg/dl to 2.8 mg/dl at age 75. This is in contrast to females, who, at age 20, have approximately the same values as males, but, as age increases, tend to rise to a value of 3.8 mg/dl (Fig. 2–1). This may reflect the withdrawal of the estrogen barrier in women, which permits parathyroid-induced bone resorption to increase and allow more bone calcium and phosphorus to enter the blood. It is also possible that mild renal failure with advancing age contributes in some part to the serum phosphorus elevation, although why this should occur in women more frequently than in men is unexplained.

**Table 2–3** SERUM PHOSPHORUS IN NORMAL AND DISEASE STATES

|              | Age (years) | Sex | n | Serum P, mg/dl (mean ± SD) |
|--------------|-------------|-----|-----|----------------------------|
| CHILDREN     |             |     |     |                            |
| Control*     | 2–8         | M   | 19  | 5.7 ± 0.9                  |
|              |             | F   | 20  | 5.3 ± 0.4                  |
|              | 8–16        | M   | 29  | 5.1 ± 0.8                  |
|              |             | F   | 28  | 4.9 ± 0.6                  |
|              | 16–20       | M   | 9   | 4.5 ± 0.8                  |
|              |             | F   | 9   | 4.3 ± 0.6                  |
| ADULTS       |             |     |     |                            |
| Control**    |             | M & F | 433 | 3.34 ± 0.50              |
| Renal failure*** |         | M   | 10  | 8.2 ± 1.2                  |
| Hypoparathyroidism |       | F   | 6   | 4.8 ± 1.7                  |

*From Arnaud et al.[2]
**From Keating et al.[3]
***From Mirahmadi et al.[4]

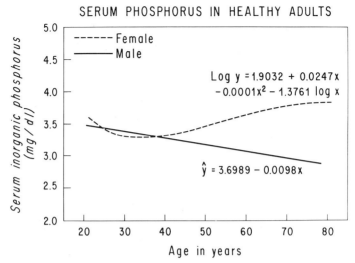

**Figure 2–1**   Variation in serum phosphorus with age in normal healthy males and females. The serum phosphorus tends to rise with age in females but not in males. (Redrawn from Keating et al.[5])

### Methods of Measurement of Serum Phosphorus

The standard method for serum phosphorus determination depends on the formation of a complex between phosphate and molybdate after trichloracetic (TCA) acid precipitation. The complex is then quantitated colorimetrically.[5, 6, 7] A variation which produces reliable results excludes the TCA precipitate and filterable step with little interference by other serum ions, such as citrates, fluorides, and so on.[8] An alternative method for non-deproteinized serum is useful, particularly in animal blood where there are large concentrations of amylase versus triosephosphate. Glycerate-1, 3-diphosphate is formed and measured colorimetrically.[9] The advantage over the protein-precipitation methods is that samples of serum as small as $20\mu$l. are adequate, and the results are accurate in the presence of amylase.

Atomic absorption spectrophotometric methods can also be used, with the advantage that calcium can be analyzed in the same sample. The addition of calcium or phosphorus to the samples has no effect on the phosphorus or calcium standards, respectively, indicating lack of interference.[10]

### CALCIUM AND PHOSPHORUS PRODUCT

It is rarely useful to look at the product of calcium and phosphorus in the serum, since, for mineralization of bone, both calcium and phosphorus must be present in relatively normal amounts. Also the product ($P_i$ 3.5 $\times$ Ca 9.4) of 33 may be as low as 23 or as high as 46, without any effect on new bone mineralization, or, in many instances, with little physiologically significant change in ionized calcium. However, it is occasionally helpful. For instance, in mild hypophosphatemia in combination with a normal or only slightly elevated serum calcium, a failure of mineralization may occur which is not present if there is frank hypercalcemia. It is obvious also that relatively small fluctuations in phosphorus will have greater impact on the product than will changes in calcium level.

Perhaps the most important consideration in the calcium-phosphorus product is soft tissue mineralization, which is particularly prone to occur when the serum phosphorus is elevated, as in renal failure.

### REFERENCES

1. Marshall, R. W., and Nordin, B. E. C.: The state of inorganic phosphate in plasma and its relation to other ions. In Hioco, D. J. (Ed.): *Phosphate et Metabolisme Phosphocalcique Regulation Normale et Aspects Physiopathologiques:* Symposium International. Paris, Laboratoires Sandoz, 1971, pp. 127–138.
2. Arnaud, S. B., Goldsmith, R. S., Stickler, G. B., McCall, J. T., and Arnaud, C. D.: Serum parathyroid hormone and blood minerals: interrelationships in normal children. Pediatr. Res., 7:485–493, 1973.
3. Keating, F. R., Jr., Jones, J. D., Elveback, L. R., and Randall, R. V.: The relation of age and sex to distribution of values in healthy adults of serum calcium, inorganic phosphorus, magnesium, alkaline phosphatase, total proteins, albumin, and blood urea. J. Lab. Clin. Med., 73:825–834, 1969.
4. Mirahmadi, K. S., Duffy, B. S., Shinaberger, J. H., Jowsey, J., Massry, S. G., and Coburn, J. W.: A controlled evaluation of clinical and metabolic effects of dialysate calcium levels during regular hemodialysis. Trans. Am. Soc. Artif. Intern. Organs, 17:118–124, 1971.
5. Fiske, C. H., and Subbarow, Y.: The colorimetric determination of phosphorus. J. Biol. Chem., 66:375–400, 1925.
6. Gomori, G.: A modification of the colorimetric phosphorus determination for use with the photoelectric colorimeter. J. Lab. Clin. Med., 27:955–960, 1942.
7. Frings, C. S., Rahman, R. and Jones, J. D.: Automated method for the determination of serum inorganic phosphorus: comparison with manual procedure. Clin. Chim. Acta., 14:563–565, 1966.
8. Goodwin, J. F.: Quantification of serum inorganic phosphorus, phosphatase, and urinary phosphate without preliminary treatment. Clin. Chem., 16:776–780, 1970.
9. Fawaz, E. N. and Tejirian, A.: A new enzymatic method for the estimation of inorganic phosphate in native sera. Z. Klin. Chem. Klin. Biochem., 10:215–219, 1972.
10. Parsons, J. A., Dawson, B., Callahan, E., and Potts, J. T.: A method for the analysis of phosphate and calcium in small samples of plasma by atomic absorption spectrophotometry. Biochem. J., 119:791–793, 1970.

# Chapter Three

# MINERAL METABOLISM: ALKALINE PHOSPHATASE

## GENERAL COMMENTS

Alkaline phosphatase in the serum is derived from a number of different sources, including the intestine, liver, placenta, lungs, and bone. Other tissues may contain minute amounts of alkaline phosphatase but not enough to make a significant contribution to circulating levels of the enzyme in the serum. Postprandial rises in alkaline phosphatase may also occur, especially in lipaemic serum, so fasting values must be evaluated.[2]

## MEASUREMENT OF ALKALINE PHOSPHATASE

Heat or urea inactivation of serum eliminates the alkaline phosphatase from sources other than bone; thus alkaline phosphatase resulting from bone abnormalities can be measured and utilized to interpret bone disorders. The units vary according to the method used; and the variation is large and can be irritating (Table 3–1). There is a real biologic variation with age, which decreases from 30 KA units in infants to 10 KA units in adults; up to the age of 17 the range is large and there are

**Table 3–1  NORMAL VALUES FOR SERUM ALKALINE PHOSPHATASE IN ADULTS**

| | |
|---|---|
| King-Armstrong Units | 3–13 (KA units) |
| Bodansky Units | 1.0–4.0 (Bodansky units) |
| Bessy-Lowry Units | 0.8–3.0 (B-L units) |
| International Units | 20–85 (IU) |
| International Units (modified) | 87–239 (IUm) |

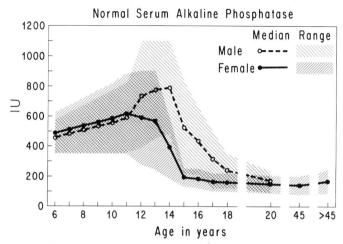

**Figure 3–1**   Normal values in male and female children and adults.

perceptible sex differences. In mild rickets in boys the values are as high as 90 KA units in infants compared with mean values of 60 KA units in girls; at age 12 the respective values are 25 and 15 KA units.[3] These measurements were made in schoolchildren in Birmingham, England, and were decreased from zero to four years of age by 40 per cent by the administration of 1.25 mg of calciferol daily, which corrected the rickets and reduced the values to normal levels.

International Units have become the most popular form of measurement.[4] Recently the method has been modified to increase sensitivity.[5, 6] In children the values show a large range, and over the age of 12 years males have both higher low and high values compared with females of the same age (Fig. 3–1). In adults males continue to have slightly higher values, and among females postmenopausal women and women taking hormones as oral contraceptives tend to have lower values. Perhaps the latter differences may be explained partly by the higher activity level of most men and premenopausal women, which would tend to stimulate bone formation, and by the well-recognized bone formation depressive effective of estrogens.

## ABNORMAL LEVELS OF ALKALINE PHOSPHATASE

The two major sources of increased serum alkaline phosphatase originating from bone are (1) a failure of mineralization and (2) increased osteoblastic activity.

**Table 3–2**   ABNORMALITIES OF ALKALINE PHOSPHATASE

| Increased bone formation | Failure of mineralization |
| --- | --- |
| Paget's disease of bone | Rickets |
| Osteoblastic carcinoma | Osteomalacia |
| Hypercalcemic hyperparathyroidism | |

Bone alkaline phosphatase is considered to be a pyrophosphatase, so it is likely to be involved in the mineralization process, being utilized as a source of phosphate. It has been histochemically localized within osteoblasts which are in the process of active bone formation. It is therefore at a high level in the serum when utilization of the enzyme is prevented by a failure of mineralization or when the mineralization process is occurring at a high level. It is not possible to distinguish between the two causes of the increased levels. For example, a patient may have an abnormally high value as a result of having osteomalacia and a fracture. The most common causes of high serum alkaline phosphatase levels are shown in Table 3–2.

## *REFERENCES*

1. Posen, S.: Alkaline phosphatase. Ann. Int. Med., *67*:183–203, 1967.
2. Warshaw, J. B., Littlefield, J. W., Fishman, W. H., Inglis, N. R., and Stolbach, L. L.: Serum alkaline phosphatase in hypophosphatasia. J. Clin. Invest., *50*:2137–2142, 1971.
3. Cooke, W. T., Swan, C. H. J., Asquith, P., Melikian, V., and McFeely, W. E.: Serum alkaline phosphatase and rickets in urban school children. Br. Med. J., *1*:324–327, 1973.
4. Bowers, G. N. Jr., and McComb, R. B.: A continuous spectrophotometric method for measuring the activity of serum alkaline phosphatase. Clin. Chem., *12*:70–89, 1966.
5. McComb, Robert B., and Bowers, G. N., Jr.: Study of optimum buffer conditions for measuring alkaline phosphatase activity in human serum. Clin. Chem., *18*:97–104, 1972.
6. Fleisher, G. A.: Personal communication, 1976.

# Chapter Four

# MINERAL METABOLISM: MAGNESIUM

## GENERAL COMMENTS

Magnesium is an essential element for a number of enzyme actions, and for this reason is necessary for the normal functioning of parathyroid hormone. The plasma level is normally 2.1 mg/dl, with a range of 1.8 to 2.4 mg/dl, and this tends to be the same in children and adults. The majority (70 per cent) is diffusible and the remainder bound to serum albumin and globulin. Only small quantities of magnesium are taken in by the diet, approximately 50 mg per day, and only about 20 mg is absorbed. This is almost completely reabsorbed from the circulation by the kidney and sequestered in bone.

In bone, approximately one third of the magnesium is surface limited and is apparently on the surface of the hydroxyapatite, since this fraction is easily eluted and is in equilibrium with the serum magnesium.[1] The majority is probably within the crystal in calcium positions and is less available for exchange.

## MAGNESIUM HOMEOSTASIS

Because of the large volume of bone, even the relatively small percentage of magnesium (0.7 per cent) forms an almost inexhaustable pool of this element (approximately 14 g). Because the renal excretion of magnesium is low, magnesium depletion causing hypomagnesemia is infrequent. If malabsorption occurs, magnesium comes out of bone to restore normal serum values in most instances while in hypermagnesemia, bone stores of magnesium increase.

Magnesium will influence the secretion of parathyroid hormone to some extent, but is much less effective than alterations in serum ionized calcium. Direct infusion of blood high in magnesium will suppress the secretion of this hormone, however, low serum magnesium levels do not result in elevated parathyroid hormone levels, despite the presence of hypocalcemia.

**Table 4–1**   STATE OF MAGNESIUM IN THE SERUM

|                      | m moles/L | % of total |
|----------------------|-----------|------------|
| Free ions            | 0.53      | 55         |
| Protein bound        | 0.30      | 32         |
| MgH PO$_4$           | 0.03      | 3          |
| Mg Cit$^{--}$        | 0.04      | 4          |
| Unknown complexes    | 0.06      | 6          |

From Walser.[3]

## Measurement Of Magnesium

Magnesium is measured by atomic absorption spectrophotometry.[2] It is an unusual measurement to carry out in some respects. However, if hypercalcemia, parathyroid malfunction, or malabsorption is evident or suspected, a serum magnesium measurement should be made. Atomic absorption measures total magnesium, despite the one-third bound fraction (Table 4–1). There appears to be no relation between magnesium and calcium and no correlation between the protein binding of calcium and magnesium.[3] Therefore, changes in the protein concentration of the blood will not affect measured values, and, since less magnesium is bound than calcium, the physiological effect of hyperproteinemia can be expected to be less.

## ACTION OF MAGNESIUM

Magnesium depletion caused by dietary insufficiency (rare) or by malabsorption and/or diarrhea (less rare) only appears to cause clinically significant hypomagnesemia in young animals or children.[4] Specific loss of magnesium resulting from malabsorption of this ion has been described very infrequently in young male babies. Presumably, in such instances, the available magnesium stores in the skeleton are not adequate to compensate for low magnesium intake or the fecal loss.

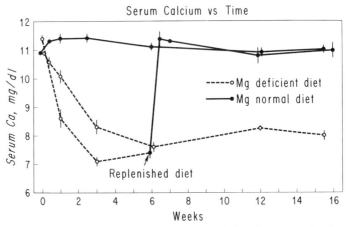

**Figure 4–1**  In young puppies on a magnesium depleted diet for six weeks, hypocalcemia develops. Half the deficient group were given magnesium, and a normal serum calcium level was restored rapidly, if the magnesium had been given IV, the return to normal serum calcium level could be expected within 15 minutes.

**Table 4–2**   OSTEOID WIDTHS IN MAGNESIUM DEFICIENCY IN PUPPIES
(microns, mean ± SE)

| Period in Weeks | Magnesium Deficient | Controls |
|:---:|:---:|:---:|
| 0 | 7.45 ± .18* | 7.71 ± .16 |
| 1 | 6.65 ± .20* | 6.66 ± .16 |
| 3 | 9.43 ± .22** | 7.39 ± .18 |
| 6 | 9.45 ± .18** | 7.25 ± .17 |
| 12 | 10.10 ± .23** | 7.83 ± .17 |
| 16 | 11.42** | 8.14 |

\*NS
\*\*P < 0.001

In hypomagnesemia hypocalcemia occurs despite adequate calcium intake and normal excretion, and tetany may develop. Serum immunoreactive parathyroid hormone levels are low or undetectable;[5] consequently the TRP% and serum phosphate are high, and urinary cyclic AMP is markedly decreased in hypomagnesemia. In fact, the syndrome resembles hypoparathyroidism, and the serum calcium levels can be restored to normal by continuous parathyroid hormone injections. Unlike hypoparathyroidism, however, the low serum calcium can also be returned to normal promptly by magnesium (Fig. 4–1). Serum parathyroid hormone also rises to normal as does the TRP% and urinary cyclic AMP; when intravenous magnesium supplement is given to depleted animals, normal parathyroid hormone levels are restored within two minutes. These rapid changes suggest that a normal magnesium level in the serum is necessary for the release of the hormone from the gland. The effect on urinary cyclic AMP and the rapidity with which this messenger system pro-

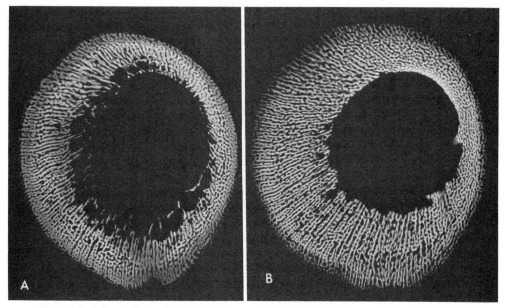

**Figure 4–2**   Microradiography of the organ sections of young chickens kept for 3 weeks on a magnesium-depleted diet. In group (a) magnesium had been repleted for 3 days and in (b) the deficient diet was maintained until the animal died. Note the increase in endosteal resorption in (a) compared with the lack of resorption and increased cortical width in (b) (magnification ×15).

Table 4-3   BONE MORPHOLOGY IN HYPOMAGNESEMIA IN PUPPIES
(mean ± SE)

| Period of Depletion | Bone Resorption (% surface) | Bone Formation (% surface) | Bone Formation Rate ($\mu$/day) |
|---|---|---|---|
| CONTROL | | | |
| week 1 | 6.70 ± 0.15 | 19.11 ± 1.45 | 3.45 ± 1.23 |
| week 6 | 7.17 ± 0.36 | 17.19 ± 0.96 | 4.10 ± 0.49 |
| Mg DEFICIENT | | | |
| week 1 | 6.20 ± 0.32 | 22.21 ± 1.28 | 3.40 ± 1.12 |
| week 6 | 4.21 ± 0.36* | 19.98 ± 1.30 | 3.09 ± 0.41* |

*Significantly different from control, $p < 0.001$.

duces appropriate responses indicate that magnesium may have an essential function in the adenyl cyclase mechanism, which is necessary for release of the hormone from the gland. In other words, magnesium prevents the parathyroid glands from "seeing" the serum calcium level and therefore from responding to decreased levels of PTH hormone.

Hypomagnesemia is accompanied by hypoparathyroidism and probably causes the failure of release of parathyroid hormone. Consequently, hypocalcemia develops, and the severity of the problem is compounded by the development of osteomalacia. In a group of young dogs, osteoid widths increased significantly after only three weeks on a magnesium-deficient diet (Table 4-2). The development of an increase in osteoid discourages bone resorption; the lack of parathyroid hormone itself also results in low bone resorption values, and the overall result is an increase in bone mass, which is particularly evident endosteally (Fig. 4-2). Although bone formation surfaces are not significantly diminished, the rate of matrix formation appears to be decreased (Table 4-3). The latter may be an effect of decreasing parathyroid hormone levels or of the essential role of magnesium in enzyme actions involved in bone formation. The increase in bone mass is thus less than would otherwise be expected.

## REFERENCES

1. Alfrey, A. C., and Miller, N. L.: Bone magnesium pools in uremia. J. Clin. Invest., 52:3019-3027, 1973.
2. Jones, J. D., and McGuckin, W. F.: Complexometric titration of calcium and magnesium by a semi-automated procedure. Clin. Chem., 10:767-780, 1964.
3. Walser, M.: Ion association. VI. Interactions between calcium, magnesium, inorganic phosphate, citrate and protein in normal human plasma. J. Clin. Invest., 40:723-730, 1961.
4. Heaton, F. W., and Fourman, P.: Magnesium deficiency and hypocalcemia in intestinal malabsorption. Lancet, 2:50-52, 1965.
5. Suh, S. M., Tashjian, A. H., Jr., Matsuo, N., Parkinson, D. K., and Fraser, D.: Pathogenesis of hypocalcemia in primary hypomagnesemia: normal end-organ responsiveness to parathyroid hormone and impaired parathyroid gland function. J. Clin. Invest., 52:153-160, 1973.
6. Reddy, C. R., Coburn, J. W., Hartenbower, D. L., Friedler, R. M., Brickman, A. S. Massry, S. G., and Jowsey, J.: Studies on mechanisms of hypocalcemia of magnesium depletion. J. Clin. Invest., 52:3000-3010, 1973.

# Chapter Five

# MINERAL METABOLISM: PARATHYROID HORMONE

## GENERAL COMMENTS[1]

Parathyroid hormone is manufactured in the parathyroid glands by the clear cells (wasserhelle cells) or the chief cells. The former type has historically been associated with "primary" hyperparathyroidism, and the latter with secondary stimulation. However, it is evident that chief cell hyperplasia can be associated with primary hyperparathyroidism, particularly since early diagnosis of this disease is common. Before parathyroid hormone assay was available, the diagnosis of the disease often rested on gland histology (Fig. 5–1). However, a great deal more is now known, about both the structure of the hormone and the mechanism of its secretion, and radioimmunoassays of the hormone are available.

In the parathyroid gland the prohormone, with a molecular weight of about 11,000, is changed to parathyroid hormone which contains 84 amino acids and has a molecular weight of 9,500; fragments account for the difference in molecular weight.[2] The hormone is secreted into the serum and rapidly cleaved into C and N fragments in the peripheral circulation. A large part of the apparent discrepancies between data from different laboratories has arisen from the difference in the immunoassay method used, and particularly in whether the C or N terminal is measured in the assay. Some assays are sensitive to the biologically active amino terminal portion of the polypeptide chain, while others measure the carboxyl terminal fragment. The latter has a long half-life, probably of some hours, and assay of this portion of the hormone will therefore give higher values than if the short-lived amino terminal part of the hormone is assayed.

The amino acid sequence of parathyroid hormone varies from species to species. This has clinical significance, since the readily available bovine hormone may cause antibody formation in other species, such as human beings and cannot be used clinically on a long term basis. In bone diseases in which parathyroid hormone treatment would be indicated, such as in post-parathyroidectomy patients, vitamin D is generally used.

23

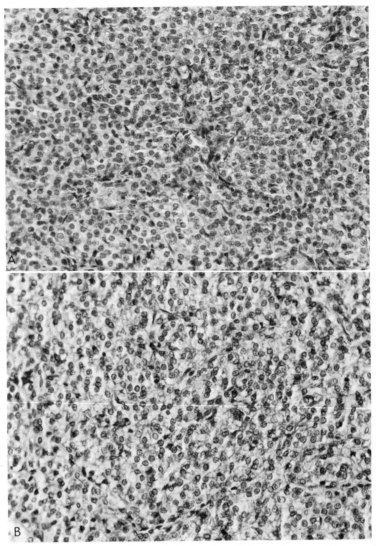

**Figure 5-1** (a) Normal parathyroid gland. (b) Parathyroid tissue showing mild hyperplasia caused by continuous hydrocortisone injections in adult rabbits. (magnification ×300). (From Adams, P., and Jowsey, J.: Effect of calcium on cortisone-induced osteoporosis: A preliminary communication. Endocrinology 81:152-154, 1967.)

A major advance in the study of the parathyroid hormone has been the development of an assay of the circulating hormone in both peripheral blood and, in some particular instances, in the venous blood exiting from the area of the parathyroid glands.[3] Levels of the hormone may be many times higher when samples are taken from the innominate vein and may help with the diagnosis of hyperparathyroidism. An assay has been developed in many laboratories for the human hormone and also for the rat, dog, and cow.[4, 5, 6] The mode of action of the hormone is through the adenyl cyclase system, and measurements of adenylcyclase are also used for evaluating the action of the hormone on target tissues. Both in bone and the kidney, high concentrations of the hormone in the blood cause a movement of calcium into the cells of the target organ, and a stimulation of 3'5'

**Table 5-1** CAUSES OF A DECREASE IN IONIZED CALCIUM

| Increased serum phosphate | Decreased serum ionized calcium |
|---|---|
| phosphate ingestion<br>decreased renal phosphate excretion<br>(renal failure) | calcium depletion, e.g. vitamin D lack, malabsorption<br>increased calcitonin (exogenous)<br>diphosphonate administration<br>increased serum phosphate |

cyclic AMP.[7, 8] The adenyl cyclase system is one common to many hormones; it is the target cells (bone and kidney) that have the specific receptors for parathyroid hormone and therefore respond specifically (see Biological Activity, p. 29).

Any state in which a low ionized calcium is produced will stimulate the parathyroid glands and cause an increase in secretion (Table 5-1). (The single exception is a lowered serum calcium in conjunction with magnesium depletion.) As a result of the parathyroid stimulation, the calcium will tend to be restored by the action of the hormone on bone, and its action on the kidney will tend to increase the renal excretion of phosphate and any serum abnormalities may well be invisible in fasting morning blood samples. The relationship between parathyroid hormone and ionized calcium is inverse, but this relationship holds only over a narrow range of serum calcium values (Figs. 5-2, 5-3).[9, 11]

## FUNCTION OF THE PARATHYROID GLAND

The parathyroid gland has two closely related functions; one of its functions is to respond to alterations in the ionized calcium level by secretions of the hormone from the gland. This feed-back mechanism is well recognized and is often the only property of the gland to receive attention. However, an equally important property is the ability to recognize the numerical value of the serum calcium and to lower or increase secretion rate above or below (respectively) a set serum calcium value.

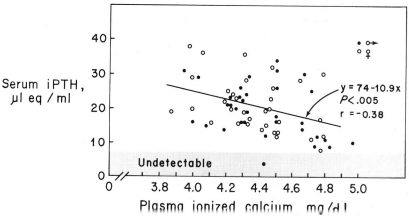

**Figure 5-2** Relationship between ionized calcium and serum immunoreactive parathyroid hormone in children. Note the wide variation in serum iPTH values for each ionized calcium value. (From Arnaud et al.[10])

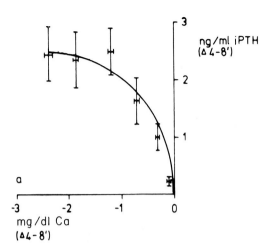

**Figure 5–3** Change in the rate of parathyroid hormone secretion, between 0 to 3 ng/ml between four and eight minutes after EGTA injection which altered the serum calcium 3 mg/dl. The study was carried out in adult Brown-Swiss cows. The response of the parathyroid hormone secretion is limited to a narrow change in serum calcium. (From: Blum et al.[11])

This is often termed the calciostat. The exact figure for the calcium appears to vary from person to person but remains fairly consistent in any one person over long periods of time (Table 5–2). It is probably a mis-setting of the calciostat that expresses itself as the disease called "primary" hyperparathyroidism.

The way in which a constant level of calcium is maintained in the serum is complex. However, the three essential factors are bone, long-term exchange, and the parathyroid glands. If the parathyroid glands are removed from an animal or person, the serum calcium falls to between 5 and 7 mg/dl; this is the equilibrium level of the exchange process between blood and bone mineral. The most easily available calcium is that which can exchange with the extracellular calcium; this lies on the surface of the hydroxyapatite crystals. There appears to be a continuous process whereby a calcium ion in the bone fluid moves onto a position in the crystal lattice in exchange for one that comes off into the fluid phase. The majority, if not all, of the rapid exchange probably occurs at the canalicular and lacunar surfaces, since these areas are in contact with the extracellular fluid. The exchange process is usually in equilibrium and involves net transfer of calcium between the bone mineral and tissue fluid. However, if a calcium depleted or deficient tissue fluid is present, there is a net transfer of calcium from bone mineral into the fluid by a physical chemical process.

The parathyroidectomized calcium level tends to be lower in young animals than in adults, presumably because any mineralization of new bone "depletes" calcium resources in a growing animal significantly, while, in adults, the amount of calcium required for mineralization is small. However, in both the growing or adult state there would tend to be a failure of mineralization at lower than normal serum calcium levels.

**Table 5–2**  UNIFORMITY OF LASTING MORNING CALCIUM VALUES IN THREE DIFFERENT NORMAL PEOPLE

| Subject | No. of Years | Mean Serum Ca mg/dl | S.D. | S.E. |
|---|---|---|---|---|
| 1 ♀ 40 | 6 | 9.2 | 0.2 | 0.04 |
| 2 ♀ 40 | 5 | 9.9 | 0.3 | 0.05 |
| 3 ♂ 30 | 5 | 10.3 | 0.2 | 0.04 |

It is possible for an adult to live asymptomatically in a parathyroidectomized state with a serum calcium maintained by mineral exchange with bone; however, any situation which would tend to lower the serum calcium further will result in hypocalcemia tetany. The same is true for children except that symptoms may be expected more frequently (see Chapter Twenty-Seven, Hyperparathyroidism).

There appears to be a limit to the amount of calcium that the bone mineral can lose by exchange; however, the total amount is significant, since the entire skeleton is affected. It has been suggested that in osteoporotic individuals the overall mineral density of the bone is less than age-matched non-osteoporotic persons (Fig. 5–4). Since only two persons with osteoporosis were included, the data must be considered tentative. Also there is only the assumption, but no proof, that the mineral density decreases, rather than that it has never attained the mineral density of non-osteoporotic persons.[11]

The maintenance of a serum calcium level above 7 mg/dl is the responsibility of the parathyroid glands. This is achieved by a feedback mechanism by which a decrease in ionized calcium stimulates parathyroid hormone release from the glands into the blood. The hormone stimulates bone cells, particularly osteoclasts, but also osteocytes and osteoblasts. The osteocytes appear to be able to resorb mineralized bone, since the lacunae increase in size and a change in the staining characteristics can be seen in individuals with hyperparathyroidism. Presumably mineral and matrix are released into the canaliculi and lacunar extracellular fluid and are carried by the extracellular fluid to the blood. The osteocyte response,

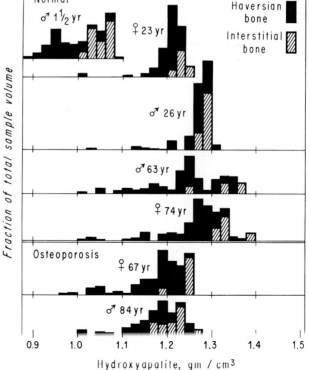

**Figure 5–4** The bone density in the two osteoporotic people is decreased compared with normal age-matched people, suggesting an overall loss of bone mineral in response to a lack of calcium.

termed osteocytic osteolysis, probably represents a rapid minute-to-minute mechanism for releasing calcium from bone to maintain higher serum calcium levels than can be achieved by long-term exchange. It also does not require cell differentiation and activation, which are necessary for osteoclastic bone resorption. Indeed, osteocytic activity may be the major cellular mechanism for maintaining serum calcium at a normal level in abnormal states such as hypothyroidism, where the population of osteoblasts and osteoclasts is low. However, in instances where bone turnover is excessively low, osteocytic osteolysis is unable to maintain a normal serum calcium level at times of stress; a common example is the tetany that develops in parturient cows.[12] The response of the osteocytes to parathyroid hormone is self-limiting in some way. Even in hyperparathyroidism associated with a bone mass decrease and fractures, the osteocyte lacunae only approximately double in size, and the bone never shows many large holes, as is seen in bone involved in mast cell disease.

Osteoclastic bone resorption is the major response to increased levels of parathyroid hormone in the serum. The specificity of this response has been established by Barnicot, who transplanted a number of different tissues adjacent to the parietal bone of a rat and observed that only parathyroid glands caused local bone resorption.[13] The gland, and also injection of exogenous hormone, result in the appearance of large multinucleate osteoclasts. These cells differentiate from blood-borne progenitor cells and migrate along mineralized bone surfaces, resorbing matrix and hydroxyapatite and therefore transferring calcium and, of course, phosphorus, hydroxyproline, and other trace elements, such as fluoride, magnesium, and citrate, into the serum. The bone loss in disorders characterized by increased levels of parathyroid hormone, such as renal failure or "primary" hyperparathyroidism, is the result of osteoclastic bone resorption rather than osteocytic osteolysis or a generalized decrease in mineral density.

Parathyroid hormone also influences the absorption of calcium in the gut indirectly through its effect on vitamin D metabolism; raised levels of the hormone cause an increase in absorption and vice versa. The renal excretion of calcium is also altered by parathyroid hormone; increased hormone levels result in an increased tubular reabsorption of calcium. Any fall in ionized calcium will be followed by a tendency to conserve calcium through the gut and kidney and to release calcium into the blood from bone. Ionized calcium will therefore return to normal, as will total serum calcium. Because maintenance of a normal serum calcium level is so essential for the continued function of a number of physiological processes essential to life, it is necessary that the parathyroids have a number of independent methods of putting calcium into the blood. Certainly a system that is independent of a dietary supply and the renal loss of calcium is necessary, since the former may be non-existent and the latter is obligatory to some degree.

## PHOSPHATE AND PARATHYROID FUNCTION

The major role of parathyroid hormone is to maintain a constant ionized serum calcium level; however, a secondary function is the prevention of hyperphosphatemia. Both hypercalcemia and high serum phosphorus are potentially life-threatening. At any time that parathyroid hormone levels are raised, calcium will be retained through absorption from the gut and kidney and by resorption from bone. The latter will also release phosphorus into the blood. Phosphorus is excreted in increased amounts in the presence of high circulating parathyroid hormone levels by a direct effect of the hormone on the kidney that inhibits tubular reabsorption of this ion. Exogenous phosphate will, by decreasing the ionized calcium by forming a calcium-phosphorus complex, also tend to increase the renal excretion of phosphate. The tubular reabsorption of phosphate (%TRP) is a comparison of the renal secretion of phosphorus in relation to the secretion of creatinine, which is constant. The value is usually subtracted from one. Therefore %TRP is $\dfrac{1-x \text{ ml/min P}}{y \text{ ml/min Creatinine}}$. Hence %TRP is a reflection of parathyroid activity and is generally low in hyperparathyroidism. The renal phosphate level is below normal; there is an increase in the hydroxylation of Vitamin D to its active form $1-25(OH)_2D_3$, and consequently an enhancement of the gastrointestinal absorption of calcium. This mechanism probably explains the effect of parathyroid hormone excess on increasing the intestinal absorption of calcium.

## BIOLOGICAL ACTIVITY

$^{125}$I-labeled parathyroid hormone has been found in bone, kidney, and liver. The half-life of the hormone in blood is very short (2 to 7 minutes). The principal organ responsible for degradation appears to be the liver.[14, 15] In the kidney the hormone appears to be deposited in the proximal tubules of the outer third of the cortex.[16] In bone the hormone is found in the cellular layers of the periosteum and in the bone cells lining the endosteum and in a lesser amount in osteocytes.[16] Since the half-life of the hormone is short, it is obvious that continual secretion of the hormone and, therefore, continual stimulation of bone and kidney cells may have different biological effects from exogenous hormone administration. The latter would result only in short-lived, peak stimulation of the cells.

Parathyroid hormone elicits its response in target cells by stimulating the adenyl cyclase system within the cells. The primary event appears to be a binding of the hormone onto receptor sites on the target cell membrane. The next event is possibly an influx of calcium across the cell membrane followed by stimulation of the adenyl cyclase, which causes an increase in the concentration of 3'-5' AMP. The 3'-5' AMP is then bound to a specific protein-releasing kinase.[1] The exact role of calcium is uncertain, since the hypocalcemia and rise in concentration of adenyl cyclase within bone cells both occur in a few minutes. However, the end result is a stimulation of bone resorption and, since parathyroid hormone affects kidney function, a rise in phosphate excretion. The correlation between the C-terminal assay and the number of osteoclasts is high (r = 0.963), while the N-terminal assay gives a poorer correlation (r = 0.669).[17] However, the N-terminal portion appears to be biologically active but has such a short half-life that a relationship between it and a differentiated active cell is hard to establish. On the other hand, the C-terminal portion of the peptide chain remains circulating for a longer time, can be measured in peripheral blood, and reflects the activity of the parathyroid gland.

## *REFERENCES*

1. Potts, J. T., and Deftos, L. J.: Parathyroid hormone, calcitonin, vitamin D bone and bone mineral metabolism. In Bondy, P. K., and Rosenberg, L. E. (Eds.): Duncan's Diseases of Metabolism, 7th ed. Philadelphia, W. B. Saunders Co., 1974, pp. 1225–1430.

2. Habener, J. F., Kemper, B., Potts, J. T., Jr., and Rich, A.: Parathyroid hormone: biosynthesis by human parathyroid adenomas. Science, *178*:630–633, 1972.
3. O'Riordan, J. L. H., Kendall, B. E., and Woodhead, J. S.: Preoperative localisation of parathyroid tumours. Lancet, *2*:1172–1175, 1971.
4. Hargis, G. K., Bowser, E. N., Henderson, W. J., and Williams, G. A.: Radioimmunoassay of rat parathyroid hormone in serum and tissue extracts. Endocrinology, *94*:1644–1649, 1974.
5. Slatopolsky, E., Caglar, S., Pennell, J. P., Taggart, D. D., Canterbury, J. M., Reïss, E., and Bricker, N. S.: On the pathogenesis of hyperparathyroidism in chronic experimental renal insufficiency in the dog. J. Clin. Invest., *50*:492–499, 1971.
6. Addison, G. M., Hales, C. N., Woodhead, J. S., and O'Riordan, J. L. H.: Immunoradiometric assay of parathyroid hormone. J. Endocrinol., *49*:521–530, 1971.
7. Aurbach, G. D., and Chase, L. R.: Cyclic 3', 5'-adenylic acid in bone and the mechanism of action of parathyroid hormone. Fed. Proc., *29*:1179–1182, 1970.
8. Parsons, J. A., Neer, R. M., and Potts, J. T., Jr.: Initial fall of plasma calcium after intravenous injection and parathyroid hormone. Endocrinology, *89*:735–740, 1971.
9. Jowsey, J.: Densitometry of photographic images. J. Appl. Physiol., *21*:309–312, 1966.
10. Arnaud, S. B., Goldsmith, R. S., Stickler, G. B., McCall, J. T., and Arnaud, C. D.: Serum parathyroid hormone and blood interrelationships in normal children. Pediatr. Res., *7*:485–493, 1973.
11. Blum, J. W., Fischer, J. A., Schwoerer, D., Hunziker, W., and Binswanger, U.: Acute parathyroid hormone response: sensitivity, relationship to hypocalcemia, and rapidity. Endocrinology, *95*:753–759, 1974.
12. Mayer, G. P., Ramberg, C. F., Jr., Kronfeld, D. S., Buckle, R. M., Sherwood, L. M., Aurbach, G. D., and Potts, J. T., Jr.: Plasma parathyroid hormone concentration in hypocalcemic parturient cows. Am. J. Vet. Res., *30*:1587–1597, 1969.
13. Barnicot, N. A.: The local action of the parathyroid and other tissues on the bone in intracerebral grafts. J. Anat., *82*:233–248, 1948.
14. Neuman, W. F., Neuman, M. W., Sammon, P. J., Simon, W., and Lane, K.: The metabolism of labeled parathyroid hormone. III. Studies in rats. Calc. Tiss. Res., *18*:251–261, 1975.
15. Neuman, W. F., Neuman, M. W., Lane, K., Miller, L., and Sammon, P. J.: The metabolism of labeled parathyroid hormone. V. Collected biological studies. Calc. Tiss. Res., *18*:271–287, 1975.
16. Neuman, W. F., Neuman, M. W., Sammon, P. J., and Casarett, G. W.: The metabolism of labeled parathyroid hormone. IV. Autoradiographic studies. Calc. Tiss. Res., *18*:263–270, 1975.
17. Arnaud, C. D., Sizemore, G. W., Oldham, S. B., Fischer, J. A., Tsao, H. S., and Littledike, E. T.: Human parathyroid hormone: glandular and secreted molecular species. Am. J. Med., *50*:630–638, 1971.

# Chapter Six

# MINERAL METABOLISM: VITAMIN D

## GENERAL COMMENTS

Exposure of the skin to sunlight and dietary ingestion of vitamin D-containing food are the two natural sources of vitamin D. The available amount varies considerably from one geographical area to another. In countries where vitamin D supplements are not added to food, sunlight exposure forms the major source of the vitamin. However, some of the earliest reports of rickets and osteomalacia come, perhaps surprisingly, not from areas with little sunshine, but from places where clothing prevents exposure to sunlight. One of the earliest studies of documented osteomalacia was in Bedouin Arab women who live in an almost cloudless climate but traditionally expose no part of their bodies, except their eyes.[1] More recently the newly-arrived Asian persons in Glasgow, who cover their skin more completely than their Scots countrymen, have been documented to have a high incidence of vitamin D deficiency.[2] Allergy to sunshine can also result in vitamin D deficiency and bone disease for the same reason; the common feature of these and other instances of environmental vitamin D deficiency is that the skin is screened from the sun by clothing.

**Environmental Adaptation.** It has been observed that skin color is darker among people native to countries near the equator and becomes progressively lighter toward the North Pole. The color is not merely a change from the familiar Negro to Caucasian; color changes from an almost purple-black at the equator, through brown, to "tanned," and to the almost albino paleness of the Finns.[3] This presumably is an adaptive device for maximum absorption of ultra-violet light when daylight hours are short, as in the north, to a role of protection in areas with long days and vertical sun rays.

## METABOLISM OF VITAMIN D[4, 5]

The vitamin D available in food and from sunlight irradiation is not metabolically active. 7-dehydrotachysterol in the skin is converted by sunlight irradiation to cholecalciferol or vitamin $D_3$. Microsomal P450 enzymes in the liver then add an OH in the 25 position forming 25-OH $D_3$ (25-hydroxycholecalciferol). 25-OH $D_3$ is then further hydroxylated in the kidney in the 1 position to form 1–25 $(OH)_2D_3$ (1–25 dihydroxycholecalciferol). Ergosterol, found in irradiated food, follows a similar pathway, as does 7-dehydrocholesterol, first to vitamin $D_2$ and then to 25–OH $D_2$. Tachysterol (AT 10) is a chemically formed compound which is converted by chemical reduction to dihydrotachysterol$_2$ (or $DHT_2$). Although not naturally occurring, the rapid and complete hydroxylation in the liver makes AT 10 and $DHT_2$ potentially useful agents in the treatment of diseases characterized by abnormalities of vitamin D metabolism, such as vitamin D-resistant rickets. Both forms of D so far mentioned, D itself and 25-OH D, are bound in plasma to albumins and alpha-globulins, apparently as a means of protection against their destruction in the serum. The metabolites can therefore be safely transported from the site of formation, that is, the skin or liver, to the next conversion site, the liver and kidney, respectively.

Early investigators noticed that when 25-OH D, which had been considered the active metabolite of vitamin D, was administered in vivo, there was a lag of a number of hours before the vitamin could be shown to have a biological effect in increasing calcium absorption in the gut. Also, large pharmacological doses of vitamin D were not completely successful in curing vitamin D-resistant rickets. In addition, actinomycin D, which inhibits nuclear function, prevented any biological effect of vitamin D. It was therefore apparent that vitamin D itself, and indeed 25-OH D, are biologically inactive, and that only the kidney-converted 1–25 $(OH)_2D$ has biological activity.[6]

The complexity of vitamin D metabolism is increased by the influence of other hormones on the rate of synthesis of the various metabolites. Retrospectively, it would be disastrous if vitamin D produced by sunlight irradiation was the active metabolite causing gastrointestinal absorption of calcium. A day in the sun might well have lethal consequences; indeed, sun exposure has been shown to result in remarkably elevated serum levels of 25-OH D (Table 6–1). Fortunately, there are a number of protective mechanisms which prevent the accumulation of excessive amounts of 1.25 $(OH)_2D$ (Table 6–2). The earliest control, in the liver, appears to be an autoregulation; there is prevention of the production of large amounts of 25-OH D by accumulation of this metabolite, which inhibits 25-hydroxylase in the liver microsomes where the first hydroxylation occurs. The second hydroxylation occurs in the kidney mitochondria, where 1–25 $(OH)_2$ D is formed. The second regulatory mechanism involves the production of this metabolite, or the inactive

**Table 6–1**   PLASMA 25-OH $D_3$ LEVELS IN VARIOUS SUBJECTS

|  | 25-OH $D_3$, (mg/dl) (mean $\pm$ SD) |
| --- | --- |
| Normals | 20.2 $\pm$  8.9 |
| Lifeguards | 73.0 $\pm$ 26.4 |
| Biliary cirrhosis | 6.1 $\pm$  2.7 |
| Uremia | 21.4 $\pm$ 10.5 |
| Sarcoidosis | 15.8 $\pm$  5.9 |

From Haddad et al.[7]

Table 6–2  FACTORS CONTROLLING THE PRODUCTION OF
1–25(OH)$_2$D IN THE KIDNEY

| Increased production | Kidney | Decreased production |
|---|---|---|
| | 1–25(OH)$_2$D | ↑ serum phosphate |
| ↑ parathyroid hormone | | ↑ serum calcium |
| | ↓ | |
| | **Intestine** | |
| low Ca diet | Ca binding protein | high Ca diet |

24–25 (OH)$_2$ D at various levels of serum calcium, phosphorus, and parathyroid hormone. DeLuca has shown that in the kidney a serum calcium below 9.2 mg/dl will permit the second hydroxylation step, while above 9.5 mg/dl the inactive metabolite 24–25 (OH)$_2$ D will be formed instead.[6] These feedback mechanisms allow efficient adaptation to a low or high calcium intake that is independent of parathyroid hormone, as well as adaptation to anything except excessively low vitamin D intake and consequent lack of this controlling system.

The final step in vitamin D metabolism occurs after the second hydroxylation by the kidney mitochondria; 1,25(OH)$_2$D is transported to the gut, where it stimulates intestinal transport of calcium from the diet into the body. Because of the delay between 1–25(OH)$_2$ D administration to deficient animals and the appearance of calcium in the serum, it has been suggested that there is further conversion to yet another metabolite, which is the active hormone for calcium absorption.[8] A specific binding protein, dependent on vitamin D, is present in the intestine, which results, through DNA, in an RNA message to form calcium binding protein (CaBP) within the cell. Calcium at the brush border is transported into the mucosal cell, probably with the help of adenosinetriphosphatase or alkaline phosphatase. The calcium is then held in mitochondria until claimed by the calcium binding protein, which transports the calcium to the serosal side of the cell. An ATP energy pump and sodium are involved in the final exit of the calcium into the blood.

The majority of intestinal calcium transported by this mechanism occurs in the duodenum and jejunum. The dietary intake of calcium can influence absorption by virtue of the fact that low calcium intake stimulates calcium absorption. In some populations, such as the colored population in South Africa, the calcium intake is estimated to be 200 mg/day, and the normal skeletal structure is explained by surprisingly low urinary and fecal calcium excretion, representing in part the adaptive possibilities of vitamin D metabolism. Adaptation of this degree of efficiency is possibly also, to some extent, a genetically acquired feature, since white persons in the USA who are lactase deficient and on a chosen 200 mg Ca/day intake, are frequently found to have abnormal skeletons and to be osteoporotic. Other populations with a high incidence of lactase deficiency, such as American Indians and Arabs, are not remarkable as characteristically presenting with osteoporosis. However, other factors may play a role, such as activity levels, age at death, and so forth.

## FUNCTION AND CLINICAL IMPLICATIONS

From the above discussion it can be seen that there are obvious consequences of a divergence from normal of any one of the many steps in vitamin D metabolism and regulation. In an intact system a high serum phosphate will depress calcium absorption by shutting off $1-25(OH)_2D$ production. Since vitamin D is a fat soluble vitamin, deficiency of the hormone will occur if dietary vitamin D is the major source in individuals with steatorrhea. Duodenectomy or jejunectomy will also cause vitamin D deficiency. Severe liver disease, with consequent impaired 25 hydroxylation, severe renal disease, or absent kidneys will, of course, prevent 1–25 hydroxylation as will absence of circulating parathyroid hormone. Fortunately, only small amounts of liver and renal tissue are necessary to prevent deficiency of the respective metabolites, and for this reason even anuretic kidneys are left in situ rather than being surgically removed.

## *REFERENCES*

1. Groen, J. J., Eshchar, J., Ben-Ishay, D., Alkan, W. J., and Ben Assa, B. I.: Osteomalacia among the Bedouin of the Negev Desert. Arch. Int. Med., *116*:195–204, 1965.
2. Gupta, M. M., Round, J. M., and Stamp, T. C. B.: Spontaneous cure of vitamin-D deficiency in Asians during summer in Britain. Lancet, *1*:586–588, 1974.
3. Loomis, W. F.: Skin-pigment regulation of vitamin-D biosynthesis in man. Science, *157*:501–506, 1967.
4. Omdahl, J. L., and DeLuca, H. F.: Regulation of vitamin D metabolism and function. Physiol. Rev.: *53*:327–372, 1973.
5. Kodicek, E.: The story of vitamin D from vitamin to hormone. Lancet, *1*:325–329, 1974.
6. DeLuca, H. F.: The kidney as an endocrine organ involved in the function of vitamin D. Am. J. Med., *58*:39–47, 1975.
7. Haddad, J. G., and Chyu, K. J.: Competitive protein-binding radioassay for 25-hydroxycholecalciferol. J. Clin. Endocrinol. Metab., *33*:992–995, 1971.
8. DeLuca, H. F. Recent advances in our understanding of the Vitamin D endocrine system. J. Lab. Clin. Med., *87*:7–26, 1976.

# Chapter Seven

# MINERAL METABOLISM: CALCITONIN

## GENERAL COMMENTS[1]

Calcitonin is a relatively recently discovered hormone. It created much excitement in the field of mineral metabolism until it was found that, in man, its effect on bone was relatively small. Calcitonin is a peptide hormone with 32 amino acids which is produced by the parafollicular, or C-cells, of the thyroid gland. Embryo-

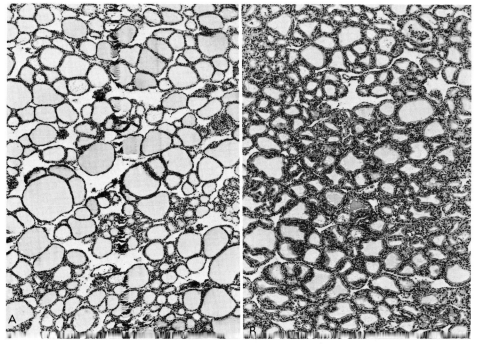

**Figure 7–1**  Thyroid gland tissue taken from a normal animal (a) and from a litter-mate puppy given calcium by intraperitoneal injection (b), which has caused hypercalcemia and a proliferation of C-cells at the expense of the follicular cells (magnification ×60).

35

logically these cells are derived from the ultimobranchial bodies; the fifth pouch becomes included in the thyroid gland in most mammals, but in the dog some parafollicular cells are found in the distal pole of the parathyroid. The cells lie around the follicle and have clear vesicular nuclei which distinguish them from thyroid hormone-producing cells (Fig. 7–1). The C-cells have also been shown to concentrate calcitonin by immunofluorescent techniques.

## THE ROLE OF CALCITONIN

It may seem strange that a hormone that appears to have a role in controlling serum calcium should remain undiscovered until 1961. At this time Copp and his associates found that dog parathyroid glands perfused with serum containing high calcium concentrations resulted in rapid systemic hypocalcemia. The fall was clearly more dramatic than the slower decline in serum calcium after parathyroidectomy.[2] Munson and his colleagues, in the rat, showed that cautery of the parathyroids, compared with excision of the parathyroids, elicited a sharper fall in the serum calcium (Fig. 7–2).[3] Both studies proved the existence of a calcium-lowering hormone, coming from the parathyroids in the dog and the thyroids in the rat. When the ultimobranchial origin of the hormone was recognized, the appearance of the hormone-producing C-cells in parathyroid tissue, thyroid tissue, and, in birds, fish, and reptiles, in separate ultimobranchial bodies was more easily understood.

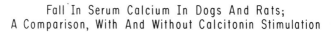

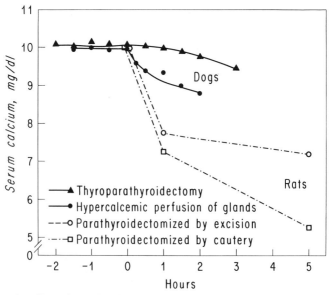

**Figure 7–2** The effect of parathyroidectomy with and without calcitonin in dogs and rats. Both hypercalcaemic perfusion and parathyroidectomy by cautery stimulate calcitonin secretion and result in a more exaggerated hypocalcemic response compared with parathyroidectomy alone. (Redrawn from Munson et al.[3])

Table 7-1  SALMON CALCIUM AND CALCITONIN IN FRESH AND SEA WATER

|  | Water calcium mg/dl | Salmon plasma calcium mg/dl | Salmon gland calcitonin unit/kg body wt |
|---|---|---|---|
| FRESH WATER | 3.6 | 16.9 | 0.39 |
| SEA WATER | 40 | 19.0 | 0.62 |

From Copp et al.[4]

Calcitonin is an essential hormone in fish which migrate from fresh water to salt water and also in birds which, during the egg-laying cycle, have to transport large quantities of calcium from intermedullary bone to the eggshell (Table 7-1).[4] Both situations would be potentially hypercalcemic, and calcitonin plays an important physiological role in preventing the hypercalcemia.

Although it is obvious from Table 7-1 that calcitonin cannot maintain a completely uniform serum calcium level, the 10 per cent rise in the serum is far less than the change in concentration in the calcium content of the water. In the turkey, Copp has reported values of 0.9 units of calcitonin, which suggests a physiological importance in this species compared with the relative unimportance in human beings, in whom the gland content is only 0.16 units per kg of body weight.[5]

In growing rats and pigs removal of the thyroid and parathyroid and, therefore, of the source of calcitonin, resulted in higher serum calcium levels after a calcium load administered by stomach tube.[6] The effect seems more dramatic in very young animals. However, in adult man, following thyroidectomy with thyroxine replacement (but with remaining calcitonin deficiency) the parathyroids appear to control the fluctuations of serum calcium satisfactorily; postprandial hypercalcemia does not develop. Indeed, when parathyroid control is abnormal, as in hyperparathyroidism or in other instances of hypercalcemia, such as sarcoidosis or malignancy, calcitonin is ineffective in preventing life-threatening and perhaps lethal hypercalcemia. The role of calcitonin in an adult man is therefore probably negligible, and it represents a residual hormone reflecting man's origin from fish.

## THE HYPOCALCEMIC EFFECTS OF CALCITONIN

While the prevention of hypercalcemia does not seem to be an effective property of calcitonin in man, even though circulating levels of the hormone are present, exogenous calcitonin will generally cause some fall in serum calcium levels by increasing the renal excretion of this ion. This is obviously part of the physiological role of the hormone in getting rid of large quantities of calcium that may have entered the blood through the environment, as in salmon migrating to salt water. Hypercalcemia in man has been treated successfully with calcitonin, although used as a temporary measure after hydration and diuretics have failed. Since a lowering of the serum calcium can also be produced by giving nephrectomized animals calcitonin, some of the effect may be the result of an inhibition of the exit of calcium from bone. The hypocalcemic effect of calcitonin may be the predominant response by the skeleton, and large doses of calcitonin have elicited secondary hyperparathyroidism in both animals and man.[7, 8]

## The Effect of Calcitonin on Phosphate

Calcitonin also increases phosphate excretion by the kidney through decreased reabsorption in the proximal tubule. Although the effect is relatively small, it is accompanied by a decrease in serum phosphate. The effect is seen in parathyroidectomized animals and is therefore not secondary to hypocalcemic-stimulated hyperparathyroidism. The hypophosphatemia is preceded by hyperphosphatemia. In animals that are thyroidectomized and the thyroxine replaced (i.e., are calcitonin deficient), calcitonin administration results in a rapid, transient rise in the serum phosphate. Since the effect occurs within minutes in fasting animals, it was suggested that calcitonin causes a transfer of phosphate from within the cells to the blood (Table 7–2).[9] Although traditionally serum phosphate is measured very infrequently compared with serum calcium, calcitonin probably has a more consistent effect in producing hypophosphatemia and phosphate excretion than the parallel effect on calcium. The reason quite possibly lies in the evolutionary need for the excretion of phosphate which has a high concentration in sea water.

## The Action of Calcitonin on Bone

Most experiments have been carried out in young, rapidly growing rats; calcitonin administration will prevent the release of $^{45}$Ca label and has even been shown to cause an increase in bone density.[1, 10] In the latter study the rats were parathyroid-intact, and it is possible that the decreased serum phosphate resulted in a raised ionized calcium and induced hypoparathyroidism. Early reports therefore claimed that calcitonin would prevent bone resorption. However, later studies in which calcitonin was administered to both adult and young animals have failed to produce osteosclerosis or increased bone density. Indeed, in patients with high circulating calcitonin levels and medullary carcinoma of the thyroid, bone density is normal or low (Table 7–3).[11] Calcitonin, possibly by depleting cells of phosphorus and limiting energy-dependent systems, decreases the activity of both bone resorbing cells and bone forming cells. This explains its effectiveness in the treatment of Paget's disease and its lack of effect in most forms of osteoporosis or bone disease where cell activity is only mildly increased.

**Table 7–2**   SERUM PHOSPHORUS RESPONSE TO CALCITONIN INJECTION IN CHRONICALLY THYROIDECTOMIZED DOGS

| Time (hours) | Serum Phosphorus (mg/dl) |
|---|---|
| $T_0$ | 3.95 |
| 5 minute injection | 4.32 |
| $T_{1/2}$ | 4.62 |
| $T_1$ | 4.70 |
| $T_2$ | 4.41 |
| $T_3$ | 3.87 |
| $T_4$ | 3.83 |
| $T_5$ | 3.89 |

From Detenbeck and Jowsey.[9]

Table 7-3   BONE MINERAL, g/cm² (mean and range)

|  | MCT (medullary carcinoma of the thyroid) | Normal |
|---|---|---|
| Females (15–52 yrs) | 0.73 (.65–.80) | 0.73 (.66–.75) |
| Males (21–68 yrs) | 0.80 (.50–.94) | 0.85 (.79–.89) |

From Melvin et al.[11]

In immobilization osteoporosis calcitonin has no mediating effect on the bone loss, although there appears to be some slight slowing of the bone losing process in experimental phosphate-induced osteoporosis. In man the results of chronic calcitonin administration to osteoporotic subjects have been unimpressive, because both osteoclastic and osteoblastic activity are slightly decreased rather than demonstrating any specific or dramatic effect on osteoclastic activity alone.[8]

## BIOLOGICAL ACTION

Calcitonin appears to have an important physiological function in animals that experience wide fluctuations in environmental calcium levels. However, except in embryonic life and in very young animals, this hormone appears to have become residual. Organ response also appears to be minimal, although kidney and bone do respond; the kidney responds in a manner similar to the response to parathyroid hormone and bone by decreasing cell activity (both osteoclastic and osteoblastic), but not dramatically.

It is obvious, therefore, that the view that calcitonin represents a hormone antagonistic to parathyroid hormone is not tenable. Its role in fish and laying fowl is explicable, and in human beings its role is probably nonexistent, although certain effects can be obtained by exogenous calcitonin administration which are reminiscent of the action of this hormone in fish.

The relationship between calcitonin and adrenal cortical hormones is discussed in Chapter Twenty-Six, Hypercortisonism. The relationship between the two hormones is not clear, but they may both be related to stress and crisis situations.

## REFERENCES

1. Potts, J. T.: Recent advances in thyrocalcitonin research. Fed. Proc., 29:1200–1205, 1970.
2. Copp, D. H., Cameron, E. C., Cheney, B. A., Davidson, A. G. F., and Henze, K. G.: Evidence for calcitonin: a new hormone from the parathyroid that lowers blood calcium. Endocrinology, 70:638–649, 1962.
3. Munson, P. L., Hirsch, P. F., Brewer, H. B., Reisfeld, R. A., Cooper, C. W., Wästhed, A. B., Orimo, H., and Potts, J. R., Jr.: Thyrocalcitonin. Recent Progr. Horm. Res., 24:589–650, 1968.
4. Copp, D. H., Brooks, C. E., Low, B. S., Newsome, F., O'Dor, R. K., Parkes, C. O., Walker, V., and Watts, E. G.: Calcitonin and ultimobranchial function in lower vertebrates. In Calcitonin, 1969 (Proceedings of the Second International Symposium, London, July 21–24, 1969). New York. Springer-Verlag, Inc., 1970, pp. 281–294.
5. Copp, D. H.: Ultimobranchial Glands and Calcium Regulation. In Hoar, W. S., and Randall, D. J. (Eds.): Fish Physiology. Vol. II. New York, Academic Press, 1969, pp. 379–398.

6. Hirsch, P. F.: Thyrocalcitonin and its role in calcium regulation in mammals. J. Exp. Zool., *178*:139–150, 1971.

7. Indech, M., and Jowsey, J.: Secondary hyperparathyroidism produced in kittens repeatedly given porcine calcitonin. Endocrinology, *88*:1489–1496, 1971.

8. Jowsey, J., Riggs, B. L., Goldsmith, R. S., Kelly, P. J., and Arnaud, C. D.: Effects of prolonged administration of porcine calcitonin in postmenopausal osteoporosis. J. Clin. Endocrinol. Metab., *33*:752–758, 1971.

9. Detenbeck, L. C., and Jowsey, J.: The effect of thyroidectomy and parathyroidectomy in the remodelling of bone defects in adult dogs. Clin. Orthop., *65*:199–202, 1969.

10. Foster, G. V.: Calcitonin, a review of experimental and clinical investigation. Postgrad. Med. J., *44*:411–422, 1968.

11. Melvin, K. E. W., Tashjian, A. H., Jr., and Bordier, P.: The metabolic significance of calcitonin-secreting thyroid carcinoma. Excerpta Medica. International Congress Series No. *270*:193–201, 1973.

# Chapter Eight

# BONE MORPHOLOGY: BONE STRUCTURE

## INTRODUCTION

Bone tissue represents the only significant store of calcium in the body; this fact has a number of consequences that will become apparent throughout this book. Both calcium and sodium are of major importance in nerve and muscle function, and for this reason effective systems have evolved to conserve and control the homeostasis of these two elements. We are concerned mainly with calcium. It has already been stressed that small changes in the amount of this element in serum and extracellular fluid profoundly affect neuromuscular activity. A decrease in serum calcium will result first in tetany and then in convulsions. High levels of extracellular calcium, at least in vitro, have been shown to produce changes in microtubules. Calcium is a key element in cell membrane transport and is essential for the transmission of messenger substances across cell walls. Calcium is also essential for blood coagulation; it functions as a cofactor in the conversion of prothrombin and thrombin.

It is obvious from the above that calcium is an essential element and also that adequate amounts of the ion must be readily available. To the average person it appears that the bone tissue that makes up the skeleton functions primarily as a supporting structure. Certainly the organization of bone along lines of stress, and the shape of the bones and joints themselves, suggest the supporting role. However, other characteristics of the skeleton suggest a primary role as a source of calcium. The continual remodeling that occurs in both trabecular and cortical bone, the intricate microscopic system of connections between the cells lying within the bone (the osteocytes) and the blood, and the possibility of responding to calcium stress both by cell activity and by physicochemical exchange between bone mineral and the intracellular fluid that flows through bone, are all characteristics suggesting a system that will respond to both acute and chronic changes in serum calcium levels.

There is no doubt that the skeleton, forming a stiff, unbending system of bones that are connected at movable joints, supports the body. However, this is a function that becomes secondary to its role as a calcium store. This may be surprising, but it is the only conclusion to be drawn from the many instances of calcium-deprived individuals who lose bone mass rather than experience hypocalcemia and tetany. The loss of bone mass may progress to a state in which skeletal support of the body is impossible and fractures develop. From the point of view of survival, a fracture is less life-threatening than hypocalcemia.

The remodeling of bone occurs in response to two kinds of stimuli. The first is the normal remodeling of the tissue as the individual bones grow and achieve their final form and then continue to remodel; to a large extent this activity appears to be independent of stimuli outside the body. A second response by bone is to lack or excess of various factors that are known to influence bone remodeling, such as hormones (cortisone and thyroxine, for example) and stress. Bone disorders largely result from the latter circumstance and from the role of the skeleton as a source of calcium. For an understanding of how bone abnormalities and mineral homeostasis occur, it is necessary to understand the structure of bone and the functions of the cells of bone.

## CORTICAL AND TRABECULAR BONE

Different bones in the skeleton have been distinguished in many ways — for example, bones can be distinguished by shape, such as long and flat bones, by whether they are formed largely from cartilage (the endochondral bones) or from the periosteum (the membrane bones), or by whether they are composed mainly of compact cortical bone or of spongy trabecular bone (the shafts of the long bones of the skeleton are largely cortical, the ends are predominantly trabecular).

Cortical bone is a solid, calcified matrix with occasional vascular channels containing blood vessels and soft tissue; approximately 80 per cent of the skeleton is cortical bone. The blood vessels and soft tissue spaces form an approximately longitudinal arrangement of tunnels, widely spaced and connected by cross branches embedded in the mineralized matrix. Although there have been few studies of the longitudinal structure of bone, most morphology is viewed in cross section; nevertheless bones, as organs, should be considered as three-dimensional structures. The major blood vessels of cortical bone spiral around each other in small groups as they move from the periosteum to the endosteum, or vice versa. The spiral is related to the axis of the bone. In the femur of the dog, in which the only study has been carried out on this aspect of microstructure, the spiral is clockwise distally in the left femur and counterclockwise in the right.[1] It is highly probable that a very intricate organization of small spirals of osteones that twist around each other, and that in turn spiral in larger bundles, are oriented in relation to stress-strain patterns in all bones. This may at first seem to be of academic interest. However, it bears on the question of early weight-bearing in fracture healing which will presumably result in early stress-related organization of bone. On the other side of the coin, it may explain the presence of fracture in osteopetrosis, where lack of bone remodeling prevents organization along stress forces.

Cancellous bone consists of scattered trabeculae in a large vascular marrow space; it constitutes less than 20 per cent of the skeleton. Within any sample of trabecular bone, the space occupied by bone varies; probably the most reliable data are from scanning electron microscopy of the vertebrae, which give a value of 23 per cent. In our laboratory, using a planimetry method, iliac crest trabecular bone

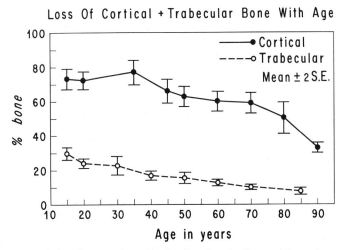

**Figure 8–1** The relative decrease in cortical and trabecular bone with age in apparently normal persons. Note the relatively rapid loss early in life in trabecular bone and comparatively little loss at this age in cortical bone: The situation is reversed after age 55.

occupies 15.4 ± SD 6.8 of the spongy bone part of the sample in 20 to 90-year-old normals. This value tends to decrease with age (Fig. 8–1). In trabecular bone the area of the bone surface is large in relation to the bone volume. This difference confers on trabecular bone certain properties not characteristically present in cortical bone. Calculations of surface-to-volume ratios have been made by different methods; the surface perimeter, in centimeters per unit area of bone, varies from 90 cm$^2$ to 165 cm/cm$^2$.[2, 3] Both of these measurements are from vertebral specimens. Lloyd has used a computerized method to study microradiographs to measure the surface-to-area or volume ratio in various areas of both cancellous and cortical bone (Table 8–1).[2]

Amstutz, using a different method, obtained a slightly higher figure for trabecular bone in a lumbar vertebra of a 40-year-old male, namely 156 ± SE, 0.58 cm$^2$/cm$^3$, in comparison with Lloyd's value of 120 cm$^2$/cm$^3$.[4] With scanning elec-

**Table 8–1**  SURFACE-TO-AREA AND VOLUME IN BONE
(figures in parenthesis are number of samples)

|  | Perimeter/area cm/cm$^2$ of bone surface (mean ± SD) | Surface/volume cm$^2$/cm$^3$ |
|---|---|---|
| TRABECULAR BONE |  |  |
| Femoral head (8) | 76 ± 4.5 | 96 ± 5.7 |
| Thoracic vertebrae (8) | 91 ± 18.0 | 116 ± 22.9 |
| Lumbar vertebrae (10) | 94 ± 9.9 | 120 ± 12.7 |
| Rib, sternal end (18) | 130 ± 37.3 | 147 ± 41.7 |
| Rib, vertebral end (17) | 70 ± 18.9 | 79 ± 21.6 |
| Iliac crest (12) | 159 ± 31.3 | 202 ± 39.9 |
| CORTICAL BONE |  |  |
| Femoral midshaft (4) | 30.3 ± 2.4 | 30.5 ± 2.9 |

From Lloyd and Hodges.[2]

**Table 8-2**  PERCENT OF BONE THAT IS TRABECULAR OR CORTICAL;
MEAN + SD

|  | Trabecular | Cortical | n |
|---|---|---|---|
| ILIAC CREST | 36.0 (12.1) | 64.0 (11.9) | 192 |
| VERTEBRA | 49.9 (6.8) | 50.1 (6.8) | 12 |
| RADIUS | 18.8 (1.5) | 81.2 (1.5) | 2 |

tron microscopy, values of 165 cm/cm² were obtained in a 26-year-old male.[3] Part of the difference in these values is real and represents variation between different individuals; part is possibly the difference in methodology.

Cortical bone, by comparison, has a small surface area and is less responsive, but it represents a large volume which proportionally increases with age; because of this, it will continue to respond to metabolic stress after trabecular bone has "burned out." It is essential therefore to include cortical bone in the evaluation of bone loss, as well as trabecular bone, especially in persons over the age of 55.

The evaluations of trabecular and cortical bone differ in relationship to the volumes of these two types of bone in a sample. Obviously a lumbar vertebra contains a high percentage of trabecular bone. However, other sites of the skeleton, which have been considered to contain "mainly trabecular bone" in fact do not. Data indicate that no area of the skeleton contains more trabecular than cortical bone (Table 8-2).

There are also changes in the proportion of trabecular and cortical bone in any one area. For example, if the percent of bone in a specimen of the iliac crest is evaluated, it is found that the cortical bone increases in percentage (and this value excludes loss by intracortical porosity), while the percentage of trabecular bone decreases with age (Fig. 8-2).

If one is searching for an area that will rapidly reflect changes in bone metabolism, then areas of the skeleton containing trabecular bone, such as the vertebrae, would be most suitable. This is true only if percentage changes in density are being

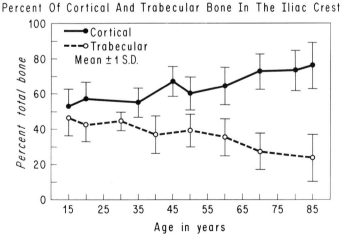

**Figure 8-2**  Changes in the proportion of cortical and trabecular bone with age. Before skeletal maturity, the volumes of these two types are nearly the same; by the age of 65 the majority is cortical bone.

measured, which is generally the case in most techniques. However, and perhaps surprisingly, if the available surface in cortical and trabecular bone in the skeleton is estimated, the values are very similar, namely, 5.4 square meters of surface in cortical bone and 5.8 square meters of surface in trabecular bone. In other words, even though the surface-to-area ratio is greater in trabecular bone, the amount of cortical bone in the skeleton is so much larger that the absolute surface in both is similar.

One other fact emerges which pushes the bone response to stimuli even further away from trabecular toward cortical bone; for some reason, cortical bone decreases in mass at a more rapid rate than does trabecular bone after age 40. This has been shown by direct measurements of bones, such as the study of long bones compared with vertebral bones by Trotter's group (Table 8–3)[5] and also by data from our laboratory (Fig. 8–2).[6]

A number of studies have shown that trabecular bone mass decreases mainly by a loss of entire trabeculae rather than by thinning of trabeculae,[7] whereas cortical bone is lost by transformation, on the endosteal surface, of compact to cancellous bone and by an increase in the number of holes in the compact midportion of the cortex.

Most trabecular bone is arranged along lines of stress, and there is a suggestion that the longitudinal arrangement of haversian systems in cortical bone is also related to stress-strain patterns. It is certainly true that the loss of bone with age conforms to the function of the skeleton as a supporting structure. In trabecular bone, the horizontal trabeculae are lost first, whereas the weight-bearing, longitudinal trabeculae remain and appear never to be entirely lost. In cortical bone, the outer third of the cortex remains. These organized processes of bone loss mean that the first bone to be lost is the least needed.

Despite the differences between cortical and trabecular bone, all bones are mixtures of these two types, and the behavior of bone as a tissue is similar, irrespective of type. For instance, cortical bone and trabecular bone have the same composition and are laid down and removed by the same mechanism; they only

**Table 8–3** REGRESSION COEFFICIENTS OF DENSITY ON AGE FOR TRABECULAR AND CORTICAL TYPE BONES IN RELATION TO SEX AND RACE; THE RATE OF BONE LOSS IS MORE RAPID IN CORTICAL BONE ($v = vertebra$)

| | | **Male** | | **Female** | |
| --- | --- | --- | --- | --- | --- |
| | | WHITE | NEGRO | WHITE | NEGRO |
| Cervical v.<br>Thoracic v.  } mean<br>Lumbar v. | | .0034 | .0015 | .0030 | .0028 |
| Humeri<br>Radii<br>Ulnae  } mean<br>Femora<br>Tibiae | | .0052 | .0040 | .0054 | .0048 |

From Trotter et al.[5]

differ in the amount of the non-bone space. The characteristics of structure, tissue turnover and cell dynamics of bone can be described in general terms and are relevant to bone throughout the skeleton.

## INCREASE IN BONE SIZE WITH AGE

There is overwhelming evidence that, in general, the majority of individuals lose things as they get older; they lose teeth, hair, strength, energy, and, of course, bone. Probably bone and teeth are the two tissues which are the least commonly lost with increasing age. When bone loss does occur, it results from disappearance of trabeculae, disappearance of endosteal bone, and increased porosity of cortical bone. There are reports suggesting that this loss is accompanied by an increase in the external dimensions of the bone, at least of the distal long bones; this means that there has been periosteal new bone deposition.[8, 9] Trotter and Peterson have studied this phenomenon carefully.[10] They have shown that part of the increase in external dimensions, measured by radiography of extremities in vivo, was exaggerated because of the increase in film-to-bone distance caused by the tendency for older individuals to have fatter thighs. A further change resulted when cleaned specimens of femur, which showed an increase of 2.2 per cent in individuals between 45 and 90 years of age, measured radiographically, decreased to 1.1 per cent when the bone width was measured directly with calipers. An increase in periosteal width does appear to occur. However, in histological examination of sections of cortical, femoral bone, new periosteal bone formation is almost never seen (evaluated histologically or by tetracycline uptake), and it is hard to account for an increase in periosteal dimension if no new bone is being laid down. An interesting point emerged from this controversy.

In any display of data in which a certain measurement is plotted against age, it is assumed that the change in the measurement, if there is one, is the result of age; however the graph is generally thought of as representing the change in a single individual as he grows older, although the data have been collected at one time from people of different ages. Thus, if external bone dimension or cortical diameter is plotted against age and there is a significant increase with increasing age, it is assumed that new bone is being laid down periosteally. There is, however, an alternative possibility, and that is that the longer ago people were born, the larger were their bones, since, in a collection of post-mortem specimens, the older individuals will have been born in earlier years. Trotter and Peterson applied cohort analysis to their data of absolute bone diameter and found that if the date of birth is taken into account, the significant relation (P less than .01) between increasing age and bone diameter disappeared and, in fact, became negative ($r = -.0746$, NS) (Table 8–4). In other words, they were able to collect a number of specimens from individuals born in 1890, 1900, 1910, and so on, who died when they were 20, 30, and 40 years old and found that, with increasing age, no increase in diameter occurred if the date of birth was the same.[11] The inference is that 50 or 60 years ago the way of life, including perhaps activity level, diet, and other factors, led to a greater bone size at the time of skeletal maturity. It may well be that cohort analysis should be applied to other age-related data in order to evaluate the importance of date of birth in relation to age at the time of measurement, and to establish if true age-related changes are occurring.

**Table 8-4** VARIABLES MEASURED IN FEMORA FROM INDIVIDUALS
BETWEEN THE AGES OF 40 AND 91
(TD = transverse diameter at the mid-point of the bone)

| Pairs of variables | Correlation coefficient, r. | Level of significance, p. |
|---|---|---|
| Age with length | −.1026 | NS |
| Length with TD | .3871 | <.01 |
| Age with TD* | .2082 | <.01 |
| Age with TD** | −.0746 | NS |

\*partial r, eliminating effect of length
\*\*partial r, eliminating effect of cohorts

From Trotter and Peterson.[11]

It is doubtful, therefore, that there is an increase in bone diameter (in the femur at least) with increasing age. It becomes likely, in fact, that the bone size is smaller in people born more recently. Therefore any bone loss that occurs represents a net loss uncompensated by any periosteal new-bone formation. This has been supported by other studies. External transverse diameter has been measured in the metacarpal and has been found not to vary with age or the presence or absence of osteoporosis, despite signficant changes in the medullary canal size.[12] However, there was a difference between sexes; the mean diameter in men was 9.7 mm (± SD 0.08), and in women it was 8.1 mm (± SD 0.09).

### REFERENCES

1. Cohen, J., and Harris, W. H.: The three-dimensional anatomy of Haversian systems. J. Bone Joint Surg., *40A*:419–434, 1958.
2. Lloyd, E., and Hodges, D.: Quantitative characterization of bone: a computer analysis of microradiographs. Clin. Orthop., *78*:230–250, 1971.
3. Dyson, E. D., Jackson, C. K., and Whitehouse, W. J.: Scanning electron microscope studies of human trabecular bone. Nature, *225*:957–959, 1970.
4. Amstutz, H. C., and Sissons, H. A.: The structure of the vertebral spongiosa. J. Bone Joint Surg., *51B*:540–550, 1969.
5. Trotter, M., Broman, G. E., and Peterson, R. R.: Densities of bones of white and Negro skeletons. J. Bone Joint Surg., *42A*:50–58, 1960.
6. Jowsey, J.: Unpublished data.
7. Wakamatsu, E., and Sissons, H. A.: The cancellous bone of the iliac crest. Calcif. Tissue Res., *4*:147–161, 1969.
8. Garn, S. M.: Human biology and research in body composition. Ann. N.Y. Acad. Sci., *10*:429–446, 1963.
9. Smith, R. W., Jr., and Walker, R. R.: Femoral expansion in aging women: implications for osteoporosis and fractures. Science, *145*:156–157, 1964.
10. Trotter, M., and Peterson, R. R.: Transverse diameter of the femur: on roentgenograms and on bones. Clin. Orthop., *52*:233–239, 1967.
11. Trotter, M., and Peterson, R. R.: Increase in the transverse diameter of the adult femur with age (abstract). Anat. Rec., *157*:334, 1967.
12. Morgan, D. B., Spiers, F. W., Pulvertaft, C. N., and Fourman, P.: The amount of bone in the metacarpal and the phalanx according to age and sex. Clin. Radiol., *18*:101–108, 1967.

# Chapter Nine

# BONE MORPHOLOGY: BONE TISSUE

Bone tissue is made up of a matrix containing calcium and phosphate; the composition is shown in Table 9–1.

### OSTEOID

The matrix is generally referred to as osteoid tissue, and, strictly speaking, only when it has been mineralized can it be referred to as bone. Osteoid is produced by osteoblasts and usually, but not always, reflects new bone formation. It is made up of collagen, glycosaminoglycans, water, and osteocytes.

**Appearance.** In demineralized sections of bone stained with hematoxylin and eosin, the new bone, formed but as yet unmineralized, appears as a pink layer, whereas the mineralized bone stains somewhat blue with hematoxylin.[2] In some "routine" preparations of this kind, it may be difficult to distinguish between bone which had never contained mineral and that which had (before the demineralization procedure); hematoxylin is not a specific stain for calcium. The use of mineralized sections avoids the problem. The sections may be left unstained or can be stained by the von Kossa technique.[1] The von Kossa stain colors insoluble phosphates and carbonates a brown-black, and, since bone mineral is made of calcium and phosphate, the von Kossa procedure is generally regarded as a stain for

Table 9–1  THE COMPOSITION OF BONE

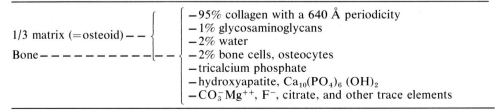

| 1/3 matrix (=osteoid) | |
| Bone | |

- —95% collagen with a 640 Å periodicity
- —1% glycosaminoglycans
- —2% water
- —2% bone cells, osteocytes
- —tricalcium phosphate
- —hydroxyapatite, $Ca_{10}(PO_4)_6 (OH)_2$
- —$CO_3^-$ $Mg^{++}$, $F^-$, citrate, and other trace elements

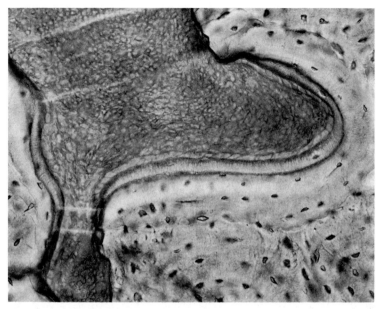

**Figure 9–1**  The narrow band of tissue marked O represents osteoid tissue bordered on the marrow side by a sheet of osteoblasts and on the bone side by the mineralization front (magnification ×250).

calcium. Unfortunately the fully mineralized bone goes black, and variations in mineralization cannot be appreciated. If the bone section is left unstained, the mineralized bone appears brown, the osteoid a pinkish yellow, and poorly mineralized bone and the mineralization front appear a darker brown (Fig. 9–1). The lack of mineral in the osteoid can be confirmed by comparing the undecalcified section with the microradiograph of the same section.

Measurements of osteoid tissue width from mineralization front to osteoid surface show a real variation from one animal species to another, but they vary only apparently in human beings owing to different methods of preparation and measurement. In contrast to demineralized, paraffin-embedded material, methacrylate embedding appears to prevent any artifactual shrinkage. Whatever the preparation technique used, the width is most commonly measured microscopically with a graduated eye-piece at a magnification of 100 times. The values in human beings when unstained methacrylate sections are used give an average figure of approximately 12 microns.[2] However, there appears to be a clearly age-related variation; at age 20 the mean value for osteoid width is 16 microns, whereas in a normal 80-year-old the value has decreased to 10 microns (Fig. 9–2). In patients with the bone disorders of osteomalacia and rickets, the osteoid border widths are 20 microns or more.

An alternative method has been developed by Woods and co-workers which makes use of polarized light. Mineralized sections are made and stained by the von Kossa technique. The polarized light produces alternate light and dark bands corresponding to lamellae of collagen. In normal persons, one to three bright bands are present, and in cases of clinically identified osteomalacia the values range from 3 to 12. This method avoids the error that may occur if the section is cut obliquely through the osteoid borders.[3]

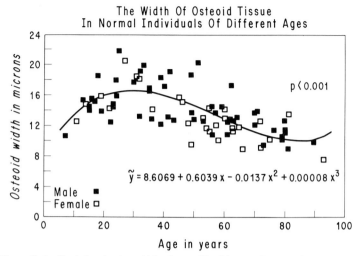

**Figure 9–2**   Variation in the width of osteoid with age. (From Johnson et al.[2]).

Although a number of studies cite values of osteoid border width that seem compatible (approximately 10 microns in normal adult men) a number of studies cite very low values. The information relating the length of surface covered by osteoid also varies, from values as low as 0 to almost 100 per cent, and it is obvious that the explanation lies in the definition of osteoid. Osteoid may be defined as active, in which case it will be 10 to 20 microns thick, have a mineralization front, and be lined by osteoblasts. Such osteoid occupies 3 per cent of the bone surface in adult man and corresponds to bone-forming surfaces. In terms of bone volume, this corresponds to approximately 0.10 per cent.[4] If inactive but recently formed osteoid is measured, the surface of bone covered by osteoid increases and the values of osteoid volume increases to about 14 per cent.[3] If the definition is taken to extend to osteoid which consists of only 1 micron thick collagen in sections of 2 microns thick viewed at high magnifications, then all surfaces of bone except those in the process of resorption are covered with "osteoid."[5] This probably extends the definition of osteoid beyond usefulness, but the presence of an all-encompassing layer of unmineralized connective tissue may constitute morphological evidence of a bone membrane that is capable of separating extracellular fluid from bone fluid.

Frost has shown that the number of osteoid borders tends to increase with age (Fig. 9–3), although this is not associated with an increase in rate of formation and refers to a mixture of cortical and trabecular bone, since the material used was human ribs.[6]

**Composition of Osteoid.**[7]   The matrix makes up about 35 per cent of the dry, fat-free weight of bone, and 95 per cent of this matrix is collagen, which is similar but not identical in structure to the collagen of other connective tissues. The remaining 5 per cent consists of glycosaminoglycans, water, and cells.

The collagen forms the connective tissue-like matrix that confers shape to bone; the mineral is deposited later, giving it rigidity. Collagen in bone is, by morphological and most chemical methods, indistinguishable from skin collagen. It is formed by osteoblasts. These cells accumulate amino acids as polypeptides on the ribosomes, which contain the messenger RNA for the formation of the proline- and lysine-rich protocollagen. Hydroxylation then occurs, and the molecules can

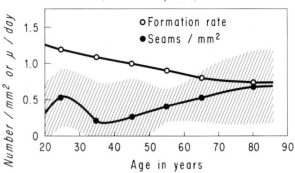

Osteoid Seams And Rate Of Formation In Normals
(from Frost, 1969)

**Figure 9–3** The volume of bone occupied by osteoid tissue and the bone formation rate in persons of different ages. (Redrawn from Frost.[6]).

then pass through the cell membrane wall to form the matrix. These molecules form a long chain called tropocollagen, which is about 2,800 Å long and 14 Å in diameter; it is made up of three strands of collagen coiled around each other and easily soluble in cold salt solutions.[8] (Of the three strands, two are similar, the $\alpha$ strands, and the third $\alpha^2$ is different.) The difference is minor and resides in the different amino acid composition.[9] Each $\alpha$-chain contains about 1,000 amino acids and has a molecular weight of approximately 95,000. The three strands form a left-handed spiral around each other to form a helix with a repetitive structure every 9.5 Å. This polypeptide chain is then wound right-handedly around a central axis.

Cross-linking occurs both between the three-stranded tropocollagen and between the different tropocollagen threads. This is less soluble and will not go into solution except by heat, enzyme action (collagenase), or other strong treatment.

Collagen is formed by the bone cells in the sequence shown in Table 9–2.

The mature collagen has a periodicity of 640 Å and, because of the regularity of its structure, will produce an x-ray diffraction pattern. It may thus be considered crystalline and, indeed, will behave like a crystal and evoke a piezoelectric effect in response to stress. This has important implications in fracture healing, since an unmineralized fracture callus is able to respond to external forces and be organized accordingly.

Proline is hydroxylated into hydroxyproline in the formation of collagen and normally forms mature collagen, which is eventually broken down and appears as peptide-bound hydroxyproline in the urine.[10] Approximately 95 per cent of the total

**Table 9–2** FORMATION OF BONE MATRIX

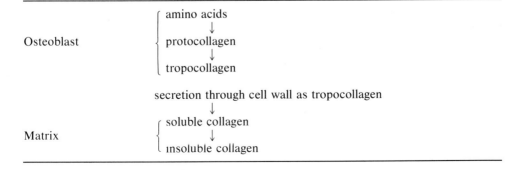

urinary hydroxyproline is bound and the amount, measured in a 24-hour urine sample, has been taken to indicate collagen breakdown.[11] Since the skeleton contains approximately 60 per cent of the body collagen, changes in urinary hydroxyproline may be taken to reflect alterations in bone destruction. Certain precautions must be borne in mind; since dietary collagen will contribute to urinary hydroxyproline, gelatin-containing food must be avoided during a hydroxyproline test period. In addition, variations in the breakdown of bone per gram of bone, as well as the total breakdown of bone in the skeleton, will be reflected in the urinary hydroxyproline values. For this reason values in infants may be between 19 and 56 mg per 24 hours or, corrected for size, 40 to 191 mg per 24 hours/$M^2$, while in 11 to 14 year old children the mg per 24 hour figures will be 63 to 180; corrected for body size they resemble the infant values, 40 to 113 mg per 24 hours/$M^2$.[8]

Both free and peptide-bound hydroxyproline may appear in the urine as a reflection of increased bone collagen synthesis. However, $^{14}$C-labeled proline incorporated into bone collagen will be excreted as $^{14}$C-hydroxyproline. Since the specific activity of the urinary and bone hydroxyproline is almost identical after three or four weeks (in experimental studies), it can be concluded that the majority of hydroxyproline in the urine is derived from degradation rather than synthesis. However, in young animals or neonates, larger proportions of urinary hydroxyproline are derived from proline that is hydroxylated but excreted before it forms mature collagen.

It is to be expected that increased urinary hydroxyproline will be associated with bone-losing diseases. Kivirikko and colleagues have shown a positive relationship between the urinary hydroxyproline and protein-bound iodine in normal and hyperthyroid patients.[12] Parathyroid hormone will also cause a rise in urinary hydroxyproline, and the same is true of Paget's disease of bone, metastatic bone disease, and fibrous dysplasia. The increased urinary hydroxyproline seen in lathyrism probably reflects the increase in the soluble fraction of collagen rather than collagen breakdown.

A number of assays have been developed for measuring urinary hydroxyproline, the majority based on a relatively early technique described by Prockop and Udenfriend,[13] in which hydroxyproline is oxidized to pyrrole, which is then quantitated colorimetrically using Ehrlich's reagent.[14] More recently, interference by other substances in human urine, such as urea and ammonium chloride, have suggested that a chromatographic purification step be added if small changes in urinary hydroxyproline must be detected.[15] $^{14}$C-proline can be used to evaluate recovery.[16]

An apparently insoluble problem exists with all these methods in that, although bone collagen is considered to be the major contributor to the hydroxyproline in the urine, skin, muscle, and connective tissue collagen also may contribute in certain disease states, such as scleroderma and dermatomyositis, which do not involve bone degradation. Recently a difference between the hydroxyproline from skin and bone collagen has been shown in that glycosylgalatosyl-hydroxyproline is found in a larger proportion in skin, while galactosyl-hydroxyproline is quantitatively more important in bone.

Ground substances of the glycosaminoglycans make up less than 1 per cent of the bone matrix and consist of chondroitin sulfate A and hyaluronic acid. These have no gross structure and have been described as amorphous, although they obviously have a microstructure. A significant fraction of water is associated partially with the ground substance. The remainder of the unmineralized fraction of bone is made up of a sparse scattering of cells, the osteocytes.

## BONE MINERAL

**Structure.** Two thirds of the weight and one half of the volume of bone is mineral in the form of hydroxyapatite, $Ca_{10}(PO_4)_6(OH)_2$. The x-ray diffraction pattern is one common to other apatites, such as fluorapatite. The latter is the only member of this family of crystal forms that has a large enough crystal for accurate structural evaluation; other apatites such as hydroxyapatite are very small but presumably have the same general structure as fluorapatite. These crystals have repeating anatomical units which combine to give a crystal 680 Å by 50 Å in size in mature bone.[17] Initial mineralization was originally considered to be a different form, the so-called amorphous tricalcium phosphate. However, the early stages of both bone and cartilage mineralization have revealed microcrystals rather than an "amorphous" precipitate, and all the mineral phase of bone can be considered as being in the form of hydroxyapatite.

The calcium-to-phosphorus ratio should be 1.67 for hydroxyapatite; the majority of chemical determinations of bone mineral result in figures below this value, suggesting that bone hydroxyapatite is calcium-poor.[18] This may be the result of substitution of other ions for calcium in the lattice or the presence of unsubstituted defects in the position of calcium. If apatite from bone is heated to 400° C, the diffraction pattern becomes clearer. A temperature of 400° C allows thermal reconstruction but not fusion, and therefore encourages the suggestion that defects are responsible for the low molar ratio of calcium to phosphorus. The defects may contain substitution ions such as sodium or magnesium which are present in bone in significant quantities.

### Mineralization of Bone

Investigations attempting to elucidate the mechanism by which bone matrix becomes mineralized have been going on for many years without providing a clear answer as to how this process occurs. Three pieces of information did, however, emerge repeatedly, which were derived from chemical studies and which indicated that the serum is supersaturated with respect to the bone mineral, hydroxyapatite. Therefore, once a crystal is formed, it will increase in size merely by being enveloped in a solution of the same approximate calcium and phosphorus activity product as serum. In vitro studies, on the other hand, repeatedly established that unmineralized bone and cartilage cannot be mineralized in solutions or in serum with the physiological concentrations of calcium and phosphorus that are found in vivo. It was evident therefore that the initiation of mineralization requires a special process that could not be satisfied by existing chemical concentrations alone. The third important fact, described in studies of cartilage mineralization, was that the process occurred extracellularly in the matrix. Originally Robison had postulated that phosphate esters were hydrolysed locally to produce high concentrations of phosphate, thus exceeding the solubility constant for hydroxyapatite and causing a small crystallite to appear![17] The mechanism of mineralization of bone remained obscure, however, until the recent work of Bonucci, Anderson, and others.[18, 19, 20] These investigators relied on morphology to describe the process by which both cartilage and bone are mineralized.

As long ago as 1949 and 1951, Gersh and Heller-Steinberg, respectively, described small spherical particles in the zone of mineralization of bone in the process of their early electron-microscopic studies.[21, 22] No one paid a great deal of attention to the findings, which are, in fact, not a great deal different from the currently accepted theories based on the formation of matrix vesicles which contain the initially formed bone mineral. The problem perhaps was that both Robison and Gersh sought to involve the collagen and its organized periodicity in the initial mineralization process; later electron-microscopic work failed to demonstrate any convincing relationship between the initial microcrystals and collagen fibers. These studies did, however, indicate that enzyme inhibitors will prevent the mineralization process, suggesting, as Robison did, that enzymatic activity was necessary. Although phosphatases are implicated in the mineralization process in matrix vesicles, alkaline phosphatase is not likely to be the enzyme involved, since it is not inactivated by fluoride or iodoacetamide, the inhibitors used. The feature that the matrix vesicle theory has in common with earlier morphological observations, and which distinguishes it from Robison's enzyme theory, is the necessity for a membrane within which high local concentrations of calcium and phosphorus can occur.

It is now clear that mineralization proceeds by the formation of vesicles which, in cartilage, are 300 Å to 1 micron in diameter. The vesicles are found in zones where mineralization is known to occur and appear in areas such as the longitudinal septa between degenerate cartilage cells. Needle-like structures are found within the vesicles and in juxtaposition to the vesicles; these crystallites are dense and, since they are removed by EDTA, they are thus highly likely to be hydroxyapatite.

The vesicles may be produced by cells, but the evidence is not conclusive. Earlier data showed electron-dense particles inside mitochondria or inside chondrocytes.[18, 19, 23] However, current data suggests that these are intercellular calcium storage particles and do not migrate. Mineral accumulates within the vesicles with the help of enzyme activity, and the crystals form. Enzymes that have been identified in the process include alkaline phosphatase and ATPase. Once formed, the concentrations of calcium and phosphorus permit growth, and the crystals burst through the vesicle membranes and grow to completion of mineralization. The sequence in bone is similar except that the dense accumulation of collagen and its orderly orientation affect the localization of the matrix vesicles and subsequent mineralization foci.[24]

The majority of the early work on matrix vesicles relied on fixed, dehydrated, and embedded material. This technique is always open to the criticism that the vesicles or crystals represent artifacts. Frozen, thin section methods and microincineration have avoided this criticism, and, although the microscopic detail is not as perfect as in the embedded sections, observations in this type of preparation are necessary for confirmation of the matrix vesicle theory of mineralization. Using frozen sections, Gay and Schraer have demonstrated the presence of electron-dense granules within the osteoblasts in areas of rapidly mineralizing bone.[24] These granules are 200 to 800 Å in size and consist of an agglomerate of smaller particles which appear, from their high electron scattering properties, to be calcium phosphate (Fig. 9–4A and B). They are contained in sac-like envelopes and are found adjacent to the boundary between the osteoblast and the matrix or osteoid. These authors' particular contribution has been the extension of the earlier work in

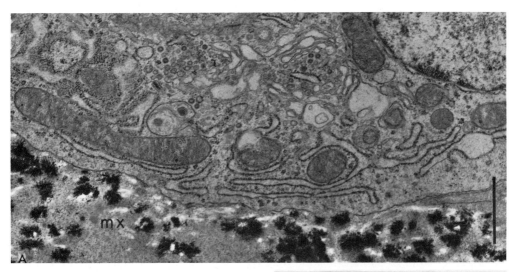

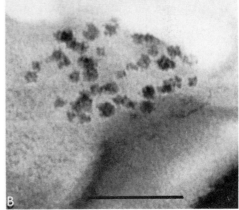

**Figure 9–4** (a) Osteoblast adjacent to the bone matrix (mx); the matrix contains aggregates of bone mineral which appear dense on the electron microscope picture. There are no mitochondrial granules (magnification x 17,800). (b) A high magnification of the matrix vesicles showing the spherical appearance. Most vesicles consist of smaller particles which are most probably calcium phosphate. (Magnification ×127,000) From: Gay and Schraer.[24]

cartilage to the study of bone tissue. The precise way in which the vesicles containing granules of calcium phosphate are extruded into the matrix and across the osteoid border to the mineralization front is not yet clear. However, it has been suggested that the particles are extruded from the osteoblasts and travel down the canaliculi to the mineralization front, where a continual supply of extracellular fluid from the canaliculi permits crystal formation and growth.[25]

The data is still incomplete, and the full story has yet to be verified in all aspects; however, the existing information is far ahead of earlier, more theoretical, approaches.

**Trace Elements.**[26, 27] Trace elements occur in varying proportions in bone mineral.[28] Magnesium, fluoride, citrate, carbonate, sodium, and potassium all occur as trace elements and can be determined in wet-ashed specimens (Table 9–3). They occur in relatively small quantities, so contamination of the sample must be carefully avoided when measurements are made. Monovalent ions such as sodium and fluoride diffuse into the hydration layer of the hydroxyapatite crystal and may enter the crystal surface. Sodium also holds a surface position on the crystal and has been used to measure crystal areas. Strontium and fluorine ($Sr^{++}$ and $F^-$) can also progress within the crystal lattice and exchange with interior ions, $Ca^{++}$ and

**Table 9–3**   TRACE ELEMENTS PRESENT IN HYDROXYAPATITE

| Element | | % present | ion displaced |
|---------|--|-----------|---------------|
| Carbonate | $CO^{2-}$ | 5.2–6.0 | $PO_4^{3-}$ |
| Citrate | $Cit^{3-}$ | 1.0 | $PO_4^{3-}$ |
| Sodium | $Na^+$ | 0.7 | $Ca^{2+}$ |
| Magnesium | $Mg^{2+}$ | 0.7 | $Ca^{2+}$ |
| Fluoride | $F^-$ | variable | $OH^-$ |
| Iron | $Fe^{2+}$ | > 0.05 | $Ca^{2+}$ |
| Zinc | $Zn^{2+}$ | 0.2 | $Ca^{2+}$ |
| Silicon | $Si^{2+}$ | 0.03 | $Ca^{2+}$ |

From Dixon and Webb.[29]

$OH,^-$ respectively. Magnesium and citrate appear to be surface bound, like sodium, but they are somewhat less frequent than sodium because of the lower concentration of magnesium and citrate compared with the high concentration of sodium in extracellular fluids.

Other ions such as chloride, although present in high concentrations in physiological fluids, do not accumulate in bone, since there is no exchange between them and crystal surface ions.

## *REFERENCES*

1. Meyer, P. C.: The histological identification of osteoid tissue. J. Pathol., 71:325–333, 1956.
2. Johnson, K. A., Riggs, B. L., Kelly, P. J., and Jowsey, J.: Osteoid tissue in normal and osteoporotic individuals. J. Clin. Endocrinol. Metab., 33:745–751, 1971.
3. Woods, C. G., Morgan, D. B., Paterson, C. R., and Gossmann, H. H.: Measurement of osteoid in bone biopsy. J. Pathol., 95:441–447, 1968.
4. Ellis, H. A., and Peart, K. M.: Quantitative observations on mineralized and nonmineralized bone in the iliac crest. J. Clin. Pathol., 25:277–286, 1972.
5. Raina, V.: Normal osteoid tissue. J. Clin. Pathol., 25:229–232, 1972.
6. Frost, H. M.: Tetracycline-based histological analysis of bone remodeling. Calc. Tiss. Res., 3:211–237, 1969.
7. Grant, M. E., and Prockop, D. J.: The biosynthesis of collagen. N. Engl. J. Med., 286:194–199; 242–249; 291–300, 1972.
8. Prockop, D. J., and Kivirikko, K. I.: Relationship of hydroxyproline excretion in urine to collagen metabolism. Ann. Intern. Med., 66:1243–1266, 1967.
9. Piez, K. A., Balian, G., Click, E. M., and Bornstein, P.: Homology between $\alpha$ 1 and $\alpha$ 2 chains of collagen. Biochem. Biophys. Res. Comm., 48:990–995, 1972.
10. Crowne, R. S., Wharton, B. A., and McCance, R. A.: Hydroxyproline indices and hydroxyproline/creatinine ratios in older children. Lancet, 1:395–396, 1969.
11. Allison, D. J., Walker, A., and Smith, Q. T.: Urinary hydroxyproline: creatinine ratio of normal humans at various ages. Clin. Chim. Acta., 14:729–734, 1966.
12. Kivirikko, K. I., Koivusalo, M., Laitinen, O., and Liesmaa, M.: Effect of thyroxine on the hydroxyproline in rat urine and skin. Acta. Physiol. Scand., 57:462–467, 1963.
13. Prockop, D. J., and Udenfriend, S.: A specific method for the analysis of hydroxyproline in tissue and urine. Anal. Biochem., 1:228–239, 1960.
14. Koevoet, A. L., and Baars, J. D.: The determination of urinary hydroxyproline. Clin. Chim. Acta., 25:39–43, 1969.
15. Pinnell, S. R., Fox, R., and Krane, S. M.: Human collagens: differences in glycosylated hydroxylysines in skin and bone. Biochim. Biophys. Acta., 229:119–122, 1971.
16. Goldsmith, R. S., Jowsey, J., Dube, W. J., Riggs, B. L., Arnaud, C. D., and Kelly, P. J.: Effects of phosphorus supplementation on serum parathyroid hormone and bone morphology in osteoporosis. J. Clin. Endocrinol. Metab., 43:523–532, 1976.
17. Robison, R.: The Significance of Phosphoric Esters in Metabolism. New York, New York University Press, 1932.

18. Bonucci, E.: Fine structure of early cartilage calcification. J. Ultrastruct. Res., *20*:33–50, 1967.
19. Anderson, H. C.: Vesicles associated with calcification in the matrix of epiphyseal cartilage. J. Cell Biol., *41*:59–72, 1969.
20. Anderson, H. C., Matsuzawa, T., Sajdera, S. W., and Ali, S. Y.: Membranous particles in calcifying cartilage matrix. Trans. N.Y. Acad. Sci., *32*:619–630, 1970.
21. Heller-Steinberg, M.: Ground substance, bone salts, and cellular activity in bone formation and destruction. Am. J. Anat., *89*:347–379, 1951.
22. Gersh, I., and Catchpole, H. R.: The organization of ground substances and basement membrane and its significance in tissue injury disease and growth. Am. J. Anat., *85*:457–521, 1949.
23. Kashiwa, H. K., and Komorous, J.: Mineralized spherules in the cells and matrix of calcifying cartilage from developing bone. Anat. Rec., *170*:119–128, 1971.
24. Gay, C., and Schraer, H.: Frozen thin-sections of rapidly forming bone: bone cell ultrastructure. Calc. Tiss. Res., *19*:39–49, 1975.
25. Rabinovitch, A. L., and Anderson, C. H.: Biogenesis of matrix vesicles in cartilage growth plates. Fed. Proc., *35*:112–116, 1976.
26. Elliott, J. C.: The problems of the composition and structure of the mineral components of the hard tissues. Clinical Orthop., *93*:313–345, 1973.
27. Bocciarelli, D. S.: Morphology of crystallites in bone. Calcif. Tissue Res., *5*:261–269, 1970.
28. Spadaro, J. A., Becker, R. O., and Bachman, C. H.: The distribution of trace metal ions in bone and tendon. Calcif. Tissue Res., *6*:49–54, 1970.
29. Dixon, M., and Webb, E. C.: Enzymes, 2nd ed. London, Longman Green, 1964.

# Chapter Ten

# BONE MORPHOLOGY: BONE CELLS

## THE PROGENITOR CELL

The bone cell population consists of osteoblasts, osteoclasts, and osteocytes. The osteoblast and the osteoclast represent different functional states and have different origins. Cell division is restricted to the progenitor cells which then differentiate into osteoblasts or osteoclasts under appropriate stimuli. The progenitor cells that will form osteoblasts and those that will become osteoclasts are distinguishable from each other. That these cells are indeed stem cells, or the cells of origin of bone cells, can be shown by autoradiography using [3]H-labeled thymidine, which is taken up only in the dividing cells. Young found that only the osteoprogenitor cells incorporated the labelled thymidine immediately after injection, and only later (at a time when the [3]H-thymidine had been cleared from the blood) did the label appear in recognizable osteoblasts that had differentiated from the progenitor cells (Fig. 10–1).[2]

The progenitor cells or osteoprogenitor cells are found on or near the surface of bone or calcified cartilage.[2] They have vesicular cytoplasm and pale-staining nuclei, are often oval, and are morphologically different from both osteoblasts and osteoclasts. Occasionally, in cortical bone, particularly in a young growing person or animal, a haversian system may be resorbing on one side and laying down new bone on the other. The surface of such a system will often show a clear picture of an active osteoclast, an inactive osteoclast, a progenitor cell and then a layer of osteoblasts. Such cells would be associated with surfaces of active resorption, inactivity, or a transition zone and an osteoid layer, respectively.

After division, the progenitor cells may remain as progenitor cells, or they may become modulated to one of the two cell types, the osteoblast or the osteoclast. The average generation time for a progenitor cell mitotic cycle is 36 hours in an area of active bone formation in a young rat and up to 200 hours in a less active area; the generation time decreases with age. In man, the generation times are probably much longer than in animals.

Both osteoblasts and osteoclasts revert to progenitor cells after the stimulus that caused their differentiation has been withdrawn.

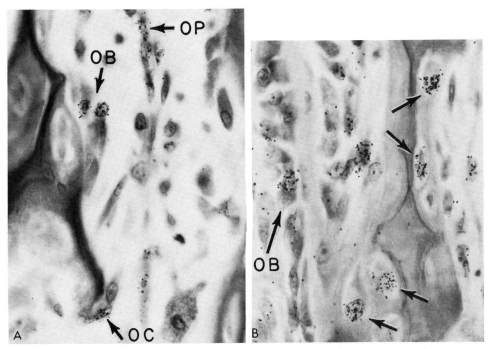

**Figure 10–1** (a) Autoradiograph of the metaphysis of a seven-day-old rat killed 33 hours after an injection of $^3$H-thymidine. Labeled cells are the osteoprogenitor cells (OP), osteoblasts (OB), and osteoclasts (OC) (magnification ×800). (b) Autoradiograph of the metaphysis of a ten-day-old rat injected with $^3$H-thymidine and killed 96 hours later. The osteoblast is labeled (OB) and the osteocytes with arrows (magnification ×800). (From Young, R. W.).[1]

An interesting observation by Owen in 1963, which was later also made by Appleton in 1969 in intestinal epithelial tissue, was the appearance of labeled thymidine in precursor cells that did not later divide, and also in the occasional osteoblast; in intestinal epithelium, post-mitotic cells that are nearly fully differentiated may take up labeled material.[3,4] It is possible, therefore, that DNA synthesis can occur at the stage of final differentiation, as well as in association with mitosis. This leads to the speculation that differentiation involves the addition of nuclear information, perhaps in relation to the newly acquired function of the cell.

## THE OSTEOBLAST

The osteoblast is a cell with a single nucleus and basophilic cytoplasm; it is generally polyhedral and is found as part of a layer of other osteoblasts lined up on bone surfaces (Fig. 10–2). These features distinguish osteoblasts from progenitor cells, which are not cuboidal and are not found in sheets or layers on bone surfaces. Tight junctions are found between the osteoblasts.[5] Although these junctions are short, they permit the existence of a very narrow layer between the osteoblasts and the matrix. This layer is isolated from the general extracellular fluid space and appears to have different properties (for example, a high collagen concentration) from the non-bone side of the osteoblasts.[6] The presence of tight junctions ap-

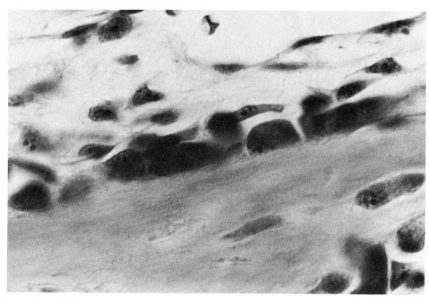

**Figure 10–2**   A layer of polyhedral osteoblasts lined up on the bone matrix surface (magnification ×750). (By courtesy of Dr. B. Boothroyd.)

pears to be related to bone-forming activity in some respects; they are decreased in adult animals, compared with immature animals. Whitson also described an increase in the number of tight junctions in estrogen-treated rabbits; however, quantitation was not attempted and the effect is not easily explained in the presence of decreased matrix formation.[7]

Electron microscopy has delineated the structure of the osteoblast itself and, to a large extent, the function of this cell. This technique, with the autoradiographic studies, has left no doubt that the osteoblast is the cell which secretes the collagen and glycosaminoglycans of the matrix. As long ago as 1959 Carneiro and Leblond used $^3$H-glycine to label new bone.[8] The isotope-labeled glycine is taken up by the osteoblasts and incorporated into the matrix components, presumably collagen. Using adult male mice and subcutaneous injection these authors showed that labeled glycine appears in the osteoblasts after 30 minutes and at 35 hours is in the newly deposited matrix. Electron microscopy, investigating structure rather than function directly, has demonstrated the osteoblast to be a protein producing cell; the cytoplasm contains large amounts of rough endoplasmic reticulum (ER), which forms cisternae, and many ribosomes whose RNA produces the basophilia seen in conventional microscopy. The ER and ribosomes are features that are generally associated with protein production. Electron dense granules are found in the cisternae, and there is a well-developed Golgi body, generally found near the nucleus. The nucleus itself has a double membrane with pores and contains one to three nucleoli, but it is otherwise unremarkable. The nucleus-to-cytoplasmic ratio is high; roughly half the volume of the cell is occupied by the nucleus, although this value may fall to less than half when the cell is in an exceptionally active matrix-producing phase, such as in Paget's disease of bone. In the cytoplasm there are both microtubules and mitochondria which may be associated with the mineralization process; electron-dense material found within the mitochrondria are thought to be calcium-rich. Although the majority of studies have been done in vitro with mitochondria from cells other than osteoblasts (Crang's studies of calciferous gland of the earthworm;[9] studies of liver mitochondria by Jones[10]), calcium containing vesicles have been demonstrated in both mineralizing cartilage and bone.[11, 12] However, the mitochondria also appear to act as storehouses of calcium; the calcium is brought into the cell as the first messenger and has to wait to be pumped out of the cell against a high concentration gradient.

The major function of the osteoblast is the production of collagen. Amino acids are congregated within the osteoblast and secreted through pores in the cell membrane. The collagen polypeptides are synthesized on the ribosomes and migrate to the cisternae of the rough endoplasmic reticulum. $^3$H-proline is localized in the ER in as short a time as five minutes after injection of this collagen precursor. The prefibrils are secreted from the osteoblast before they arrive at any degree of structural complexity by which collagen is usually recognized.[13] Once outside the cell, tropocollagen is formed, and this aggregates to produce collagen with the typical 640Å crossbanding, which can be demonstrated by the electron microscope.

Attempts have been made to measure the productivity of osteoblasts. Although the studies have been carried out in a rapidly growing bone system (young rats), and the actual values are probably much higher than would be found in man, at least they give the upper limits of matrix production rate. The surface covered by a single osteoblast is approximately $150 \mu m^2$, and each cell produces$^{470}$ $\mu m^3$ of matrix.[14] Owen used young rabbits and found that each osteoblast produces two or three times its own volume of matrix per day.[3] This would be somewhat higher than the value reported by Jones; however, in the rabbit model the bone surface was being formed rapidly at the rate of $170 \mu$ per day. This is approximately 170 times faster than the rate of apposition in secondary haversian bone in man; it may therefore be calculated that osteoblasts in the adult person are producing $100 \mu^3$ of matrix per day, based on their size and a rate of appositional bone formation of approximately $1 \mu$ per day.

The osteoblast secretes collagen in sheets on the bone surface, each sheet having a slightly different orientation of the collagen fibers with respect to the long axis of the bone. Each of these sheets of oriented collagen fibers is a lamella and is about 10 microns in thickness. The lamellae may be arranged around the endosteal or periosteal surfaces of the bone, or around trabeculae, or it may be oriented concentrically around the central vascular canal of the primary or secondary haversian canal. The lamellar pattern can be seen with polarized light or by phase contrast illumination (Fig. 10–3). Electron microscopic pictures suggest that the orientation of the collagen fibers in the lamellae are more usually somewhat vertical or parallel to, rather than horizontal to, the long axis of the canal. Since the majority of haversian canals with their circumferential lamellae run approximately parallel to the long axis of the bone, this lamellar arrangement probably has strength properties above that of a system with no degree of organization, such as exists in woven bone.

Glycosaminoglycans, or the ground substance of bone, are also produced by osteoblasts. $^{35}$S-sulfate and $^3$H-fucose have been demonstrated in osteoblasts which are actively forming bone; both these compounds are utilized in glycosaminoglycan production. The Golgi apparatus appears to be active in the process, since the $^{35}$S and $^3$H labels appear to be concentrated in these areas.[15]

Electron microscopic evidence of osteoblastic production of material identifiable as a protein-polysaccharide is absent, presumably because the ground sub-

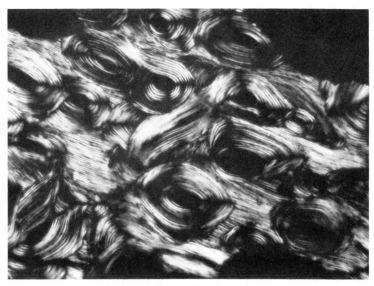

**Figure 10–3**  A polarized light picture of secondary haversian bone showing the circular arrangement of the lamellae around haversian canals and some longitudinally arranged lamellae in the interstitial bone (magnification ×100).

stance of bone has no gross structure. Histochemistry also confirms the presence of glycosaminoglycans in osteoblasts using the periodic acid-Schiff stain (PAS); the stain density of the reaction varies from cell to cell but is present in all osteoblasts to some degree.

Initially the organic matrix or osteoid is unmineralized and remains so for a period of approximately 15 days in man. Since the osteoblasts produce matrix at a rate of about 1 micron per day, there is a border of unmineralized bone about 15 microns wide on surfaces where normal bone formation is taking place. At the end of 15 days, a histologically demonstrable change occurs in the matrix, and it becomes mineralizable. Calcium and phosphorous are deposited at the mineralization front in the form of calcium phosphate in vesicles, and this is later converted to larger hydroxyapatite crystals (Fig. 10–4).

It is obvious perhaps that the amount of new bone formed per unit of time depends on the rate of matrix production per cell and the percentage of the bone surface covered by bone cells. The overall rates can vary tremendously, probably over a thousand-fold depending on the bone site and age of the animal.[16, 17] In adult man the appositional rate is about $1\mu$ per day in most instances, although it can be as high as $2.5\mu$ per day in children or in patients with Paget's disease of bone (Table 10–1).[17, 18]

The major factor in variations in the amount of bone formed is the number of osteoblasts, which of course also means the length of surface covered by osteoblasts.

Osteoid borders can be easily demonstrated in undemineralized sections. It is essential not to demineralize the material, since the osteoid matrix must be compared with the mineralized bone for identification. The material may either be stained or unstained. Villaneuva and colleagues, in a group of 134 normal individuals between the ages of 1 month and 84 years, showed a fall in childhood from 1.4

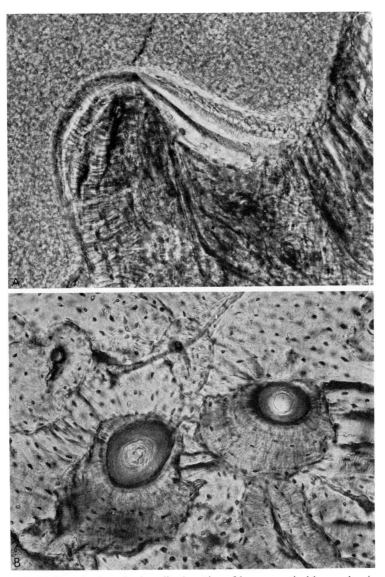

**Figure 10-4** (a) Unstained, undemineralized section of human cortical bone, showing an osteoid border covered by osteoblasts. Between the osteoid and the new bone is a normal mineralization front (magnification x 250). (b) Undemineralized, unstained section showing two osteones in cortical bone of adult cats given EHDP. The mineralization front appears as a granular deposit in the matrix, grossly broadened because of the effect of the diphosphonate in preventing the conversion of the initial mineral deposit into mature bone crystals (magnification ×200).

osteoid borders per mm² of bone to a low value at age 35 of less than 0.2; between 35 and 65 the values rise about two-fold (Fig. 10–5).[19, 20] The measurements were made in both rib and clavicle and include both cortical and trabecular bone. Villaneuva felt that these osteoid borders represented bone formation, since they were associated with osteoblasts. Similar data were found using iliac crest material, although in this data the rise in osteoid borders was accompanied by a slight decrease in the rate of matrix production (see Fig. 9–3).

**Table 10–1**   APPOSITIONAL BONE FORMATION RATE, $\mu$/DAY (mean ± SD)

|  | Trabecular bone | Cortical bone |
| --- | --- | --- |
| Puppy (3 mo old)[16] | 2.5 ± 0.3 | 2.0 ± 0.3 |
| Adult dog (1–2 yrs old)[16] | 1.5 ± 0.3 | 1.4 ± 0.1 |
| Old dog (? age)[16] | – | 1.0 ± 0.1 |
| Man (2 yr old, rib)[17] | – | 0.8 ± 0.4 |
| Man (4 yr old)[17] | – | 1.3 ± 0.3 |
| Man (20 yr old)[18] | – | 1.2 ± 0.6 |

From Lee.[16, 17] from Frost.[18]

Using just trabecular bone of the iliac crest Merz and Schenk arrived at similar results, namely, a slight fall at age 40 and thereafter a slight rise to age 65 followed by subsequent decrease.[21] However, these authors chose, perhaps somewhat arbitrarily, to eliminate from the data all individuals with high values in the older age groups and later confirmed these earlier conclusions that bone formation, identified by osteoblasts, decreases from 5 per cent in 30 to 40 year old persons to 3 per cent in 60 to 70 year old persons (although no statistical analysis or confirmation of this observation was made). The data appear to reflect a difference between trabecular and cortical bone which becomes more marked with age. Microradiographic studies of bone formation in iliac crest specimens, which included both cortical and trabecular bone, showed no fall with age, while if cortical bone was excluded, the trabecular bone showed a tendency to fall, although the slope did not show a significant regression.

## THE OSTEOCYTE

As osteoid is laid down, osteoblasts become included in the matrix at regular intervals in a lacuna or space and are subsequently buried in the mineralized bone.

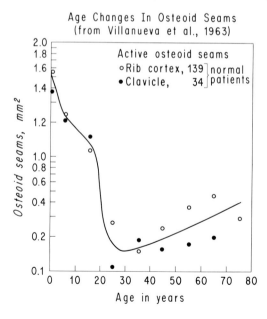

**Figure 10–5**   The number of osteons containing osteoid borders related to age. Human cortical bone was used for these determinations. (Redrawn from Villanueva et al.)[20]

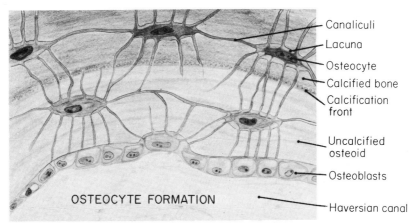

Canaliculi
Lacuna
Osteocyte
Calcified bone
Calcification front
Uncalcified osteoid
Osteoblasts
Haversian canal

OSTEOCYTE FORMATION

**Figure 10–6** Diagram of an osteoblast about to become incorporated into the unmineralized osteoid as an osteocyte. The canalicular projections already exist between osteocytes within mineralized matrix and those in the osteoid. From the most recently incorporated osteocytes, the canaliculi connect to the surface of the osteoid. (From Jowsey, J.: Autoradiographic and microradiographic studies of bone. In Zipkin, I. (ed.): Biological Mineralization of Bone. New York, John Wiley and Sons, 1973, pp. 297–333).

The cell is then called an osteocyte (Fig. 10–6). Labeling methods have indicated that a period of time (2 or 5 days in six-day or six-week-old rats, respectively) must elapse before [3]H-thymidine appears in osteocytes that are surrounded by matrix. Osteoblasts, which are the cells initially labeled, must therefore spend a certain time as osteoblasts before becoming osteocytes.[1, 8] In man, an osteocyte is approximately 10 by 10 microns in height and depth and 15 microns in length, housed in a lacuna that is only a little larger than the cell itself. Each osteocyte is connected to its neighbors in each direction by tunnels in the mineralized bone called canaliculi. The canaliculi are about 0.7 to 1.0 micron in diameter and contain projections from the cytoplasm of the osteocyte. The canaliculi eventually connect with the vascular spaces in bone, either through the osteoid or through the bone if the osteoid has become mineralized. They form a radiating network of canals throughout bone tissue and link haversian bone to the vascular spaces; they also cross cement lines and therefore connect haversian systems with one another (Fig. 10–7). Extracellular fluid of some kind separates the cell membrane from the lacunar and canalicular walls. Cooper and associates in 1966 thought the space contained only fluid; others have considered it to be rich in a protein-polysaccharide.[22, 23]

Some osteocytes may look like osteoblasts with an active endoplasmic reticulum and Golgi bodies; others, which are found in more mature bone, have only vaguely discernible cell inclusions.

For a long time it was thought that the osteocytes were unresponsive cells, merely functioning to transport various nutritive elements to the deep part of the bone. However, observations of increased or decreased lacunar size in various disease states or in response to drug administration have forced a change of view. Duriez has shown an increase in the mean osteocyte surface area in osteoporosis compared with normal and has also demonstrated a rapid response to calcitonin by a decrease in the mean surface area.[24] The variation is large, mainly because not all lacunae are affected. It may be more meaningful to compare the numbers of os-

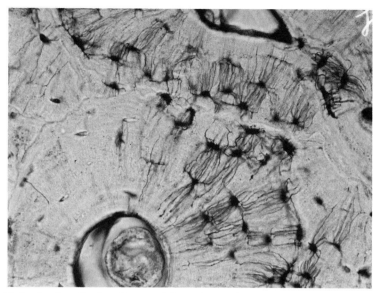

**Figure 10–7**  A mineralized section, partially embedded in methylmethacrylate. Air-filled lacunae and canaliculi demonstrate the intricate radiating system of canaliculi that links the osteons with each other and each osteocyte with its neighbor providing a nutrient network throughout the bone (magnification ×400).

teocytes which are above normal size; this would be zero in a 20-year-old normal person but would rise as bone disease develops.

Ruth in 1954 was probably one of the earliest authors to point out the relationship between a change in the osteocyte and a physiologic stimulus; rats fed a calcium-free diet developed rings of modified basophilic matrix around the osteocytes.[25] Later work by Belanger, Meunier, and others has confirmed that the osteocyte is a responsive cell and reacts to stimuli by resorbing the bone surrounding it (Fig. 10–8).[26, 27] The terms osteocytic osteolysis or osteolysis (less accurate) are used to describe this phenomenon. The stimuli are almost always those which also produce increased osteoclastic activity, such as parathyroid hormone. The presence of a stimulus, increased size of the lacuna, and the staining ring around the lacuna are associated with electron microscopically demonstrable changes; lysosomes predominate and the outline of the lacunae is rough rather than smooth. Bone formation, as well as resorption, appears possible by osteocytes, since the presence of a prominent endoplasmic reticulum and Golgi body with a layer of immature, unmineralized collagen fibers in the periosteocytic space suggests that the osteocytes can form bone, albeit in small quantities.[23]

The physiologic role of the osteocyte is apparent. It is a cell in an ideal position for the short-term regulation of calcium, since there are many thousands of them in bone, and, with their canalicular surface, they constitute a vast cell-to-mineralized bone interface. However, long-term calcium homeostasis and the maintenance of normocalcemia is obviously the function of the osteoclast. This is evident because the osteocytes only appear to increase in size a certain amount, and even under strong stimulus (such as secondary hyperparathyroidism) the dimensions are hardly bigger than in "primary" hyperparathyroidism (Fig. 10–9). In both

# Osteocytic Osteolysis

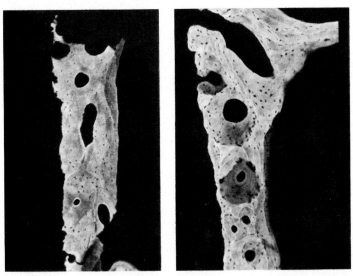

**Figure 10–8** Enlarged osteocyte lacunae are seen in a microradiograph from a patient with hyperparathyroidism. They are irregularly distributed and by no means all osteocytes are affected (magnification ×70). (From: Jowsey, J.: The microradiographic assessment of bone structure. Triangle, *12*:93–101, 1973.)

of these diseases, the significant bone loss is by increased osteoclast number and activity.

It is important to distinguish between osteocytic osteolysis and the large, irregular osteocyte lacunae that are found normally near calcified cartilage in woven bone, fracture callus, and other areas of rapidly forming bone (Fig. 10–10). The

Osteocytic Osteolysis
(from P. Meunier, 1971)

**Figure 10–9** The dimensions of osteocyte lacunae in normal, osteoporotic and hyperparathyroid individuals. The characteristically increased levels of parathyroid hormone in secondary hyperparathyroidism do not result in any increase in osteocyte size compared with "primary" hyperparathyroidism. (Drawn from Meunier et al.)[27]

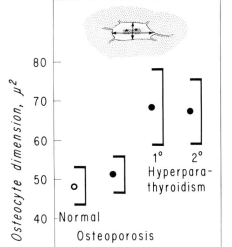

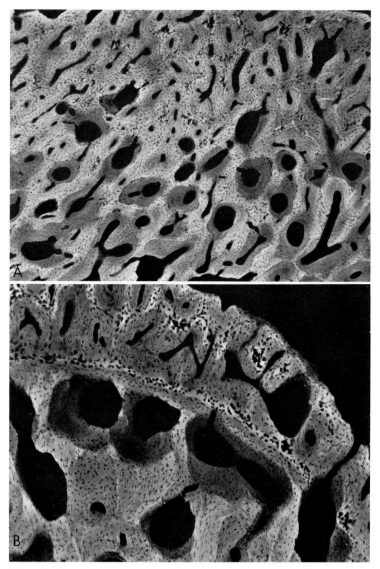

**Figure 10-10**   (a) Microradiograph of metaphyseal bone in a normal rabbit showing the large size and irregular dimensions of the osteocyte lacunae adjacent to the cartilage (magnification ×50). (b) Microradiograph of the diaphysis of a young normal monkey; rapid periosteal new bone deposition has resulted in woven bone formation of high mineral content, which contains large and irregular osteocytes (magnification × 75).

problem, of course, is one familiar to all morphologists and anatomists, that of interpreting appearances in terms of function. Because the osteocytes are large it must be confirmed that it is either certain or highly likely that they were once small before osteocytic osteolysis can be established.

In rickets and hypoparathyroidism, a different phenomenon is seen which probably represents poor mineralization and is morphologically distinguishable from osteolysis (Fig. 10–11). The mineral density around the osteocyte is low, but the matrix dimensions are not changed.

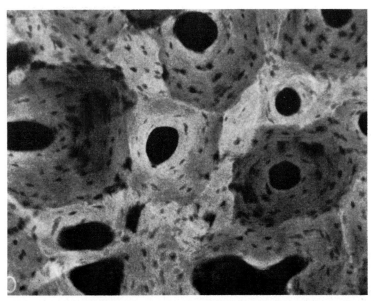

**Figure 10–11** Microradiograph of the cortical bone from a child with rickets, many of the osteocytes appear enlarged and have poorly distinguished lacunar borders; however the phenomenon only appears in the microradiograph and therefore represents a mineralization defect rather than disappearance of both mineral and matrix (magnification ×250).

## THE OSTEOCLAST

The osteoclast[28] is morphologically different from the osteoblast; it is large, often multinucleate, and has a large volume of vacuolated, acidophilic cytoplasm. Unlike the osteoblast, it varies significantly in both size and shape; there are also differences in the number of nuclei in each cell which have been related to cell activity. Osteoclasts that are recently differentiated and beginning to resorb bone, or that are just finishing resorption and dedifferentiating, have darkly-staining nuclei and cytoplasm and tend to be oval in shape, whereas actively resorbing osteoclasts have a large volume of cytoplasm in contrast to the nuclear volume, the cytoplasm is pale and vacuolated (often described as "foamy"), and there are many nuclei (Fig. 10–12). The nuclei are generally round or oval and have one or occasionally two nucleoli. They are less densely stained than the nucleoli in osteoblasts, and the nuclei tend to lie in the center and frequently on the non-bone side of the cell. The nucleus may be indented, but mitosis has not been observed in osteoclasts.

Other cell inclusions include mitochondria, which are generally numerous and lie in the cell cytoplasm on the side away from bone. There is a Golgi body but apparently little or no endoplasmic reticulum, in contrast to osteoblasts; this can be explained by the lack of protein manufacture in osteoclasts as opposed to osteoblasts, which are making protein. The other, perhaps more striking, microscopic difference between the osteoclast and osteoblast is the presence of many vacuoles and vesicles of various sizes in the osteoclast that usually lie close to the bone; these also reflect a functional difference between the two cells, since the vesicles play a role in the bone resorption process.

[3]H-labeled thymidine autoradiographic studies have shown that osteoclasts are formed by fusion of unicellular precursor cells, the osteoprogenitor cells.[29] The os-

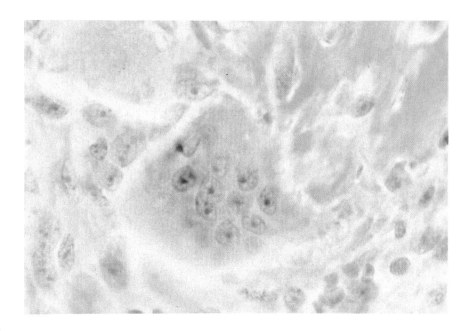

A

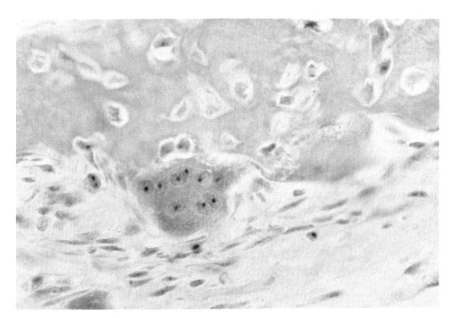

B

**Figure 10–12**  (a) A stained section of a large, multinucleate osteoclast lying adjacent to the blue-stained bone tissue (magnification ×250). (Courtesy of Dr. B. Boothroyd.) (b) A stained section of two osteoclasts lying on the bone surface. The vacuoles and projections of the cells are seen adjacent to the mineralized bone (magnification ×160). The stain used was Masson's Trichrome stain. (Courtesy of Dr. B. Boothroyd.)

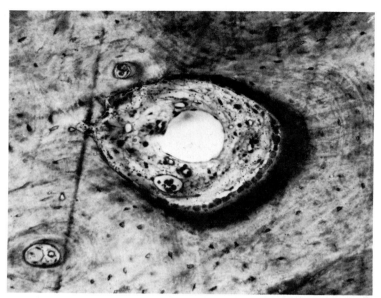

**Figure 10–13**  An undemineralized, stained section of cortical human bone showing a layer of osteoblasts on the right. On the upper left of the vascular canal is an osteoclast and between it and the osteoblast layer is a progenitor cell (magnification × 64).

teoclasts grow in size and can accumulate more nuclei as they become more active. After they cease functioning, they dedifferentiate into progenitor cells and eventually into fibroblasts. Osteoclasts do not divide to form more osteoclasts. Incorporation of $^3$H-thymidine has been observed in osteoclasts occasionally, but since neither nuclear division nor cell division has been observed, this must be interpreted in terms of the accumulation of nuclear material rather than mitosis. Nor do osteoclasts split up into osteoblasts. The cell inclusions, staining properties, and characteristic appearance of the osteoclast are too different from those of an osteoblast to allow one to miss such a direct transformation, if such did occur. On the other hand, an area of active osteoclastic activity close to an area of active osteoblastic activity is separated by an inert zone in which can be found dedifferentiating osteoclasts and progenitor cells. This zone is approximately 800 $\mu$m in longitudinal section but may be only 100 $\mu$m in cross section (Fig. 10–13). In most of the bone in adult man the progenitor cells revert to fibroblasts and seem to disappear; most bone surfaces lack any type of bone cell but are covered by or are adjacent to a layer of marrow tissue (endosteum), connective tissue (periosteum), or the components of a vascular canal.

Unlike osteoblastic function, which can be proved by autoradiographic as well as by tetracycline-labeling experiments, the function of the osteoclast is derived from observing these cells in places where resorption is known to be occurring, such as the periosteal metaphysis and the marrow cavity end of the spongiosa. Conclusive evidence of the resorbing function of the osteoclast comes from electron microscopic descriptions. In addition, cinephotography of live cell cultures has dramatically shown the osteoclasts actually gobbling up mineralized bone.[30] The cells therefore come to lie in osteoclast-sized depressions called Howship's lacunae (Fig. 10–14).

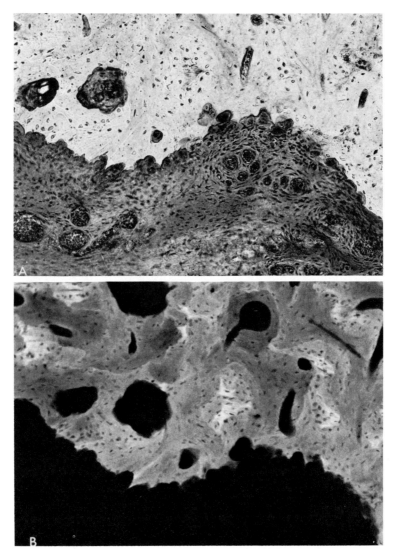

**Figure 10–14** (a) Paragon stained mineralized section with large multinucleate osteoclasts lying along the pale staining bone surface (magnification × 90). (b) Microradiograph of the same area of bone as seen in (a), showing the eaten-out Howship's lacunae in the areas of osteoclastic resorption (magnification × 90). (From Jowsey, J., and Gordan, G.: Bone turnover and osteoporosis. In Bourne, G. H. (ed.): The Biochemistry and Physiology of Bone, 2nd edition, Vol. III. New York. Academic Press, 1971, pp. 201–238.)

When an osteoclast is actively resorbing bone, the side of the cell adjacent to the bone forms the ruffled border (or brush border). This term was originally based on the light microscope appearance of the cell; electron microscopy has now shown that the brush border consists of a number of villus-like projections from the osteoclast toward the bone. Pieces of bone broken up into crystals (or aggregates of crystals) and collagen fragments are found between the folds of the villae. Crystals and pieces of collagen are also found in vesicles or vacuoles in the cytoplasm of the osteoclast. This provides definitive evidence that the osteoclast is phagocytosing bone fragments as well as breaking it up into these fragments.[28] However, the osteoclast is not a macrophage; a macrophage will phagocytose collagen, trypan blue, carbon particles, and dead bone, but an osteoclast will only resorb bone.

The ruffled border appears to be essential for the proper function of this cell. In a study of IA rats (rats with inherited osteopetrosis and "incisors absent"), the number of cells and their enzyme content appeared to be normal; however, the ruffled border of the osteoclasts was found to be absent, and there were no extracellular lysosomal enzymes.[31] This implies an abnormality of function both in the inability to form a resorbing cell surface and in the membrane permeability of this surface. Earlier work with this and other strains of osteopetrotic animals (the microophthalmic rabbit and the grey lethal mouse) had already excluded an abnormality of "insolubility" of bone, absence of osteoclasts, or any aberration in parathyroid hormone secretion as being the cause of this bone disorder.[32, 33] Recently, Walker has reversed the disorder by subcutaneous parabiotic union between an affected and an unaffected sibling and thus caused resorption of bone tissue. This study implicates the functional properties of the osteoclast directly as the cause of the disease.[34] Presumably a normal mesenchyme or stem cell travels across the parabiotic union and becomes the progenitor cell for normal differentiation into normal osteoclasts. This may be significant in the treatment of osteopetrosis in man.

Resorption of bone appears to be achieved by the production of enzymes from lysosomes that lie within the cytoplasm of the osteoclast. Acid phosphatase has been identified in the osteoclast by histochemical techniques; more recently, Walker has developed a micro-imprint technique, by which he isolates and identifies osteoclasts from bone-marrow imprints of very young rats. He has confirmed and quantitated the presence of acid phosphatase and also lactate and malate dehydrogenase, the latter two increasing in amount in the cells after parathyroid extract.[35] These two enzymes are involved in citrate production, and citric acid may well be responsible for mobilization of mineral from bone.[36]

Bone sections will almost always contain many osteoblasts compared with the number of osteoclasts. In systems in which the rates of deposition and removal of bone are known and the mass of bone is constant, it is possible to draw conclusions of the relative rate of work of these two cells. Owen has used the growing rabbit and has found that the ratio of the two cells was 22 osteoblasts to 1 osteoclast.[29] Assuming that nuclear number in each cell is related to activity, the ratio is still in favor of the osteoblast by 6 to 1. Therefore, it is not unreasonable to assume that the osteoclast is working more efficiently (perhaps six times more efficiently) than the osteoblast. Cell-counting methods, therefore, may be in error in that it is incorrect to equate cell number with cell activity; as a result, resorption is underestimated by such methods. Jaworski attempted to evaluate this factor directly in animals.[37] Three one-year-old, nearly mature, dogs were given tetracycline, and longitudinal "tunneling" or remodeling was observed. The rate at which the osteoclast dug the tunnel (the longitudinal erosion rate) and the rate at which they enlarged the tunnel (the radial erosion rate) were measured by means of tetracycline markers, with the assumption that the distance between the end of the tunnel and the beginning of the zone of formation was a constant. The assumption proved to be correct by direct measurement; therefore, the rate of longitudinal osteoid deposition is about the same as the longitudinal rate of resorption. Radial bone resorption rate appeared to be about 7 microns per day, a figure that compares well with

**Table 10–2**  RATES OF OSTEOCLASTIC RESORPTION AND MATRIX
DEPOSITION IN IMMATURE DOGS

| Resorption Rate in Dogs, $\mu$/day | |
|---|---|
| RADIAL | LONGITUDINAL |
| 7.1 ± (SD 2.9) | 39.2 ± (SD 13.7) Jaworski[37] |
| 9.2 ± (SE 0.5) | 43.6 ± (SE 1.0) Jaworski[38] |

| Formation Rate in Dogs, $\mu$/day | |
|---|---|
| RADIAL | LONGITUDINAL |
| 2.0 ± (SD 0.3) Lee[16] | 44.4 ± (SD 12) Jaworski[37] |
| 1.4 ± (SD 0.1) Lee[16] | 43.6 ± (SE 0.7) Jaworski[38] |

From Lee;[16] from Jaworski.[37, 38]

the estimate of Owen's. Jaworski thought that the resorption rate would be lower in
man than in the dogs he studied, since the rate of formation in man is less (Table
10–2). However, the discrepancy remains, and it is therefore reasonable to multiply
osteoclast numbers by three to approach the cell-to-activity ratio of the osteoblast.
There is also evidence from tritiated glucosamine studies that active resorption is
occurring on bone adjacent to osteoclasts. Owen estimated that 70 per cent of a
resorbing surface may be free of cells but in the process of active destruction.[29]
Other studies have also shown a discrepancy between the numbers and rate of
resorption of bone. Parathyroid-induced changes in the electron-microscopic appearance of osteoclasts and the associated accelerated bone loss were linked with no
change in osteoclast numbers but presumably by an increase in activity.[39]

Osteoclasts are responsible for the following two major functions: (1) the
remodeling of bone to form the adult skeleton in conjunction with osteoblasts, and
(2) the maintenance of serum calcium under the control of parathyroid hormone.
The normal remodeling of bone is also to some extent under the control of the
parathyroids, since parathyroidectomy produces a failure of remodeling in growing
animals. Otherwise control of normal bone growth and turnover remains somewhat
of a mystery. All that can be said is that piezoelectricity and an inborn pattern of
remodeling are both involved. Of the two functions, the maintenance of normal
serum calcium takes predominance over the continued remodeling process.

There are sporadic reports in the literature of cells, other than osteoclasts, that
resorb bone. Mast cells can be produced in excessive numbers by procedures that
are known to stimulate bone remodeling, in particular the bone resorptive aspect of
remodeling. Fracture, administration of beta-amino-propionitrile (BAPN, active
principle of the sweet pea, Lathyrus odoratus), and excessive parathyroid hormone
secretion, induced by a low calcium diet, will all increase mast cell numbers. Since
these cells are found in direct contact with the bone surfaces, it is not unlikely that
they are involved in resorption of mineralized tissue through the production of
lysosomal enzymes.[40] Mast cell disease can produce a picture not unlike, but yet
distinguishable from, osteocytic osteolysis, again suggesting that this cell can in-
dulge in active resorption (Fig. 10–15). In patients with osteoporosis, mast cells
have not been a repeated finding. However, in a study directly attacking this ques-

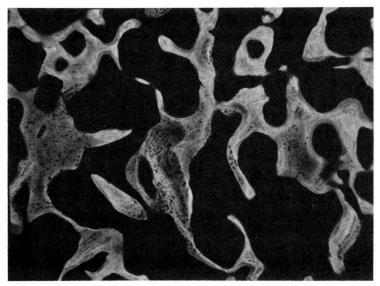

**Figure 10–15** Microradiograph of trabecular bone from a patient with mast cell disease. Many osteocyte lacunae in specifically defined locations are enlarged resembling osteocytic osteolysis, although the latter is characterized by a random scattering of the enlarged lacunae (magnification × 50).

tion. Frame and Nixon found a significant increase in mast cells in patients with osteoporosis in contrast to those with no clear skeletal disease (Fig. 10–16).[41] Mast cell resorption of bone is a different phenomenon than the osteoclast-stimulating agents which act by causing differentation and activity of osteoclasts.

In our laboratory we have observed cells lying in Howship's lacunae in spaces in cortical bone in the occasional young patient with osteoporosis. The cells are plump, mononuclear, and have a relatively large cytoplasmic volume. Their role in

**Figure 10–16** The number of mast cells in individuals with and without osteoporosis. Those with symptomatic disease frequently fall into the categories which in the bone marrow cell count contains more mast cells. (Drawn from Frame and Nixon[41]).

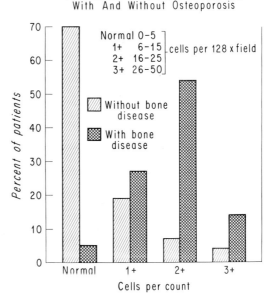

bone resorption is incriminated only by their presence in patients with rapid, progressive bone loss and their appearance in the scalloped-out indentations or Howship's lacunae of mineralized bone, a position where one would expect to find a typical osteoclast (Fig. 10–14).

Myeloma cells also appear to cause bone erosion directly. Certainly most patients with myeloma develop osteoporosis; they are probably not severely affected by this disease because the majority die of the myelomatous process before the bone loss has had time to progress to any great extent. The work of Trummel and co-workers would suggest that an osteoclast activating factor (OAF) may be produced by lymphocytic or myeloma cells.[42] Prostaglandins may also mediate bone resorption.[43]

Despite these exceptions it is probably accurate to say that the majority of bone resorption is the result of parathyroid hormone mediated osteoclastic bone resorption. The exceptions quoted above are of interest in that they clearly indicate that other cells are able to resorb mineralized tissue and because they infer that the absence of osteoclasts does not necessarily imply absence of resorption.

## *REFERENCES*

1. Young, Richard W.: Cell proliferation and specialization during endochondral osteogenesis in young rats. J. Cell Biol., *14*:357–370, 1962.
2. Kember, N. F.: Cell division in endochondral ossification. J. Bone Joint Surg., *42B*:824–839, 1960.
3. Owen, M.: Cell population kinetics of an osteogenic tissue. I. J. Cell Biol., *19*:19–32, 1963.
4. Appleton, T. C., Pelc, S. R., and Tarbit, M. H.: Formation and loss of DNA in intestinal epithelium. J. Cell Science, *5*:45–55, 1969.
5. Weinger, J. M. and Holtrop, M. E.: An ultrastructural study of bone cells: the occurrence of microtubles, microfilaments and tight junctions. Calcif. Tissue Res., *14*:15–29, 1974.
6. Neuman, W. F.: The milieu interieur of bone: Claude Bernard revisited. Fed. Proc., *28*:1846–1850, 1969.
7. Whitson, S. W.: Tight junction formation in the osteon. Clin. Orthop., *86*:206–213, 1972.
8. Carneiro, J., and Leblond, C. P.: Role of osteoblasts and odontoblasts in secreting the collagen of bone and dentin, as shown by radioautography in mice given tritium-labelled glycine. Exp. Cell Res., *18*:291–300, 1959.
9. Crang, R. E., Holsen, R. C., and Hitt, J. B.: Calcite production in mitochondria of earthworm calciferous glands. Bioscience, *18*:299–301, 1968.
10. Jones, A. R.: Mitochondria, calcification and waste disposal. Calcif. Tissue Res., *3*:363–365, 1969.
11. Bonucci, E.: Fine structure of early cartilage calcification. J. Ultrastruct. Res., *20*:33–50, 1967.
12. Martin, J. H., and Matthews, J. L.: Mitochondrial granules in chondrocytes. Calcif. Tiss. Res., *3*:184–193, 1969.
13. Ross, R.: The connective tissue fiber forming cell. In Gould, B. S. (Ed.): Treatise on Collagen. New York, Academic Press, 1967, Vol 2, Part A, pp. 2–82.
14. Jones, S. J.: Secretory territories and rate of matrix production of osteoblasts. Calcif. Tissue Res., *14*:309–315, 1974.
15. Weinstock, A., Weinstock, M., and Leblond, C. P.: Autoradiographic detection of ³H-fucose incorporation into glycoprotein by odontoblasts and its deposition at the site of the calcification front in dentin. Calcif. Tissue Res., *8*:181–189, 1972.
16. Lee, W. R.: Appositional bone formation in canine bone: a quantitative microscope study using tetracycline markers. J. Anat., *98*:665–677, 1964.
17. Lee, W. R.: A quantitative microscopic study of bone formation in a normal child and two children suffering from osteogenesis imperfecta. In Calcified Tissues. L'Université de Liège, Symposium, *31*:451–463, 1964.
18. Frost, H. M.: Tetracycline-based histological analysis of bone remodeling. Calcif. Tiss. Res., *3*:211–237, 1969.
19. Johnson, K. A., Riggs, B. L., Kelly, P. J., and Jowsey, J.: Osteoid tissue in normal and osteoporotic individuals. J. Clin. Endocrinol. Metab., *33*:745–751, 1971.
20. Villanueva, A. R., Sedlin, E. D., and Frost, H. M.: Variations in osteoblastic activity with age by the osteoid seam index. Anat. Rec., *146*:209–213, 1963.

21. Merz, W. A., and Schenk, R. K.: A quantitative histological study on bone formation in human cancellous bone. Acta Anat., *74*:44–53, 1969.
22. Cooper, R. R., Milgram, J. W., and Robinson, R. A.: Morphology of the osteon. J. Bone Joint Surg., *48A*:1239–1271, 1966.
23. Baud, C. A.: Submicroscopic structure and functional aspects of the osteocyte. Clin. Orthop., *56*:227–236, 1968.
24. Duriez, J.: Les modifications calciques péri-ostéocytaires; etude microradiographique à l'analyseur automatique d'images. La Nouvelle Presse Medicale; *3*:2007–2010, 1974.
25. Ruth, E. B.: Further observations on histological evidence of osseous tissue resorption (abstract). Anat. Rec., *118*:347, 1954.
26. Bélanger, L. F.: Osteocytic resorption. In Bourne, G. H. (Ed.): The Biochemistry and Physiology of Bone, Vol. 3, 2nd ed. New York, Academic Press, 1971, pp. 239–270.
27. Meunier, P., Bernard, J., and Vignon, G.: La mesure de l'élargissement périostéocytaire appliquée au diagnostic des hyperparathyroïdies. Pathol. Biol. (Paris), *19*:371–378, 1971.
28. Hancox, N. M.: Biology of Bone. London, Cambridge University Press, 1972, pp 113–145.
29. Owen, M.: Cellular dynamics of bone. In Bourne, G. H. (Ed.): The Biochemistry and Physiology of Bone, Vol. 3, 2nd ed., New York, Academic Press, 1971, pp. 271–298.
30. Goldhaber, P.: General phenomenon of bone resorption. 16 mm film. Harvard School of Dental Medicine, 1962.
31. Schofield, B. H., Levin, L. S., and Doty, S. B.: Ultrastructure and lysosomal histochemistry of ia rat osteoclasts. Calcif. Tissue Res., *14*:153–160, 1974.
32. Barnicot, N. A.: Some data on the effect of parathormone on the grey-lethal mouse. J. Anat., *79*:83–91, 1945.
33. Barnicot, N. A.: The supravital staining of osteoclasts with neutral red, their distribution on the parietal bone of normal growing mice, and a comparison with the mutants grey-lethal and hydrocephalus-3. Proc. Roy. Soc. Lond. (Biol), *134*:467–485, 1947.
34. Walker, D. G.: Congenital osteopetrosis in mice cured by parabiotic union with normal siblings. Endocrinology, *91*:916–920, 1972.
35. Walker, D. G.: Enzymatic and electron microscopic analysis of isolated osteoclasts. Calcif. Tissue Res., *9*:296–309, 1972.
36. Krane, S. M., Shine, K. I., and Pyle, M. B.: Citric acid metabolism in slices and homogenates of cortical bone. In Greep, R. O., and Talmadge, R. B. (Eds.): The Parathyroids. Springfield, Illinois, Charles C Thomas, 1961, pp 298–309.
37. Jaworski, Z. F. G., and Lok, E.: The rate of osteoclastic bone erosion in Haversian remodeling sites of adult dog's rib. Calcif. Tissue Res., *10*:103–112, 1972.
38. Jaworski, Z. F. G., Lok, E., and Wellington, J. L.: Impaired osteoclastic function and linear bone erosion rate in secondary hyperparathyroidism associated with chronic renal failure. Clin. Orthop., *107*:298–310, 1975.
39. Cameron, D. A., Paschall, H. A., and Robinson, R. A.: Changes in the fine structure of bone cells after the administration of parathyroid extract. J. Cell Biol., *33*:1–14, 1967.
40. Severson, A. R.: Mast cells in areas of experimental bone resorption and remodeling, Br. J. Exp. Pathol., *50*:17–21, 1969.
41. Frame, B., and Nixon, R. K.: Bone marrow mast cells in osteoporosis of aging. N. Engl. J. Med., *279*:626–630, 1968.
42. Trummel, C. L., Mundy, G. R., and Raisz, L. G.: Release of osteoclast activating factors by normal human peripheral blood leukocytes. J. Lab. Clin. Med., *85*:1001–1007, 1975.
43. Kelin, D. C., and Raisz, L. G.: Prostaglandin: stimulation of bone resorption in tissue culture. Endocrinol., *86*:1436–1440, 1970.

# Chapter Eleven

# BONE MORPHOLOGY: TYPES OF BONE TISSUE

**General Comments.**[1] Bone tissue has various appearances, which are related mainly to the function of the different types. The major divisions are lamellar and non-lamellar bone. All types are formed of the same composition of mineral and matrix and are laid down by the same cells, the osteoblasts, and resorbed by the same cells, the osteoclasts (Fig. 11–1).

## APPEARANCE OF BONE TISSUE

In non-lamellar bone the osteoblasts lay down the collagen in a haphazard way, with the collagen fibers unoriented to the surface on which they are deposited. As a result there is no polarized light appearance of alternating dark and light bands. When osteoblasts become incorporated in the matrix, the osteocytes and their lacunae tend to be larger and more irregular than in lamellar bone, and they are also more numerous. Non-lamellar bone is often referred to as woven bone because of the criss-cross arrangement of the collagen; it may be more deeply staining with stains that are specific for glycosaminoglycans, and it also contains a higher concentration of hydroxyapatite.[2] It is generally true that the greater the ratio of glycosaminoglycans to collagen, the higher the concentration of bone mineral. Woven bone is limited to the tissue laid down around the calcified cartilage struts that remain after chondrocyte death and chondroclasis, adjacent to the physis. The woven bone to some extent smooths the irregular surface of the cartilage bars, and, when the zone of secondary spongiosa is reached, the bone becomes lamellar and orderly. Woven bone is also found in fracture callus and occasionally in pathological states such as hyperparathyroidism, both "primary" and secondary. It appears in cross section in bone laid down early on in the formation of bones or in callus, and it is usually associated with cartilage (Fig. 11–2). It is generally of a temporary nature and seldom remains in the adult bone.

The majority of bone is lamellar, the layers of collagen being arranged in orderly sheets parallel to the bone surface on which the bone is deposited. Primary

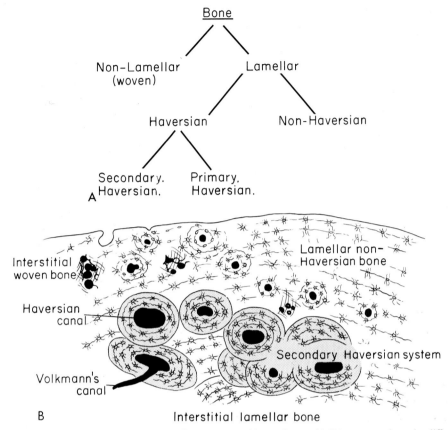

**Figure 11–1** (a) The names of the different types of bone tissue. (b) Diagram to show the different types of bone which are illustrated in Figures 11–2 to 11–5. (From Jowsey, J.: Autoradiographic and microradiographic studies of bone. In Zipkin, I. (Ed.): Biological Mineralization of Bone, New York, John Wiley and Sons, 1973, pp. 297–333.)

haversian bone is laid down on top of the woven, bone-covered cartilage rods; as the trabeculae thicken, the lamellae are arranged around a central hole or tunnel carrying blood vessels (Fig. 11–3). Primary haversian bone is found in the trabecular and cortical bone in the metaphysis and may also be formed subperiosteally when rapid bone formation is occurring. The haversian systems are somewhat small and indistinct, mainly because they are not surrounded by a cement line.

Lamellar non-haversian bone is deposited on the endosteum and periosteum of both long and flat bones (Fig. 11–4). It is arranged parallel to these surfaces and in some instances may constitute the majority of the cortex. When this happens, it is often because haversian remodeling has not taken place and the non-haversian bone has remained; this occurs most frequently in animals and not in human beings, in whom haversian remodeling begins early in life. Nevertheless, even in animals, the non-haversian lamellar bone tends to disappear with age.

Secondary haversian systems constitute the major remodeling role, fulfilling both biomechanical and calcium homeostasis functions. After bone is in its mature form, and generally after the cartilage plate has ceased growth and has been remodeled, the cortex of the long bones continue to undergo secondary haversian

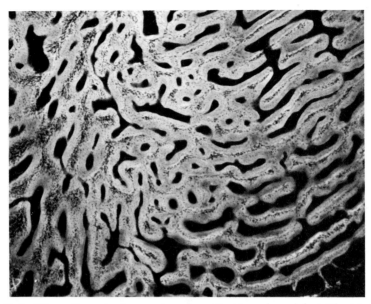

**Figure 11-2**   Microradiograph of woven bone in cortical bone in an infant. The woven bone lies mainly in the center of the somewhat dense trabeculae; it is highly mineralized and contains irregular, large osteocytes which are more numerous than in non-woven lamellar bone (magnification ×40).

system formation. Tunnels are dug continually through the bone by osteoclasts, and, after a period of time which may vary from a few days to a few months, the tunnel is filled in with regularly arranged collagen lamellae (Fig. 11-5). Because haversian systems or osteones formed in this way replace bone, they are called secondary and are easily distinguishable from primary haversian systems by the cement line that surrounds them. The cement line forms the boundary of the old tunnel wall where destruction of the bone ceased and new bone was deposited. It is morphologically identifiable because it contains slightly less collagen and more glycosaminoglycans than the surrounding bone and contains slightly more mineral.

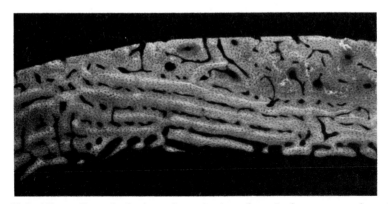

**Figure 11-3**   Microradiograph of primary haversian bone from the femur cortex of an adult rabbit. In the upper right the osteones have been cut in cross-section and in the lower left, in longitudinal section. The areas of high mineral density are calcified cartilage or woven bone (magnification ×40).

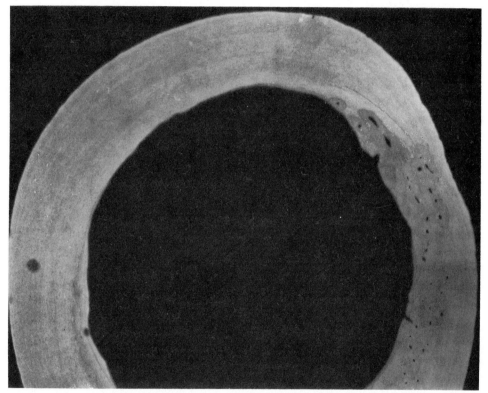

**Figure 11–4** Micrograph of lamellar non-haversian bone in a young monkey. Some haversian systems are seen on the right, but the majority of the bone has not been remodeled (magnification ×5).

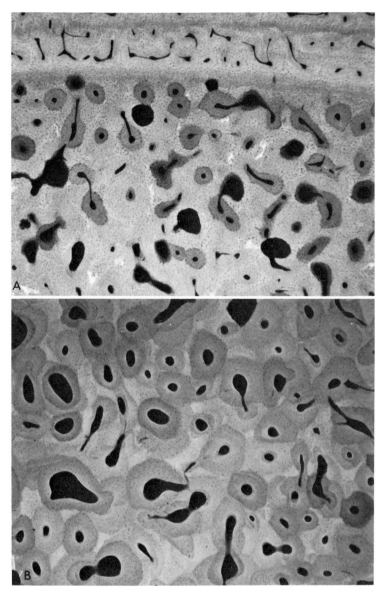

**Figure 11-5** (a) Micrograph of secondary haversian system formation in cortical bone of an adult cow. The outer limits of the haversian systems or osteones are clearly delineated by cement lines and the osteones are varying degrees of mineral density (magnification ×40). (b) Microradiograph of continued secondary haversian system remodeling seen in cortical bone of an adult man. In contrast to (a), the majority of the bone consists of secondary osteones and there are interstitial bone fragments between them. Volkmann's canals link one osteone to another in a few areas (magnification ×40).

Although the cement line is only 1 micron in thickness, it is easily visible in a stained section (Fig. 11–6). In a microradiograph the cement line is occasionally thick enough to be visible as a line of increased density; however, secondary haversian systems are most clearly identified in such a preparation by the arrangement of the surrounding bone. Since the resorbing tunnel is dug through both non-haversian bone and other haversian systems, the surrounding lamellae are at an angle to the new osteone and in this way delineate its boundaries.

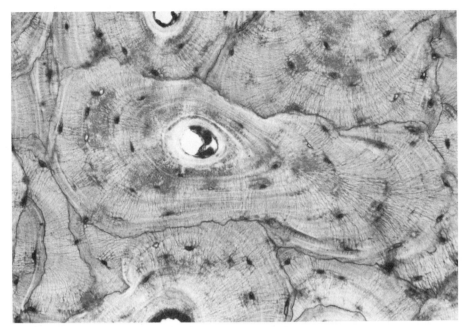

**Figure 11–6** The cement lines surrounding secondary haversian systems. The systems are irregular, and between them lie fragments of interstitial bone with no central haversian canal (magnification ×220). (From Steendijk, R., et al.: Microradiographic and histological observations in primary vitamin D: resistant rickets. In Calcified Tissues. Heidelberg, Springer-Verlag, 1966, pp. 175–178.)

Secondary haversian systems are connected to each other by Volkmann's canals, which are channels through the bone at approximately right angles to the haversian canals. Like the latter they contain blood vessels, but they are not surrounded by concentric lamellae of bone.

Haversian remodeling continues for the life span of the bone, and tertiary and quartiary systems are formed. As this process continues, pieces of osteones may remain without their central canal (Fig. 11–1b). These and the occasional bit of non-haversian lamellar bone form interstitial bone fragments, which remain viable because of the efficient osteocyte and canalicular system that exists throughout bone and which connect the haversian systems with each other and with the interstitial lamellae.

## REFERENCES

1. McLean, F. C., and Urist, M. R.: Bone. Chicago and London, The University of Chicago Press, 1961.
2. Owen, M., Jowsey, J., and Vaughan, J.: Investigation of the growth and structure of the tibia of the rabbit by microradiographic and autoradiographic techniques. J. Bone Joint Surg., *37B*:324–342, 1955.

# Part II

# Methods of Evaluation

Chapter Twelve

# CALCIUM BALANCE

## INTRODUCTION

An enormous number of different techniques are used to evaluate one or another aspect of bone. Probably more than any other tissue, bone uniquely lends itself to analysis by such methods as quantitative radiology as well as the more general methods of histology, tissue chemistry, and so on. The techniques can be divided into the following three kinds: (1) they may measure the amount of bone by radiation methods, or more directly by chemical determination; (2) they may measure bone activity by quantitating bone cell numbers; or (3) they may be directed to more peripheral factors that reflect bone activity, such as serum calcium, parathyroid hormone, and others.

So many investigators limit themselves to using the techniques they are familiar with that it is often irrelevant to indicate by what means the appropriate methods should be chosen for any particular study. However, the methods themselves clearly indicate what information will be derived from them. Once certain information has been obtained, it must always be remembered that every method gives somewhat different results, and great care must be taken not to compare noncomparable results. For example, the results from tissue culture should not be expected to be the same as the results of in vivo studies, and results from analysis of trabecular bone will not give the same numerical data as those from cortical bone.

## CALCIUM BALANCE STUDIES

**Dietary History of Calcium and Phosphorus Dietary Intake.** A dietary history relevant to mineral metabolism should include an estimation of calcium and phosphorus intake, and also some evaluation of other substances that affect mineral metabolism, such as vitamin D intake and exposure to the sun. Commonly only the calcium and, less frequently, the phosphorus intake are quantitated.

The amount of these two elements in the food is obviously important to the state of the skeleton, since two thirds of its mass is composed of these two elements. Most calcium in the diet is in the form of dairy products—milk, butter, cheese, and ice cream. An individual who avoids dairy products, although his diet may be quite adequate otherwise, will generally have an intake of less than 200 mg of calcium per day;[1] most of this will be in the form of leaf vegetables. In an average diet of an individual in the United States who drinks milk and eats cheese and ice cream, the intake is about 650 mg of calcium per day. However, this figure varies enormously from person to person, and in a group of normal persons it can range from 100 mg to 2000 mg per day. The variation is largely the result of the total amount of food consumed per day, a factor that will affect mainly the phosphorus, protein, and carbohydrate intake and, to a somewhat lesser extent, the calcium intake. Persons who have a low dietary calcium intake are generally those who avoid dairy food products and may be lactose intolerant (see Chapter Twenty-eight, Osteoporosis). Reports in the literature show that calcium intake also varies a great deal as a result of geographic variations in the diet. In England, bread and flour contain added calcium, and a significant amount of milk is consumed in tea by the adult population. In the United States, in contrast, coffee without milk, alcoholic beverages, and soft drinks are the major liquids ingested; these, of course, do not contain calcium. Among the Eskimos are a number of tribes who eat largely meat — either fish or seal and walrus meat — which is high in phosphorus and low in calcium.[2]

Calcium intake appears to decrease with age (Fig. 12–1). This is largely the result of dietary habits, which in the pre-20-year-olds includes ice cream sodas and generally a significant amount of milk. This is altered in the adult, who is more conscious of calories and cholesterol, and who replaces milk-shakes and the like in favor of black coffee. Although this has not been documented, it is possible that dietary calcium levels are also decreasing in general at all ages.

Phosphorus is a major component of most food and is high in those commonly eaten, such as bread, potatoes, and meat; it is also high in the dairy products that contain calcium. An estimate of the phosphate intake in a relatively random selection of individuals is 1600 mg per day, which is over twice the calcium intake, and this may well be an underestimate. Therefore, although dietary calcium deficiency can be a real phenomenon and may result in bone disease in children and possibly in adults, dietary phosphate deficiency is probably nonexistent; even poor diets, such as those consisting of rice alone (Japan and China) or mealies (Africa), provide a large amount of phosphorus, although they may be low in protein and are certainly low in calcium.

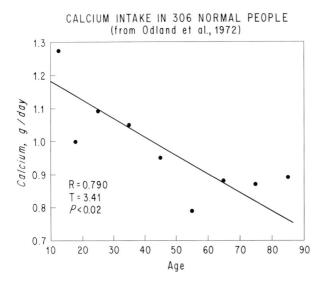

CALCIUM INTAKE IN 306 NORMAL PEOPLE
(from Odland et al., 1972)

R = 0.790
T = 3.41
P < 0.02

Calcium, g / day

Age

**Figure 12–1** There is a marked decrease in the calcium intake with increasing age. (Drawn from Odland et al.[3])

Recent investigations have suggested that the important factor in bone and mineral metabolism is the ratio of dietary calcium to phosphorus, rather than the absolute amount of each.[4] It is, therefore, necessary to evaluate the intake of both of these elements; in the past this has rarely been done, and this may account for some of the discrepancies in the results of different reports.

**Dietary History.** The major problem in obtaining any dietary history is that it is based on accurate recall by the patients of what they habitually eat. The calcium and phosphorus contents of the food are then obtained from a handbook. Probably the most complete one is in the U.S.A. Handbook 8.[5] However, it consists of collected data from different laboratories, and the last issue, dated 1963, is incomplete in some respects. The dietary intake may also vary at different times; there is often a considerable difference between the diet consumed at home and food eaten away from home. Dietary intake may also vary periodically with time. For instance, many habitual non-milk drinkers may present with osteoporosis (one third of our patients have a history of disliking milk and not drinking it). However, some such patients have been told by their physicians, or have been persuaded by what they have read, to drink milk; therefore, they present with the bone disease and a recent history of high dietary calcium intake. In such instances, the present history may be misleading in terms of the cause of the bone disease and of the calcium intake in earlier life.

In general, it is important to obtain a dietary history in order to unveil any dietary peculiarities, but probably only grossly peculiar habits will appear to be significant in terms of skeletal status. An interesting speculation here is the role of the traditional Masai diet of a mixture of milk and blood as the staple food. Meat is only occasionally ingested. This may well be the only example of a dietary intake after weaning in which the calcium content is higher than the phosphorus intake. It is tempting to mention the unusual height of the Masai at this point, and to wonder if it is related at all to the high calcium intake and the high calcium-to-phosphorus ratio of the diet.

Heavy milk drinkers (frequently ulcer patients) will have a high calcium intake, but since the calcium-to-phosphorus ratio is 1.2:1, the phosphorus intake will also be high. This is, of course, true for all dairy products. Cheese, ice cream, and butter all contain considerable amounts of phosphorus as well as calcium. In fact, processed cheese has phosphate added to such an extent that the calcium-to-phosphorus ratio is less than 1. Most cheese, therefore, cannot be recommended as a calcium supplement.

A recently emerging cause of potentially misleading information is the use of additives in processed food. These are commonly phosphate salts or may be ethylenediamenetetraacetic acid (EDTA); both complex calcium and, in dairy products, result in solubilization of the casein and a softening of texture, apparently a desirable property in the food-marketing world. The phosphate content of the commonly used emulsions (cream whip, salad dressing, etc.) is high; however, the amount has not been documented, and people seldom record the amount of these types of food dressings in a dietary history. It may be safely assumed, therefore, that estimates of the average dietary intake of phosphorus represent a significant underestimate of the actual intake.

The recommended calcium intake is 800 mg per day for an adult. It has already been pointed out that the calcium-to-phosphorus ratio is more relevant to bone metabolism than the absolute amount of either element, and in the average

Western diet this ratio is 0.5 or less. Furthermore, it is apparent from animal studies that the calcium-to-phosphorus ratio in the diet should be at least 1. Studies have also been carried out in man given calcium supplements. It is relevant that Heaney[6] recently reported that a regression line of dietary calcium intake on calcium balance crossed the zero point of the calcium balance at about 1.4 g of dietary calcium intake. From these data, a calcium intake of less than 1.4 g per day could be considered inadequate and would be expected to result in a gradual loss of bone with age.

## Calcium Balance Studies

**General Comments.**    Balance studies are performed to find out whether an individual is losing or retaining calcium. The principle on which balance studies are founded is that what goes in must either stay in or come out. If elements such as nitrogen, sodium, or phosphorus are used, a balance study will give empiric information, but it will not be possible to interpret the data accurately in terms of the metabolism of turnover of a specific tissue. This is so because these elements occur in almost all tissues and metabolites. Other elements, such as iodine (thyroid) and calcium or fluorine (bone), have a relatively specific target tissue; still other elements or compounds may be unmetabolized and are merely retained (perhaps in a specific tissue) or excreted. An example of this would be the synthetic diphosphonates with bone as the target tissue.

For a balance study to be meaningful, all intake and excretion must be measured. Any substance that is not excreted in the urine or feces is difficult to measure accurately. Measuring excretion in the breath, as would be necessary for a carbon balance study, is very difficult. Water balance is also essentially impossible to measure because of loss in breath and sweat, unless large changes are occurring and the effect is mainly through the urine (such as the effect of diuretics).

Calcium balance generally reflects bone metabolism. In general, a positive balance represents an increase in bone mass, whereas a negative balance implies a loss of bone tissue. The "calcium balance" of an individual is the sum of the calcium intake, which is almost always the dietary content of calcium, and the calcium lost in the urine, feces, and sweat. For most investigations, the sweat calcium is ignored because it is small, approximately 10 to 15 mg per day in temperature climates. Most calcium is lost in the feces, and this calcium comprises the dietary calcium that has not been absorbed (the exogenous calcium) and the endogenous calcium that is secreted into the intestine and remains unreabsorbed (the endogenous calcium).

## Technique and Interpretation

Calcium balance studies consist of measuring the calcium content of the food, which is done by taking measured samples of the food the subject is ingesting, subjecting them to chemical analysis, and measuring the total amount of calcium in the urine and stool for the same period of time over which ingestion is measured. A difficulty arises because of the variable amount of time between the ingestion of the food and the arrival of that food in the expelled feces. Food consumed on the first day of the study may not be excreted for 24 hours or more, and the elimination in the feces is more variable than the secretion in the urine. For this reason, a non-metabolized marker, red carmine, is given with the food at the beginning and end of the balance study period, and only the stools excreted with marker or between two markers are collected. If chromium sesquioxide is used, the stools can be analyzed for chromium, and only those containing chromium are used; because chromium is not metabolized, an idea of the completion of collection can be obtained. All the injected chromium should be retrieved in the feces.[7]

Most balance studies are done over a five-day period. However, the longer the period, the more accurate the data. The balance study must also be carried out when the individual is in equilibrium with his or her dietary intake. In practical terms, this means that if the patient is on the same diet before and during the study period, that is, if he remains on his habitual dietary intake, a balance study is meaningful. However, if the diet is altered, then the study may be meaningless, or it may mean something quite different from the former measurement. This means not only that, for a calcium balance study, the calcium content should be constant but also that all substances that might alter calcium absorption and excretion should be kept constant; this would include phosphorus, vitamin D, acid or alkali content, fat, and such substances as calcium-complexing agents (for example, phytates and oxalates). Theoretically, exercise, sun exposure, and consumption of alcohol should be maintained at the accustomed level. However, although exercise is often maintained at the habitual level, it would be surprising if there were a single published study that included the material aspect of the "happy hour," and yet it is unlikely that all balance studies have been carried out on "abstainers."

The most meaningful balance studies, therefore, are those in which the patients remain on their habitual intake or are carried out on chronically "institutionalized" individuals whose intake has been controlled for a long time. The studies by Spencer and colleagues[8] in Veterans' Administration Hospital inmates are meaningful for this reason. Conversely, balance studies carried out while the patient is put on very low calcium intake should be interpreted with caution. Dent has expressed the view that such studies are useless.[9] In terms of how the individual habitually handles normal dietary calcium, this is certainly true; however, with strict regard to the explanation of the data, the information may be relevant to the way different individuals handle calcium stress.

In this regard, it is frequently meaningful to plot the dietary absorption of calcium in relation to calcium balance. For example, using radiocalcium tracer methods, individuals with osteoporosis tend, on their habitual diet, to malabsorb calcium in comparison with normal individuals on the same habitual dietary calcium level; if the patients are placed on a low calcium intake, this difference disappears (Fig. 12–2).[10, 11] The same cautionary words apply to balance studies in persons given a high calcium intake. The key to the problem is that we do not know how long a person takes to adapt to a new dietary regimen. Studies, such as those with fluoride, suggest that a year or longer is a good approximation of the equilibrium time.

Urinary calcium is relatively fixed in amount, although it may decrease somewhat on a grossly calcium-restricted diet and will increase in response to vitamin D or a raised calcium intake. Fecal calcium tends to vary more widely. After the samples have been collected, the calcium levels in the urine, feces, and food are

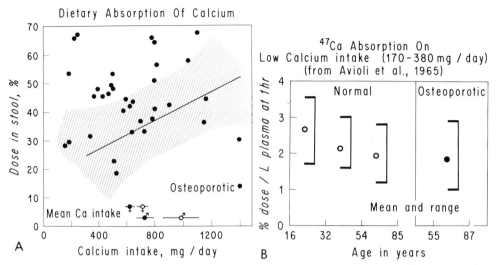

**Figure 12–2** (a) The calcium absorption in 34 osteoporotic patients compared with the absorption in age-matched and calcium-intake matched normal persons. Both patients and normal volunteers remained on their estimated habitual dietary intake. Approximately half the patients malabsorbed calcium, compared with the normal volunteers in this study. (From Riggs et al.[10]) (b) Calcium absorption in osteoporotic patients and in normal individuals who have been placed on a low calcium intake. The ability of osteoporotic and normal individuals to absorb calcium on a deficient diet is the same for age-matched groups. (Drawn from Avioli et al.[11])

currently measured by spectrophotometric methods, after ashing if appropriate (feces and food).

The last cautionary note regarding calcium balance studies refers to the initial statement that a calcium balance represents the status of the skeleton. It very well may, but it may not. All that can be said is that a positive balance represents a retention of calcium by the body. In some instances, the calcium may well be deposited in soft tissues. Muscle, skin, and connective tissue constitute approximately 50 per cent of body weight (30 kg in an average adult). If the calcium content of the tissue increases only five-fold from normal (0.2 mg/g to 1.0 mg/g), this would represent an addition of 240 g of calcium to the body. This would be a significant amount in a balance study, but it would be invisible by any techniques except chemical analysis of soft tissue. Balance studies in phosphate-supplemented persons are probably an instance in which soft-tissue calcium deposition accounts for the larger proportion of net calcium retention.[12]

Balance study data are displayed conventionally in a way that was used first by Dr. Fuller Albright. A graph is made of the amount of calcium in milligrams, the amounts increasing upward negatively from zero and downward positively from zero on the ordinate, while the weekly periods are plotted along the abscissa (Fig. 12–3).[13] The dietary calcium intake is marked on the ordinate on the positive side, downward from the zero; the fecal calcium is marked upward from the dietary intake line and the urine calcium above that. If the combined fecal and urinary calcium adds up to more than the intake, then obviously the figure will be above the zero line and represent a negative calcium balance. The reverse is true if the combined excretion is less than the intake; then the column will fall below (on the positive side) of the zero and represent net calcium retention.

Calcium balance studies, or any balance studies, are both tedious and time-consuming. They are also likely to be inaccurate to some degree and probably are meaningful only if large abnormalities in calcium metabolism exist. Balance studies

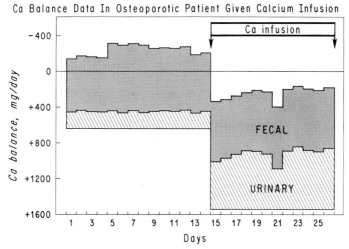

**Figure 12–3**  Dietary calcium intake during the first period was about 600 mg per day, and urinary and fecal loss resulted in a negative calcium balance of approximately 200 mg per day. Calcium infusion raised the intake to about 1600 mg per day and because the fecal and urinary excretion was not proportionally increased, the patient went into positive calcium balance. (Redrawn from Pak et al.[13])

should probably be done only in special instances and must be interpreted with caution.

### Calcium Absorption

The other major component of the calcium balance study, besides the dietary history and calcium excretion measurements, is the absorption of dietary calcium in the gut. By measuring dietary calcium and fecal calcium, the net absorption can be calculated; this is the absorption of the dietary calcium plus the difference between the calcium secreted into the gut from the body (the endogenous fecal calcium) and the calcium reabsorbed from the gut, the reabsorbed endogenous calcium.

The intestinal absorption of calcium occurs mainly in the duodenum and becomes progressively less throughout the small intestine. This obviously has important implications in the consequences of gastric surgery on calcium-deprivation bone disease; a duodenectomy (Billroth II) would be expected to result in more severe calcium depletion than an ileectomy because the duodenum appears to be the primary site of vitamin D-induced calcium absorption. The calcium is absorbed by a calcium-binding protein mechanism that is dependent on an active metabolite of vitamin D, 1, 25-dihydroxycholecalciferol. Of course, lack of the original hormone, vitamin D, will impair calcium absorption, as will liver or kidney disease severe enough to prevent the conversion of vitamin D to its first metabolite, 25-hydroxycholecalciferol, and its active form, 1, 25 = $(OH)_2D$.

Calcium absorption is also influenced, through the vitamin D mechanism, by calcium deficiency. There is evidence in animals that a decrease in calcium intake results in an increase in the 1,25-dihydroxycholecalciferol-induced absorption. However, in man, not all individuals adapt to a low calcium intake by increased absorption.

Other factors have already been mentioned; calcium binding substances, such as phytates, oxalates, and fats, will decrease the availability of calcium for absorption, as will achlorhydria, which results in a failure of acidification of the stomach contents. Adrenocortical steroids also impair calcium absorption, and this may be a factor in the osteoporosis of hyperadrenocorticosteroidism.

The absorption of dietary calcium is generally estimated two hours after oral ingestion of a dose of $^{47}$Ca; at this time, absorption of dietary calcium is significant and secretion of endogenous calcium is low. The net absorption can be calculated by measuring stool radioisotope content, stool collections being made until less than 1 per cent of the administered dose appears in a 24-hour collection. The normal absorption generally varies between 10 and 50 per cent, with a mean of 30 per cent. Absorption can differ greatly in bone disease; for example, absorption is high in hyperparathyroidism (up to 80 per cent) and low in untreated osteomalacia (15 per cent).[14] The dietary calcium level also influences calcium absorption. On a low calcium intake of 200 mg per day, the per cent absorbed increases in normal individuals up to an average of about 50 per cent.[11] The reverse is true of a high calcium intake, and absorption decreases. However, despite the low percentage of absorption, most individuals on a high calcium intake are in positive calcium balance, and those on a low calcium intake are generally in negative calcium balance. Therefore, although adaptation does occur, a high intake will positively affect calcium balance.[9]

Most absorption studies are carried out at short intervals after oral ingestion if radioisotope methods and serum levels are used. The serum $^{47}$Ca levels at both two and four hours are negatively related to the cumulative fecal $^{47}$Ca, perhaps obviously, since they both reflect calcium absorption. However, at intervals longer than four hours after the oral dose, the plasma or serum $^{47}$Ca levels will begin to fall because of loss into the urine and as part of endogenous loss, and these levels then cease to reflect dietary absorption.[15] Although calculation of the endogenous calcium secretion can be made, a direct measurement can be carried out by means of an oral $^{47}$Ca load given at the same time as an intravenous $^{45}$Ca injection; the arrival of the $^{45}$Ca in the feces will indicate endogenous calcium loss.[16]

Radioactive strontium has also been used; however, strontium differs from calcium in its absorption and secretion rates and, therefore, gives quantitatively slightly different data.[17] An additional caution in absorption measurements is related to the availability of the calcium in the diet; isotope-labeled milk is generally thought to be a good reflection of the average availability of calcium in foods, but high phytate levels in food or lactase deficiency would obviously alter availability.

Data on calcium absorption have been relatively consistent, assuming that the stable calcium levels in the study are uniform. A study conducted in 1965 showed that older individuals tend to absorb less calcium than young people.[11] A more recent study has shown that the first metabolite of vitamin D formed in the liver (25-hydroxycholecalciferol) can markedly influence the absorption of calcium in Cushing's disease, in which calcium absorption is low.[18] It is unlikely that this will result in clinical improvement in this disease, but this is unproven.

### REFERENCES

1.  Birge, S. J., Jr., Keutmann, H. T., Cuatrecasas, P., and Whedon, G. D.: Osteoporosis, intestinal lactase deficiency and low dietary calcium intake. New Engl. J. Med., 276:445–448, 1967.

2. Mazess, R. B.: Bone density in Sadlermiut Eskimo. Hum. Biol., *38*:42–49, 1966.

3. Odland, L. M., Mason, R. L., and Alexeff, A. I.: Bone density and dietary findings of 409 Tennessee subjects. II. Dietary considerations. Am. J. Clin. Nutr., *25*:908–911, 1972.

4. Jowsey, J., and Balasubramaniam, P.: Effect of phosphate supplements on soft tissue calcification and bone turnover. Clin. Sci., *42*:289–299, 1972.

5. Watt, B. K., and Merrill, A. L.: Composition of foods. Agriculture Handbook No. 8 (Consumer and Food Economics Research Division). Agricultural Research Service, United States Department of Agriculture, revised December, 1963.

6. Heaney, R. P., Recker, R. R., and Saville, P. D.: Calcium balance and calcium requirements in middle-aged women (abstract). Clin. Res., *22*:649A, 1974.

7. Rose, G. A.: Experiences with the use of interrupted carmine red and continuous chromium sesquioxide marking of human feces with reference to calcium, phosphorus and magnesium. Gut, *5*:274–279, 1964.

8. Spencer, H., Menczel, J., Lewin, I., and Samachson, J.: Effect of high phosphorus intake on calcium and phosphorus metabolism in man. J. Nutr., *86*:125–132, 1965.

9. Dent, C. E.: General principles of metabolic balances as illustrated in particular by calcium balance determinations. Sonderdruck aus Klinische Ernährungslehre (Wissenschaftliche Veröffentlichungen der Deutschen Gesellschaft für Ernährung Band 13) Dr. Dietrich Steinkopff, Darmstadt Verlag, 1963, pp. 10–22.

10. Riggs, B. L., Kelly, P. J., Kinney, V. R., Scholz, D. A., and Bianco, A. J., Jr.: Calcium deficiency and osteoporosis. J. Bone Joint Surg., *49A*:915–924, 1967.

11. Avioli, L. V., McDonald, J. E., and Lee, S. W.: The influence of age on the intestinal absorption of [47]Ca in women and its relation to [47]Ca absorption of postmenopausal osteoporosis. J. Clin. Invest., *44*:1960–1967, 1965.

12. Goldsmith, R. S., Richards, R., Dube, W. J., Hulley, S. B., Holdsworth, D., and Ingbar, S. H.: Metabolic effects and mechanism of action of phosphate supplements. In Hioco, D. J. (Ed.): Phosphate et Métabolisme Phosphocalcique: Régulation Normale et Aspects Physiopathologiques; Symposium International. Paris, Laboratoires Sandoz, pp. 271–291, 1971.

13. Pak, C. Y. C., Zisman, E., Evens, R., Jowsey, J., Delea, C. S., and Bartter, F. C.: The treatment of osteoporosis with calcium infusions. Clinical Studies. Am. J. Med., *47*:7–16, 1969.

14. Parsons, V., Veall, N., and Butterfield, W. J. H.: The clinical use of orally administered [47]Ca for the investigation of intestinal calcium absorption. Calcif. Tissue Res., *2*:83–92, 1968.

15. Spencer, H., Lewin, I., Fowler, J., and Samachson, J.: Influence of dietary calcium intake on Ca[47] absorption in man. Am. J. Med., *46*:197–205, 1969.

16. DeGrazia, J. A., Ivanovich, P., Fellows, H., and Rich, C.: A double isotope method for measurement of intestinal absorption of calcium in man. J. Lab. Clin. Med., *66*:822–829, 1965.

17. Samachson, J.: Plasma values after oral [45]calcium and [85]strontium as an index of absorption. Clin. Sci., *25*:17–26, 1963.

18. Caniggia, A., and Gennari, C.: Effect of 25-hydroxycholecalciferol (25-HCC) on intestinal absorption of [47]Ca in four cases of iatrogenic Cushing's syndrome. Helv. Med. Acta, *37*:221–225, 1973.

# Chapter Thirteen

# BONE DENSITY MEASUREMENTS

## MASS AND VOLUME DETERMINATIONS

The choice of a method of measuring bone density depends on what sort of information is desired. If the density of the whole bone is measured, any differences between "control" and "experimental" will reflect loss of cortical and trabecular bone and also total loss of bone in enlargement of the medullary cavity. Only weight (generally dry, fat-free weight, after ether-acetone extraction of the fat and alcohol dehydration and equilibrium to room temperature) and volume measurements are necessary. Weight poses no problem; the bone is weighed to "constant weight," that is, until there is no change in weight on two consecutive occasions. Volume measurements are a little difficult because displacement of fluids produces meaningful differences in volume, depending on the fluid used. Water and other fluids (oil, mercury) will soak into the bone and marrow cavity and give a volume measurement of the mineralized tissue (and some holes, depending on which have been filled; this is generally not very meaningful data, since bone density at the milligram level is rarely different even in obviously diseased states). The bone may be coated with wax or plastic to form a layer impervious to the water, and volume measurements may then be made which are exaggerated only by the amount of wax on the bone surface. This method is probably the most satisfactory for small bones, such as small animal bones or bones of the human foot and hand. It can also be used for larger bones such as vertebra. Dunnill used this technique to measure external bone volume in males and females.[1] His results show quite clearly that the technique can be used to measure bone size changes by expressing the results as displaced water volume; by dividing by weight, the density can be measured (Fig. 13–1).

There is a technique that avoids the waxing process for the volume determination, namely, the displacement of millet seed. This was first described by Trotter and associates in 1958[2] and is a simple method with margin of error of between 1.1 and 3.2 per cent. The millet seed is allowed to fill the marrow cavity and is the right size to fit into all major indentations, but it will not penetrate the holes of the haversian systems themselves. The method provides interesting information on the densities of bone with age, race (black versus white), and sex. For example, the humeri lose weight at a more rapid rate than any other bone, whereas the vertebrae lose bone least rapidly with age, although the latter start out with less bone at age 30 (Fig. 13–2).

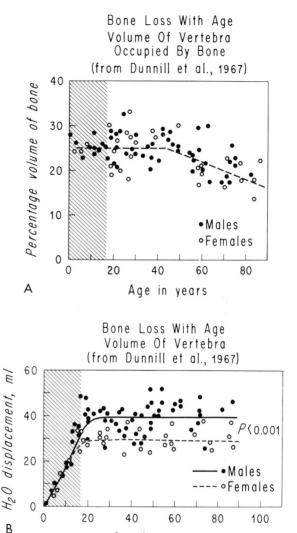

**Figure 13–1** (a) Volume of bone excluding the marrow space and therefore measuring the trabecular and endosteal bone loss. (b) Bone volume of vertebrae in which the external whole bone is coated with wax and only external size measured. Female vertebrae tend to be smaller at maturity and remain smaller than male vertebrae. In neither sex is there a significant loss of periosteal size with increasing age. (Drawn from Dunnill et al.[1])

## THE FEMORAL TRABECULAR INDEX: SINGH INDEX

Evaluation specifically and exclusively of trabecular bone would have the advantage of looking at what is evidently the more "sensitive" type of bone, compared with cortical bone when evaluating changes in bone mass. By "sensitive" is meant the degree to which the tissue responds to metabolic changes. A method has recently been developed of assigning grades I to VII to the arrangement of trabeculae in the femoral head.[4] The index, called the Femoral Trabecular Index by the senior author, Dr. Manmohan Singh, and the Singh Index by his co-authors, is a numerical indication of the degree of bone loss and is therefore considered to reflect degrees of normality or osteoporosis.[5]

The basis of the Singh Index is the observation that the bundles of trabeculae in the femoral head, and probably also in other areas of predominantly trabecular

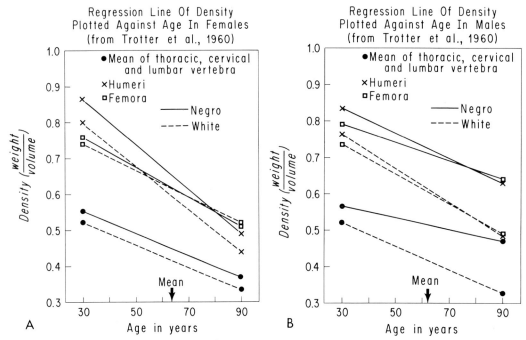

**Figure 13–2** (a) Values for bone density loss with age in white and Negro females measured by displacement of millet seed. Vertebral bone tends to lose bone less rapidly than the cortical bone of the humeri and femora. (b) Loss of bone density with age in white and Negro males. Vertebrae tend to lose bone more slowly than the cortical bones. (Drawn from Trotter et al.[3])

bone, are arranged in relation to stress patterns. Koch used mathematical principles to define the forces in the femur; his analysis enabled him to predict the variations in tensile and compressive stress in a normal femur loaded with 100 lb on the femur head and simulating an upright standing position.[6] The computed highest maximum compressive stress (+1310 lb/in²) lies on the internal cortex of the femoral neck. The values decrease down the femur shaft and are significantly lower in the distal third. The maximum tensile stress is at the external cortex of the femoral neck (−976 lb/in²) and is also the highest figure at any point on the femur. Although this work is now perhaps only of historical interest because of the advent of more sophisticated biomechanical methods, the sites where fracture is predicted most likely to occur according to the Singh Index, are in fact, the areas where they occur most frequently and in the predicted manner. Thus, femoral neck fractures with the femur head displaced distally are the most common fractures of that bone.

The predictions Koch made were derived from observations of the distribution of the trabeculae in the femur. In the head and neck of the femur an anteroposterior x-ray view shows the following three major bundles of trabeculae: the principal compressive, the principal tensile, and the secondary compressive and tensile trabeculae. These are lost one after the other, rather than all disappearing at the same time. In a normal young adult, all three bundles are present as well as a number of somewhat randomly arranged trabeculae that fill Ward's triangle. Such an x-ray is graded VII by the Singh method. These random trabeculae disappear first, Ward's triangle appears empty, and the x-ray is graded VI. The secondary compressive trabeculae disappear next at the outer femoral cortex end, then at the inner cortex end; next, the secondary tensile trabeculae disappear and then the primary tensile trabeculae in grades V, IV, and III, respectively. Grades II and I show only the principal compressive trabeculae, and eventually a decrease is seen in these as well (Fig. 13–3).

The method requires only an x-ray of the pelvis, which should be taken with the feet in 15° internal rotation to obtain a good view of the head and neck of the femur. The method is simple and, although there will obviously be instances in which different individuals will differ in their evaluation, inter-observer differences are generally small.

A good correlation exists between the Singh Index and clinical and radiologic indications of osteoporosis. A comparison showed that 89.7 per cent of people with clinical osteoporosis and spinal fractures had a Singh Index of grade III, II, or I, whereas 90 per cent of individuals who did not have any symptomatic or radiologic evidence of osteoporosis had a Singh Index of grades V to VII.[7] The overlap between clinically normal and clinically abnormal individuals is less than in any other method that attempts to distinguish this disease from normal (Fig. 13–4).[8]

In a study of osteoporotic patients and subjects with osteoarthritis, Roh and colleagues found that 12 out of 14 males and 15 out of 23 females with osteoporosis had Singh Indices of four or less.[9] The separation between normals and osteoporotic subjects, including grade IV as an osteoporotic one, is 80 per cent, which is not as clear a separation as that reported by Singh and colleagues.[7] When only grades I to III were considered osteoporotic, only 51 per cent of the patients had osteoporotic grades. It is possible that a number of the patients with osteoporosis had also osteomalacia, a common complication of osteoporosis in the northern part of Europe, and the presence of osteomalacia would prevent the bone loss that leads to a decreasing Singh Index; the poorer discrimination in women

## Trabecular Grading Patterns (Singh)

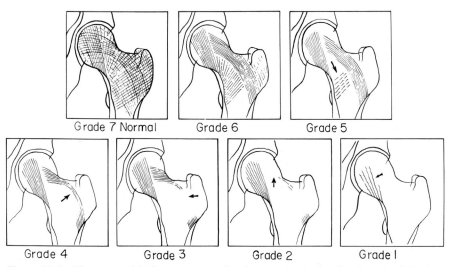

Figure 13–3 The sequential disappearance of trabeculae in the head and neck of the femur as progressive bone loss occurs. The loss of trabeculae has been divided into seven grades. (From Jowsey, J.: Osteoporosis: Its etiology and treatment. Sandoz Medical Services Dept., Sandoz Pharmaceuticals, Division of Sandoz (Canada) Ltd, Dorval, Que.)

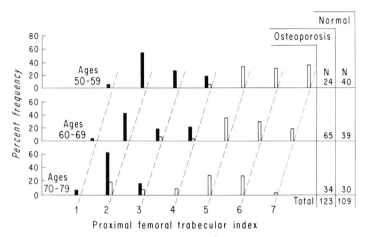

**Figure 13–4**   If the Singh Index of grades 1 to 3 are indicative of osteoporosis, there is almost complete separation of osteoporotic individuals from normal individuals. (From Wahner et al.[8])

compared with men could also be explained on this basis, since a mixture of the two bone diseases is common in women. The relation between the Singh Index and osteoarthritis was low or negative, which confirms the clinical impression that osteoporosis rarely accompanies this joint problem.

The Singh Index differs from all other methods of quantitating bone in that it is independent of the size of the skeleton. All normal people, that is, people without known bone disease after ambulation to age 20, have a Singh Index of VII, irrespective of body size. Methods such as the Cameron-Sorenson densitometer and the quantitative radiographic scanning methods all measure the amount of bone in a given area or scan path. Thus the bigger the individual, the larger the bone mass number compared with that of a small, slight person, although both the large and small person may have completely normal bone densities and will have the same Singh Index.

It should perhaps be mentioned, therefore, that no relationship may be expected to exist between the Singh Index and measurements of bone mass.[10] This may seem obvious, but, since some investigators have erroneously drawn such a comparison, it is necessary to make the point.[11]

The Singh Index has been most useful in separating osteoporotic from normal individuals and in evaluating the amount of bone in non-osteoporotic individuals. Since trauma of some type is a predisposing factor in symptomatic osteoporosis, and since the definition of the disease is clinical and depends on the existence of a fracture, the Singh Index is of potential value in deciding whether asymptomatic individuals have "osteoporosis"—that is, bone loss to a degree that would put them into a fracture-risk category. It may also be useful for evaluating skeletal status in instances where bone disease is suspected. For example, in a group of 91 adult outpatients with epilepsy who had received treatment with phenobarbital, the Singh Index was found to be less than in a control group of age-matched people (Fig. 13–5).[12] In a group of 11 teenagers with Scheuermann's kyphosis, ten had indices of less than VII compared with 200 control subjects between 4 and 20 years old who all had an index of VII (Fig. 13–6). This suggested that bone loss might have played a part in their spinal abnormalities.[13]

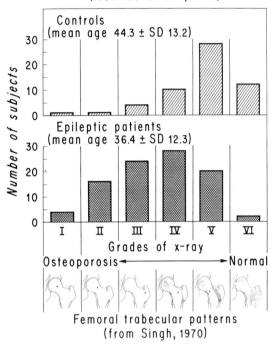

Radiological Changes
Resulting From
Anticonvulsant Therapy
(from Sotaniemi, 1972)

**Figure 13-5** In relatively young individuals, those treated with phenobarbital for epilepsy had a lower Singh Index than untreated patients. This early paper uses only six grades as described by Singh et al. in 1970. (Redrawn from Sotaniemi et al.[12])

The method may or may not be useful in longitudinal studies. A decrease in the Singh Index has been seen in an individual with immobilization osteoporosis. However, it has not yet been established whether the technique will reflect increases in bone density. If it does, this would suggest that the "disappearance" of trabecular bundles is a loss of trabeculae to a level at which they are radiologically "absent" but "reappear" as they thicken with increased bone formation. This may well occur, since reappearance of trabeculae has been seen in x-rays of the vertebral bodies in response to fluoride and calcium.

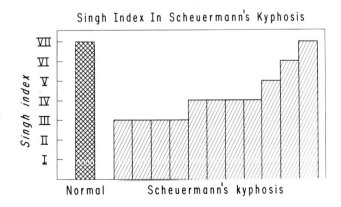

Singh Index In Scheuermann's Kyphosis

**Figure 13-6** In patients with Scheuermann's kyphosis, the Singh Index was found to be low in all except one patient when compared with normals of the same age. (Bradford et al.[13])

## CORTICAL THICKNESS

In 1960 Barnett and Nordin described a method of measuring the thickness of the femoral and second metacarpal cortex, and lumbar vertebrae (usually L3), and deriving a numerical value in each of these areas which they added to make a score that they believed could be used to distinguish normal from abnormal bone.[14] The technique utilizes an x-ray and thickness measurements are made with calipers on the x-ray film. In the femur, the sum of the width of the thickness of the two cortices in the midshaft is divided by the total external diameter of the cortex and multiplied by 100. The same is done for the metacarpal (Fig. 13–7). These values reflect the loss of bone endosteally and correctly assume that there has been no loss of bone from the periosteum. However, increase in the porosity of the cortex is not appreciated in the measurement.

In the spine, the vertical height of the middle of the vertebral body is divided by the vertical height of the maximum anterior height and multiplied by 100. This reflects the "ballooning" of the intervertebral disk. Since there appears to be no correlation between the peripheral (femur and metacarpal) values and the spinal values, these were considered separately; a total peripheral score of 88 or less was believed to indicate peripheral osteoporosis, whereas a spinal score of 80 or less indicated spinal osteoporosis. The method may provide a quantitative estimation of the radiographic appearance. However, some individuals with incontrovertible osteoporosis have normal scores, and the method has proved only slightly more useful than a non-quantitative evaluation by a radiologist of the lumbar and cervical spine, with comments on the degree of biconcavity and number of crush fractures.

As an indication of bone mass, the cortical thickness of long bones, particularly the metacarpal, is probably most often used and has probably yielded the most meaningful results. The bones measured include the metacarpals, phalanges, humerus, and, less often, the clavicle. The measurements are generally of the thickness of the cortex at a point equidistant from the two ends of the bone or at some other predetermined point. Both cortices are measured and the values are added to give cortical thickness or what is sometimes referred to as combined cortical thickness (CCT), meaning the sum of the thickness of the two cortices.[15] The errors may be significant, both between observers and to a lesser extent between two measurements by the same observer. The main problem seems to be the precise determination of the inner border of the cortex, which, with severe disease, becomes more and more indistinct and arbitrary.[16]

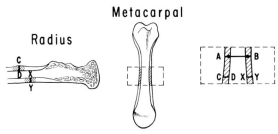

**Metacarpal**

**Radius**

CD + XY = combined cortical thickness

$$\frac{CD + XY}{AB} = \text{cortical thickness index}$$

**Figure 13–7** The cortical thickness measurements in the metacarpal and radius. The index, which includes the external size of the bone, has not usefully added to the precision or meaning of the measurement.

Cortical thickness measurements made in the clavicle have shown that gastrectomy accelerates bone loss (Fig. 13–8).[17] Meema and Meema, using a lateral x-ray, measured the cortical thickness of the humerus just below the condyles and added values for both cortices to give the CCT. This method was used extensively to evaluate attempts at therapy in osteoporosis as well as to follow normal changes of bone mass with age.[18] CCT measurements also appear to be higher in elderly women with diabetes compared with non-diabetic controls. Non-diabetics with a low body weight are more often osteoporotic; that is, they have vertebral fractures and also low CCT measurements and bone loss.[19]

More recently, Bloom and Laws[20] made measurements more or less in the center of the humerus from an anteroposterior radiograph; this view and site they felt to be more accurate than those used by Meema's group because the bone was more uniform in thickness at this point. The metacarpal and phalanx have also been used to measure cortical thickness. In these methods no attempt is made to correct for body size by measuring the outside diameter of the bone, in the way Barnett and Nordin did.[14] In fact, Morgan and associates showed that there was no correlation between cortical thickness and diameter; using a diameter correction factor to produce the "metacarpal" index appeared to confuse the data, and a simple cortical thickness measurement is thought to be the most reliable measure of bone loss.[16]

Using the third metacarpal, Shimmins and Smith found that the quantitative radiographic methods (next section) are superior to the cortical thickness measurements.[21, 22] This conclusion was derived from the better correlation ($r = +0.88$) between the aluminum equivalency and bone ash than between cortical thickness and bone ash ($r = 0.70$). This is to be expected, since x-ray density measurements include evaluation of cortical bone porosity, whereas cortical thickness measurements do not.

**Figure 13–8** The cortical thickness of the clavicle shows the development of bone loss in patients after gastrectomy. (Redrawn from Fujita et al.[17])

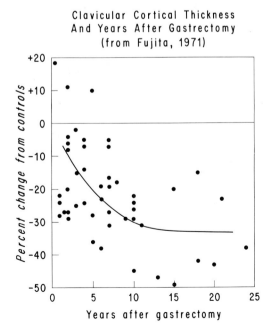

## DENSITOMETRIC MEASUREMENTS OF THE X-RAY

This term generally refers to techniques that quantitate bone mass by measuring its absorption of an x-ray or energy beam. The methods all have in common two imperfections that also apply to some extent to the cortical thickness measurements just described. First, in any sampling technique the piece evaluated may not be truly representative of the skeleton as a whole. In females, bone density of multiple samples from four different areas showed a high correlation, but for some reason, in males the only correlation was between distal femur and lumbar vertebra; it is possible that manual labor in the upper extremities in males increased bone mass locally.[23, 24] Secondly, it is not possible to correct the value for body size. As mentioned previously, the information generally desired relates to whether the amount of bone an individual has is normal or abnormal. Bone densitometry data, therefore, should be a good way of comparing an individual with himself at two different times but will not be ideal for evaluating skeletal status at any one time in an individual except at the extremes of bone disease. Therefore, although the techniques described below are not ideal, they are used because a better method has not been available and they have proved useful. The precise methods are many and varied, but they can be divided into those using a step-wedge and x-ray of a bone and those using absorption of energy from an isotope. It may be true to say that the many bones (ulna, radius, os calcis, femur, vertebrae) and the many methods reflect the lack of complete success of any one method.

## QUANTITATIVE RADIOGRAPHY OF THE OS CALCIS AND HAND

A roentgenogram is made of the os calcis (laterally) or of the hand, with an aluminum wedge placed beside the bone to be analyzed (Fig. 13–9). The beam qualities and kilovoltage are standardized as much as possible. Single multiple scans of the radiograph are made over the bone and the step-wedge, and the results are expressed in terms of aluminum equivalency. This value can be turned into hydroxyapatite by suitable reference measurements. The early methods relied on a single scan of the metacarpal or the os calcis.[25, 26] Mayo pointed out that the frequently encountered problem with this and any other quantitative evaluation of bone mass is that of the very large variation between different individuals.[27] This makes any differences that should be evident, such as between males and females or between foot soldiers and hospital staff, disappear. If the method is sensitive, then variations in bone mass which avoid individual differences should be meaningful—that is, studies in a single individual with time. Multiple scans should also improve sensitivity.

Vogel, Donaldson and co-workers, and Mack have obtained the most useful data using multiple scans of the os calcis in volunteers or subjects, concentrating mainly on the effect of weightlessness, non-weight-bearing, and ambulation.[26, 28, 29] The method has also proved useful in evaluating therapy under admittedly somewhat experimental conditions.

Perhaps the most interesting data have come from a study of bone loss in the os calcis in the astronauts on the Gemini IV, V, and VII flights.[30, 31] High losses of up to 23 per cent in the 4- and 8-day flights were reported. The change decreased to approximately 3 per cent in the longer 14-day flight in which the calcium intake

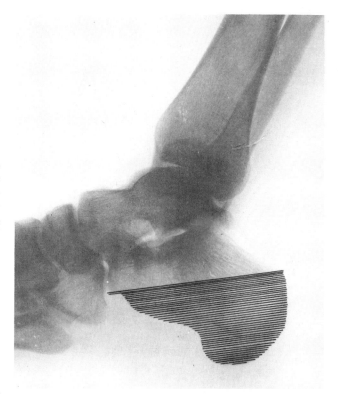

**Figure 13–9** An x-ray of the os calcis with an adjacent aluminum wedge. The sites of the scan by the densitometer are shown by the dark lines crossing the x-ray of the os calcis. (Courtesy of G.P. Vose.)

was increased to 1 g per day (Table 13–1). Comparable losses occurred in the hand. However, there are some difficulties. If the high losses in the astronauts occurred throughout the skeleton, then the total calcium losses were tremendous and seem to defy excretion. Although vertebral radiography showed that the correlation between the aluminum equivalency and the ash content of vertebral samples from cadavers was high ($r = 0.93$), on the other hand, an individual placed on a calcium diet that varied from 450 to 800 mg per day showed an increase of 520 mg of calcium in one month in the vertebral body measured, and there is at present no evidence that a high dietary intake of calcium will increase skeletal mass at all.

**Table 13–1** THE EFFECTS OF VARYING CALCIUM INTAKES ON BONE MASS

| Subjects | Calcium Intake mg/day | Duration (days) | Bone Mass, % change | |
| --- | --- | --- | --- | --- |
| | | | Os Calcis | Hand, Phalanx |
| Space Pilots | 600–700 | 4 | −9.1 | −9.05 |
| Bed Rest Patients | 600–700 | 210 | −3.47 | −1.02 |
| Space Pilots | 300 | 8 | −12.0 | −20.09 |
| Bed Rest Patients | 300 | 210 | −7.41 | −1.19 |
| Space Pilots | 1000 | 14 | −2.38 | −7.31 |
| Bed Rest Patients | 1000 | 210 | −4.76 | −1.05 |

From Mack and LaChance.[29]

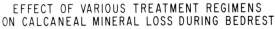

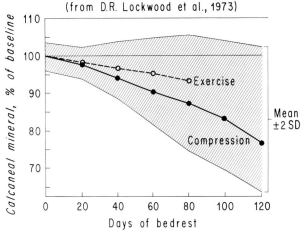

**Figure 13–10** Using young volunteers, densitometry of the os calcis showed that exercise and compression in bed failed to alter the rate of bone loss seen in untreated individuals. (Redrawn from Lockwood et al.[33])

The results of studies on the effect of exercise in immobilization and weightlessness were variable. In the Gemini VII flight, planned exercise appeared to reduce the bone loss, and this was also found in bed rest volunteers by the same authors, Mack and LaChance.[29] However, other investigators, also using the os calcis, came to different conclusions. Hantman and co-workers[32] evaluated the effect of various forms of therapy, including exercise and longitudinal compression on disuse osteoporosis in healthy men, and other investigators have come to the same conclusions; the bone loss is marked and, in studies in which calcium balance was measured, the bone loss was accompanied by significant fecal and urinary calcium loss, which was unchanged by exercise or compression in bed and only reversed by weight-bearing ambulation (Figs. 13–10, 13–11).[28, 33]

The relationship between compressive breaking strength and the mineral content of the bone measured either directly or radiologically has indicated the practical usefulness of the technique. Comparing three lumbar vertebrae (L–3, L–4, L–

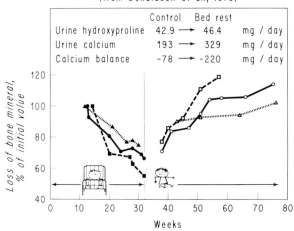

**Figure 13–11** Using densitometry of the os calcis, weight-bearing ambulation restored the bone mass seen before immobilization in normal volunteers. (Drawn from Donaldson et al.[28])

5) and calcaneal ash weights with compressive strength, Weaver and Chalmers[23] found a high correlation (r = 0.827 for the vertebrae and 0.811 for the calcaneus) between strength and ash weight. However, when compressive strength was related to age, the relationship was less apparent, particularly in the calcaneus. The authors attributed this to a differential effect of exercise on the calcaneus and the variability of the amount of activity in different people.

Keane in 1959 and Doyle in 1961 reported a method of assessing ulnar density in which an aluminum step-wedge was used with a water bath to standardize soft tissue mass.[34, 35] The peculiarity of the technique is the use of multiple determinations along the long axis of the shaft of the ulna. The x-ray density is expressed in terms of aluminum equivalency and is divided by the ulnar thickness determined from an x-ray taken at right angles. The advantage of the method is that a profile of density is obtained which varies with the area and, presumably, with the relative amount of cortical and trabecular bone. The profile is different in different diseases. The technique has been applied by others and related to bone ash and strength. A relationship has been obtained that indicates that bone density of the ulnar (by Doyle's modification of Keane's method) is biologically meaningful in terms of bone strength and "failure."

New methods will probably take the place of the quantitative radiological techniques described above as instrumentation becomes more sophisticated. Videodensitometric analysis of an x-ray may prove to be more useful than routine densitometry, while computerized axial tomography (CAT) holds promise of being able to determine bone density accurately.

## VIDEODENSITOMETRY

The problem inherent in all densitometric measurements of the bones thus far described, except the CAT method, is the relatively small volume of any one bone that is evaluated. Even when multiple scans are used the values represent only a small proportion of the bone that needs to be evaluated. Recently a method has been utilized in which a television scan coupled with a light pen allows evaluation of the bone density of the whole bone or any part of one. The x-ray itself, or a print, perhaps enlarged, is used as the image. The light pen allows the operator to outline the desired area to be measured, such as a single metacarpal, the tibia, or part of a bone, and this area is recorded. The image is then scanned by the television, which records 256 different levels of density over the area at 52,000 different points.[36] Of course, the number of density levels and the number of separate points evaluated will vary with the particular system available, but the possibilities are good for obtaining accurate data of large areas of trabecular bone, cortical bone, or both.

The method can be used to measure the amount of bone versus non-bone in a microradiograph or stained section by setting a discrimination point between the bone and soft tissue by a gray level thresholding technique, and then counting the number of points that fall above or below this threshold. The values are usually expressed as a percentage and represent bone mass in the section. Repeat measurements on 13 different days gave a reproducibility of 1.2 in two different sections. The method applied to an x-ray rather than a section appears to be equally promising.

## PHOTON ABSORPTION METHODS

Inherent in all quantitative radiologic methods are variations in the x-ray beam characteristics, film response, and variables in emulsion development. These can be overcome by the use of the aluminum or ivory step-wedge. However, variation in the density of the beam across the film is difficult to control, and perhaps this is why alternative techniques such as the scan methods, using a monoenergetic beam from a radioisotope, have been developed. Iridium-192 was probably the first source to be used, and the bone chosen, sensibly, was a lumbar vertebra; sensibly, because this bone is one that is affected in osteoporosis. Water is used to maintain a constant "soft tissue" mass, and the results in a small group appeared promising.[37] From the thickness of the bone, a "density" in g/cm² was obtained. For some reason, Gershon-Cohen and his co-workers did not publish further.

Later, Americium-241 and Iodine-125 were used as the source of photons; the most commonly scanned site is the radius.[38, 39] This technique was developed by Cameron and Sorenson and will be referred to as the Cameron-Sorenson bone densitometry method. The beam from the isotope is collimated and passed through the forearm, which is surrounded by tissue-equivalent material, rather than water, to maintain a constant soft tissue thickness. The source of energy, the radionuclide, and the energy detector (a scintillation detector pulse-height analyzer system) are linked together and more transversely across the forearm, producing a record of the energy absorbed over the scan path. The values represent total bone mass when soft tissue is eliminated (Fig. 13–12).

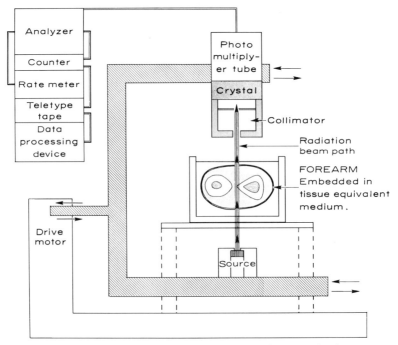

**Figure 13–12** Diagram of the Cameron-Sorensen apparatus for measuring bone mass. The bone scan covers a path of approximately two millimeters across the radius. A distal scan, near the wrist, or a mid-radial scan or both are used. (From Riggs, B. L., Jowsey, J., Kelly, P. J. and Wahner, H. W.: Special procedures for assessing metabolic bone disease. Med. Clin. North Am., *54*:1061–1070, 1970.)

The bone mineral content may be divided by the width of the bone measured from the scan path, although an arbitrary bone diameter value for all subjects has also been used.[40] The scatter for the Cameron-Sorenson bone densitometer data is enormous; this is not a reflection of accuracy or of reproducibility but of the variation in body size in different individuals (Figs. 13–13, 13–14).[41, 8] The problem is one of comparing a large, hefty man or woman with a slight, "bird-boned" person. The same problem is true of quantitative radiological methods. However, longitudinal studies have proved useful in some instances when changes in bone mass would be expected, as in renal failure and lactating females and in metabolic bone disease (Fig. 13–15).[38, 43] The method appears successful in some investigator's hands and less so in others', both for separating normal from abnormal and for longitudinal studies. By adding bone diameter Evens has improved the discrimination, although the total diameter is not a reflection of bone loss but rather of an initially smaller skeleton (Fig. 13–16).[43] In general, the method has proved disappointing in that increases in density seen radiographically have not been reflected in Cameron-Sorenson densitometry values.[44] The major problem may be that even the distal radius is composed mainly of cortical bone (Fig. 13–17). The iliac crest or vertebrae are preferable sites, but they are more difficult to use as scanning sites.

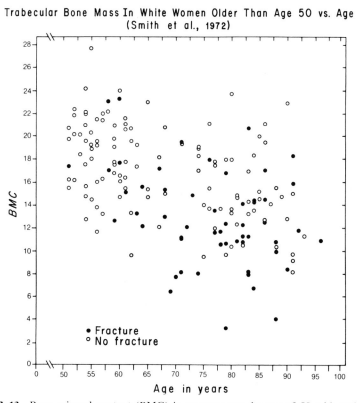

**Figure 13–13** Bone mineral content (BMC) in women over the age of 50 with and without vertebral fractures. Although persons with fractures tend to fall in the lower part of the graph, the overlap is large. The spread in persons both with and without fractures is also large. (Redrawn from Smith et al.[41])

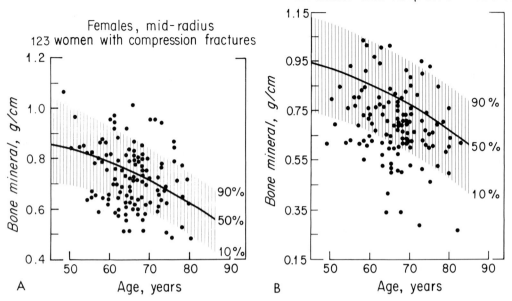

**Figure 13–14** (a) Cameron-Sorenson densitometer values in 153 normal, healthy women shown in the hatched area compared with the values in 123 women with fractures of the spine. It can be seen that there is essentially no separation between fracture and non-fracture patients. The measurement has been made in the mid-radius. (b) The same group and comparison as in Figure 13–14(a). The measurement has been made in the distal radius. 81 per cent of osteoporotic women fell below the fiftieth percentile and 24 per cent below the tenth percentile. However the majority of osteoporotic individuals (76 per cent) still fall above the tenth percentile of normal. (From Wahner et al.[8])

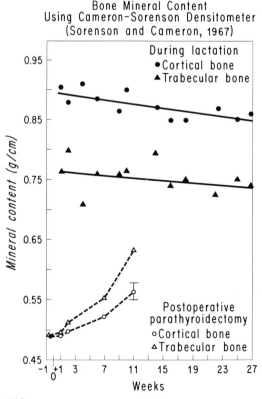

**Figure 13–15** Bone mineral content in a lactating female shows a slight decline in bone mass over the six months of lactation. The increase in mineralized bone mass in a patient with primary hyperparathyroidism after parathyroidectomy; the increase suggests mineralization of osteoid because it is so rapid. (Redrawn from Sorenson and Cameron.[38])

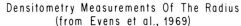

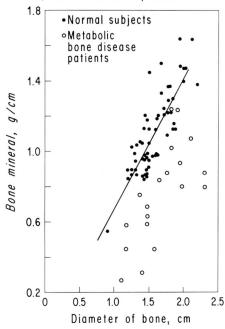

Densitometry Measurements Of The Radius
(from Evens et al., 1969)

**Figure 13-16** Bone mineral content and diameter measurements in normal subjects and in patients with bone disease. Bone mineral values alone give a 50 per cent overlap between persons with and without bone disease; however, the addition of bone diameter adds a parameter that improves the discrimination. (Redrawn from Evens et al.[43])

Using two isotope sources together allows the preferential absorption of one beam for evaluation of soft tissue and the absorption of the second energy beam preferentially for hard tissue. It is therefore possible to subtract and obtain values for relatively small amounts of bone within large volumes of soft tissue, which is the situation in the vertebrae. Hansson and co-workers have proved the usefulness

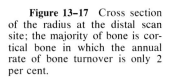

**Figure 13-17** Cross section of the radius at the distal scan site; the majority of bone is cortical bone in which the annual rate of bone turnover is only 2 per cent.

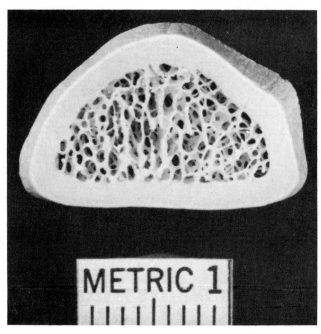

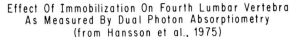

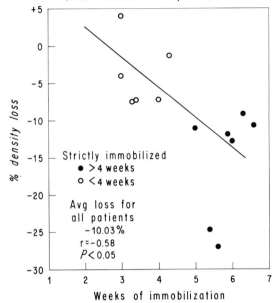

Figure 13–18  Bone mass, measured as the percentage change with time, shows a rapid rate of loss with the length of time of immobilization. (From Hansson et al.[45])

of this technique by evaluating patients immobilized in a plaster cast for correction of scoliosis (Fig. 13–18).[45]

The various methods of bone densitometry, excluding the double energy method described by Hansson, have been analyzed by Goldsmith and colleagues.[46] It was concluded that the distal radius measured by the Cameron-Sorenson densitometer was the best site for measurement, at least as far as reflecting osteoporosis. However, there still remains the problem of the differences in individual body size and the problem of the definition of osteoporosis. To differentiate osteoporosis from normal, the Singh Index appears to be the most useful. The grading system usually used, of 0 to 3 or 0 to 4 signifying the presence of bone disease, is clinically useful if it is recalled that a fractured bone depends on both the amount of bone and the amount of stress. Two individuals may have the same amount of bone, but one may be a cautious person living in a labor-saving type of house, whereas the second may be active and perhaps reckless and prone to fracture.

Variations on the theme of the Cameron-Sorenson densitometer have been devised; an x-ray beam with continual standardization has been found promising, avoiding as it does the problem of purchasing a radionuclide source every six months.[47] The reproducibility appears good, but sensitivity has yet to be demonstrated.

## REFERENCES

1. Dunnill, M. S., Anderson, J. A., and Whitehead, R.: Quantitative histological studies on age changes in bone., J. Pathol., *94*:275–291, 1967.
2. Broman, G. E., Trotter, M., and Peterson, R. R.: The density of selected bones of the human skeleton. Am. J. Phys. Anthropol. *16*:197–211, 1958.
3. Trotter, M., Broman, G. E., and Peterson, R. R.: Densities of bones of white and Negro skeletons. J. Bone Joint Surg., *42A*:50–58, 1960.

4. Singh, M., Nagrath, A. R., and Maini, P. S.: Changes in trabecular pattern of the upper end of the femur as an index of osteoporosis. J. Bone Joint Surg., *52A*:457–467, 1970.
5. Singh, M., Riggs, B. L., Beabout, J. W., and Jowsey, J.: Femoral trabecular pattern index for evaluation of spinal osteoporosis: A detailed methodologic description. Mayo Clinic. Proc., *48*:184–189, 1973.
6. Koch, J. C.: The laws of bone architecture. Am. J. Anat., *21*:177–298, 1917.
7. Singh, M., Riggs, B. L., Beabout, J. W., and Jowsey, J.: Femoral trabecular-pattern index for evaluation of spinal osteoporosis. Ann. Intern. Med., *77*:63–67, 1972.
8. Wahner, H. W., Riggs, B. L., and Beabout, J. W.: Diagnosis of osteoporosis: comparison of value of photon absorptiometry at the radius with an index based on trabecular structure of the proximal femur. J. Nucl. Med. In press, April, 1977.
9. Roh, Y. S., Dequeker, J., and Mulier, J. C.: Trabecular pattern of the upper end of the femur in primary osteoarthrosis and in symptomatic osteoporosis. J. Belge. Radiol., *57*:89–94, 1974.
10. Singh, M., and Riggs, B. L.: Letter to the editor. J. Bone Joint Surg., *55A*:888–889, 1973.
11. Kranendonk, D. H., Jurist, J. M., and Lee, H. G.: Femoral trabecular patterns and bone mineral content. J. Bone Joint Surg., *54A*:1472–1478, 1972.
12. Sotaniemi, E. A., Hakkarainen, H. K., Puranen, J. A., and Lahti, R. O.: Radiologic bone changes and hypocalcemia with anticonvulsant therapy in epilepsy. Ann. Intern. Med., *77*:389–394, 1972.
13. Bradford, D. S., Brown, D. M., Moe, J. H., Winter, R. B., and Jowsey, J.: Scheuermann's kyphosis: a form of juvenile osteoporosis? Clin. Orthop., *118*:10–15, 1976.
14. Barnett, E., and Nordin, B. E. C.: The radiological diagnosis of osteoporosis: A new approach. Clin. Radiol., *11*:166–174, 1960.
15. Meema, H. E.: Cortical bone atrophy and osteoporosis as a manifestation of aging. Am. J. Roentgenol. Radium Ther. Med., *89*:1287–1295, 1963.
16. Morgan, D. B., Spiers, F. W., Pulvertaft, C. N., and Fourman, P.: The amount of bone in the metacarpal and the phalanx according to age and sex. Clin. Radiol., *18*:101–108, 1967.
17. Fujita, T., Okuyama, Y., Handa, N., Orimo, H., Ohata, M., Yoskikawa, M., Akiyama, H., and Kogure, T.: Age-dependent bone loss after gastrectomy. J. Am. Geriat. Soc., *19*:840–846, 1971.
18. Meema, H. E., and Meema, S.: Prevention of postmenopausal osteoporosis by hormone treatment of the menopause. Canad. Med. Assoc. J., *99*:248–251, 1968.
19. Meema, H. E., and Meema, S.: The relationship of diabetes mellitus and body weight to osteoporosis in elderly females. Canad. Med. Assoc. J., *96*:132–139, 1967.
20. Bloom, R. A., and Laws, J. W.: Humeral cortical thickness as an index of osteoporosis in women. Br. J. Radiol., *43*:522–527, 1970.
21. Shimmins, J., Anderson, J. B., Smith, D. A., and Aitken, M.: The accuracy and reproducibility of bone mineral measurements "in vivo." Clin. Radiol., *23*:42–46, 1972.
22. Smith, D. A., Anderson, J. B., Shimmins, J., Speirs, C. F., and Barnett, E.: Changes in metacarpal mineral content and density in normal male and female subjects with age. Clin. Radiol., *20*:23–31, 1969.
23. Weaver, J. K., and Chalmers, J.: Cancellous bone: its strength and changes with aging and an evaluation of some methods for measuring its mineral content. I. Age changes in cancellous bone. J. Bone Joint Surg., *48A*:289–299, 1966.
24. Aitken, J. M., Smith, C. B., Horton, P. W., Clark, D. L., Boyd, J. F., and Smith, D. A.: The interrelationships between bone mineral at different skeletal sites in male and female cadavers. J. Bone Joint Surg., *56B*:370–375, 1974.
25. Anderson, J. B., Shimmins, J., and Smith, D. A.: A new technique for the measurement of metacarpal density. Br. J. Radiol., *39*:433–450, 1966.
26. Vogel, J. M., and Anderson, J. T.: Rectilinear transmission scanning of irregular bones for quantification of mineral content. J. Nucl. Med., *13*:13–18, 1972.
27. Mayo, K. M.: Quantitative measurement of bone mineral content in normal adult bone. Br. J. Radiol., *34*:693–698, 1961.
28. Donaldson, C. L., Hulley, S. B., Vogel, J. M., Hattner, R. S., Bayers, J. H., and McMillan, D. E.: Effect of prolonged bedrest on bone mineral. Metabolism, *19*:1071–1083, 1970.
29. Mack, P. B., and LaChance, P. L.: Effects of recumbency and space flight on bone density. Am. J. Clin. Nutr., *20*:1194–1205, 1967.
30. Mack, P. B., LaChance, P. A., Vose, G. P., and Vogt, F. B.: Bone demineralization of foot and hand of Gemini-Titian IV, V and VII astronauts during orbital flight. Am. J. Roentgenol. Radium Ther. Nuc. Med., *100*:503–511, 1967.
31. Vose, G. P., Hoerster, S. A., Jr., and Mack, P. B.: New technic for the radiographic assessment of vertebral density. J. Med. Electronics, *3*:181–188, 1964.
32. Hantman, D. A., Vogel, J. M., Donaldson, C. L., Friedman, R., Goldsmith, R. S., and Hulley, S. B.: Attempts to prevent disuse osteoporosis by treatment with calcitonin, longitudinal compression and supplementary calcium and phosphate. J. Clin. Endocrinol. Metabol., *36*:845–858, 1973.

33. Lockwood, D. R., Lammert, J. E., Vogel, J. M., and Hulley, S. B.: Bone mineral loss during bedrest. Excerpta Medica, International Congress Series No. *270*:216–265, 1973.
34. Keane, B. E., Spiegler, G., and Davis, R.: Quantitative evaluation of bone mineral by a radiographic method. Br. J. Radiol., *32*:162–167, 1959.
35. Doyle, F. H., III: Ulna bone mineral concentration in metabolic bone diseases. Br. J. Radiol., *34*:698–712, 1961.
36. Robb, R. A., Johnson, S. A., Greenleaf, J. F., Wondrow, M. A., and Wood, E. H.: An operator-interactive computer-controlled system for high-fidelity digitization and analysis of biomedical images. Proc. Soc. Photo-Optical Instrumentation Engineers Seminar on Quantitative Imagery in the Biomedical Sciences-II, San Diego, California (August 27–29), *40*:11–26, 1973.
37. Gershon-Cohen, J., Cherry, N. H., and Boehnke, M.: Bone density studies with a gamma gauge. Radiat. Res., *8*:509–515, 1958.
38. Cameron, J. R., and Sorenson, J.: Measurement of bone mineral in vivo: an improved method. Science, *142*:230–232, 1963.
39. Sorenson, J. A., and Cameron, J. R.: A reliable in vivo measurement of bone mineral content. J. Bone Joint Surg., *49A*:481–497, 1967.
41. Smith, D. M., Johnston, C. C., Jr., and Yu, P. L.: In vivo measurement of bone mass. JAMA, *219*:325–329, 1972.
42. West, R. R., and Reed, G. W.: The measurement of bone mineral in vivo by photon beam scanning. Br. J. Radiol., *43*:886–893, 1970.
43. Evens, R. G., Pak, C. Y. C., Ashburn, W., and Bartter, F. C.: Clinical investigation in metabolic bone disease: quantitative measurements of bone mineral. Invest. Radiol., *4*:364–369, 1969.
44. Kyle, R. A., Jowsey, J., Kelly, P. J., and Taves, D. R.: Multiple myeloma bone disease: the comparative effect of sodium fluoride and calcium carbonate or placebo. New Engl. J. Med., *293*:1334–1338, 1975.
45. Hansson, T. H., Roos, B. O., and Nachemson, A.: Development of osteopenia in the fourth lumbar vertebra during prolonged bed rest after operation for scoliosis. Acta Orthop. Scand., *46*:621–630, 1975.
46. Goldsmith, N. E., Johnston, J. O., Ury, H., Vose, G., and Colbert, C.: Bone mineral estimation in normal and osteoporotic women: a comparability trial of four methods and seven bone sites. J. Bone Joint Surg., *53A*:83–100, 1971.
47. Archer-Hall, J. A., Carpenter, P. B., Edwards, J. P. N., and Francois, P. E.: A new method of bone mineral estimation using a conventional x-ray set. Br. J. Radiol., *46*:375–380, 1973.

Chapter Fourteen

# RADIOISOTOPE
# METHODS

## BONE SCANNING

### $^{18}$F and $^{85}$Sr

The general principle of bone scanning using injected radioisotopes is to administer to a patient a radioisotope that produces either a particle or energy that can be detected externally. The data are displayed geographically, and various parts of the skeleton will show increases in concentration of the isotope and reflect alterations from the normal, that is, from pictures of normal people displayed in a similar way.

The common denominator in the elements used for bone scanning is that they are bone-seekers, which means that they are taken up from blood by mineralized bone tissue rather than by muscle, skin, fat, or other soft tissue. The choice of radioisotope rests mainly on its characteristic emission, half-life, and, to a lesser extent, on expense, availability, and other such factors.

Fluorine is a "bone-seeker" which exchanges with the hydroxyl ion on the hydroxyapatite lattice and therefore is taken up in mineralized bone in the hydroxyapatite crystal. Fluorine-18 emits a 0.65 mev positron that has a 17-hour half-life, and the positron annihilation provides 0.51 mev photons that can be seen on a scanning device.[1] The isotope can be given orally or intravenously; the blood levels produced by the two means of administration are different but comparable. The main use has been in the recognition of the presence of bone lesions. However, in most reported series, there is only a small percentage of patients who have positive scans and a negative x-ray; in addition, any soft tissue tumor or chrondrosarcoma will be missed on the scan because of the lack of mineral in the abnormal area.[2]

$^{85}$Sr-Strontium is very like calcium in its behavior in the body and substitutes for calcium in the hydroxyapatite crystal. It is a gamma emitter with an energy of 0.51 mev. The results using strontium are similar to the findings using fluorine, although the number of positive scans in patients with skeletal malignancies and no positive radiologic findings has been greater than for $^{18}$F, even though as with fluorine, in many instances the scan has merely confirmed the radiologic findings.[3] $^{85}$Sr has a long half-life (64 days), and the total dose to bone is therefore greater.

$^{85}$Sr has also been used for the prediagnosis of alterations in bone adjacent to joints. People with painful knees but who demonstrate no abnormality by x-ray study may show hot spots or areas of increased concentrations of the isotope, which would indicate the development of what may later become a definite defect.[4] The usefulness of this to the orthopedist depends on whether early treatment or operation has a distinct advantage over waiting and later therapy.

### $^{99m}$Tc-Technetium

$^{99m}$Tc-Technetium has a short half-life of 6 hours and is produced by the decay of molybdenum-99; it forms a firm complex with a number of different substances that are bone-seekers, such as a diphosphonate or polyphosphate. While $^{18}$F and the strontium isotopes are both bone-seekers and radioactive, the $^{99m}$Tc method utilizes the $^{99m}$Tc as the radioisotope and the polyphosphate as the bone-seeker, which carries the label along with it.[5] Its ready availability makes it a convenient isotope to use. The gamma rays are essentially monoenergetic and have an energy of 140 kev. As with $^{18}$F and strontium isotopes, a scan of the body gives a geographic localization of the technetium polyphosphate, and high concentrations indicate abnormalities such as skeletal metastases and fracture healing (Fig. 14–1).

There has been much argument as to the physiologic or chemical mechanism responsible for the uptake of polyphosphate. Fluorine and strontium have

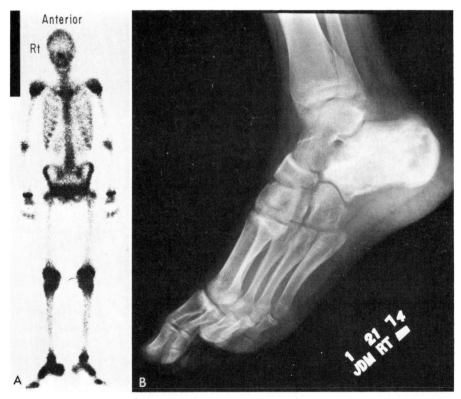

**Figure 14–1** (a) $^{99m}$Tc-polyphosphate scan of a 14 year old male showing high concentrations of the isotope at the joints, which is normal in a growing person. However there is a unilateral and abnormal concentration of the isotope in the right heel. (b) X-ray of the right foot of the patient whose $^{99m}$Tc scan is shown in (a). There is obvious osteosclerosis of the os calcis which accounts for the increased concentration of the isotope.

been positively identified by in vivo and in vitro methods as substituting for ions or elements in the hydroxyapatite crystal. In studies of $^{99m}$Tc, autoradiography of $^{14}$C-labeled diphosphonate at short times after injection (four hours) showed that it is localized on all mineralized bone surfaces. Later work on the polyphosphates using higher-resolution autoradiography showed the $^{99m}$Tc at the mineralization front of bone to a somewhat higher degree than at inactive or resorbing surfaces.[6] In vitro work with diphosphonates showed that they coat bone crystal surfaces; unlike strontium, which is highly concentrated in actively mineralizing bone, the deposition appears to be on all mineralized surfaces as well as on the new bone-forming surfaces.

The mechanism of uptake of polyphosphate appears to be passive diffusion through the cell layer of the bone and deposition on all mineralized surfaces, with a preference for the areas where mineralization of new bone is taking place. Presumably this reflects the large crystal surface available at the mineralization front, rather than any participation of the diphosphate or polyphosphate in the normal process of mineralization.

A degree of controversy has centered on the importance of the vascular supply. It is obvious, grossly obvious, that if there is no blood supply or a much reduced one, even the most exaggerated bone abnormality will not show an increased uptake of the isotope-labeled material, merely because there is no way for the isotope to reach the involved area. Also, if the blood supply is well developed (for example, a healing fracture) but no mineral is being deposited (as in osteomalacia), no increase in uptake will occur. The interpretation of the scan picture should be made with this in mind. For instance, in Paget's disease of bone, successful treatment may show decreased density of the uptake in the scan area compared with before treatment, both because of a decreased blood supply and a decrease in the bone abnormality, or by either alone.[7]

## KINETIC ANALYSIS

Disappearance of bone-seeking isotopes from the blood into bone and also into feces and urine may be used to reflect activity of the skeleton. Heaney and Whedon, in 1958, described a model that consisted of a single compartment system with two routes of loss from blood after injection of an isotope: the urinary and endogenous fecal excretion represented complete loss of isotope from the body, and incorporation into the bone by several different routes constituted the second pathway.[8] After a single intravenous injection (approximately 10 $\mu$Ci) of a calcium or strontium radioisotope, the isotope equilibrates with the miscible pool of calcium, which is generally called E and is expressed in grams. This pool slowly loses isotope and becomes "cooler" (that is, the specific activity, $^{45}$Ca to $^{40}$Ca ratio, decreases) as the isotope exits into the endogenous calcium in the gut and into the urine, and is taken up in bone. The slope of the blood specific activity curve will reflect the disappearance of the isotope into the bone, assuming that gut and renal excretion rates are normal, and can be evaluated and subtracted from the disappearance into bone. These can be measured by urine and fecal collection and the content of isotope can be quantitated directly after acid digestion of the samples. The A or bone accretion value is obtained by extrapolating the exchangeable portion of the curve to zero time and dividing the isotope concentration by the dose

## Radiocalcium metabolism

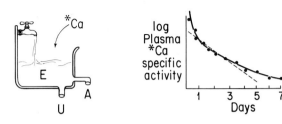

**Figure 14–2** Diagram to explain the derivation of an A value representing bone mineral accretion rate. E is the exchangeable pool, T is time and U is the fecal and endogenous loss.

1 $E(mg) = \dfrac{Dose\,(cps)}{Sp\ act\,(cps/mg)}$

2 $k = \dfrac{0.693}{T\frac{1}{2}\,(days)}$

3 $T(mg/day) = kE$

4 $A(mg/day) = T-U$

administered (Fig. 14–2). The bone accretion rate may be calculated from the fractional loss of isotope from the pool into the skeleton. This can be shown by the following formula:

K (fractional loss from pool) $= K_u + K_f + K_b$, the loss into the urine, feces, and bone. Since K can be derived from the blood disappearance curve directly by measuring the slope from about one hour to five days (this is $E + K_b$), the exchangeable pool and bone accretion rate are generally related.[9] Both, for example, are high in Paget's disease of bone and low in hypoparathyroidism (Table 14–1). The accretion rate A has been equaled with new bone formation. Values for adult normal human beings give an exchangeable pool of approximately 6 g of calcium and a "bone formation rate" of approximately 500 mg of calcium per day. This figure is larger than that derived from the bone turnover and exchange figures (104 mg calcium per day of bone formation + 250 mineral exchange = 350 mg Ca per day), but the values are not disturbingly different.

At this point it is evident that the bone formation rate of Heaney and Whedon or the Vo + and A or accretion value of others[10, 11, 12] is not identical to the real rate of deposition of newly mineralized bone tissue. Heaney and Whedon recognized this and described the isotope entering the bone in the following three different ways: (1) rapid exchange with a small fraction of bone calcium, which is the exchangeable calcium that is defined as being in equilibrium with the blood and therefore having

**Table 14–1**   RESULTS OF Ca[45] TRACER STUDIES

| Age and Sex | Diagnosis | E (mg/Ca/kg) | BFR or A (mg/Ca/kg/day) |
|---|---|---|---|
| 65 M | Control | 93 | 9.53 |
| 40 F | Hypoparathyroidism (surgical) | 67 | 2.69 |
| 62 F | Hypoparathyroidism (idiopathic) | 68 | 6.29 |
| 52 (5F) (1M) | Osteoporosis | 79 | 9.4 |
| 56 F | Paget's disease of bone | 398 | 154.0 |
| 63 M | Paget's disease of bone | 438 | 102.0 |

From Heaney and Whedon, 1958.[8]
(BFR = "bone formation rate")

the same specific activity and time curve as blood; (2) non-exchangeable calcium, which represents mineralization of new bone and therefore quantitatively represents new bone formation; and (3) long-term exchange with the stable bone calcium (Fig. 14–3). Since rapid exchange can be excluded by waiting for a complete mixing time with this compartment, bone formation rate measured from the slope of the blood curve remains as a mixture of mineralization of new bone and long-term exchange. Some attempts have been made to quantitate the amount of calcium entering the bone by long-term exchange. Data in man are sparse because of the complications of injecting human beings with radioactive isotopes in sufficient quantity to produce the autoradiographs necessary to make this calculation. However, the long-term exchange has been estimated to be responsible for at least 50 per cent of the total skeleton calcium retention in normal individuals. The radium autoradiographic studies of Rowland showed a large variation in the percentage in the exchange and new bone compartments even in the comparatively normal radium dial-painters, and the percentage may vary even more in people with bone disease. In such instances the true bone formation rate would be impossible to evaluate.[13]

Nevertheless, mineral accretion values are useful and, in contrast to bone biopsies, do not require invasive techniques (apart from blood sampling) and do evaluate the whole skeleton. However, the values should perhaps be regarded as empirical information, and certainly should not be considered as being numerically equal to new bone deposition.

## NEUTRON ACTIVATION ANALYSIS

This technique differs from the previous two in that no radioactive isotope is injected into the body. It is also the only available method for measuring the total

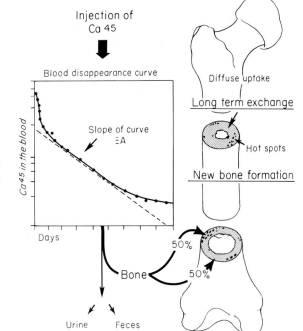

**Figure 14–3** Diagram of the behavior of injected calcium[45] radioisotope, and the relation of the blood curve to the physiological destination of the calcium.

amount of bone in a person. The method involves neutron activation of the body and subsequent analysis of the induced gamma activities. When elements are irradiated with neutrons, a proportion may be transformed into the unstable radioactive forms of the element, which can then be measured. Neutrons react with stable $^{48}Ca$ to produce $^{49}Ca$, which has an 8.8 minute half-life. The neutron flux used for the irradiation of the person must be of uniform density through the whole body; this is generally achieved by multiple irradiation sources on both sides of the body. Special attention is paid to the geometry of the body to achieve uniform irradiation. The technique involves very extensive and elaborate equipment, including an irradiation chamber and a whole body counter. The neutron source is placed at regular intervals above and below the patient, and polyethylene moderators surround the patient. A neutron generator may be used; however, the Brookhaven total body neutron activation chamber has 14 sources of neutrons produced by $^{238}PuO_2$-Be, each approximately 27 cm apart. Measurements of the neutron flux density can be obtained by using an anthropomorphic phantom.[14]

After irradiation, the patient is rapidly removed from the irradiation source or sources and placed in a whole body counter. Such counters consist of a chamber made up of material with a low content of radioactivity and containing sodium iodide crystals that measure the amount and energy of the gamma rays emitted by the patient. As with the neutron sources, the crystals must be placed around and along the body so as to receive representative signals from the whole body. A computer program can be used to analyze the gamma ray spectrum and a phantom used for calibration. $^{49}Ca$ has an energy of 3.1 mev; $^{24}Na$ and $^{38}Cl$ are also counted. The methods report accuracies of $\pm 1.0$ per cent (Brookhaven)[14] and 2.0 per cent.[15] Since a considerable amount of equipment is required, with all the paraphernalia that must accompany such a large amount of radiation, the technique has only been set up and used by a small number of institutions. It has nevertheless provided some interesting information on total body calcium. In a number of normal subjects, the total body calcium varied from 933 to 1361 g and was less in patients with bone disease (Table 14–2). In both normals and patients with metabolic bone disease there is a close relationship between the total body calcium and body height, so that a correction can be made for height by multiplying by one fifth of the cube of the height in meters in order to compare two individuals. In a study in patients with bone disease, osteoporotic patients before and after growth hormone treatment showed

Table 14–2   TOTAL BODY CALCIUM-TBNAA (or TB-Ca)

|  | Normal Males | Male Patients with Osteopenic Disease* | Female Patients with Osteoporosis** |
|---|---|---|---|
| AGE (yr) | | | |
| Mean | 33.5 | 41.8 | 65 |
| Range | 22–41 | 35–52 | 55–75 |
| N | 8 | 5 | 32 |
| BODY CALCIUM (g) | | | |
| Total | 1093 | 750.2 | 682 |
| Range | 933–1361 | 664–865 | 468–895 |

*Nelp et al.[16]
**Chestnut et al.[17]

**Table 14–3** TBNAA IN OSTEOPOROSIS AFTER TREATMENT WITH
GROWTH HORMONE (GH)

|  | Time (mo) | Grams (mean ± SD) | |
| | | Na | Ca |
|---|---|---|---|
| 2 U GH/day | 0 | 60.0 ± 6.2 | 640 ± 104 |
|  | 6 | 59.1 ± 9.3 | 643 ± 90 |
| Approximately 9 U GH/day | 6 | 60.6 ± 9.3 | 661 ± 84 |
|  | 12 | 61.6 ± 8.1 | 638 ± 104 |

From Aloia et al.[18]

no change, a finding which was supported by the bone morphometric findings
(Table 14–3).[18] In another study, in untreated osteoporotic patients, a loss of 5.2
per cent in total body calcium was shown to occur over a 13 to 22 month period.

There is no doubt that the method of neutron activation of body calcium represents the most accurate means of measuring bone mass, mainly because it is
measuring precisely the calcium and also because it is measuring all the calcium in
the body, so that small changes are easily discernible.

Besides evaluating bone disease, total body neutron activation analysis
(TBNAA) has been useful in evaluating the accuracy and credibility of other, less
precise, methods. In a group of patients with renal disease, a comparison of bone
mineral content by the Cameron-Sorenson photon absorption method and the
TBNAA showed a good correlation (Fig. 14–4). However, a similar comparison in
a group of patients, some untreated and some treated either successfully or unsuc-
cessfully for bone disease, demonstrated no correlation between the change in bone

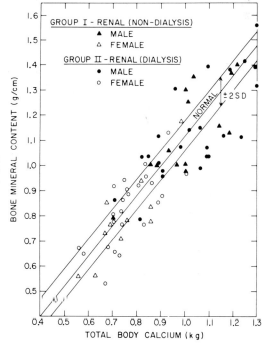

**Figure 14–4** The correlation between bone mass measured by the Cameron-Sorenson and TBNAA methods. The correlation coefficient is 0.906. (From Cohn et al.[19])

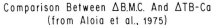

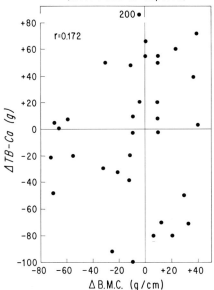

**Figure 14–5** The comparison between the change in bone mass measured by TBNAA and the Cameron-Sorenson method. There is essentially no relationship (redrawn from Aloia et al.).[20]

mass shown by the two methods (Fig. 14–5). Since the TBNAA method is indubitably the most accurate and is also very sensitive, it must be concluded that the Cameron-Sorenson technique, though useful for reflecting bone mass, is not of value in measuring small changes in mass in the skeleton.

A modification of total body calcium measurements has been developed by Catto and colleagues in which the hand is irradiated by a cylinder, 3 cm in diameter and 10 cm long, containing 25 ci americium-241 and beryllium-9, which provide a neutron source. $^{48}$Calcium is activated to $^{49}$calcium and counted using sodium iodide crystals.[21] A calibration curve between $^{49}$calcium and the weight of calcium gave a correlation of 0.9995. A study was conducted on patients undergoing dialysis using a dialysis bath concentration of 5.3 to 5.5 mg/dl calcium. The patients had been dialyzed for 6 months to 5 years and were studied for the final 26 weeks of that period; all except the patient on dialysis for only 6 months showed a clear loss of calcium, as would be expected with a dialysis bath calcium concentration of 5.5 mg/dl or less. Other methods, such as the bone densitometer (Cameron-Sorenson) and radiographic assessment, proved far less sensitive. Although overall sensitivity of this method must be expected to be less than total body calcium measurements, the hand has proved to be an area of the skeleton that reflects bone loss, and the technique is certainly a great deal more possible to develop than the enormously expensive total body method.

## *REFERENCES*

1. Moon, N. F., Dworkin, H. J., and LaFluer, P. D.: The clinical use of sodium fluoride F 18 in bone photoscanning. JAMA, *204*:974–980, 1968.
2. Blau, M., Nagler, W., and Bender, M. A.: Fluorine-18: a new isotope for bone scanning. J. Nucl. Med., *3*:332–334, 1962.

3. Parsons, V., Williams, M., Hill, D., Frost, P., and Lapham, A.: Strontium-85 scanning of suspected bone disease. Br. Med. J., *1*:19–23, 1969.
4. Tong, E. C. K., and Rubenfeld, S.: The strontium[85] bone scan in myeloma. Am. J. Roentgenol. Radium Ther. Nucl. Med., *103*:843–848, 1968.
5. Subramanian, G., McAfee, J. G., Bell, E. G., Blair, J., O'Mara, R. E., and Ralston, P. H.: [99m]Tc-labeled polyphosphate as a skeletal imaging agent. Radiol., *102*:701–704, 1972.
6. Tilden, R. L., Jackson, J., Jr., Enneking, W. F., Deland, F. H., and McVey, J. T.: [99m]Tc-Polyphosphate: histological localization in human femurs by autoradiography. J. Nucl. Med., *14*:576–578, 1973.
7. Russell, A. S., and Lentle, B. C.: Mithramycin therapy in Paget's disease. Can. Med. Assoc. J., *110*:397–400, 1974.
8. Heaney, R. P., and Whedon, G. D.: Radiocalcium studies of bone formation rate in human metabolic bone disease. J. Clin. Endocrinol. Metab., *18*:1246–1267, 1958.
9. Bronner, F., and Harris, R. S.: Absorption and metabolism of calcium in human beings, studies with calcium.[45] Ann. N.Y. Acad. Sci., *64*:314–325, 1956–57.
10. Neer, R., Berman, M., Fisher, L., and Rosenberg, L. E.: Multicompartmental analysis of calcium kinetics in normal adult males. J. Clin. Invest., *46*:1364–1379, 1967.
11. Marshall, J. H.: Measurements and models of skeletal metabolism. *In* Comar, C. L., and Bronner, F. (Eds.): Mineral Metabolism, Vol. III, New York and London, Academic Press, 1969, pp. 1–122.
12. Aubert, J. P., Bronner, F., and Richelle, L. J.: Quantitation of calcium metabolism. Theory. J. Clin. Invest., *42*:885–897, 1963.
13. Rowland, R. E., and Marshall, J. H.: Radium in human bone: the dose in microscopic volumes of bone. Radiat. Res., *11*:299–313, 1959.
14. Cohn, S. H., Shukla, K. K., Dombrowski, C. S., and Fairchild, R. G.: Design and calibration of a "broad-beam" [238]Pu, Be neutron source for total-body neutron activation analysis. J. Nucl. Med., *13*:487–492, 1972.
15. Nelp, W. B., Palmer, H. E., Murano, R., Pailthorp, K., Hinn, G. M., Rich, C., Williams, J. L., Rudd, T. G., and Denney, J. D.: Measurement of total body calcium (bone mass) in vivo with the use of total body neutron activation analysis. J. Lab. Clin. Med., *76*:151–162, 1970.
16. Nelp, W. B., Denney, J. D., Murano, R., Hinn, G. M., Williams, J. L., Rudd, T. G., and Palmer, H. E.: Absolute measurement of total body calcium (bone mass) in vivo. J. Lab. Clin. Med. *79*:430–438, 1972.
17. Chestnut, C. H., Nelp, W. B., Denney, J. D., and Sherrard, D. J.: Measurement of total body calcium (bone mass) by neutron activation analysis: applicability to bone wasting disease. Excerpta Medica International Congress Series No. *270*:50–54, 1973.
18. Aloia, J. F., Zanzi, I., Ellis, K., Jowsey, J., Roginsky, M., Wallach, S., and Cohn, S. H.: Effects of growth hormone in osteoporosis. J. Clin. Endocrinol. Metab., *43*:992–999, 1976.
19. Cohn, S. H., Ellis, K. J., Caselnova, R. C., Asad, S. N., and Letteri, J. M.: Correlation of radial bone mineral content with total body calcium in chronic renal failure. J. Lab. Clin. Med., *86*:910–919, 1975.
20. Aloia, J. F., Ellis, K., Zanzi, I., and Cohn S. H.: Photon absorptiometry and skeletal mass in the treatment of osteoporosis. J. Nucl. Med., *16*:196–199, 1975.
21. Catto, G. R. D., McIntosh, J. A. R., MacDonald, A. F., and MacLeod, M.: Haemodialysis therapy and changes in skeletal calcium. Lancet, *1*:1150–1153, 1973.

# Chapter Fifteen

# BONE GROWTH MARKERS

The longitudinal growth of bones was first measured accurately by placing radio-opaque pins in the side of the shaft of a long bone of a growing animal, just beneath the epiphyseal plate. As the physis continued to grow the pins "moved" further and further away from the plate.[1] The method involved radiographs of the bones and represented a gross measurement of long bone growth.

**Alizarin.** The marking of bone by dyes was described by Bélchier in 1736.[2] He observed that the oral ingestion of madder (alizarin) was followed by the appearance of a red dye in the bone. Many investigators subsequently have used alizarin red-S to measure the rate of bone deposition.[3] The dye forms a lake with calcium and is deposited in high concentrations at the mineralization front and also in lower concentrations through the mineralized bone. The dye appears in bone rapidly within one hour, as would be expected of any blood-borne label. The usual dose is 20 to 50 mg per kg, given either intraperitoneally or intravenously in an 0.45 per cent sodium chloride solution. This will result in a narrow band of red, or in several bands if more than one dose is given a few days apart. Alizarin can be excited by a mercury lamp to give a red fluorescence. High doses are toxic, and in tissue culture very high doses have been shown to slow bone growth.[4]

**Chloro-S-Triazines.** These dyes are less well known, but they have been used in a number of animal studies. They are Procion M dyes and may be yellow, orange, blue, or red.[5] Like alizarin, they will stain tissue after in vivo administration; because different colors are available, sequential markers will not be confused. The dyes are generally mixed with 5 per cent dextrose (without boiling) to give a 2 per cent solution and given intravenously at a dose level of 1.0 mg per 100 gm body weight; higher doses are toxic. The dyes bind to collagen, and decalcified sections can therefore be prepared.

Since the Procion M dyes are toxic and cannot be sterilized by boiling, their use in human beings is contraindicated. They would also have the dramatic but cosmetically unacceptable effect of turning the sclera and other exposed collagen yellow, orange, blue, or red.

## TETRACYCLINE

Since the advent of tetracycline in 1957, alizarin and the Procion dyes have been less commonly used, for obvious reasons. The tetracyclines are far less toxic and have a huge advantage in that they can be administered to human beings.[6] They bind to mineralized tissue only and are preferentially taken up at the mineralization front. Mineralized sections must be prepared, as with alizarin. Intermittent administration will result in a series of bands in the mineralized bone, making it possible to measure the rate of new bone deposition accurately (Fig. 15–1). The rate is the thickness of collagen formed per unit surface per unit time. In a group of normal individuals, Frost found that the average rate of bone deposition, using tetracycline, is 1.5 microns per day in young children and falls to 1.0 micron in the adult; he demonstrated a further decline to 0.72 micron per day in people in their 70's and 80's.[8]

Unfortunately, tetracycline is used so commonly to treat infection and as a pre-operative protective agent that the majority of people, particularly people with diseases, and a large number of animals have many labels of tetracycline in their bone which may be difficult to distinguish from the markers given by the investigator. For this reason it is preferable to have other criteria of bone formation, such as an osteoblast layer, to identify the "experimental" tetracycline bands before using them to measure bone formation rate.

Since tetracycline, as well as alizarin, is deposited in bone with calcium, osteomalacia, rickets, or any failure of mineralization will prevent the uptake of these markers in a discrete line; rather, either they will be deposited diffusely, particularly in incompletely mineralized areas of bone, or they will not be localized to any extent.

As with calcium, radium, and other minerals that can be labeled as radioactive elements, there is an exchange phenomenon which occurs throughout mineralized bone and which is independent of new bone mineralization. In a section this can be

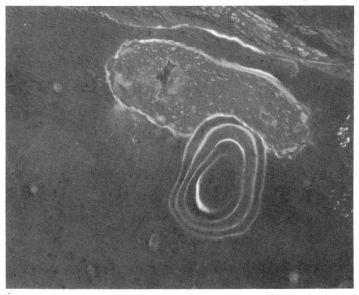

**Figure 15–1** Four intermittent injections of tetracycline have produced four concentric rings of fluorescence in an osteone that was being formed during the time of injection. Mineralized inactive bone surfaces take up the substance also to a lesser extent (×120). (Jowsey, J.: Autoradiographic and microradiographic studies of bone. In Zipkin, I. (ed.): Biological Mineralization of Bone. New York. John Wiley and Sons, 1973, pp. 297–333.)

**TABLE 15-1**   MICRORADIOGRAPHIC AND TETRACYCLINE DATA

| CASE | Microradiographic Measurement, % GROWTH SURFACE | Tetracycline Reading, mm³ IN GROWING OSTEONES* | TOTAL TETRACYCLINE** |
|:---:|:---:|:---:|:---:|
| 1 | 1.3 | 1.0 | 4.3 |
| 2 | 1.5 | 1.2 | 3.6 |
| 3 | 4.4 | 2.9 | 6.5 |
| 4 | 4.2 | 2.1 | 4.0 |
| 5 | 4.6 | 3.0 | 6.0 |
| 6 | 7.8 | 3.5 | 5.2 |
| 7 | 9.0 | 3.7 | 10.6 |

*For significance of difference from % growth surface: $r = 0.939$, $t = 6.11$, $p < .005$.
**For significance of difference from % growth surface: $r = 0.76$, $t = 2.63$, $p < .05$.

seen as an over-all yellow tint in the bone after tetracycline administration, which occurs in areas distant from the discrete mineralizing lines. The importance of this "exchange" uptake is that it precludes the use of extraction and measurement of total bone tetracycline as an accurate means of measuring new bone formation. While extraction using demineralizing solutions and quantitation of the tetraycline with a fluorimeter is possible, the data will represent new mineralization *and* exchange. There is experimental verification of this in man, where an attempt was made to evaluate the extent of the diffuse uptake. Plugs of bone were removed from the lateral side of the proximal femoral shaft in eight females with fractured femoral necks: tetracycline had been given 24 hours before the bone sample was removed. The new bone containing the concentrated band of tetracycline was separated from the mature bone containing the "diffuse" deposit by microdissection, the two pools of bone demineralized, and the fluorophore measured. Table 15-1 shows that the tetracycline associated with new bone mineralization is clearly associated with new bone formation as evaluated microradiographically, with a high correlation of 0.94. However, the total amount of tetracycline is less closely related to formation because the proportion in the diffuse component is variable.

In general, bone markers such as tetracycline have given valuable and accurate data on bone formation rates that were not available in man and only approximated, using radioisotopes, in animals.

### REFERENCES

1. Sarnat, B. G.: Growth of bones as revealed by implant markers in animals. Am. J. Phys. Anthropol., *29*:255–286, 1968.
2. Bélchier, J.: An account of bones of animals being changed to a red color by aliment only. Philosoph. Trans., *39*:287–299, 1736.
3. Vilmann, H.: The in vivo staining of bone with alizarin red S. J. Anat., *105*:533–545, 1969.
4. Paff, G. H., and Eksterowicz, F. C.: The selective stoppage of bone growth in tissue culture. Anat. Rec., *108*:45–55, 1950.
5. Goland, P. P., and Grand, N. G.: Chloro-s Triazines as markers and fixatives for the study of growth in teeth and bones. Am. J. Phys. Anthropol., *29*:201–218, 1968.
6. Milch, R. A., Rall, D. P., and Tobie, J. E.: Bone localization of the tetracyclines. J. Natl. Cancer Inst., *19*:87–93, 1957.
7. Finerman, G. A. M., and Milch, R. A.: Interaction of tetracycline with mineral salts and calcified matrices (abstract). J. Bone Joint Surg., *44-A*:1023, 1962.
8. Frost, H. M.: Tetracycline-based histological analysis of bone remodeling. Calcif. Tissue Res., *3*:211–237, 1969.

# Chapter Sixteen

# AUTORADIOGRAPHY

## GENERAL PRINCIPLES

A radioactive element is an unstable atom which emits some form of energy or a particle. The energy can be in the form of x-rays or gamma rays, while the particles are generally beta or alpha particles. A beta particle is an electron, may be negatively or positively charged, and has a very small mass, while the alpha particle is a helium atom with a large mass. Both the energy from the gamma rays or the particles can be geographically visualized by laying a photosensitive emulsion over the source or tissue containing the radioisotope. The process is called autoradiography[1] and has been used to "tag" elements and compounds, to follow time-related events, and to investigate cell dynamics.

The majority of radioactive isotopes emit a mixture of particles and energy. However, some general distinctions can be made; the elements at the beginning of the periodic table emit beta particles, while the heavy elements produce alpha particles. Elements common in the body, such as carbon and hydrogen, are beta-emitters, as are calcium and phosphorus, while elements such as radium are alpha-emitters. Radioisotopes can be purchased as solutions, such as $^{45}CaCl_2$, or as labeled compounds (e.g., $^3H$-proline). The specific activity, that is, the concentration of the radioactive label with respect to the non-radioactive or stable isotope of the same element, can vary. If all the element is radioactive (e.g., a solution of $Na^{35}SO_4$ with no $NaSO_4$), then the solution is said to be carrier-free; alternatively, quite a large percentage of the stable isotope may be present.

In bone tissue, the general procedure for preparation of an autoradiograph is to inject an animal with the radioactive tracer, wait for some time period dictated by the question that is being asked, kill the animal, remove the bones, and make sections. These may be demineralized if the organic matrix is the tissue of interest, but they must be prepared as mineralized sections if the bone mineral is to be investigated. Mineralized sections must also be prepared if the element or compound is leached by the demineralization process, such as citrate. The sections are then placed on a slide coated with an emulsion and held in place by pressure (contact autoradiography); or the section, mounted on a slide, may be covered with an emulsion (generally backed by a layer of gelatin) by the stripping film technique. The mounted section may also be dipped in warm liquid emulsion which then solidifies on cooling and coats the section. The emulsions are generally a mixture of silver halide crystals of various sizes suspended in a gelatin film. The radioisotope, which is now localized somewhere in the bone, emits particles or energy which travel through the emulsion; when they hit a silver halide crystal they create a latent

**127**

image in the crystal. This turns into metallic silver on development and appears as a dot on the emulsion. After the particles collide with the silver halide crystals they lose energy but may travel on through the emulsion, repeating this procedure. A beta particle is so small that it will pass through a standard emulsion with only a 50 per cent or smaller chance of hitting a silver halide crystal; this means that more events have occurred within the tissue than are represented by the number of dots in the emulsion. An alpha particle, because of its large mass, will have a high chance of hitting a silver halide crystal and will also lose energy doing so, and will proceed and bump into another crystal and so on, losing speed rapidly. The result is a "track" in the emulsion, consisting of dots which are successively closer together as the end of the path is reached.

Resolution depends on the ability of the emulsion to separate two points in the underlying section which contain the radioactive element. The resolution will be high, depending on the following four factors: (1) the energy of the particle, which should be low; (2) the distance between the section and the emulsion, which should be zero and probably is, except in contact autoradiography; (3) the thickness of the section, which will be unimportant if the energy of the particle is low; and (4) the emulsion thickness, with the same reservations as for (3). For these reasons a thin, 5-micron demineralized section containing a low energy beta emitter such as $^3$H (0.018 mev) will give excellent resolution, while an autoradiograph of a thick mineralized section containing $^{32}$P (1.70 mev) or $^{90}$Sr (0.61 mev) will be of poor resolution (Fig. 16–1).[2, 3]

If the emulsion is left in contact with the section (which is mandatory in the dipping, optional in the stripping, and impossible in the contact methods), the localization of the isotope with respect to a biological structure can be made microscopically. The section may be stained through the emulsion, or if this is a problem, the section may be temporarily removed and then replaced exactly.[4]

If the material of interest is soluble in water, contact autoradiography should be used, or the stripping film method can be adapted to a contact method by stripping off the film and pressing it directly onto the specimen.[5]

By using the electron microscope rather than the light microscope, and using a small piece of eponembedded tissue and thin (1 micron) sections, resolution can be further improved.[6] Elements or labeled compounds may be associated with intracellular structures such as the Golgi apparatus or the endoplasmic reticulum (Fig. 16–2).[7]

## QUANTITATIVE AUTORADIOGRAPHY

Occasionally it is necessary to know not only where but also how much of a radioisotope is retained by a specific tissue. This is achieved by exposing standards alongside the section when the emulsion is placed in contact with the material. The standards are usually plaster of Paris (calcium sulfate), which has approximately the same mass absorption coefficient as bone and can be mixed as a powder with water containing known and varying amounts of $^{45}$Ca. When this hardens, standards of known specific activity allow calibration of the unknown amounts of radioactive calcium in the adjacent specimen. Because exposure and development are all carried out at the same time and on the same plate, there will be no discrepancy caused by variations in emulsion characteristics or development.

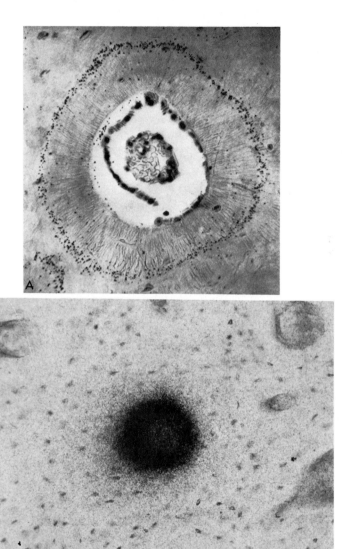

**Figure 16–1** (a) Autoradiograph of a bone section from a rabbit given $^3$H some days before killing the animal. The hydrogen has been taken up by the collagen and forms a necklace of dots around the haversian canal. The resolution is high because of the low energy of $^3$H $\beta$ particles, 0.018 mev (magnification ×1250). (b) Autoradiograph of a bone section containing $^{90}$Sr with a $\beta$ particle energy of 0.61 mev. The resolution is so poor that the central haversian canal can hardly be seen (magnification ×250).

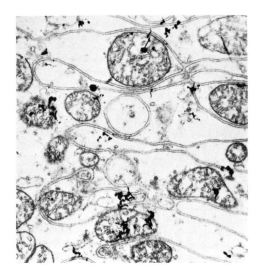

Figure 16-2 Parathyroid hormone labeled with $^{125}$I, localized in kidney tissue. (Courtesy of a friend.)

The method has been applied to contact autoradiography in which depressions are made in the plates which hold the section. The depressions are filled with the plaster of Paris standards (Fig. 16-3).

Quantitation of darkening of the autoradiograph can be carried out by viewing the autoradiograph through a microscope and counting the number of grains or tracks; the method is tedious, although reasonable for alpha tracks. The most common technique for evaluating the degree of darkening involves the use of a densitometer, in which the interruption of light by the darkened film is measured, the degree of light absorption ultimately being related to radioisotope concentration.[8] Dye precipitation may be used instead of a densitometer, with the advantage that irregular, chosen areas of emulsion can be quantitated rather than the generally circular area specified by the densitometer.[9]

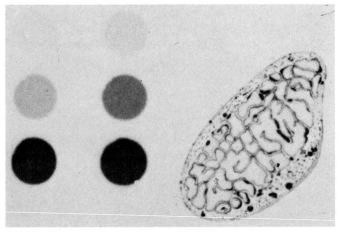

Figure 16-3 Autoradiograph of a rib containing $^{45}$Ca and six adjacent standards, each containing different amounts of $^{45}$Ca mixed with plaster of Paris. The latter can be used to quantitate the degree of film darkening in terms of the amount of $^{45}$Ca (magnification x 4). From Jowsey, J.: Autoradiographic and microradiographic studies of bone. In Zipkin, I. (ed.): Biological Mineralization of Bone. New York, John Wiley and Sons, 1973, pp. 297–333.

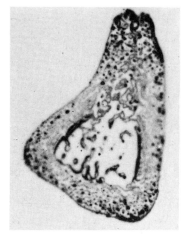

**Figure 16-4** ⁴⁵Ca uptake in a cross section of the tibia of a puppy. Many areas of bone are in the process of formation and mineralization (magnification ×55).

## THE USES OF AUTORADIOGRAPHY

**The Localization of an Element.** As an example of this use of autoradiography, the disappearance of calcium from blood after intravenous injection can be related to the appearance of the isotope in bone, using autoradiographic methods (Fig. 16–4), and also to the presence in the feces and urine, where it will be measured radiochemically. The localization of elements not commonly found in bone, such as plutonium or radium, may also be followed by autoradiography. Radium, in fact, behaves much like calcium (see below), while plutonium and other rare earth elements are located on mineralized surfaces. (Fig. 16–5).

**The Localization of a Labeled Compound.** Tritium (³H) and carbon (¹⁴C) are popular isotopes with which to label compounds and which can then be followed by autoradiography. ³H-thymidine is used in following nuclear dynamics, and ³H-proline to label collagen precursors. ¹⁴C has been used to label ethane-1-hydroxy-1,

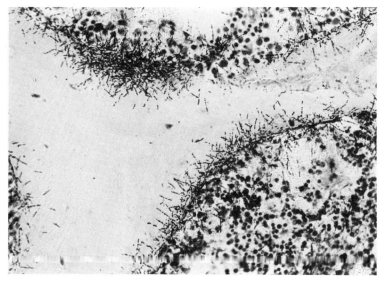

**Figure 16–5** The uptake of plutonium on the bone surface of a trabeculum surrounded by cellular marrow. As an alpha-emitter the autoradiographic image is a band of tracks (magnification ×350).

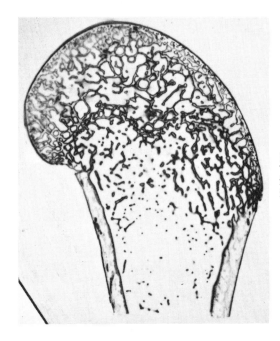

**Figure 16–6**   The deposition of $^{14}$C labeled EHDP (ethane-1-hydroxy-1, 1-diphosphonate). The isotope was injected into a cat 4 hours before killing it. The EHDP appears to be localized on all bone surfaces (magnification ×4).

1-diphosphonate (EHDP), one of the diphosphonates, and to establish its presence in bone (Fig. 16–6).

**The Metabolism of Bone.**   To some extent, this overlaps with the localization of an element. However, if the rate of mineralization of bone is to be investigated or the effect of agents such as estrogens or fluoride on bone, autoradiography may be helpful. For instance, estrogen administration to rats results in metaphyseal sclerosis; this could occur as a result of an increase in new bone or a failure of bone resorption. If $^{45}$Ca is given as a label of newly formed mineralized bone, followed by estrogen administration for a week, a failure of resorption will result in retention of the heavily labeled bone in the metaphysis, while normal resorption and increased formation will produce a picture of less densely labeled bone (Fig. 16–7).

Occasionally investigators have taken bone tissue sections and placed them in a solution containing a radioisotope. If a mineralized section of bone is put into a solution containing $^{45}$Ca, exchange will occur between the radioisotope and the stable calcium, and an autoradiograph may be made of this section.[11] The localization of the isotope will be a reflection of physical chemical exchange, however, and may not be related in any way to the in vivo metabolism of the element. In vitro autoradiography may therefore be misleading and unenlightening in terms of bone physiology.

## BONE TURNOVER RATE

Three major contributions to the study of bone metabolism have been achieved using autoradiography. One such contribution is the long-term rate of bone turnover, the second is the exchange of mineral, and the third is sequence of bone cell differentiation from pre-bone cells.

Bone turnover rate is the amount of bone removed from the skeleton minus the amount of bone added to the skeleton per unit time. To be able to evaluate such questions as the daily calcium requirements, the effect of treatment in osteoporosis,

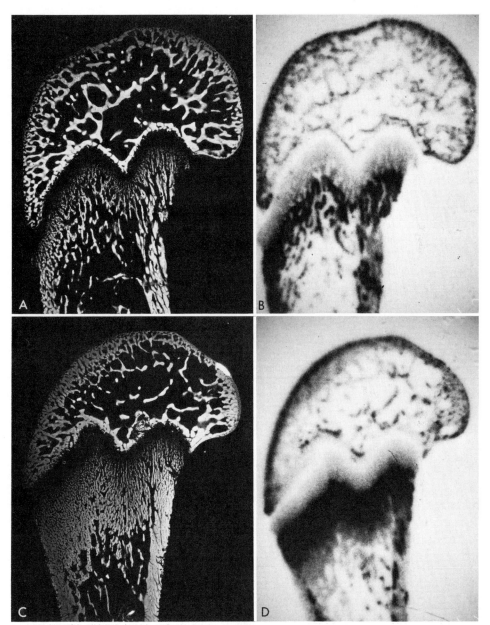

**Figure 16–7** (a) Microradiograph and (b) autoradiograph of the distal femur of a rat given $^{45}$Ca eight days before killing the animal. Rat (c) microradiograph and (d) autoradiograph received estrogen. The estrogen causes a failure of resorption, depicted in the dense metaphyseal bone seen in the microradiograph and in the dense concentration of primary $^{45}$Ca uptake in the autoradiograph (magnification ×10).

and the like, it is useful to know how much bone is being remodeled in a day or a year. The most reliable information comes from studies of radium uptake and long-term retention in the skeleton.

In the 1930's the watch-dial and airplane instrument-panel industry used $^{226}$Ra as a source of energy to make fluorescent paint luminescent. The mixture of the radioactive radium isotope and the fluorescent material was normally painted on the hands and the numbers of the dials, the workers using paint brushes. During this procedure, partly by "tipping their brushes" and partly by using the paint "extramurally" (painting their fingernails and teeth with it on Important Occasions, for example), they ingested significant quantities of the isotope $^{226}$Ra. The workers were mainly 18- to 22-year-old girls, and the majority worked only for a short time in the factories. Thirty years later some samples of bone were available from a few of these people, and, in a large number, the total body burden of radium was estimated by external counting.[12] In some individuals bone specimens were available, and autoradiography showed small patches of bone, which was less heavily labeled than the rest and therefore corresponded to bone laid down after the worker had left the dial-painting industry (Fig. 16–8). By measuring the area of this bone and dividing it by the number of years between the time the worker left the factory and the time the bone specimen was obtained, accurate, long-term values for turnover in both cortical and trabecular bone were derived (Table 16–1). The rate derived in this manner will be a low estimate by the amount of resorption which occurs, and is not followed by new bone formation. Similar data can be derived by calculating the rate at which osteones must have been labeled when the radium was originally deposited (when the workers were 20 years of age) in order to leave the observed number labeled when the autoradiographs were made 30 years later. Of course, the rate must be low enough so that continued turnover does

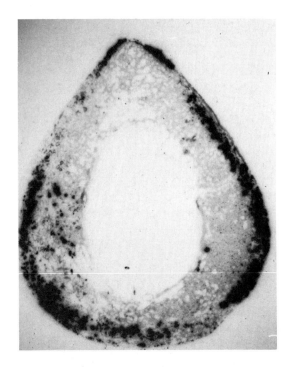

**Figure 16–8** Autoradiograph of a cross section of the femur from a radium-burdened person. The hot-spots of high density represent radium taken up in osteones at the time the radium was ingested. The "empty" spots are areas of bone formed after exposure to radium had stopped (magnification ×3).

**Table 16-1**  BONE REMODELING RATES DERIVED FROM
RADIUM-BURDENED HUMAN BONE

| Case | Bone | Resorption Rate from Radium-Free Bone (% per year) | Growth Rate from Radium Hot Spots (% per year) |
|------|------|------|------|
| 1 | Cortical tibia | 0.30 | 0.43 |
| 2 | Cortical femur | 0.66 | 0.83 |
| 3 | Cortical tibia | 0.78 | — |
|   | Trabecular tibia | 0.93 | — |
| 4 | Cortical humerus | 1.12 | 2.1 |
| 5 | Cortical femur | 3.03 | 2.56 |
|   |   | mean ± SD 1.1 ± 1.0 | mean ± SD 1.5 ± 1.0 |

From Rowland.[12]

not result in rapid resorption of all the labeled osteones; yet it must also be high enough to label a significant number so that some (the observed percentage) remain in the terminal sample. The rate which satisfies both these requirements gives values very close to those calculated from the resorption rate (Table 16–1). Two per cent per year is a realistic figure for adult human bone turnover.

At a rate of 2 per cent per year, and using a value of 10 per cent for the percentage of body weight that is bone, 104 mg of calcium is being deposited and removed per day in the process of cellular turnover (excluding exchange) in adult human beings. This is the best data available on bone turnover in the human being; it is the same as the figure of 104 mg reported by Frost in 1963, using tetracycline,[13] and it comes close to the figure of 40 per cent of the "accretion" value recorded by Heaney;[14] 40 per cent of the accretion value gives a figure of 124 mg. Marshall also derived a figure of 120 mg per day for the bone turnover rate (Table 16–2).[15]

## MINERAL EXCHANGE

Because of the ubiquitousness of phosphorus in the human body, mineral exchange studies in bone have centered on calcium. In 1956 Arnold pointed out that there was autoradiographic evidence of retention of calcium in an area of bone that was not increasing its mineral content.[16] Marshall later made quantitative estimations of $^{45}Ca$ autoradiographs in dogs of different ages and found that the uptake of isotope corresponds to a loss of stable calcium; this explained the lack of calcium increment in the presence of isotope retention.[15] The exchange of mineral, exclusive of new bone formation and bone resorption, is termed long-term exchange. Long-term exchange of calcium occurs throughout all mineralized bone and represents a physical-chemical exchange of a calcium atom from the extracellular fluid bathing the bone with the calcium of hydroxyapatite. The calcium atom that has just moved onto the crystal is not exchanged back off the crystal immediately or even soon, merely because the amount of calcium in bone is so much more than the amount in the extracellular fluid compartment (2500 grams of calcium in bone, 0.5 gram in blood and extracellular fluid). If the exchange is random, then

**Table 16–2**  BONE FORMATION RATES IN MAN DETERMINED BY DIFFERENT INVESTIGATORS (mineral accretion by the skeleton)

| Author | Term | mg, Ca per day | Mechanisms |
|--------|------|----------------|------------|
| Rowland[12] | turnover rate | 104 | bone formation |
| Frost[13] | bone formation | 104 | bone formation |
| Heaney[14] | "accretion" | 335 | bone formation and long-term exchange |
| Marshall[15] | long-term exchange | 250 | long-term exchange |
| Marshall[15] | bone formation | 120 | bone formation |

there will be only a 1 in 5000 chance for immediate exchange off into the extracellular fluid and blood. The chance will increase with increasing time of residence of the originally exchanged atom.

Calculations have been made of the amount of calcium in the long-term exchange pool, and this is somewhat more than that involved in bone formation. If bone turnover stops, such as in hypothyroidism, then a flow of calcium between blood and bone will still occur through the long-term exchange mechanism. Calculations have shown that this is equal to about 250 mg of calcium per day in an adult human being.[15] The actual figures vary somewhat but are surprisingly consistant when the mechanisms acting to produce the measured rate are taken into account (Table 16–2).

## CELL CYCLES

$^3$H-thymidine is a specific percursor of DNA, and thymidine will only be incorporated into cells undergoing DNA synthesis; there is no turnover of DNA after synthesis, and injected $^3$H-thymidine is rapidly removed from the blood and either utilized, degraded, or excreted. All dividing cells can be identified during different phases of their division, and these phases have been divided into four periods. $G_2$ is the short phase before mitosis; M is the mitosis or genetic duplication phase; $G_1$ is the period after completion of mitosis; the S phase is when synthesis of new DNA occurs. The whole cycle ($T_c$) is expressed by the following equation: $(G_2 + M + G_1 + S) = T_c$. Only during the S phase does $^3$H-thymidine become incorporated into DNA, so that, in a population of dividing cells, the time between injection of the labeled thymidine and the appearance of the label in mitoses is the $G_2$ period.

The time between injection and the appearance of label in 100 per cent of the dividing cells is an estimate of the maximum length of the periods ($G_2 + M$). At longer periods after injection there will be an increase in unlabeled cells, as the S period occurs at a time when the blood has been cleared and the thymidine is no longer $^3$H-labeled. The time including the period at which 50 per cent of the cells are first labeled to when they fall back to 50 per cent labeling (after 100 per cent labeling) is an estimate of the duration of DNA synthesis.

[3]H-thymidine has been used to measure bone cell cycles and bone cell activity. Quantitative studies using [3]H-thymidine have shown that osteoblasts can produce 2 to 3 times their own volume of matrix at times of very active bone formation.[17] [3]H-thymidine has also been used to label the osteoclast and osteoblast precursor the progenitor cell and follow the label into the two differentiated, active cell types. Since a single intravenous injection of the nuclear label results in simultaneous arrival of the tagged label in both cell types, it is obvious that these cells are derived from separate precursors;[14] they are not derived one from the other.

## REFERENCES

1. Rogers, A. W.: Techniques of Autoradiography, 2nd ed. Amsterdam, Elsevier Publishing Co., 1973.
2. Mankin, H. J., Revak, C., and Lippiello, L.: Ribonucleic acid in the epiphyseal plate of the rat: an autoradiography study. Bull. Hosp. Joint Dis., 29:111–118, 1968.
3. Jowsey, J., Owen, M., Tutt, M., and Vaughan, J.: Retention and excretion of [90]Sr by adult rabbits. Br. J. Exp. Pathol., 36:22–26, 1955.
4. Hoecker, F. E., Wilkinson, P. N., and Kellison, J. E.: A versatile method of microautoradiography. Nucleonics, 11:60–64, 1953.
5. Fitzgerald, P. J., Ord, M. G., and Stocken, L. A.: A dry mounting autoradiographic technique for the localization of water soluble compounds. Nature, 189:55–56, 1961.
6. Salpeter, M. M., Bachmann, L., and Salpeter, E. E.: Resolution in electron microscope radioautoradiography. J. Cell. Biol., 41:1–20, 1969.
7. Rogers, A. W.: Recent developments in the use of autoradiographic techniques with electron microscopy. Philos. Trans. R. Soc. Lond. (Biol. Sci.), 261:159–171, 1971.
8. Riggs, B. L., Marshall, J. H., Jowsey, J., Heaney, R. P., and Bassingthwaighte, J. B.: Quantitative [45]Ca autoradiography of human bone. J. Lab. Clin. Med., 78:585–598, 1971.
9. Jowsey, J.: Densitometry of photographic images. J. Appl. Physiol., 21:309–312, 1966.
10. Linquist, B., Budy, A. M., McLean, F. C., and Howard, J. L.: Skeletal metabolism in estrogen-treated rats studies by means of Ca[45]. Endocrinology, 66:100–111, 1960.
11. Amprino, R.: Rapporti fra processi di ricostruzione e distribuzione dei minerali nelle ossa. II. Ricerche con metodo autoradiografico. Z. Zellforsch, 37:240–273, 1952.
12. Rowland, R. E.: Resorption and bone physiology. In Frost, H. M. (Ed.): Bone Biodynamics. Boston, Little, Brown and Co., 1964, pp. 335–351.
13. Frost, H. M.: Measurement of human bone formation by means of tetracycline labeling. Can. J. Biochem., 41:31–42, 1963.
14. Heaney, R. P.: Calcium tracers in the study of vertebrate calcium metabolism. In Zipkin, I. (Ed.): Bone Mineralization. New York, John Wiley & Sons, 1973, pp. 829–844.
15. Marshall, J. H.: Theory of alkaline earth metabolism. J. Theor. Biol., 6:389–412, 1964.
16. Arnold, J. S., Jee, W. S. S., and Johnson, K.: Observations and quantitative radioautographic studies of calcium[45] deposited in vivo in forming Haversian systems and old bone of rabbits. Am. J. Anat., 99:291–314, 1956.
17. Owen, M.: Cell population of an osteogenic tissue. I. J. Cell Biol., 19:19–32, 1963.

# Chapter Seventeen

# MORPHOLOGY

The majority of methods that quantitate bone are "black box" with respect to bone metabolism; they observe the net result of cell activity, that is, increased or decreased mass, but they cannot identify the cause. For example, is the osteosclerosis of osteopetrosis the result of a failure of resorption or of excessive formation of new bone? For this sort of information the bone tissue itself must be observed and, if possible, the observations quantitated.

## BIOPSY

Bone biopsy is the first step. This immediately introduces the first disadvantage, that of a potentially painful procedure with the possibility of infection. However, the development of a bone trephine and the choice of a biopsy site beneath the superior aspect of the anterior iliac spine have proved to be relatively pain-free, and complications are few.[1]

The second disadvantage of the bone biopsy is that it is a sampling technique, and its use depends on the relationship between the findings in trephine biopsy and those in the rest of the skeleton. This is not peculiar to biopsy techniques; it is true of all sampling techniques; radioisotope kinetic analysis, total body counting, and neutron activation analysis are exceptions among methods for evaluating the skeleton, since they are not sampling methods. To some extent the problem has been answered by taking bone samples from autopsy specimens in a number of different sites and comparing the results from site to site. The results suggest that a single biopsy does indeed represent the findings in the whole skeleton; the values are different from site to site, but the figures change in the same direction in the same skeleton (Table 17–1).

Almost all bone biopsies are taken from the anterior iliac crest. However, the rib has been used and yields a good sample with a mixture of both cortical and trabecular bone, although after a rib biopsy the patient may have pain associated with his "fractured" rib.[2] The iliac crest has a number of advantages as a biopsy site. It is not a weight-bearing bone and therefore will not fracture. It contains both cortical and trabecular bone, and if the sample is taken beneath the superior spine, where there are no muscle attachments to the bone, and if the muscle is divided and not removed with the bone core, the procedure can be almost painless.

Two investigators have used whole cross sections of rib in studies of bone disease.[2, 3] All others, including these two, have used the anterior iliac crest; however, with two exceptions, only trabecular bone has been analyzed. The sample may be taken from the superior aspect or laterally, and approximately the same

138

**Table 17-1** CORRELATION BETWEEN RESORPTION AND FORMATION IN DIFFERENT AREAS OF THE SKELETON

|  | Correlation Coefficient, r | No. of Samples |
|---|---|---|
| RESORPTION |  |  |
| Anterior iliac crest vs femur | 0.85 | 35 |
| Anterior iliac crest vs vertebra | 0.73 | 10 |
| Posterior iliac crest vs rib | 0.74 | 14 |
| FORMATION |  |  |
| Anterior iliac crest vs femur | 0.83 | 35 |
| Anterior iliac crest vs vertebra | 0.81 | 10 |
| Posterior iliac crest vs rib | 0.79 | 14 |

From Jowsey et al.[6]

trabecular bone sample is obtained. The difference is that the superior specimen size is limited laterally by the walls of the trephine, while, in the lateral specimen, the superoinferior size is limited by the walls of the trephine. Trephine sizes also vary from one investigator to another (Fig. 17–1).

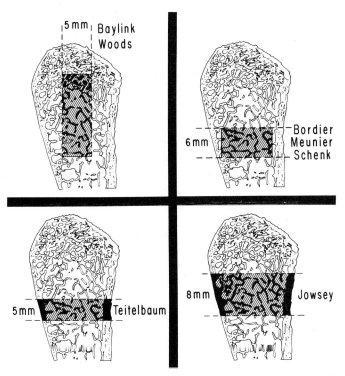

**Figure 17-1** Different biopsy sites used by various investigators using bone biopsy techniques. The areas analyzed are colored black.

## HISTOLOGY

The trabecular and cortical bone samples are prepared by routine histologic methods, although in current practice they are more frequently embedded undemineralized and cut with a microtome or saw.

Paraffin or celloidin embedding of the biopsy tissue is used for demineralized material.[4, 5] Methacrylate or polyester resin are used for mineralized sections.[6, 7, 8] Alternatively, fresh, unembedded material may be used,[9] although this technique may result in loss of material in the grinding process because no embedding material is used to hold the trabeculae in the section. For trabecular bone, microtome sections can be cut, using a heavy and often motor-driven knife. The resulting sections are thin (10 microns), but they are often fractured. It is not possible for material as hard as bone to slide up the surface of the V-shaped knife without breaking the trabeculae and occasionally tearing out pieces of the centers (Fig. 17–2). For both trabecular and cortical bone, a motor-driven saw or blade produces sections that are of uniform thickness and are not broken (Fig. 17–3).[6, 10] The disadvantages are that the equipment is expensive, the sections are thicker (not always a disadvantage), and material is lost as "sawdust"; this loss is not important when large samples are available, but it can be if small biopsies (2 mm) are used.

The resultant sections can be stained as is,[9, 11] or the plastic material can be removed and the section then stained. Paraffin and celloidin sections are stained without removal of the embedding material.

A number of different staining techniques are suitable for bone cells. The Goldner stain distinguishes unmineralized (red) from mineralized (green) bone and also stains cells nicely.[11] The only disadvantage is that the staining procedure is long. The Von Kossa technique also distinguishes mineralized from unmineralized bone. It stains calcium-phosphate-citrate complexes; it is not specific for calcium but is so for calcium citrophosphates.[12] A stain that specifically colors calcium has been developed for both soft tissue and bone. Glyoxal bis (2-hydroxyanil) or GBHA will only stain free calcium and not the calcium in hydroxyapatite.[13] The method has proved useful for studying calcium-containing secretory granules. The advantage of the Paragon stain is that it will stain plastic-embedded mineralized sections without removal of the plastic.[14]

The most usual method of tissue morphologic quantitation involves the use of a grid, and bone morphology is no exception. The grids vary from the conventional square of squares to lines with points or wavy lines. Basically two kinds of measurements can be made. The first is a measurement of the number of cells on the bone surface, the cells being the osteoblasts and osteoclasts that are forming and resorbing bone. Since bone is a hard substance and formation and resorption occur on the surfaces of the trabeculae, the measurements are generally made by evaluating the type of activity occurring at the point at which a grid line intersects a bone surface.[15] The number of points will depend on the number of lines that intersect a surface, and the "events" will be osteoclastic resorption, osteoblastic formation, or nothing, the last being the most frequent. Secondly, the area of bone per unit area of the biopsy can be quantitated by using a grid of squares, or one with lines with intersecting points on the grid, or one with the lines in the grid intersecting bone surfaces. Commonly, the measurements are made at a magnification of 100 times, and in 20 to 50 grid areas; the results are expressed as a percentage of bone formation or resorption per unit surface or area of bone sample.[16, 17]

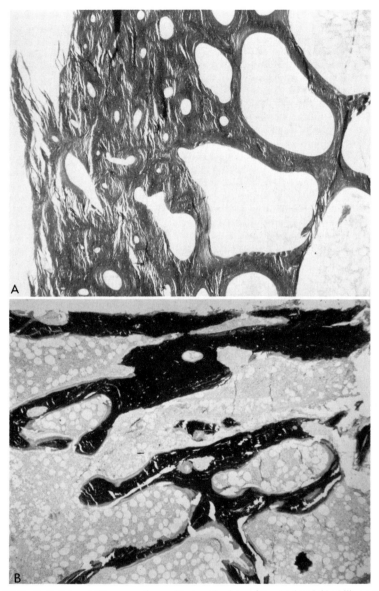

**Figure 17-2** Both (a) and (b) are sections of trabecular bone from undecalcified iliac crest sections. The sections have been cut with a microtome knife and illustrate the microfractures in the hard, mineralized tissue (magnification ×40).

Osteoid tissue, fibrous connective tissue in the marrow, inactive Howship's lacunae, and other features can also be measured.

No two investigators use precisely the same technique, and the results are often at variance; however, when biopsies from individuals with bone disease are compared with normal bone, the conclusions regarding the abnormality of the bone disease are usually the same.

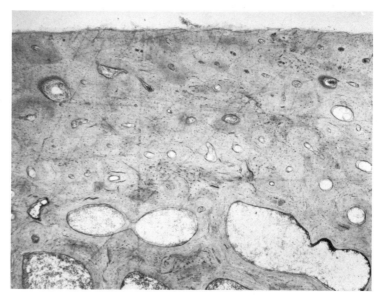

**Figure 17–3**　Undecalcified section of cortical human bone cut by a circular saw. The bone is not fractured or broken because the section is not bent during the cutting procedure (magnification ×40).

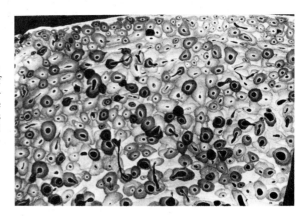

**Figure 17–4**　A microradiograph of a cross-section of the femur cortex of a 50-year-old woman. There is considerable variation in the density of the haversian systems, the darker osteones representing those most recently formed and still incompletely mineralized (magnification ×21).

## MICRORADIOGRAPHY

An alternative to counting cell numbers is the evaluation of surfaces of bone by the appearance on a micro-x-ray or microradiograph. A mineralized bone section is exposed on a very fine-grain emulsion to a beam of soft x-rays. Copper is generally used as the target material, since this produces an x-ray beam at between 10 and 20 kv, which is absorbed by hydroxyapatite in preference to soft tissue.[18] A tungsten target has also been used.[19] An aluminum, beryllium, or a nickel window in the tube filters the beam so that it is essentially monoenergetic.

The bone section is placed on the emulsion, which is on film or on glass slides, and close contact is made with the section. The exposure time will vary with the section thickness and the voltage and amperage of the x-ray equipment; in general, the amperage of the machine is the limiting factor. At 20 kv, 20 ma, and a thickness of 100 microns, five minutes gives an adequate exposure; however, if low amperage

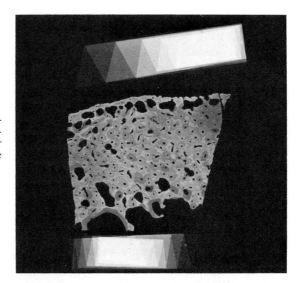

**Figure 17–5** Microradiograph of cortical bone from a young person with aluminum step-wedges above and below for evaluation of mineral density of the bone (magnification ×7). (From Jowsey, J.[22])

equipment is used (3 ma) the exposure time may be as long as one hour or more.[19] After exposure, the emulsion is developed in a high-contrast developer such as D19b (Kodak), although there may well be times when a low-contrast developer will produce a more appropriate microradiograph. The resulting image portrays the variations in mineral density of the microradiograph (Fig. 17–4).

One exclusive use of microradiography is to evaluate mineral density. It is possible to microdissect osteones, interstitial bone, and lamellar bone and make microchemical determinations of calcium content, but this is tedious.[20] Microradiographic analysis of mineral density is easier and more accurate than microanalysis. The degree of absorption of the x-ray beam is related to the density of the bone; in fact, most of the absorption of the beam at the energy used is by the calcium.

The relationship between the absorption of the beam by the calcium and the density of the emulsion can be evaluated with the use of an aluminum step-wedge (Fig. 17–5), similar to the way the whole-limb x-ray is analyzed.[21] The darkening of the emulsion is measured by absorption of light by means of a densitometer and compared with the darkening related to a known thickness of aluminum.

**Table 17–2** THE VARIATION IN BONE MINERAL DENSITY IN DIFFERENT ANIMALS

|         | Low Density | | High Density | |
|---------|-------------|-------------|--------------|-------------|
|         | g Ca/cm$^3$ | g HA/cm$^3$ | g Ca/cm$^3$  | g HA/cm$^3$ |
| Rat     | 0.565       | 1.41        | 0.678        | 1.70        |
| Rabbit  | 0.556       | 1.39        | 0.612        | 1.53        |
| Mouse   | 0.476       | 1.22        | 0.550        | 1.38        |
| Dog     | 0.460       | 1.15        | 0.554        | 0.39        |
| Cow     | 0.444       | 1.11        | 0.600        | 1.50        |
| Man     | 0.420       | 1.00        | 0.530        | 1.33        |

From Rowland et al.[23]

The area measured is generally a circle 30 μm in diameter; this will include canaliculi but exclude osteocyte lacunae. An alternative method can be used which avoids the densitometer and instead quantitates dye precipitation,[22] its advantage is that irregular areas of bone, such as whole cross sections, osteones, or the irregular contour of a fracture callus, can be evaluated. Videodensitometry also has potential use in quantitating bone mineral.

From quantitation of the microradiograph, it is evident that there are considerable differences between the mineral density of different animals (Table 17–2).[23] The data show a decline in the mineral density of osteones with increasing age,[18]

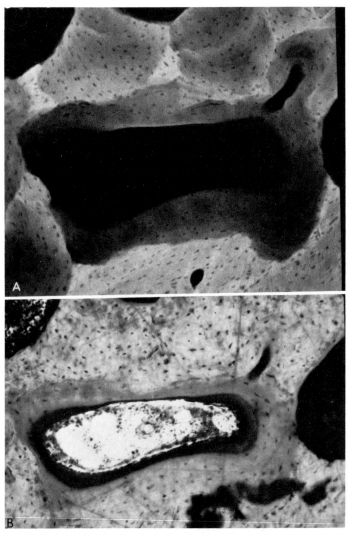

**Figure 17–6** (a) Microradiograph of a newly deposited osteone of low mineral density. The majority of the surface is of continual low density; however, a short length above is sclerotic and indicates cessation of bone formation (magnification ×160). (b) Stained, mineralized section of the same area as seen in the microradiograph with osteoid and osteoblasts on the surface of low mineral density and no active cells on the surface which appears sclerotic in the microradiograph (magnification ×160).

and also in people with osteoporosis. This suggests that mineral exchange throughout compact bone, which has been suggested as a mechanism for maintaining serum calcium, may in fact be a substantial cause of generalized mineral loss from bone; this assumes that individuals are in negative calcium balance and are experiencing a tendency toward hypocalcemia.

Bone formation and resorption can be quantitated from a microradiograph using the appearance of the surfaces to distinguish between formation, resorption, and inactivity.[24] Forming surfaces are of low mineral density and smooth, while resorbing surfaces are uneven and microscopically crenated (Figs. 17–6 and 17–7).

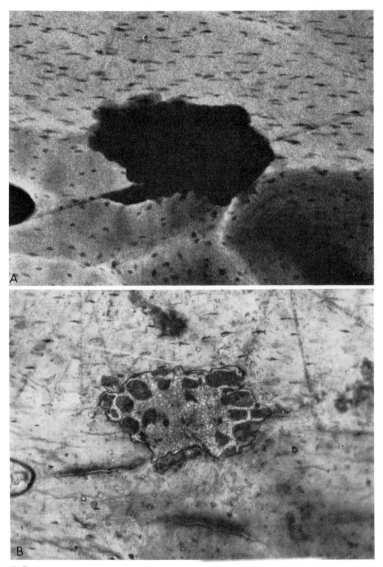

**Figure 17–7** (a) Microradiograph of a small resorption cavity with the scalloped surface of Howship's lacunae (magnification ×250). (b) Stained mineralized section of the same area of bone as above, showing the numerous osteoclasts (magnification ×250).

When both formation and resorption activities cease, a line of high mineral density appears on the microradiograph, indicating a cellularly inert surface (Figs. 17–6 and 17–8). With the recent use of the Paragon stain, it has been possible to correlate the appearance of cells with the appearance of the surface in the microradiograph. The best information is derived from both the microradiograph and the histologic preparation together. Only when the histology (cell detail) is poor, as in some postmortem material, is the microradiograph the major source of data.

It is important to remember the following three points when reading papers referring to bone morphology:

**1.** Cell number or surface activity may not reflect cell activity; in other words, if the surface occupied by osteoblasts and osteoclasts is the same, bone destruction

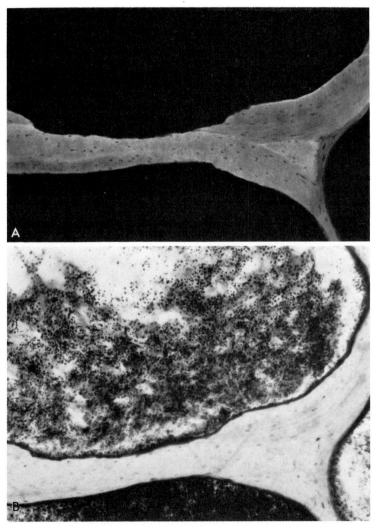

**Figure 17–8** (a) Microradiograph of a trabeculum of bone to show the smooth surface with a narrow sclerotic line where resorption has ceased and the bone is inactive (magnification ×160). (b) Stained section of mineralized bone of the same area, showing lack of osteoclasts and presence of only the marrow elements (magnification ×160).

may still be in excess of deposition, or vice versa, because of a difference in activity per unit cell.

2. There is a real difference in sampling sites. The major difference is that the majority of investigators sample trabecular bone, whereas, currently, only Jowsey and Teitelbaum evaluate cortical and trabecular bone. The results are bound to be different, and it is unreasonable to compare data from the two types of bone and expect the values to be the same.

3. The patient population may be different. Controls may be unselected, large city morgue deaths or highly selected "normals" from which abnormals have been excluded by history and pathologic report. Patients may be ambulatory people living at home, who are seen only in a clinic, or they may be bed patients in a hospital, or patients already on treatment. (In some instances, the treatment may not be expected to alter bone metabolism when, in fact, it does.)

Viewed with these points in mind, bone morphology is a useful tool for evaluating bone turnover and is the only way to answer precisely and quantitatively a number of questions of cell activity.

## ELECTRON MICROSCOPY

An electron microscope (EM) technique has permitted greater detail of bone structure to be appreciated than is possible by light microscopy.[25] Basically the technique consists of passing a beam of parallel, focused electrons through a section onto a fluorescent screen. The screen fluoresces in proportion to the number of electrons hitting it, so the resulting picture represents variations in electron density. Preparation of the material requires special consideration; the piece of tissue must be taken immediately after death of the animal or person, or else taken in vivo, and the sample should be no more than 1 mm in one dimension. The tissue must be placed immediately in an appropriate fixative (usually osmium tetroxide buffered with cacodylate) and processed. The reason for the special procedures is that detailed cell morphology is the object, and autolysis must be prevented at all costs by rapid and complete fixation. The material is embedded in methacrylate or Epon and cut with a glass or diamond knife into thin sections, generally less than 1 micron in thickness (e.g., 800Å).

Robinson has been largely responsible for developing the technique of electron microscopy for bone, and Cooper has further extended the method.[26, 27] These authors have described unmyelinated nerves which lie in the osteones of compact bone; they lie adjacent to the capillaries within the canal. Frequently, two capillaries are found in a single canal and may subsequently branch off in a Volkmann's canal to another osteone. There is often little difference between morphological appearance of the two capillaries; however, one may be more thick-walled and may possibly be an artery, the other representing a vein. There are gaps in the endothelium of the capillary wall that allow escape of the vascular fluid through the basement membrane to the osteoblasts and bone.

Electron microscopy has also nicely pictured the new collagen filaments being produced by the osteoblasts and the later development of hydroxyapatite mineral in the matrix. The spherical nature of the initial stages of mineralization has been clearly outlined by electron microscopy. In 1965, Hancox, using wet preparations, first illustrated the small spherical islands of mineral that appeared within the matrix.[28] These appeared to be vesicles containing mineral, and Hancox described them in areas distant from the collagen fibrils and, therefore, first divorced the process of mineralization from those that described the initial process as being associated with "seeding" on specific sites on collagen fibrils. It is more likely that the appearance in the EM on which such theories rested was the result of fixation artefact.

The processes from the osteoblasts into the matrix and mineralized bone are below the resolution of the light microscope, but the morphologic structure is clearly visible on EM. The cytoplasm from the cell proceeds down the canalicular channel and meets the cytoplasmic process from an adjacent osteocyte to make a cellular interstitium from the bone-soft tissue surface into the most remote parts of mineralized bone (Fig. 17–9). In all EM preparations there is a gap between the cytoplasmic process of the osteocyte and the wall of the matrix. This area is presumably filled with extracellular, extravascular fluid and permits nutrition, removal of metabolic waste, and mineral exchange throughout the bone in the absence of a permeating vascular system. A vascular bed, in the form of the haversian systems and Volkmann's canals, is a necessary part of the maintenance of bone tissue. However, it is an error to believe that proximity to a blood vessel is essential for the survival of bone; the canalicular and osteocyte system will provide an adequate means of supplying the tissue over many square millimeters of mineralized cortex. The distance between the canaliculi is in the order of five microns, a distance which is small enough to permit relatively efficient exchange of ions by the process of diffusion.

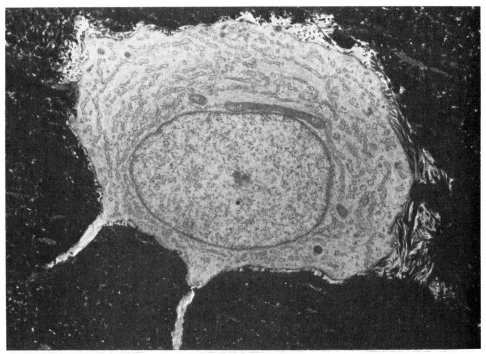

**Figure 17–9**  Electron microscopic appearance of an osteocyte with two canaliculi projecting from the cell cytoplasm (magnification ×10,000). (Courtesy of Dr. B. Boothroyd.)

**Table 17–3**  THE CELL INCLUSIONS IN THE DIFFERENT TYPES OF
BONE CELLS

| Bone Cells | Progenitor Cell | Osteoblast | Osteocytes | Osteoclasts |
|---|---|---|---|---|
| Nucleus | One | One | One | Many (not always) |
| Organelles | Few | One | Variable | Few |
| Cytoplasm | Not dense | Dense | Variable | Vacuolated |
| Rough endoplas-<br>mic reticulum | Scant | Abundant | Variable | Scant |
| Mitochondria | Abundant | Abundant | Variable | Abundant |
| Lysosomes | Few | Occasional | Few | Many |
| Ribosomes | – | Abundant | Occasional | – |
| Golgi body | Well developed | Well developed | Variable | – |
| Special features | Large | Cell processes extending to bone; adjacent collagen fibers | Cell processes; large nuclear cytoplasmic ratio | Brush border |

Cell types have also been well described by electron microscopy (Table 17–3).
Because of the careful fixation, details of cell morphology are probably recorded
more accurately than in conventionally, formalin-fixed material where large pieces
of tissue are prepared for histological examination. Osteoclasts contain vesicles
which engulf both the mineral and collagenous phases of the bone (Fig. 17–10). Osteoblasts contain an abundant endoplasmic reticulum and, like osteocytes, demonstrate cell processes which become the canalicular projections. They can be seen
to form a curtain over the bone surface, which may behave as a bone-non-
bone membrane,[29] although apparently it is relatively permeable, since tight junctions do not exist between the cells.

One of the most definitive contributions of electron microscopic studies of
bone has been the demonstration of the process of mineralization. As already mentioned, Hancox in 1965 showed mineralization spheres; more recently Matthews
has shown calcium-rich granules in the mitochondria of osteoblasts where bone
mineralization is taking place.[30] These are absent in vitamin D deficiency and led to
the thesis that mitochondria are capable of concentrating this cation and form the
nidus for mineralization. However, since they are present in osteoclasts which are
not involved in mineralization, as was mentioned in Chapter Nine, it is possibly
more likely that the calcium represents accumulation as a result of the messenger
system involving calcium transport across the cell membrane and stimulation of the
adenyl cyclase system. The mitochondria may retain the calcium at times of stimulation until it can be pumped out of the cell. The initiation of mineralization is most
probably by the formation of extracellular matrix vesicles.

## SCANNING ELECTRON MICROSCOPY (SEM)

Sawed or fractured bone surfaces can be scanned by an electron microscope to
give a three-dimensional picture of bone; whole bone can be used, or the cell and
organic material can be removed with hot ethylene diamine. The mineral remains in
an exact microscopic replica of the whole bone structure.[31] The surface may also be
prepared by polishing with silicon carbide.[32] The exact method used depends on the
information desired. The beam of electrons impinges on the bone surface and the

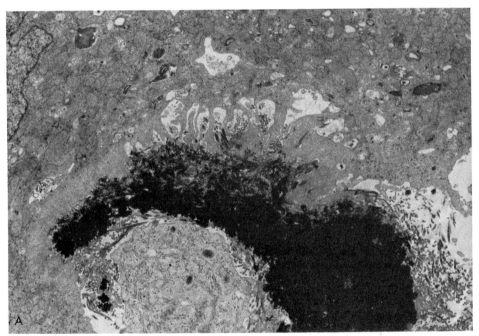

**Figure 17–10** (a) An osteoclast adjacent to a bone surface showing the irregular border which constitutes the ruffled surface or brush border (magnification ×8700). (Courtesy of Dr. B. Boothroyd.)

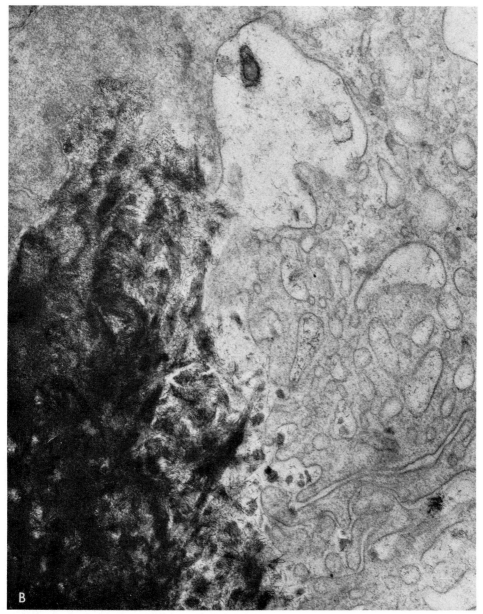

**Figure 17–10** (*Continued*)  (b) An electronmicrograph of an osteoclast at high power. Both hydroxyapatite crystals and collagen can be seen in the vesicles that have formed in the cytoplasm (magnification ×60,000). (Courtesy of Dr. B. Boothroyd.)

resultant current of low energy secondary electrons is used to produce a picture on a cathode ray screen. Low magnification of about ten times can be used to give general information on bone structure somewhat above the level of the dissecting microscope (Fig. 17–11). Higher magnification can span the gap from this level up to that of the electron microscope; depth of focus is maintained even at high magnifications, unlike optical microscopes.

The majority of studies consist of morphological descriptions of bone surfaces and of trabecular and cortical bone. The lamellae in mature bone are clearly seen, and an excellent three-dimensional appearance of osteocyte lacunae and Howship's lacunae can be appreciated.[33] Quantitative measurements of bone surface-to-volume ratios in trabecular bone have also been derived and are probably the most accurate data available. They agree well with the same information obtained by other methods (see Chapter Eight) (Table 17–4).

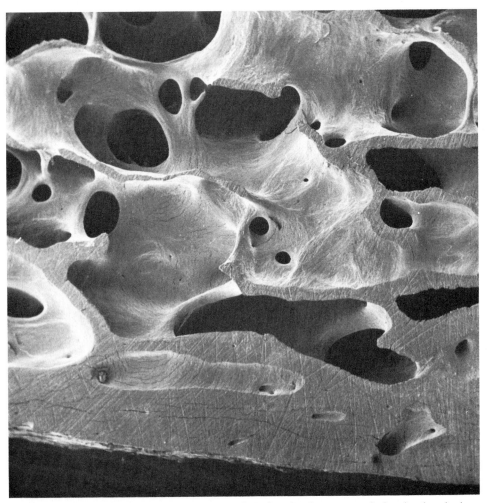

**Figure 17–11**  Scanning electron micrograph of the junction between cortical and trabecular bone (magnification ×30). (From Whitehouse, W. J.: Scanning electron micrographs of cancellous bone from the human sternum. J. Pathol., *116*:213–224, 1975.)

**Table 17–4**  SCANNING ELECTRON MICROSCOPE STUDIES OF
TRABECULAR BONE FROM A HUMAN VERTEBRAL BODY
(mean ± SD)

| % Volume | Perimeter (cm/cm²) | Bone Marrow Surface Area (cm²/cm³) (calc) |
|----------|-------------------|-------------------------------------------|
| 14.5 ± 2.3 | 22.2 ± 4.3 | 28.1 ± 5.5 |

From Whitehouse et al.[32]

Collagen orientation can also be nicely portrayed by this method and shows the lamellar orientation changing every five micra. If this observation is carried into the polarized light method, then each bright and dark band measures approximately ten microns, and this value can be used to derive quantitative data for osteoid width.

Resorption and formation surfaces can also be identified, mainly on the basis of the collagen orientation but also by changes in mineral density.[34] Forming surfaces are microscopically irregular because mineralization occurs somewhat unevenly in the newly formed bone. Several layers of collagen with different orientation can be seen at the sites of resorption, as can the presence of well-defined dense borders.

## ELECTRON PROBE

This method has recently been applied to bone to quantitate in very small areas the amount of calcium, phosphorus, and other elements in bone. The specimens consist of dehydrated, plastic embedded material which has a smooth, cut and polished surface. Such preparations appear to be preferable to thin sections. The surface of the bone must be rendered electrically conductive; this is achieved by evaporating a layer of carbon 400 Å thick onto the block. The surface is then scanned by a minute beam of highly accelerated electrons, which are absorbed by the surface layers of the specimen, and the atoms are excited to a raised energy state. Energy is then released from each particular atom in the form of an x-ray, the energy and wave-length of the x-ray being characteristic for each atom. The type of atom, i.e., calcium, phosphorus, or magnesium, and the amount, can be analyzed by using the diffraction angle for the spectral lines of the elements and comparing the line intensity with that of a known standard for measuring the quantity of the element.

The method is non-destructive, and although chemical analysis of bone will give the same data, microprobe analysis will accurately relate the proportions of the various elements with the anatomical site in the bone. Small specimens may also be analyzed accurately, and the method is sensitive to as little as $5 \times 10^{-7}$ microgram of calcium or phosphorus. It is therefore much more sensitive than the technique of microradiography for quantitation of bone mineral. By using a beam diameter of 3 to 4 microns, some significant variations in the calcium-to-phosphorus ratio can be found in bone of different maturity. In vertebral specimens from one-month-old infants, values are given of 1.63 to 1.67 for the molar ratio of

**Table 17–5** CALCIUM-PHOSPHORUS RATIO IN DIFFERENT TYPES OF BONE.
ANALYZED BY THE ELECTRON PROBE

| Specimen | Calcium-Phosphorus Ratio |
|---|---|
| Young human, trabecular* | 1.63–1.71 |
| Adult human, trabecular* | 1.72–1.78 |
| Bovine bone—femur cortex** | 2.31 |
| Weanling rat—tibia cortex** | 1.6 |
| Rats—femur cortex*** | 1.7 |

\*From Mellors.[35]
\*\*From Wergedal and Baylink.[36]
\*\*\*From Sissons et al.[37]

calcium to phosphorus, values embracing the theoretical 1.67 molar ratio of perfect
hydroxyapatite.[35] In mature bone the amount of calcium rises to 1.75 (Ca/P) (Table
17–5). The same kind of results can be obtained in cortical bone; however, the
densities reported are somewhat lower.[38] Lack of more exciting data probably stems
from the fact that bone tends to be relatively constant in its composition both with
respect to the mineral-to-organic ratio and also for the calcium-to-phosphorus ratio.
The calcium concentration is higher in animal bone in relationship to phosphorus
than in human bone, a finding not unexpected in view of earlier microradiographic
data.

High resolution analysis has enabled investigators to plot the rise in the calcium-to-phosphorus ratio as mineralization proceeds at the mineralization front.[36]
This had been accomplished previously using densitometric methods applied to
microradiographs.[37] However, the resolution with the electron probe is far superior,
and calcium and phosphorus can be specifically quantitated rather than relying on
density which is interpreted by means of the x-ray beam characteristics used to
make the microradiograph and the composition of hydroxyapatite.

Initial mineralization occurs very rapidly, approximately 50 per cent of the calcium being deposited within half a day; from this time onwards the accretion of mineral is approximately exponential (Fig. 17–12). Wergedal and Baylink found that by

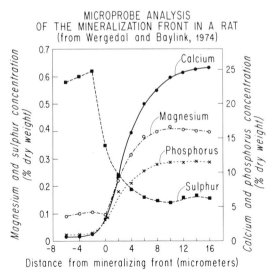

MICROPROBE ANALYSIS
OF THE MINERALIZATION FRONT IN A RAT
(from Wergedal and Baylink, 1974)

Distance from mineralizing front (micrometers)

**Figure 17–12** Electron probe analysis
of the mineralization front in a rat. 0 is the
initiation of mineralization and minus figures
represent values in the unmineralized matrix.
The phosphorus appears to reach a plateau,
approximately four microns before calcium,
which indicates the increase in Ca:P in bone
with maturity. (Redrawn from Wergedal and
Baylink.[36])

four days, in young rats, the final mineral density had been achieved; this corresponds to a distance of about 14 to 16 microns from the mineralization front.[36] These investigators also reported a loss of sulfur from the area of mineralization, which implies an involvement of organic constituents in the process of mineralization. Within the bone high concentrations of calcium have been found in the osteocyte, and these concentrations increase upon treatment with vitamin D.[39]

The microprobe is at a resolution that encourages its use in studies of mineralization, and of mineral fluxes that occur within the canalicular network.[40]

## REFERENCES

1. Johnson, K. A., Kelly, P. J., and Jowsey, J.: Percutaneous full technique, iliac crest biopsy. Clin. Orthop., April, 1977.
2. Jett, S., Wu, K., and Frost, H. M.: Tetracycline-based histological measurement of cortical-endosteal bone formation in normal and osteoporotic rib. Henry Ford Hosp. Med. J., *15*:325–344, 1967.
3. Barer, M., and Jowsey, J.: Bone formation and resorption in normal human rib: a study of persons from 11 to 88 years of age. Clin. Orthop., *52*:241–247, 1967.
4. Pearse, A. G. E.: Histochemistry, Theoretical and Applied. London, Churchill Ltd., 1953, pp. 81–98.
5. Lillie, R. D.: Histopathologic technic and practical histochemistry, 3d ed. New York, McGraw-Hill, 1965.
6. Jowsey, J., Kelly, P. J., Riggs, B. L., Bianco, A. J., Scholz, D. A., and Gershon-Cohen, J.: Quantitative microradiographic studies of normal and osteoporotic bone. J. Bone Joint Surg., *47A*:785–806, 1965.
7. Rijke, A. M., McCoy, S., and McLaughlin, R. E.: A rapid embedding technic for the preparation of undecalcified bone and tooth sections. Am. J. Clin. Pathol., *56*:766–768, 1971.
8. Kwan, S. K.: Sticky wax infiltration in the preparation of sawed undecalcified bone sections. Stain Technol., *45*:177–181, 1970.
9. Villaneuva, A. R., Hattner, R. S., and Frost, H. M.: A tetrachrome stain for fresh, mineralized bone sections, useful in the diagnosis of bone diseases. Stain Technol., *39*:87–94, 1964.
10. Cochran, G. V. B., Pawluk, R. J., and Bassett, C. A. L.: Electromechanical characteristics of bone under physiologic moisture conditions. Clin. Orthop., *58*:249–270, 1968.
11. Goldner, J.: A modification of the Masson trichrome technique for routine laboratory purposes. Am. J. Pathol., *14*:237–243, 1938.
12. Bills, C. E., Eisenberg, H., and Pallante, S. L.: Complexes of organic acids with calcium phosphate: the von Kossa stain as a clue to the composition of bone mineral. Johns Hopkins Med. J., *128*:204–207, 1971.
13. Kashiwa, H. K.: Calcium in cells of fresh bone stained with glyoxal bis (2-hydroxyanil). Stain Tech., *41*:49–55, 1966.
14. Paragon stain. C. & C. Paragon Co., Inc., 190 Willow Ave., Bronx, N.Y. 10454.
15. Schenk, R. K., Merz, W. A., and Muller, J.: A quantitative histological study on bone resorption in human cancellous bone. Acta Anat., *74*:44–53, 1969.
16. Bordier, P. J., Miravet, L., and Hioco, D.: Young adult osteoporosis. Clin. Endocrinol. Metabol., *2*:277–292, 1973.
17. Meunier, P., Courpron, P., Eduoard, C., Bernard, J., Bringuier, J., and Vignon, G.: Physiological senile involution and pathological rarefaction of bone. Clin. Endocrinol. Metabol., *2*:239–256, 1973.
18. Sissons, H. A., Jowsey, J., and Stewart, L.: Quantitative microradiography of bone tissue. In Engstrom, A., Cosslett, V., and Pattee, H. (Eds.): X-ray Microscopy and X-ray Microanalysis. (Proc. Sec. Int. Symp., Stockholm, 1959). Amsterdam, Elsevier Publishing Co., 1960, pp. 199–205.
19. Dunn, E. J., Bowes, D. N., Rothert, S. W., and Greer, R. B., III: Microradiography of undecalcified bone: a simplified, relatively inexpensive technique. Johns Hopkins Med. J., *135*:106–113, 1974.
20. Strandh, J.: Microchemical studies on single haversian systems. II. Methodological considerations with special reference to the Ca/P ratio in microscopic bone structures. Exp. Cell Res., *21*:406–413, 1960.
21. Owen, M., Jowsey, J., and Vaughan, J.: Investigation of the growth and structure of the tibia of the rabbit by microradiographic and autoradiographic technique. J. Bone Joint Surg., *37B*:324–342, 1955.

22. Jowsey, J.: Densitometry of photographic images. J. Appl. Physiol., *21*:309–312, 1966.
23. Rowland, R. E., Jowsey, J., and Marshall, J. H.: Microradiographic measurements of mineral density. Radiat. Res., *10*:234–242, 1959.
24. Jowsey, J.: Microradiography: A morphologic approach to quantitating bone turnover. Exerpta Medica, International Congress Series No *270*:114–123, 1972.
25. Hayat, M. A.: Principles and Techniques of Electron Microscopy, Vols. I, II, and III. New York, Van Nostrand Reinhold Co., 1970.
26. Cameron, D. A., Paschall, H. A., and Robinson, R. A.: The EM ultrastructure of bone cells. In Frost, H. M. (Ed.): Bone Biodynamics. Boston, Little, Brown and Company, 1964, pp. 91–104.
27. Cooper, R. R., Milgram, J. W., and Robinson, R. A.: Morphology of the osteon. J. Bone Joint Surg., *48A*:1239–1271, 1966.
28. Hancox, N. M., and Boothroyd, B.: Electron microscopy of the early stages of osteogenesis. Clin. Orthop., *40*:153–161, 1965.
29. Robinson, R. A.: Observations regarding compartments for tracer calcium in the body. In Frost, H. M. (Ed.): Bone Biodynamics. Boston, Little, Brown and Company, 1964, pp. 423–439.
30. Matthews, J. L.: Ultrastructure of calcifying tissue. Am. J. Anat., *129*:451–458, 1970.
31. Boyde, A., and Hobdell, M. H.: Scanning electron microscopy of lamellar bone. Z. Zellforsch., *93*:213–231, 1969.
32. Whitehouse, W. J., Dyson, E. D., and Jackson, C, K.: The scanning electron microscope in studies of trabecular bone from a human vertebral body. J. Anat., *108*:481–496, 1971.
33. Nixon, W. C.: Scanning electron microscopy. Contemp. Physiol., *10*:71–96, 1969.
34. Hobdell, M. H., and Boyde, A.: Microradiography and scanning electron microscopy of bone sections. Z. Zellforsch., *94*:487–494, 1969.
35. Mellors, R. C.: Electron microprobe analysis of human trabecular bone. Clin. Orthop., *45*:157–167, 1966.
36. Wergedal, J. E., and Baylink, D. J.: Electron microprobe measurements of bone mineralization rate in vivo. Am. J. Physiol., *226*:345–352, 1974.
37. Sissons, H. A., Jowsey, J., and Stewart, L.: The microradiographic appearance of normal bone tissue at various ages. In Engstrom, A., Cosslett, V., and Pattee, H. (Eds.): X-ray Microscopy and X-ray Microanalysis. (Proc. Sec. Int. Symp., Stockholm, 1959). Amsterdam, Elsevier Publishing Co., 1960, pp. 206–215.
38. Ortner, D. J., and Von Endt, D. W.: Microscopic and electron microprobe characterization of the sclerotic lamellae in human osteons. Isr. J. Med. Sci., *7*:480–482, 1971.
39. Remagen, W., Höhling, H. J., Hall, T. A., and Caesar, R.: Electron microscopical and microprobe observations on the cell sheath of stimulated osteocytes. Calcif. Tissue Res., *4*:60–68, 1969.
40. Thorogood, P. V., and Gray, J. C.: Demineralization of bone matrix: observations from electron microscope and electron-probe analysis. Calcif. Tissue Res., *19*:17–26, 1975.

# Chapter Eighteen

# ORGAN AND TISSUE CULTURE

## CHEMICAL DETERMINATIONS OF BONE

The four major constituents of bone are calcium, phosphorus, collagen, and glycosaminoglycans. It is sometimes, but not often, useful to know the proportions of these in bone, since, with few exceptions, bone is of unaltered chemical composition and in the few instances where the composition is changed, morphological visualization of the abnormality is generally far more sensitive than a chemical measurement. The majority of chemical investigations have been directed at answering questions concerning the basic composition of bone matrix and bone mineral.

Bone is generally either wet or dry-ashed in a muffle furnace. In dry-ashing the mineral, calcium and phosphorus, can be isolated from the organic matrix by heating in a furnace at 800° C. The organic material is burnt off, and the mineral remains as a white ash, hence the term "ashing" for this procedure. Alternatively, low temperature ashing after pulverizing the bone mechanically can be used, and this avoids the possibility of any loss of calcium, which occurs in the high temperature ashing methods.[1, 2] Ethylene diamene extraction, generally accomplished by using a reflux condenser, will also solubilize and remove the organic matrix and leave the mineral. Prolonged boiling in water will also tend to remove organic matrix but not as completely as ethylene diamene.[3] "Wet-ashing" methods are alternatives which allow retention of elements that are not part of the organic matrix and that would be volatile and therefore lost in the furnace method.[4] The remaining bone mineral extracted in these ways is then dissolved in a known quantity of acid, generally 20 per cent hydrochloric acid, and the calcium and phosphorus are measured in the resulting solution by the methods used for serum calcium and phosphorus in acid solutions. The ratio of calcium to phosphorus is constant, with few exceptions. The majority of results report the calcium content alone, which is expressed in terms of the nitrogen content, or the original wet or dry weight of the bones. This ratio (Ca:N) will be decreased if (a) mineralization is defective and there is a significant increase in the amount of osteoid, or (b) if there has been significant bone loss, and mineralized tissue is replaced by connective tissue, as in osteitis fibrosa. Large changes in bone morphology are necessary to produce any differences from normal, and the method is not frequently useful or used. In addition the method cannot distinguish between situations (a) and (b).

The collagen content of bone is measured by dissolving bone and quantitating the hydroxyproline content.[5] Since collagen exists in soluble (before cross linking) and less soluble forms (after cross linking) some idea of the amount of new bone being formed will be derived from the soluble-to-insoluble hydroxyproline ratio. (For a further discussion of hydroxyproline estimation, see Chapter Nine.)

The glycosaminoglycans can be measured by digestion and quantitation of hexosamine.[6]

## ORGAN AND TISSUE CULTURE

Investigations may be divided into two large groups. The first, and most usual, is concerned with observing normal and diseased states; the second involves studying experimentally perturbed states. For instance, one might observe the renal excretion and bone changes in patients with hyperparathyroidism, and at the same time give animals parathyroid extract and look at the same parameters. Both approaches contain one unknown: is it the hormone increase that is directly causing the observed changes or some secondarily stimulated factor? This problem can often be avoided by using tissue culture, in which the bone is isolated from the influence of secondarily induced hormonal response. For this reason (it must be stressed) in vitro and in vivo results are *different*. For example, phosphate given to an intact animal will produce increased parathyroid hormone secretion and increased bone resorption and bone loss; in vitro phosphate added to tissue culture will result in a retention of calcium by the bone. With this point in mind, it may be said that tissue and organ culture techniques have contributed significantly to our knowledge of bone.

**Organ Culture.**  Organ culture of bone involves the removal of limb bones from embryonic animals and their culture in horse serum, Tyrode's solution, or another tissue culture medium. The bones must have an intact periosteum; they are laid on a stainless steel grid in the culture medium, and the hormone, chemical, or other substance is added to the medium. The bones are observed for four to eight days generally, and the culture medium is changed every two days. The femurs of embryonic chicks have been used by Fell and colleagues;[7] these are removed from four to 14 days after the egg is laid, and the in vitro culture system differs little from real-life development, except that it is hormone-free. Gaillard uses cultures from the humerus of 16-day-old mice,[8] whereas Raisz uses embryonic rat limb bones.[9] Flat rather than cylindrical embryonic bones have also been used; generally these are bones of the skull, either calvaria, frontal, or parietal bones.[10]

Growth, incorporation of amino acids, labeled proline, and calcium all occur in these preparations, and the cells remain viable and stain normally. The whole limb rudiment will undergo considerable anatomic development while in culture, and it will change from a wholly cartilaginous blastema to a recognizable bone made up of cartilage and unmineralized bone with an appropriate shape. Lack of stress, however, prevents the bone from developing completely normally.

Organs in tissue culture remain viable, in contrast to similar culture procedures carried out in mature samples, for example, human iliac crest trephine biopsies or adult rabbit bone.[11, 12] In the latter, careful examination showed that the osteocytes did not survive more than 30 minutes when kept in saline for six hours after vascular occlusion in vivo. In other words, once a bone has become dependent on a well-developed blood supply, removal from that blood supply will result in death of the specimen. For this reason, tissue and organ culture procedures are carried out in incompletely developed embryonic tissue.

Conventional methods are used for the analysis of the effect of the added substance on bone metabolism. The length of the bone can be measured on consecutive days as a bone becomes longer; the bone can be removed and weighed (wet) and returned to the medium also for sequential measurements. Alternatively, bones may be "sacrificed" at intervals and subjected to chemical analysis for glycosaminoglycans, collagen, or bone mineral, or they may be processed for histologic procedures, electron microscopy, and so on.

A fruitful technique has been to pre-label the bones with $^{45}$Ca or $^3$H-labeled proline in vivo before removing the embryo from the mother. In this way the release of the isotope from the bone during the culture period can be used as a measure of mineral and collagen release from the explanted limb bone. The effect of parathyroid hormonal addition to the medium results, not surprisingly, in an increase in the release of $^{45}$Ca and $^3$H-hydroxyproline and suggests increased bone resorption.[9] Recent data have uncovered a bone-resorbing factor, not in osteoclasts but in myeloma cells, suggesting that cells which, clinically at least, resorb bone can directly mediate bone resorption without becoming conventional osteoclasts.[13] Antibody and complement directed against cell membranes have also been shown to cause cartilage degradation and bone resorption.[14]

Culture of bone calvaria have been used in a somewhat different way by Jacobsen and Goldhaber and others to evaluate the action of cells on bone;[10] these investigators cultured gingival cells from male patients and put them or the broken cells in the culture medium and measured the disappearance of the bone visually. In some, $^{45}$Ca release from pre-labeled bone was correlated with the visual scoring method. The resorption activity resided in the epithelial rather than the fibroblast cells and was related to the cell concentration added to the medium. These findings showed that osteoclast-mediated resorption is not the only way that mineralized bone is resorbed.

If the limitations of the method are kept in mind, and particularly if morphology and the release of labeled compounds are correlated, organ culture can be a useful and informative technique.

**Tissue Culture.**   Once the periosteal membrane is removed from the bone or the bone is split or cut so that the naked bone is exposed to the medium, then quite a different situation exists. Citrate production stops, mineralization of the tissue becomes dependent on culture medium,[8] and bone potassium content decreases.[15] If bone pieces are cultured, the bone cells escape and proliferate as fibroblasts, and the preparation degenerates into a mass of connective tissue or cartilage, depending on the oxygen concentration of the medium.[16]

### REFERENCES

1. Kato, Y., and Ogura, H.: Low-temperature ashing of bovine dentine. Calcif. Tissue Res., *18*:141–148, 1975.
2. Abu-Samra, A., Morris, J. S., and Koirtyohann, S. R.: Wet ashing of some biological samples in a microwave oven. Anal. Chem., *47*:1475–1477, 1975.
3. Hilleman, H. H., and Lee, C. H.: Organic chelating agents for decalcification of bones and teeth. Stain Technol., *28*:285 287, 1953.
4. David, D. J.: Determination of calcium in plant material by atomic-absorption spectrophotometry. Analyst, *84*:536–548, 1959.

5. Neuman, R. E., and Logan, M. A.: The determination of hydroxyproline. J. Biol. Chem., *184*:299–306, 1950.
6. Boas, N. F.: Method for the determination of hexosamines in tissues. J. Biol. Chem., *204*:553–563, 1953.
7. Fell, H. B.: The effect of environment on skeletal tissue in culture. Embryologia (Nagoya), *10*:181–205, 1969.
8. Gaillard, P. J., Moskalewski, S., Verhoog, M. J., and Wassenaar, A. M.: The effect of parathyroid extract on the aggregation and the secretion of isolated chondrocytes. Kon. Nederl. Akademie van Wetenschappen, Proc. Series, C, *72*:521–536, 1969.
9. Raisz, L. G.: Bone formation and resorption in tissue culture. Arch. Intern. Med., *126*:887–889, 1970.
10. Jacobsen, J., and Goldhaber, P.: Bone resorption in vitro induced by products of human gingival cells in culture. J. Periodont. Res., *8*:171–178, 1973.
11. Nelson, C. L., and Haynes, D. W.: The survival of cells in human bone after exposure to air and saline correlated with deoxyribonucleic acid abnormalities. Calcif. Tissue Res., *6*:260–264, 1970.
12. Rösingh, G. E., and James, J.: Changes in cell nuclei of the ischemic femoral head. Calcif. Tissue Res., 2, Suppl:38, 1968.
13. Mundy, G. R., Raisz, L. G., Cooper, R. A., Schechter, G. P., and Salmon, S. E.: Evidence for the secretion of an osteoclast stimulating factor in myeloma. N. Engl. J. Med., *291*:1041–1046, 1974.
14. Lachmann, P. J., Coombs, R. R. A., Fell, H. B., and Dingle, J. T.: The breakdown of embryonic (chick) cartilage and bone cultivated in the presence of complement-sufficient antiserum. III. Immunological analysis. Int. Arch. Allergy, *36*:469–485, 1969.
15. Ramp, W. K., and Neuman, W. F.: Bone mineralization in tissue culture. Calcif. Tissue Res., *11*:171–175, 1973.
16. Stern, P., Glimcher, M. J., and Goldhaber, P.: The effect of various oxygen tensions on the synthesis and degradation of bone collagen in tissue culture. Proc. Soc. Exp. Biol. Med., *121*:869–872, 1966.

# Part III

# Metabolic Bone Disease

## INTRODUCTION

Disease implies pain and discomfort. In metabolic bone disorders, it implies that a fracture or deformity of the bone has occurred to cause the subsequent pain and discomfort. Most metabolic bone disease is characterized by bone loss, which eventually produces a skeleton of a mass so decreased that any sudden stress will result in fracture of the bone. It has been pointed out that bone is very intricately designed microscopically and grossly, and that it is organized to withstand most efficiently the normal stresses and strains that are put upon the skeleton. The constant turnover of bone allows some adaptation to these stresses, such as the increase in mass that occurs with increased exercise. Any disorder of bone, therefore, leading to a fracture, or even partial fracture as in osteomalacia, will result from a combination of decreased bone mass and stress. It is obvious from the characteristic areas where fractures occur—the lower part of the spine, the femoral neck, and the distal end of the forearm, when this is stressed by a fall—that these areas are prone to fracture because of their biomechanical relationship to excessive or unusual stress.

Therefore, most metabolic bone disease is diagnosed as a result of the fracture, frequently many years after the bone disorder has been in existence and causing the bone loss. In some instances the cause of the bone disorder is also associated with some other visible indication not associated with the skeleton. For instance, hypercortisonism may result in the moon-face and abdominal striae, and sometimes increase in fat deposition in the dorsal region and abdomen, a characteristic appearance which may frequently present before any symptoms related to bone occur. The same may be true of hyperthyroidism; although bone loss is associated with increased thyroxine secretion, weight loss, nervousness, tachycardia, and fatigue are seen very commonly as presenting symptoms. This section on metabolic bone disease will make no attempt to describe the biochemistry of the disease, or the non-skeletal symptoms, but will concentrate on the relationship between the hormone abnormality and its effect on bone turnover and the pathologic processes it produces.

It has already been mentioned that bone disease is almost always associated with bone loss; the presence of too little bone in itself is not symptomatic, and only when fractures or deformity occur do pain and disease accompany the skeletal abnormality. However, two types of bone disease are discussed which are not bone-losing or osteopenic. The first is Paget's disease of bone, which may be either osteosclerotic or osteoporotic but which is not a metabolic bone disease; the other is osteosclerosis, which most frequently presents as osteopetrosis or so-called marble bone disease. Hypothyroidism and hypoparathyroidism are also two metabolic bone diseases which are not characteristically associated with bone loss and fracture, but these are included as part of a discussion of the effects of hormones on bone.

Chapter Nineteen

# PAGET'S DISEASE
# OF BONE

## PAGET'S DISEASE OF BONE: GENERAL COMMENTS

Sir James Paget originally described this bone disease, believing it to be a form of chronic bone inflammation, possibly because of the warmth that is generally associated with the affected area. Since the bone is also abnormal in external contour in most chronic cases, Sir James named the disease osteitis deformans; however, Paget's disease of bone is the term most commonly used. In contrast to other bone diseases discussed in this volume, it is not a metabolic bone disease and is not generalized, but local. Paget's disease of bone can probably be most usefully considered a neoplastic disease, since a number of individuals with the disease go on to develop frank osteogenic sarcomata.

Paget's disease is uncommon in persons under 40 and increases steadily in both men and women with age (Fig. 19–1). There is a hereditary factor which has suggested that the mutant was common in England, since the English, Australians, and New Zealanders (the latter two largely English immigrants) have a high incidence of the disease, while in Asians and Africans the disease is very rare. The symptoms also appear to be more severe in the populations in which the incidence is high.[3]

Sir James originally noted that two of his five cases of osteitis deformans also had bone tumors. Since then, in a large series of Paget's disease, patients have been reported with malignant bone tumors occurring 25 times more frequently than in patients without Paget's disease.[4] The tumors are either osteosarcomas or fibrosarcomas and are found in the sites commonly affected by the osteitis.[3] The tumors are also more malignant than osteogenic sarcomas normally are, and the patients have a decreased survival rate compared with sarcomas in non-Pagetoid patients;

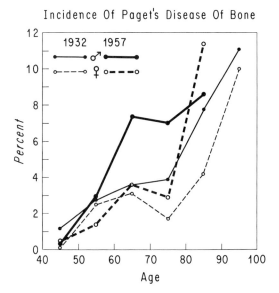

**Figure 19–1**  The incidence of Paget's disease of bone in 1932 and 1957 in men and women. The incidence resembles that of osteogenic sarcoma in that there is an increase with age. Men are more frequently affected than women. (Redrawn from Schmorl[1] and Pygott.[2])

Harris and Krane reported only a 4 per cent survival rate longer than one year.[5] The Pagetoid process itself involves rapid differentiation and a high activity rate of these cells, and there is no reason to suppose that these features of the Pagetoid state are not passed onto the sarcomatous state, resulting in the rapid development of the bone tumors.

**Radiography.**  The x-ray picture is generally easy to diagnose in a patient who has developed enough discomfort to seek medical aid. There is a local area, commonly the pelvis, spine, skull, or a bone of the lower extremity, which has abnormally large periosteal dimensions and appears patchily sclerotic and osteolytic (Fig. 19–2). The pain is most commonly associated with joint involvement, and indeed the sclerotic or early phases of the disease may be asymptomatic. An early and now classic case describes a man who had Paget's disease of the skull and noticed that his hat size got larger and larger. This is a feature of most patients with skull involvement, provided of course that they wear hats.

In the distal limbs particularly, bony involvement will often be accompanied by increase in temperature of the skin. There may also be fractures of the affected bones. This at first appears strange when the radiological picture is most often of sclerosis. The sclerosis is particularly apparent in the trabecular bone and often occurs at the expense of the cortical bone[6] (Fig. 19–3). The shape of the whole bone and the lack of arrangement of the trabeculae result in a loss of biomechanical strength. Microscopically the orientation of the bone and the collagen within the bony fragments contribute to the fragility and loss of elasticity.

**Morphology.**  The earliest phase is one of osteoclastic bone erosion; this occurs rapidly and involves a large percentage of the bone surface in the affected area. The osteoclasts are not only numerous but large and frequently contain many

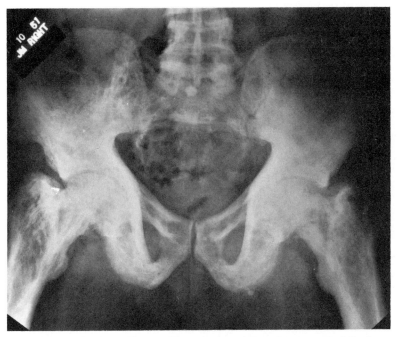

**Figure 19–2**  X-ray of Paget's disease of bone in the pelvis and upper end of the femurs; there is generalized sclerosis and coarsening of the trabeculae and some deformity of the external contours of the bones.

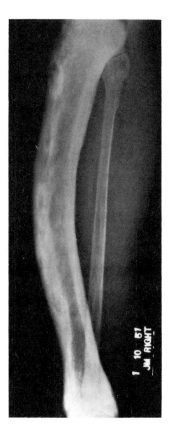

**Figure 19-3** X-ray of Paget's disease of the tibia. One cortex is involved extensively and the cortical bone appears patchily sclerotic and the entire bone is bowed in contrast to the fibula which appears relatively unaffected and undeformed.

nuclei (Fig. 19-4). Compared with other bone disorders (with the exception of secondary hyperparathyroidism in which there is much bone resorption), in Paget's disease the resorption is not two or three times normal, but 10 or 20 times normal[7] (Table 19-1). Although the early phase is of bone resorption, this is soon followed by, and mixed with, osteoblastic bone formation. Both the resorption and formation occur in small areas frequently adjacent to each other (Fig. 19-5). In an area of active Pagetoid involvement 100 per cent of the bone surface may be covered by osteoblasts or osteoclasts; this is a dramatic increase compared with the amount of active surface in normal bone, approximately 2 per cent in the adult. After the osteoclastic phase, the predominantly osteoblastic phase causes the involved bone, which is osteolytic on x-ray and probably of relatively normal external contour, to show the features more typical of the Pagetoid process. When the osteoblastic phase becomes relatively more important, the trabeculae thicken irregularly and new periosteal bone forms, both without any apparent control by piezoelectric forces. The result is an increase in external size of the bone, a porous cortex, and irregular, sclerotic trabeculae (Fig. 19-6).

The diagnosis of Paget's disease on a bone biopsy is usually straightforward and difficult to confuse with any other bone abnormality. Because bone formation and bone resorption are rapid and adjacent processes, small pieces of bone, rather

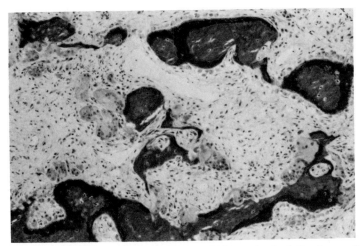

**Figure 19-4** Histological stained section of Pagetoid bone, in the lytic phase with many large osteoclasts containing a large number of nuclei. There are also surfaces of bone covered with dark-staining osteoid and osteoblasts (magnification ×80).

than complete osteones, are formed which have a haphazard appearance, especially when viewed by microradiography or in polarized light (Fig. 19–7). The irregular bone formation and resorption give the bone a patchwork or marquetry appearance during the active phase and also later when both formation and resorption have become less active (Fig. 19–8).

When bone formation exceeds bone resorption and the external deformation becomes visible, there may be neurological symptoms resulting from the bone pressing on the cranial and spinal nerves, causing deafness or neurological weakness distal to the spinal cord involvement. If the skull is markedly lytic, platybasia may occur. The fractures generally are associated with the lytic phase of the disease but may occur at any time because of lack of proper trabecular and cortical bone orientation. The fractures may be partial and frequently occur on the convex side of the bone, unlike the fractures of osteomalacia. If fractures occur and the patient is immobilized, the immobilization itself causes decreased formation and increased resorption and, in association with the high turnover of the Pagetoid bone, may result in hypercalcemia and hypercalciuria.

**Table 19-1  BONE FORMATION AND RESORPTION SURFACES IN PAGET'S DISEASE**

|  | % Formation | % Resorption |
|---|---|---|
|  | mean ± SD | |
| PAGET'S (n = 9) | 10.9 ± 7.0 | 18.0 ± 9.0 |
| CONTROLS (n = 58) | 1.9 ± 1.3 | 3.8 ± 1.3 |

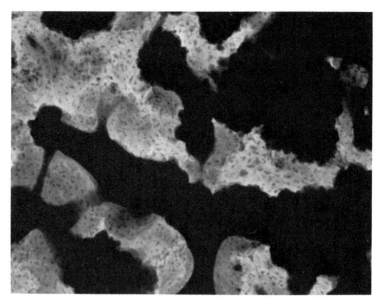

**Figure 19–5** Microradiograph of an area of active Paget's disease. The majority of bone surfaces are in process of active bone formation or resorption (magnification ×75).

The marrow space of an area of Pagetoid bone generally contains many fibroblasts and progenitor cells as well as the osteoclasts and osteoblasts, giving the appearance of mild osteitis fibrosa. As in secondary hyperparathyroidism, it is tempting to speculate that these cells have differentiated and are waiting to become

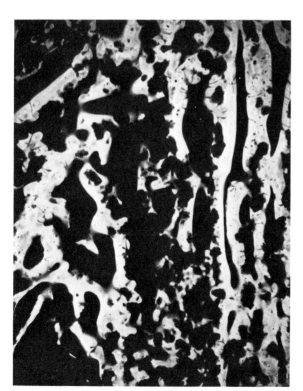

**Figure 19–6** Microradiograph of the lytic phase of Paget's disease of bone during the resorptive activity. The trabeculae are disoriented and fragmentary and the cortex has become largely porous with only a few normal patches of cortical bone remaining (magnification ×13).

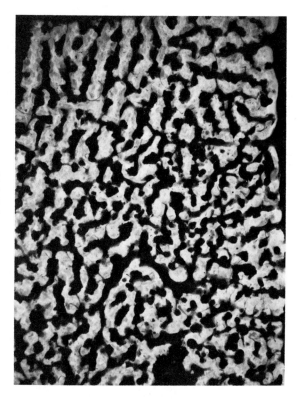

**Figure 19-7** Microradiograph of cortical bone of advanced Paget's disease of bone during the sclerotic phase. Again notice the lack of orientation of the bone (magnification ×12).

active osteoblasts or osteoclasts, since they are especially associated with active formation and resorption areas. The marrow also contains many small blood vessels, which explains the increased temperature of a Pagetoid bone and also the high cardiac output that is characteristic of this disease, particularly when many bones are involved.

**Treatment.** Unlike hyperthyroidism or hypercortisonism, in Paget's disease the offending endocrine gland cannot be removed. Treatment has historically been as unscientific as the understanding of the etiology. Corticosteroids and aspirin have been used with some benefit, based perhaps on the thesis that Paget's disease is an inflammatory reaction. However, the doses required produced undesirable side effects. One of the earliest forms of therapy has been fluoride. A total of 22 patients treated by three different groups of investigators reported relief of symptoms or a fall in urinary hydroxyproline as a result of ingestion of 50 to 60 mg per day of fluoride. A total of three patients treated with 30 mg of fluoride did not show such consistently good results.[8] The use of fluoride is therefore controversial but, on the whole, promising. The action of the fluoride appears to be to stimulate osteoblastic activity, and in the absence of additional calcium for mineralization of the new bone there is an increase in the width and length of the surface of bone occupied by unmineralized osteoid. Osteoclastic activity and osteoblastic activity, indeed, not only activity but the number of cells present, are inhibited by osteoid. As a result, the high cell activity is eventually decreased. It is preferentially decreased in the Pagetoid areas because the osteoblasts rapidly lay down matrix over a large per cent of the surface in such an area; this matrix will remain unmineralized, and therefore bone remodeling will decrease.

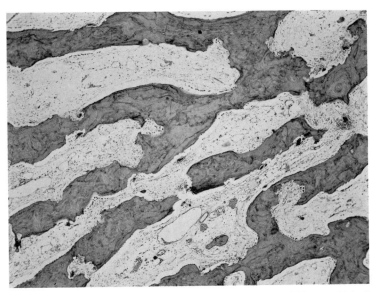

**Figure 19–8**   Demineralized haematoxylin and eosin stained Pagetoid bone which shows relative cellular inactivity but which also shows the marquetry pattern typical of the disease. The cement lines are frequent and irregular and the trabeculae are thick (magnification ×30).

A similar mechanism is the basis of the success of the diphosphonates. The chief difference is that there is no osteoblast stimulation but merely a physical-chemical prevention of all new matrix mineralization, except for the earliest stage of this process, the matrix vesicle formation. Russell and co-workers and Khairi and associates have treated over 100 patients with symptomatic Paget's disease with ethane-1-hydroxy 1–1-diphosphonate (EHDP) in varying doses.[9, 10] Unfortunately, in the first study the initial biochemical values varied such that those on the high doses of EHDP (20 mg/kg/day) had alkaline phosphatase and total urinary hydroxyproline that were about double those of patients on placebo or the low doses.[9] However, the percentage changes bore out the findings of Khairi's investigations that only at 5 mg/kg/day or more of EHDP was there any significant fall in the biochemical parameters or any improvement in the radioactive bone scans. Quantitative morphological studies have invariably shown increases in unmineralized osteoid tissue.[8, 9] Increased amounts of osteoid will obviously also develop in the non-Pagetoid part of the skeleton, but because turnover of bone is much slower in the normal bone, the accumulation of osteoid will be slow. However, the development of osteomalacia must be recognized as a side effect of both fluoride and diphosphonate therapy.

A particular aspect of the development of the osteomalacia is the complication of callus formation if a fracture occurs. The callus will remain unmineralized as long as EHDP treatment is continued, and it will only mineralize when administration of the drug is stopped.

The most commonly used treatment for Paget's disease is calcitonin. Now that salmon calcitonin is available, its use has become practical. The effect of the hormone appears to be on the bone cells, which decrease in activity and therefore result in a depression of the Pagetoid process. There is evidence that osteoclasts, osteoblasts, and therefore surfaces of newly formed osteoid are decreased. These changes are accompanied by a decrease in alkaline phosphatase.[12] Calcitonin also produces hypocalcemia, and a number of studies have demonstrated the development of a secondary hyperparathyroidism with "therapeutic" levels of calcitonin.[13] The osteoclastic and osteoblastic depressive effect of calcitonin must therefore be considered a direct one. Nausea, antibody formation, and the necessity of frequent intramuscular injections are side effects or complications of calcitonin in the treatment of this disease.

It has been mentioned that individuals with Paget's disease frequently develop bone tumors. For this, and for the treatment of Paget's disease itself, mithramycin is possibly the treatment of choice, although its potential toxicity has not made it a popular choice. Alkaline phosphatase and urinary hydroxyproline decrease, as does bone cell activity in the involved areas.[11] Fluoride bone scans and x-rays show improvement. The marked advantage is that the side effects are minimal and remission continues for up to a year after a ten-day infusion of 15 to 25 mg/kg/day of mithramycin. Transient hepatic and renal toxicity are observed in some patients during transfusion but disappear when drug treatment is stopped at the end of the transfusion process. At doses of 25 mg or lower no bleeding has been encountered, although the high doses of mithramycin used for neoplasms have resulted in hemorrhage. The lack of more widespread use of mithramycin lies partly in its universal unavailability and perhaps partly as the result of a fear of the use of a cytotoxic agent in a disease that does not initially present as cancer.

## REFERENCES

1. Schmorl, C.: Über ostitis deformans Paget. Virchows Arch. (Pathol. Anat.), *283*:694–751, 1932.
2. Pygott, F.: Paget's disease of bone. The radiological incidence. Lancet, *1*:1170–1171, 1957.
3. Evans, R. G., and Bartter, F. C.: The hereditary aspects of Paget's disease. JAMA, *205*:900–902, 1968.
4. Price, C. H. G., and Goldie, W.: Paget's sarcoma of bone. J. Bone Joint Surg., *51B*:205–224, 1969.
5. Harris, E. D., Jr., and Krane, S. M.: Paget's disease of bone. Bull. Rheum. Dis., *18*:506–511, 1968.
6. Meunier, P.: La maladie osseuse de Paget. Histologie quantitative, histopathogenie et perspectives thérapeutiques. Lyon Medical, *233*:839–853, 1975.
7. Jowsey, J.: Quantitative microradiography; a new approach in the evaluation of metabolic bone disease. Am. J. Med., *40*:485–491, 1966.
8. Riggs, B. L., and Jowsey, J.: Treatment of Paget's disease with fluoride. Semin. Drug Treat., *2*:65–68, 1972.
9. Russell, R. G. G., Smith, R., Preston, C., Walton, R. J., and Woods, C. G.: Diphosphonates in Paget's disease. Lancet, *1*:894–898, 1974.
10. Khairi, M., Rashid, A., Johnston, C. C., Jr., Altman, R. D., Wellman, H. N., Serafini, A. N., and Sankey, R. R.: Treatment of Paget's disease of bone (osteitis deformans). Results of a one-year study with sodium etidronate. JAMA, *230*:562–567, 1974.
11. Ryan, W. G., Schwartz, T. B., and Perlia, C. P.: Effects of mithramycin on Paget's disease of bone. Ann. Int. Med., *70*:549–557, 1969.
12. Kanis, J. A., Horn, D. B., Scott, R. D. M., and Strong, J. A.: Treatment of Paget's disease of bone with synthetic salmon calcitonin. Br. Med. J., *3*:727–731, 1974.
13. Haddad, J. G., Jr., Birge, S. J., and Avioli, L. V.: Effect of prolonged thyrocalcitonin administration on Paget's disease of bone. N. Engl. J. Med., *283*:549–555, 1970.

# Chapter Twenty

# OSTEOPETROSIS

Osteopetrosis is also called "marble-bone disease" or Albers-Schönberg's disease. It is uncommon, although it may be asymptomatic, and it is therefore difficult to be sure of the frequency.

**Radiology.** The skeletal appearance of osteopetrosis is one of increased bone density which is generally marked (Fig. 20–1). The bones are not only dense but thickened and lack to some extent the remodeled appearance seen in the normal skeleton. This is particularly evident in the long bones, where the cortices are thickened by lack of periosteal remodeling at the metaphyses and lack of endosteal remodeling, which results in a straight bone with often an almost non-existent marrow cavity. One of the accompanying features of osteopetrosis is an enlarged spleen, which attempts to take over the role of the marrow. This is frequently only partially successful, with the result that patients with the disease often appear pale and anemic.

The failure of remodeling may also result in hydrocephalus, exophthalmos, optic nerve entrapment, and consequent blindness. Osteomyelitis is also a common finding in osteopetrosis. Even in the asymptomatic form found in the adult, a failure of remodeling is evident (Fig. 20–2).

Fractures are common in osteopetrosis, a feature which seems difficult to explain in a disorder of increased bone density (Fig. 20–3). However, it appears that remodeling and the ability of the skeleton to be organized along lines of maximum stress and tension are most important. Without this ability the skeleton is structurally weak, despite its increased mass.

**Etiology.** In man two genetic variants have been described which are, on close scrutiny, mainly separable because one is inherited as an autosomal recessive trait while the other is dominant. These two genetic patterns have been called "malignant" and "benign." The malignant, recessive form frequently presents at birth and frequently causes fatal complications, the most common being cranial nerve palsy. The benign form is frequently asymptomatic. If a failure of bone resorption is taken to be the underlying abnormality in both forms of osteopetrosis, the differences may be explained by the exaggerated importance of growth in a disorder characterized by a failure of resorption, which represents as important a part of skeletal development as new bone deposition. Evidence to support this thesis can be seen in the classical case report described by Dent and his colleagues.[1] Symptoms were present at age three weeks, and a radiological diagnosis confirmed at age three months. Treatment consisted of a low calcium intake, dietary vitamin D restriction, and both cortisone and prednisolone. The patient's anemia was treated by blood transfusions. At age four years, cellulose phosphate was

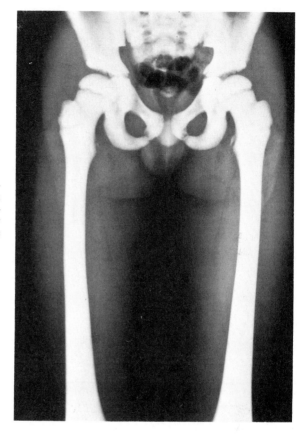

**Figure 20–1** Radiological appearance of the femurs and pelvic girdle of a patient with osteopetrosis. There is almost complete absence of the marrow cavity and lack of remodeling of the femoral neck and acetabulum.

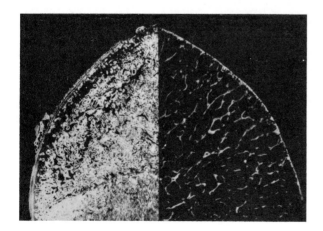

**Figure 20–2** Microradiographs of half a normal femoral head (right) and half a femoral head from a 60-year-old male with asymptomatic osteopetrosis. The increased density, compared with normal, is obvious; remains of an unremodeled epiphyseal plate are also evident. All signs of the physis would normally have disappeared by the age of 25 years (magnification ×1). (From Jowsey, J.: Variations in Bone Mineralization with Age and Disease. In Frost, H. F. (ed.): Bone Biodynamics. Boston, Little, Brown and Company, 1964.)

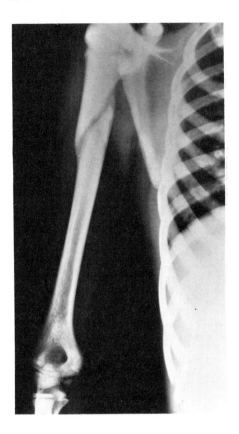

**Figure 20–3** An x-ray of a fracture of the proximal end of the humerus in a 12-year-old boy with osteopetrosis. The fracture has occurred through a dense, sclerotic area of bone, and was caused by the boy throwing a ball in a game at home.

added to his dietary calcium restriction, and for the first time the patient went into negative calcium balance and eventually developed hypocalcemic tetany. The tetany was corrected by injection of large doses of Parathormone and small amounts of vitamin D.[2] The skeleton at age five years showed dramatic bands of dense and relatively normal bone, corresponding to calcium restriction and cellulose phosphate when prednisolone had been withdrawn and a growth spurt had resulted. This single case appeared to show successful treatment of this disease, partly perhaps because of the energetic treatment. Calcium intake was frequently restricted to less than 100 mg daily, and on occasion this was accompanied by 10 g of cellulose phosphate. Later studies, in which two infants were placed on a limited calcium intake, were less successful because the therapy was less aggressive and always accompanied by prednisone, which restricts growth and therefore contradicts any calcium restricted regime. A report from Australia also tends to support the contention that severe calcium restriction (50 mg per day) and cellulose phosphate are a successful form of treatment.[3] It appears, therefore, that the malignant form can be induced to become relatively benign by aggressive therapeutic measures. The most successful form appears to stimulate bone resorption, the failure of which is the underlying cause of this disorder.

   **Morphology.**   Bone from both infants and adults with osteopetrosis appears dense, with thickened cortices containing remnants of mineralized cartilage and many trabeculae. Failure to resorb and replace the epiphyseal growth plate by trabecular bone is also evident (Figs. 20–2 and 20–4). Histologically, there are many osteoclasts present, which seems strange in a disorder characterized by a

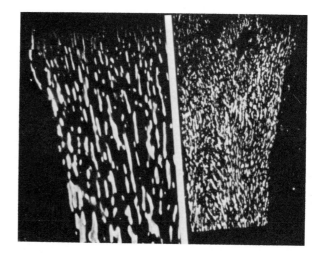

**Figure 20–4** Microradiographs of the proximal end of the tibia of a normal infant (left) and an infant with osteopetrosis (right). There has been a failure of remodeling of the primary spongiosa into secondary spongiosa (magnification ×10). (From Jowsey, J.: Variations in Bone Mineralization with Age and Disease. In Frost, H. F. (ed.): Bone Biodynamics. Boston, Little, Brown and Company, 1964.)

lack of bone resorption (Fig. 20–5). Elegant electron microscopic studies have now shown that the basic defect is that the osteoclasts lack a brush border and are unable to resorb bone. Early theories that osteopetrosis is a disease of increased calcitonin secretion have not been substantiated either by a failure to find increased calcitonin levels in patients with osteopetrosis or by the failure of individuals with medullary carcinoma of the thyroid and high circulating calcitonin hormone levels to exhibit any evidence of increased bone density.

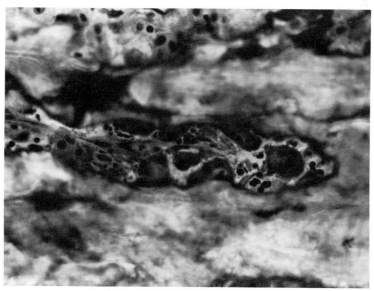

**Figure 20–5** Stained histological section of a patient with early, symptomatic osteopetrosis. The area is from the metaphysis in the zone of the primary spongiosa. There are many multinucleate osteoclasts which are apparently ineffective in resorbing bone (magnification ×400).

**Treatment.** At present the regime used by Dent and co-workers[1] is undoubtedly the most promising. Severe calcium restriction by a low calcium intake and cellulose phosphate administration appears in some way to stimulate osteoclastic activity. Prednisone, since it restricts growth, should probably only be used intermittently. Optic nerve decompression, splenectomy, and blood transfusions have also been used to treat the side effects of the bone disorder.

Many animal models of osteosclerosis exist, including the IA rats, microophthalmic mice, and grey-lethal mice.[4] In osteopetrotic mice, Walker has shown that reversal of the bone changes can be achieved by infusion of bone marrow cells or parabiotic union.[5, 6] Pre-osteoclasts or progenitor cells are presumably transferred from the unaffected to the affected animal and are capable of functioning normally under the influence of the normal hormonal environment present. Ultimately this should become the preferred treatment for osteopetrosis.

## OSTEOSCLEROSIS IN HYPERPARATHYROIDISM

Parathyroid hormone has induced osteosclerosis when given chronically to very young animals. The response is independent of calcitonin and occurs in parathyroidectomized animals; it therefore cannot be the result of endogenous parathyroid suppression.[5] Parathyroid hormone administration results in restoration of normocalcemia after tetany, indicating a response of the bone by a release of calcium.[7]

Although hyperparathyroidism in man is almost invariably associated with increases in resorption of bone and bone loss, occasional cases of what appears to be hyperparathyroidism have been reported in which the radiological picture is one of generalized radiological osteosclerosis (Fig. 20–6). The microradiographic appearance is one of increased cortical thickness and an increase in the number of trabeculae, which is most marked when compared with bone from a patient with "conventional" hyperparathyroidism (Fig. 20–7). The four patients described who had generalized osteosclerosis all presented with hypercalcemia and a decreased serum phosphorus.[8, 9] In instances where serum immunoreactive parathyroid hormone was measured, the values were high normal or above normal, while surgery has revealed parathyroid adenomas (Table 20–1). Serum calcium and phosphorus values fell after removal of the adenomas, and the histology of the glands showed chief cell hyperplasia. It is difficult to avoid a diagnosis of hyperparathyroidism.

Why sclerosis rather than porosis develops in the skeleton is puzzling. It is possible that episodes of chronic, mild hyperparathyroidism in the past in these persons resulted in sustained, though mild, hypophosphatemia, which in turn resulted in a failure of mineralization of bone and osteomalacia; this is borne out by the increased osteoid width found in three of the four cases at the time of biopsy and by the low calcium-phosphorus product. Resorption of unmineralized osteoid is only very slowly carried out by osteoclasts, and these cases may represent the osteosclerosis of osteomalacia; in three of the four patients osteomalacia may have been exaggerated by thiazide and Dilantin treatment.[9] However, the amount of osteoid is not great, and the alternative explanation rests on the finding that parathyroid hormone also has an anabolic effect, which has been shown in dogs.[10] On the other hand, it may be that certain fragmentation of the parathyroid hormone or cell response to the hormone is abnormal in these individuals and results in osteo-

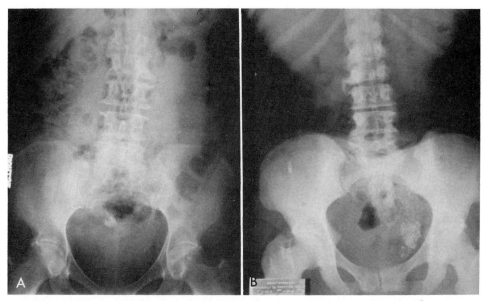

**Figure 20–6** (a) X-ray of the pelvis and lumbar spine of a normal 58-year-old female. (b) X-ray of the pelvis and lumbar spine of a 62-year-old female patient with generalized osteosclerosis associated with hyperparathyroidism. In contrast to osteopetrosis, bone remodeling appears normal. (From Connor et al.[9])

sclerosis. When hypercalcemia develops, the bone cell activity represents the findings typical of hypercalcemic hyperparathyroidism and presumably differs from the cell activity present during the non-symptomatic phase when the osteosclerosis developed.

## OTHER BONE DISORDERS RESULTING IN OSTEOSCLEROSIS

### Hypophosphatasia

Hypophosphatasia is characterized by a low serum alkaline phosphatase with rachitic-like lesions appearing in the skeleton radiologically and histologically. The disease is an autosomal recessive and, although common in some populations (in southern Hungary and the Canadian Mennonites), is generally a rare disorder affecting only 0.001 per cent of individuals. The most severely affected individuals are children, born often with fractures in utero and frank rickets; such infants are sick, and most will die at an early age. Other forms are rare and are characterized by later onset of the disorder and milder expression of the rickets. The only symptoms may be early loss of the deciduous teeth and poor enamel, which leads to cavities.

The biochemical abnormalities are limited to hypophosphatasia, sometimes hypercalcemia with accompanying hypercalciuria, and the presence of phosphoethanolamine in the urine. Serum phosphate and the tubular reabsorption of phosphate is normal. Urinary pyrophosphate is increased and with the low alkaline phosphatase suggests that the etiology of the disease is a failure of the mineralization

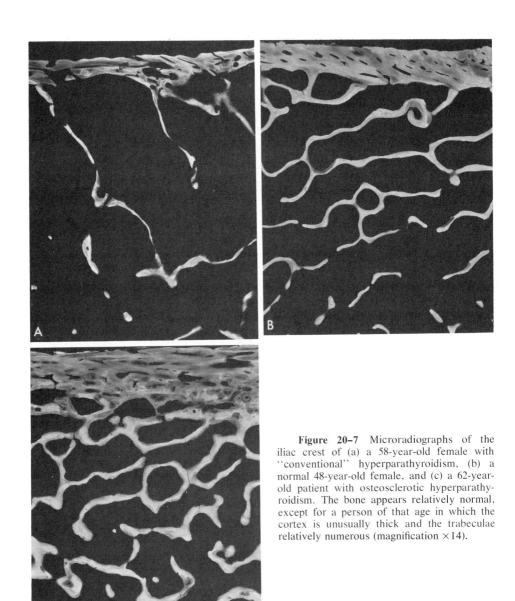

**Figure 20-7** Microradiographs of the iliac crest of (a) a 58-year-old female with "conventional" hyperparathyroidism, (b) a normal 48-year-old female, and (c) a 62-year-old patient with osteosclerotic hyperparathyroidism. The bone appears relatively normal, except for a person of that age in which the cortex is unusually thick and the trabeculae relatively numerous (magnification ×14).

**Table 20–1** BIOCHEMICAL AND BONE HISTOLOGICAL CHANGES IN OSTEOSCLEROTIC HYPERPARATHYROIDISM

| | Patient 1 62 ♀ | Patient 2 55 ♀ | Patient 3 38 ♀ | Patient 4 53 ♀ | Normal |
|---|---|---|---|---|---|
| Serum Ca (mg/dl) | 11.3–12.2 | 10.3–11.2 | 10.3–11.2 | 11.5 | 8.6–10.4* |
| Serum P (mg/dl) | 2.2– 3.0 | 1.4– 3.1 | 1.9– 3.0 | 2.6 | 2.8– 4.3* |
| Parathyroid gland (wt, mg) | 1200 | 1400 | 760 | 900 | — |
| Parathyroid hormone (ng/dl) | 1.5– 2.9 | 1.3– 1.8 | 0.5– 1.0 | — | 0–0.9* |
| Bone resorption (% surface) | 11.8 | 12.0 | 15.6 | 9.3 | 5.1 ± 1.9** |
| Bone formation (% surface) | 1.0 | 0.8 | 3.8 | 5.6 | 2.5 ± 1.5** |
| Osteoid width (microns) | 19.2 | 18.0 | 23.3 | 10.4 | 14.8 ± 2.0** |

  *Range
**Mean ± SD

mechanism which is not dependent on lack of calcium or phosphorus. Bone appears histologically to have wide osteoid borders; the new matrix lacks a mineralization front[11] (Fig. 20–8). The hypercalcemia and hypercalciuria probably reflect the normal or high absorption and lack of deposition of these elements in bone and

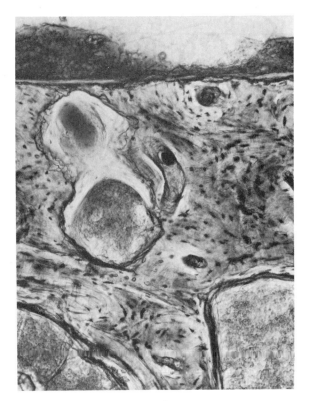

**Figure 20–8** Undemineralized bone section, unstained to show the pale lining of wide osteoid, from an adult patient with hypophosphatasia. The width of the tissue is three or four times normal, and no mineralization front lies between it and the cement line (magnification ×160).

cartilage. The bone biopsy also shows increased amounts of bone resorption, which may account for some proportion of the hypercalcemia and hypercalciuria (Fig. 20–9). The resorption may also be a response to some degree of inactivity secondary to pain and fracture, rather than being an expression of the hypophosphatasia itself.

Corticosteroids and phosphate supplements have been attempted as forms of treatment for no apparent reason and with no success. Gradual spontaneous recovery appears to occur in the late onset forms.

## Melorheostosis

This disorder may present at any age and is seen radiologically as a thickening of the bone.[12] This occurs mainly subperiosteally, although obliteration of the marrow cavity may also occur. One or more bones may be affected, unlike osteopetrosis, and the increased density and thickness of the bone is the result of the deposition of new bone on top of the normal bone beneath. The bone is primitive in appearance and consists in the early stages of metaplastic cartilage; this gradually ossifies and produces bone which is made up mainly of primary haversian systems (Fig. 20–10). The deposition begins at the proximal end of the bone and proceeds distally, somewhat like a massive periosteal reaction (Fig. 20–11).

The disorder is rare and is painful; symptoms generally precede diagnosis and occur most commonly in children and young adults. The etiology is unknown, although injury to a limb in utero has been suggested and would be a reasonable assumption, since melorheostosis occurs frequently at birth.

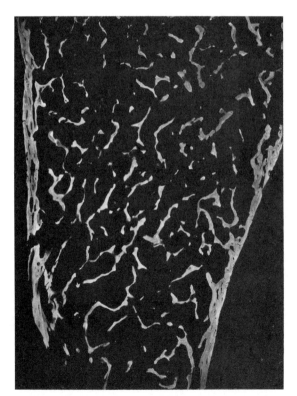

**Figure 20–9** Microradiograph of the iliac crest of a patient with hypophosphatasia. There is evidence of extensive bone resorption and bone loss (magnification ×7).

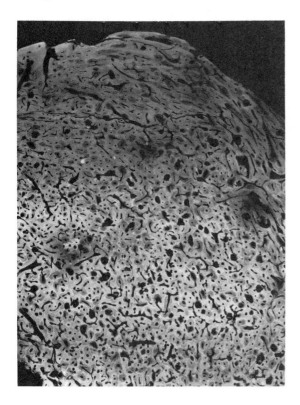

**Figure 20–10** Microradiograph of a cross section of cortical bone of the femur of a patient with melorheostosis. The bone consists mainly of primary haversian bone, particularly on the periosteal surface (magnification ×10).

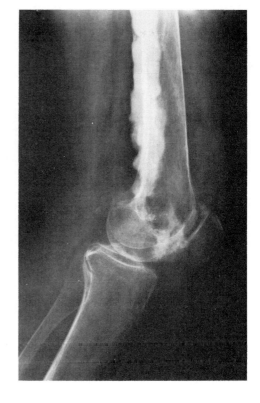

**Figure 20–11** X-ray of the distal femur of the same patient shown in Figure 20–10. The posterior cortex of the femur demonstrates the proliferation of new bone, and the thickened cortex can be seen in the center of the sclerotic mass (magnification ×⅓).

## Osteopoikilosis

The characteristic radiologic appearance of this disorder is one of small dense spots of bone appearing randomly throughout the skeleton, which is otherwise normal. Histologically, the dense bone areas are compact bone. Occasionally, osteopoikilosis may resemble melorheostosis or perhaps present together with this disease. It is an uncommon familial disorder which is inherited as an autosomal dominant. The condition clinically appears painless and uncomplicated.[13]

## Engelmann's Disease

Engelmann's disease of bone, also referred to as hereditary diaphyseal dysplasia, is rare; only 90 cases have been reported, and the sex incidence is equal. The symptoms in some respects resemble those of osteomalacia. There is bone pain and a waddling gait associated with decreased muscle mass, and hypocalcemia has been reported.[14] However, the distinguishing feature is a thickening of the cortices, both on the periosteal and endosteal surface. In two of three cases presented, the father was mildly affected, but familial relation is not apparent in all instances. There may be a failure to grow, and blood abnormalities, such as low hemoglobin, may reflect obstruction of the hematopoietic tissue of the marrow cavity by bone; there may be hepatosplenomegaly on the same basis.

The cortical bone in involved areas show an increase in porosity, although there is an overall increase in cortical width. A large proportion of the bone is immature primary bone (Fig. 20–12). There appears to be an increase particularly in endosteal new bone formation.

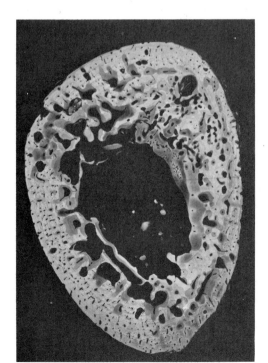

**Figure 20–12** Microradiograph of a cross section of the fibula of a nine-year-old boy with untreated Engelmann's disease. Some periosteal bone and patches of endosteal bone are composed of primitive, primary haversian bone (magnification ×10). (From Allen et al.[15])

Steroids have been used for treatment with success. Large doses of 50 mg per day are often used initially and then rapidly decreased to approximately 5 mg per day.[15] On this regime the muscle weakness disappears, as do the bone pain and morphological abnormalities; secondary haversian systems are formed and the bones remodeled normally. Muscle strength increases and symptoms disappear. Since 5 or 10 mg of steroids per day represents a large dose in a child of 1 to 5 years of age, chronic administration may very well result in steroid osteoporosis and should be carefully monitored. Prevention of the osteoporosis may be necessary if long-term treatment is required.

## Pachyostosis

The term means thick bones, and the radiological picture resembles osteopetrosis except that the "abnormality" represents an adaptation to environment, not a disease. During early evolution, some time after terrestrial life had become well developed, there appeared to be some degree of pressure from a high population density, and a number of mammals returned to the ocean to live. Having developed the mammalian characteristics of warm-bloodedness, they were faced with the problem of heat loss in the relatively cold sea water. Body fat was therefore increased and restricted to sub-dermal sites. The result of increased fat reduced the density of the animal as a whole, and, since the food supply was in the water rather than on top of it, it was necessary for the animals to go down into the sea to find food. A secondary evolutionary adaptation, therefore, was to increase body density; this was achieved by increasing bone mass at the expense of the marrow cavity (Fig. 20–13).

Unlike osteopetrosis, the bone appears to be relatively normal, but, like osteopetrosis, hematopoiesis is carried on primarily in the spleen. Bone is the most dense tissue in the body, and, as a result, the animal becomes heavier and is therefore well adapted to an aquatic life. Whales, dugongs, and manatees are the most common species still living that are pachyostotic, while partially aquatic animals, such as otters, show some degree of pachyostosis, with a narrow marrow cavity which is still functional, rather than one almost completely obliterated, as in

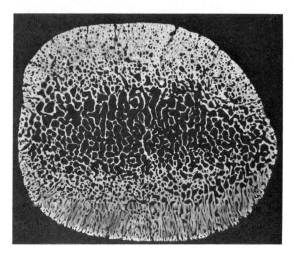

**Figure 20–13** Microradiograph of a cross section of the rib of a dugong. The medullary cavity is almost completely obliterated by trabecular bone (magnification ×4).

the whale; semi-aquatic animals do not sequester all their body fat subcutaneously, but have a normal fat distribution.

The main interest in this phenomenon lies in the ability of the bone to adapt to environmental needs. The more familiar adaptation is the very light bones of birds with intracortical air sacs in addition to the marrow cavity spaces (Fig. 20–14). The adaptation here obviously represents a need to decrease the body weight for easier flight.

Other causes of increased bone density, such as osteomalacia, fibrogenesis imperfecta ossium, and hypoparathyroidism, are discussed in the chapters on osteomalacia and parathyroid bone disease.

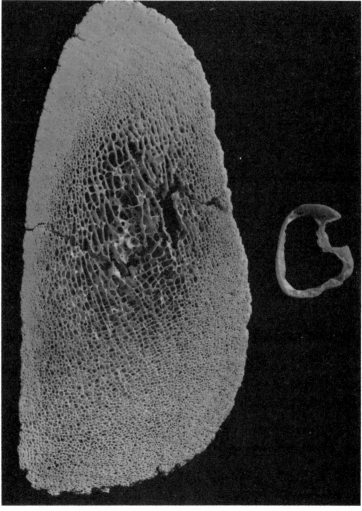

**Figure 20–14**   Macerated thick sections from the rib of a whale, left, and the ulna of a pelican. The whale bone shows almost no medullary cavity, while the pelican has thin cortices with air-spaces within the cortices (magnification ×1.3).

## REFERENCES

1. Dent, C. E., Smellie, J. M., and Watson, L.: Studies in osteopetrosis. Arch. Dis. Child., *40*:7–15, 1965.
2. Moe, P. J., and Skjaeveland, A.: Therapeutic studies in osteopetrosis. Acta Paediatr. Scand., *58*:593–600, 1969.
3. Yu, J. S., Oates, R. K., Walsh, K. H., and Stuckey, S. J.: Osteopetrosis. Arch. Dis. Child., *46*:257–263, 1971.
4. Brown, D. M., and Dent, P. B.: Pathogenesis of osteopetrosis: a comparison of human and animal spectra. Pediatr. Res., *5*:181–191, 1971.
5. Walker, D. G.: Bone resorption restored in osteopetrotic mice by transplants of normal bone marrow and spleen cells. Science, *190*:784–785, 1975.
6. Walker, D. G.: Osteopetrosis cured by temporary parabiosis. Science, *180*:875, 1973.
7. Kalu, D. N., Pennock, J., Doyle, F. H., and Foster, G. V.: Parathyroid hormone and experimental osteosclerosis. Lancet, *1*:1363–1366, 1970.
8. Genant, H. K., Baron, J. M., Straus, F. H., II, Paloyan, E., and Jowsey, J.: Osteosclerosis in primary hyperparathyroidism. Am. J. Med., *59*:104–113, 1975.
9. Connor, T. B., Freijanes, J., Stoner, R. E., Martin, L. G., and Jowsey, J.: Generalized osteosclerosis in primary hyperparathyroidism. Trans. Am. Clin. Climatol. Assoc., *85*:185–201, 1973.
10. Reit, B., Rafferty, B., and Parsons, J. A.: Chronic effects of parathyroid hormone infused to dogs at near-physiological rates. In Kuhlencordt, F., and Kruse, H. P. (Eds.): Calcium Metabolism, Bone and Metabolic Bone Diseases. Berlin, Springer-Verlag, 1975, pp. 362–366.
11. Birtwell, V. M., Jr., Riggs, B. L., Peterson, L. F. A., and Jones, J. D.: Hypophosphatasia in an adult. Arch. Intern. Med., *120*:90–93, 1967.
12. Morris, J. M., Samilson, R. L., and Corley, C. L.: Melorheostosis. J. Bone Joint Surg., *45A*:1191–1 06, 1963.
13. Abrahamson, M. N.: Disseminated asymptomatic osteosclerosis with features resembling melorheostosis, osteopoikilosis, and osteopathia striata. J. Bone Joint Surg., *50A*:991–996, 1968.
14. Stegman, K. F., and Peterson, J. C.: Progressive hereditary diaphyseal dysplasia. Pediatrics, *20*:966–973, 1957.
15. Allen, D. T., Saunders, A. M., Northway, W. H., Jr., Williams, G. F., and Schafer, I. A.: Corticosteroids in the treatment of Engelmann's disease: progressive diaphyseal dysplasia. Pediatrics, *46*:523–531, 1970.

# Chapter Twenty-One

# OSTEOGENESIS IMPERFECTA

## INTRODUCTION

Osteogenesis imperfecta is transmitted as a dominant autosomal trait, although the bone abnormality in this disease varies and has been the basis for dividing affected individuals into a congenita or tarda group.[1] In the congenita form, the skeleton is so severely affected that multiple fractures occur in utero and at birth (Fig. 21–1).[2] In the tarda variety fractures occur generally after weight-bearing and may be associated with trauma; the only consistent finding is the slender bones (Fig. 21–2). More recently, patients with osteogenesis imperfecta have been divided into three, rather than two, groups—mild, moderate, and severe. A cynical observer might suggest that there is in fact a continuum from severely affected neonates born dead with multiple fractures to individuals so mildly affected that they are indistinguishable from the normal population until they sustain a fracture as a result of surprisingly mild trauma.

## CLINICAL, RADIOLOGICAL, AND BIOCHEMICAL FINDINGS

Osteogenesis imperfecta is not uncommon; including both the congenita and the tarda groups the frequency is 0.004 per cent in the general population. The skeletal abnormalities are characterized by thin, slender bones with pencilled cortices, a picture superficially like rickets except that there is no flaring or cupping at the metaphysis, no widening of the epiphyseal plate, and the bones are narrow. In the severely affected cases there are fractures and healing fractures. The fractures heal adequately, with callus formation out of proportion to the small, thin bones, but perhaps normal for fractures of normal bones. The ability to respond to the stimulus of fracture and the equipment to do so appear normal, which contrasts sharply with the abnormal bone metabolism. The vertebrae are frequently decreased in height, either symmetrically or show anterior wedging, not unlike the spinal changes in osteoporosis. As a result, the trunk height is frequently decreased. The skull may be flattened posteriorly, producing the characteristic Tam-o'-Shanter skull.

There are associated clinical findings in this disease, including deafness and poor teeth (dentinogenesis imperfecta), which are related to the general mineral and skeletal abnormalities. Blue sclera have been associated with osteogenesis imper-

**186**

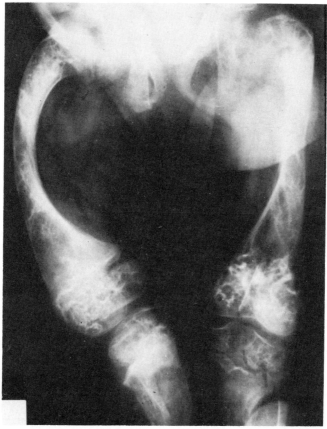

**Figure 21–1**   Radiograph of the lower limbs of a child who has suffered from the malignant form of osteogenesis imperfecta since birth. There are healed and unhealed fractures present and gross deformity of the bone. (From Jaffee.[2])

fecta; however, close examination indicates that although blue sclera are more common in patients with osteogenesis imperfecta than in the general population, blue sclera are most common in mildly affected individuals, occurring in only a little more than 50 per cent of the severe group reported by Bauze,[3] although other investigators have found blue sclera a more common finding.[4]

Loose ligaments and hyperextensible joints are also common in osteogenesis imperfecta patients and, with the blue sclera, suggest a collagen deficiency as the basic defect in this disease. However, definitive proof of such an abnormality is still lacking. Some investigators have demonstrated normal values for urinary and bone hydroxyproline, while others report these values to be above or below normal. Possibly some of the lack of consistency results from the variation in the severity of the disease and from the presence or absence of a recent fracture, since fracture healing occurs effectively and with abundant callus in these patients, and since it is probable that hydroxyproline excretion will reflect the recent incident of a fracture rather than alterations in bone metabolism. Serum parathyroid hormone levels are normal or low normal, nor is any other hormonal abnormality evident.[4] Serum and urine values are normal, as are ascorbic acid and phosphatases.[5]

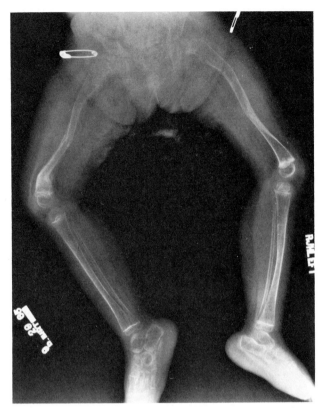

**Figure 21-2**    Radiograph of the lower extremities of a child with osteogenesis imperfecta. The bones are slender and the cortices excessively thin; both femurs have incurred fractures which are partially healed although deformity still exists.

Collagen microstructure appears to be relatively normal in both bone and tissue samples taken from the cornea and sclera of patients with osteogenesis imperfecta with blue sclera. The only demonstrable abnormality appears to be the poor organization of the collagen in the cornea; lamellar structure is poor or absent and the fibers are narrower than normal.[4] Both these findings suggest a primitive and immature form of collagen, and it is tempting to interpret the extraskeletal findings in this way, since the bone morphology is also usefully and realistically explained by a lack of bone maturity.

**Morphology.** While the biochemistry of this disease has yielded nothing definitive, the bone biopsy investigations clearly indicate abnormal bone turnover. Iliac crest bone samples demonstrate many large osteocyte lacunae, a large proportion of primary woven bone, and a marked lack of secondary haversian systems, which is more pronounced in severely affected cases (Fig. 21-3).[4] The presence of primary woven bone is responsible for the large osteocyte lacunae; these have been misinterpreted as representing increased resorption by the osteocytes. The data regarding bone turnover are controversial; Villanueva and Frost reported high bone formation rates using tetracycline labeling, while Riley and co-workers, using histological and microradiographic methods, concluded that bone formation is somewhat low.[4, 6] In any event, either the rate is low or the bone is formed at a nor-

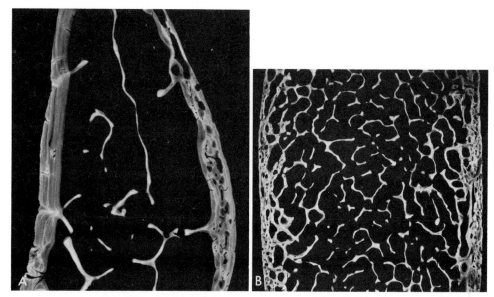

**Figure 21–3** Microradiographs of the iliac crest of (a) a 20-year-old male with osteogenesis imperfecta (tarda). The periosteal dimensions are small, the majority of the cortices consist of unremodeled non-haversian bone and the trabeculae are sparse. (b) A normal 20-year-old male (magnification x 7). (From Riley et al.[4])

mal or high rate but is of an immature kind. The osteoblasts are abnormal in appearance; they are densely staining and are somewhat fibroblastic in appearance, while sheets of connective tissue often lie adjacent to new bone-forming sites (Fig. 21–4). Osteoid border widths are also somewhat diminished (Table 21–1). The impression supported by the bone turnover and collagen data shown in Table 21–1 is

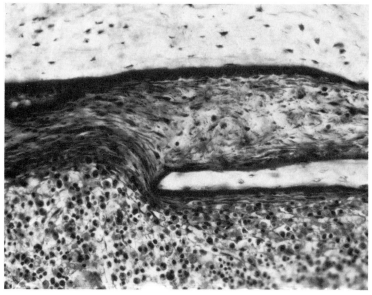

**Figure 21–4** Stained section of the endosteal surface of the cortex from a four-year-old child with osteogenesis imperfecta tarda. The osteoblasts are flattened, darkly staining and look somewhat like fibroblasts. Sheets of fibroblasts and connective tissue lie adjacent to the bone (magnification x 200). (From Riley et al.[4])

**Table 21–1**  BONE MORPHOLOGICAL FINDINGS IN
OSTEOGENESIS IMPERFECTA

|                                    | Normal        | Osteogenesis Imperfecta |
|------------------------------------|---------------|-------------------------|
| Age, years                         | 2–22          | 2–22                    |
| No. osteones/section[*4]           | 78.0 ± 20.1   | 8.6 ± 1.5               |
| Bone formation[*4] % surface       | 4.9 ± 0.7     | 3.6 ± 0.7               |
| Osteoid width[*4] microns          | 14.4 ± 1.3    | 9.5 ± 0.9               |
| Bone resorption[*4] % surface      | 9.8 ± 1.4     | 8.9 ± 1.0               |
| Osteoid fiber width[**7] % control width | 100 ± 3.5 | 28.7 ± 1.32            |

Values mean ± SE (n = 3[**] or n = 11[*])

From Riley et al.[4] and Teitelbaum et al.[7]

that the bone cells lack the messenger system necessary to respond to changes in environment and to stress and that they continue to manufacture, rapidly or slowly, the kind of bone that is laid down only in the early months of uterine life.[4, 6] In the tarda variety the maturity of the bone gradually increases but lags behind that for normal age-matched persons.

**Treatment.** Individuals with osteogenesis imperfecta tarda generally "grow out" of their symptoms as they mature, at which time the bone turnover findings are less abnormal.[4] They are less abnormal partly because remodeling has somewhat increased, but mainly because normal bone turnover is decreased at age 20 compared with age 10. Normal children undergo an intensely active bone remodeling phase characterized by high formation and resorption rates up to the age of 14, a phase which children with osteogenesis imperfecta appear to avoid.

Treatment has proved disappointing.[7, 8] No clearly defined biochemical or hormonal abnormality can be used as a base for some form of treatment; however, all likely therapeutic agents have been investigated.[8] Calcitonin appears to be ineffective, while anabolic steroids, estrogens, and ascorbic acid have been suggested on the basis (wrongly in the case of anabolic steroids and estrogens) that they will stimulate bone formation.[9] They appear to be ineffective. Solomons and colleagues suggested the use of magnesium oxide based on high serum and urinary pyrophosphatase values reported in their patients.[10] No other investigators have been able to reproduce their work or provide evidence of any beneficial effect of magnesium in this disease.

Fluoride has also been used by several investigators and, perhaps surprisingly, has proved totally ineffective.[4, 8] It would appear therefore that the osteoblasts lack the ability to respond to this potent agent as well as to other stimuli, such as stress, normal growth, and maturation. In this light it should be recalled that fracture healing is normal, and the only effective form of treatment still rests on surgical intervention and the production of numerous fractures and intermedullary nailing.

Since the characteristic feature of osteogenesis imperfecta is lack of response to stimuli, such as growth and stress, it is tempting to suggest that there is a deficiency in the cell messenger system. Since fracture healing, a local phenomenon, appears to be normal, it is possible that an intercellular abnormality exists, possibly in the adenyl cyclase system.

## *REFERENCES*

1. McKusick, V. A.: Heritable Disorders of Connective Tissue. St. Louis, C. V. Mosby Co., 1972.
2. Jaffee, H. L.: Metabolic, Degenerative and Inflammatory Disease of Bones and Joints. Philadelphia, Lea and Febiger, 1972.
3. Bauze, R. J., Smith, R., and Francis, M. J. O.: A new look at osteogenesis imperfecta. J. Bone Joint Surg., *57B*:2–12, 1975.
4. Riley, F. C., Jowsey, J., and Brown, D. M.: Osteogenesis imperfecta: morphologic and biochemical studies of connective tissue. Pediatr. Res., *9*:757–768, 1973.
5. Currarino, G., and Brooksaler, F.: Osteogenesis imperfecta. Prog. Pediatr. Radiol., *4*:346–374, 1973.
6. Villanueva, A. R., and Frost, H. M.: Bone formation in human osteogenesis imperfecta, measured by tetracycline labeling. Acta Orthop. Scand., *41*:531–538, 1970.
7. Teitelbaum, S. L., Kraft, W. J., Lang, R., and Avioli, L. V.: Bone collagen aggregation abnormalities in osteogenesis imperfecta. Calcif. Tissue Res., *17*:75–79, 1974.
8. Castells, S.: New approaches to treatment of osteogenesis imperfecta. Clin. Orthop., *93*:239–249, 1973.
9. Winterfeldt, E. A., Eyring, E. J., and Vivian, V. M.: The effect of ascorbic acid on hydroxyproline excretion in metabolic bone disease (abstract). Fed. Proc., *29*:295, 1970.
10. Solomons, C. C., and Styner, J.: Osteogenesis imperfecta: effect of magnesium administration on pyrophosphate metabolism. Calif. Tissue Res., *3*:318–326, 1969.

# Chapter Twenty-Two

# RICKETS AND OSTEOMALACIA

## INTRODUCTION

Rickets is essentially osteomalacia occurring in children,[1] so the two disorders will be considered together, as the patient's age is frequently the only distinguishing feature. In contrast to osteoporosis, in rickets and osteomalacia the bone tissue is qualitatively abnormal in that there are excessive amounts of unmineralized osteoid and, in rickets, also unmineralized cartilage. The deposition of mineral in cartilage and bone requires the presence of adequate amounts of both calcium and phosphorus; serum values for either of these elements that are generally considered abnormally low will result in a failure of new bone mineralization (i.e., serum calcium levels of less than 8.5 mg/dl and serum phosphorus levels of less than 2.5 mg/dl). As a result of lack of bone mineralization the skeleton may become soft in advanced disease, and deformity fractures, or pseudofractures, may occur. The single consistent histological feature is an accumulation of osteoid tissue which replaces normal bone. The osteoid tissue contains a high concentration (95 per cent) of collagen and therefore produces an x-ray image that is denser than that of soft tissue (Fig. 22–1). In addition, resorption of unmineralized osteoid is decreased because osteoclastic resorption of matrix is inhibited and therefore accumulates in abnormal amounts. As a result, the x-ray density of bone in osteomalacia may be increased in some cases, and this is called osteosclerotic osteomalacia. In rickets this is rarely so, because a normal amount of bone has seldom had time to accumulate and because the patient has a combination of osteoporosis and osteomalacia.

## OSTEOPOROSIS AND OSTEOMALACIA

Since the majority of patients with rickets or osteomalacia have developed a mineralization failure as a result of a lack of adequate levels of calcium in the serum, stimulation of the parathyroid glands must be expected. This can occur before, during, or after the development of osteomalacia. When calcium deprivation first occurs, then the serum calcium will fall transiently. Most frequently the fall will be a drop in total serum calcium if vitamin D is implicated, but it may be the result of a decrease in ionized serum calcium if phosphate is involved. The transient fall in ionized serum calcium will stimulate parathyroid hormone secretion,

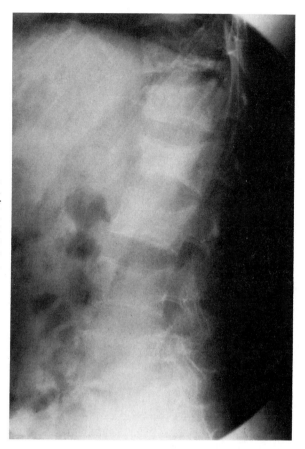

**Figure 22–1** Radiograph of the lumbar and thoracic spine of a 27-year-old male with osteomalacia. A number of the vertebral bodies are collapsed, indicating osteoporosis, but in contrast to osteoporosis, the vertebral bodies are filled with a diffused, somewhat structureless substance and lack the pencilled outline of osteoporosis.

and an increase in bone resorption will return calcium and phosphorus to the blood. Because parathyroid hormone also increases the renal excretion of phosphate, any decreased serum phosphate will be negated by the phosphate coming out of bone. The decreased serum calcium will be compensated for by the release of calcium from bone. The net result will be normal serum and phosphorus values but at the expense of loss of bone. This is the mechanism of the development of osteoporosis (Fig. 22–2). If the calcium deprivation is excessive, as, for example, in a person with a gastrectomy and consequent vitamin D and calcium deficiency, then the parathyroids may not be able to maintain the serum calcium; consequently the serum calcium values fall below that necessary to mineralize bone. Osteomalacia then develops. For this reason, individuals with osteomalacia almost invariably have a previous history, or perhaps just the morphological findings, of osteoporosis (Fig. 22–3). To illustrate this sequence Bloom and colleagues took adult egg-laying hens on a normal diet (i.e., produced a moderately calcium deprived chicken); osteoporosis developed. In an identical group of adult hens, egg-laying was continued, and they were fed a calcium deficient diet. These hens developed osteoporosis and osteomalacia as a result of the excessive calcium loss resulting from a low calcium intake and the necessity of depleting their skeleton for the calcification of the eggshell (Fig. 22–4).[2]

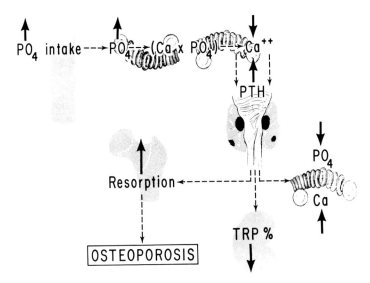

**Figure 22–2** Diagrammatic representation of the mechanism of development of osteoporosis. A high phosphate intake results in postprandial rises in serum phosphate, which eventually cause bone loss.

This has clinical significance, since patients with osteomalacia, in whom the mineralization defect is corrected, will very likely have osteoporosis, even after successful treatment for osteomalacia. The exception is hypophosphatemic osteomalacia, in which the mineralized bone mass may be normal. Unless the individual has a chronic mineralization defect, for example, vitamin D-resistant rickets, the disease may be non-symptomatic as far as the bone is concerned until a significant proportion of bone is composed of osteoid and stress fractures occur.

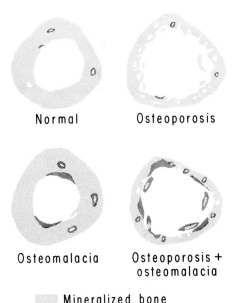

**Figure 22–3** Diagram representing the development of osteoporosis and osteomalacia. The vast majority of symptomatic osteomalacic patients have first developed osteoporosis.

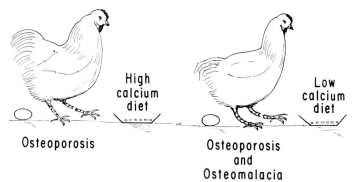

**Figure 22–4** Illustrative description of the comparison of osteoporosis and osteomalacia. Osteoporosis, shown by the fractured leg, may develop in the chicken laying eggs daily on a high or normal calcium intake. If a low calcium intake is substituted the osteoporosis will develop and be followed by osteomalacia, shown by the fracture of one leg and the bowing of both.

## Osteomalacia

**Clinical Presentation.** Patients most frequently present with bone pain and may have a waddling gait, particularly if they are heavy. Indeed, the somewhat overweight osteomalacic or rachitic patient may present with symptoms before biochemical evidence of the disease is present; however, this rarely occurs, and symptoms are generally accompanied by an elevated alkaline phosphatase and other biochemical abnormalities. Muscle weakness, probably the cause of the waddling gait, can be pronounced and associated with proximal limb girdle myopathy. Since the weakness responds very dramatically to vitamin D treatment, it has been suggested that it is the result of ionized calcium deficiency combined with lack of vitamin D, which may be responsible for transferring calcium across muscle cell membranes.[3]

X-rays of rachitic patients show a failure of mineralization of cartilage at the physes and the joint surfaces, which are consequently widened (Fig. 22–5). Lack of mineral in the cartilage prevents osteoclastic or chondroclastic resorption of the hypertrophic zone of the cartilage, with the result that hypertrophic cartilage accumulates in large amounts. Even after mineralization of the cartilage occurs, followed by remodeling and ossification, islands of unremodeled cartilage frequently remain in the metaphyseal bone (Fig. 22–6). On the x-ray this results in a patchy, lytic appearance in the metaphysis and occasionally in horizontal bars of high mineral density, which represent partially mineralized cartilage. The x-ray also illustrates the point made in Figure 22–3, that there is associated osteoporosis; a failure of resorption on the periosteal surface of the cortex gives an appearance of flaring. Increased resorption is responsible for the thinness of the cortices and the sparse appearance of trabeculae in areas of spongy bone. Osteoporosis, resulting in an attempt by the parathyroids to maintain the serum calcium at a normal level, almost invariably precedes the development of the osteomalacia. When clinical osteomalacia eventually develops and the parathyroids can no longer maintain a normal serum calcium, osteoid is formed and results in a lack of both calcium and phosphorus being released from bone, therefore permitting the hypophosphatemia resulting from the effect of parathyroid hormone on the kidney to become biochemically evident. At this stage the phe-

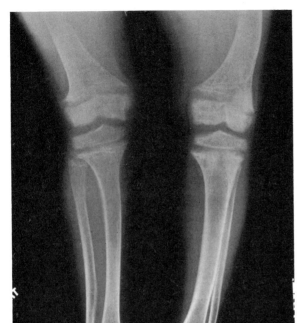

**Figure 22–5** Radiograph of an eight-year-old boy with rickets, showing the widened physes and flared periosteal surface. The cortices are thin and there are signs of bowing of both femurs. The pencilled cortices are a typical radiological feature of osteoporosis, while the normal width of the bones distinguish the appearance of rickets from osteogenesis imperfecta.

nomenon is graced with the name "secondary hyperparathyroidism." The christening depends on the arrival of abnormal biochemical findings and generally gross histological abnormalities.

In both rickets and osteomalacia, the osteoporosis, followed by the accumulation of large volumes of unmineralized osteoid, results in weakened bones. Stress produces the typical partial fractures of Looser zones (also called Milkman pseudofractures). The fractures may go completely across both cortices, but if they only cross one, it is almost invariably the concave side of the bone. The defects are often bilaterally symmetrical, appearing most frequently in the ribs (20 per cent), femoral neck (18 per cent), femoral shaft and pubic rami (15 per cent), and scapulae (10 per cent).[4] (The percentage figures represent the frequency with which the fractures occur in each site.)

Nutrient arteries and veins go through the cortices at this point, and it is very likely that the small hole through which the vessels travel is just wide enough to make such a point comparatively weak. The whole bone is weakened by the osteomalacic process, and the hole is the "last straw." The bone collapses at this point, producing the rather unusual features of the fracture with a sclerotic margin and often the protruded lips at the periosteal surfaces. These two features represent the compression of the bone along the stress line (Fig. 22–7).

Looser zones or pseudofractures heal slowly because the two processes necessary for bone remodeling are absent — the resorption of the collapsed fragments and the mineralization of any new osteoid that is deposited in the fracture callus. The

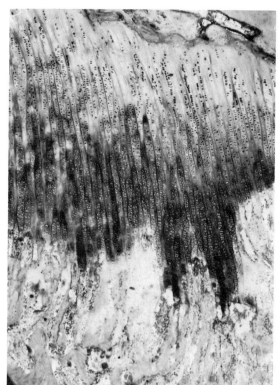

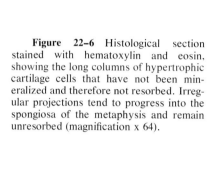

**Figure 22-6** Histological section stained with hematoxylin and eosin, showing the long columns of hypertrophic cartilage cells that have not been mineralized and therefore not resorbed. Irregular projections tend to progress into the spongiosa of the metaphysis and remain unresorbed (magnification x 64).

resorption is prevented by the newly deposited callus, consisting of unmineralized osteoid tissue which inhibits osteoclastic activity. The failure of mineralization also prevents the callus from appearing as an area of increased density on the x-ray.

**Biochemical Features.** The biochemical abnormalities include an elevated serum alkaline phosphatase and often a low serum phosphate (Table 22-1). Alkaline phosphatase is involved in the mineralization of bone in a way still not completely understood, and a failure of mineral deposition results in an accumulation of alkaline phosphatase in the serum, resulting in high values in the majority of patients. The serum phosphate decrease is the result of increased parathyroid hormone secretion and consequently an increase in the renal excretion of phosphate, which is expressed also in the low TRP%. As long as the bone has a reasonable proportion of mineralized surface tissue, the serum calcium remains normal. However, when significant accumulation of osteoid occurs, then the serum calcium tends to fall and may be low normal or below normal. The values that are within the normal range may, in fact, be abnormally low for that particular individual, although still above the level considered abnormally low for the laboratory values of a particular hospital. The low calcium occurs in the face of parathyroid hormone and hypophosphatemic-induced stimulation of the hydroxylation of 25-OH vitamin D to the metabolite 1-25 (OH) vitamin D, which would tend to increase the intestinal absorption of calcium. This adaptive mechanism is obviously unable to function in the absence of vitamin D, therefore the patient with vitamin D deficiency osteomalacia is the one most prone to present with hypocalcemia.

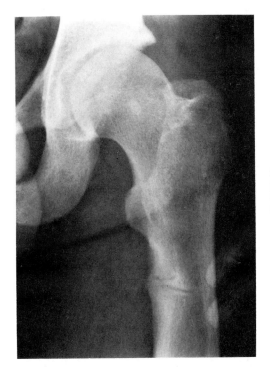

**Figure 22–7** Radiograph of a femur of an individual with osteomalacia and a pseudofracture on the medial side of the femoral shaft. Bone adjacent to the fracture lines is sclerotic representing collapse of bone.

Persons who have had osteomalacia for some time frequently have a low urine calcium because of the effect of parathyroid hormone on calcium retention by the kidney, and also because the available mineral reservoir is "depleted" both by osteoporosis and by the covering of the bone by osteoid.

Urinary hydroxyproline may be elevated; this is a reflection of the stimulated parathyroid gland activity and consequent bone resorption.

**Bone Morphology.** Osteomalacia is one of the clearest diagnoses to make from a bone biopsy, provided an undemineralized section is available. Demineralized bone, even if very carefully and incompletely demineralized, can be misleading because the lighter pink borders may represent newly formed bone matrix that either was, or was not, mineralized before the sample was put in the demineralizing fluid. A stained or unstained mineralized section leaves no doubt as to the area that contains no mineral and, in addition, a mineralization front will be apparent, if present.

The following four stages in the development of osteomalacia are chronologically evident as the failure of mineralization persists:

1. The disappearance of the mineralization front occurs first, since that is the zone of new bone mineralization. The border between the osteoid and the mineralized bone loses the granular line where the initial mineralization step is taking place and is replaced by a hard line separating the unmineralized and completely mineralized old bone tissue.

2. As the osteoblasts continue to produce osteoid which remains unmineralized, the second stage, an increase in osteoid border width, occurs. In normal individuals osteoid width is 15 microns, with a maximum reading rarely above 20 microns. In patients with symptomatic osteomalacia the osteoid border width is frequently more than 20 microns in width and also lacks a mineralization front (Fig. 22–8).

**Table 22–1** BIOCHEMICAL VALUES IN OSTEOMALACIA; ALL HAD
SYMPTOMS AND MORPHOLOGICAL EVIDENCE OF OSTEOMALACIA

| | Normal Value (Mean & Range) | No. of Patients | Value in Osteomalacia (Mean & Range) | % Above Normal (Mean) | % Below Normal (Mean) | % Normal (Mean) |
|---|---|---|---|---|---|---|
| **SERUM** | | | | | | |
| Alkaline phosphatase, U/L | 48 (23–65) | 44 | 113 (30–470) | 79.5 | 18.1 | 2.3 |
| Phosphorus, mg/dl | 3.5 (2.5–4.5) | 44 | 2.9 (1.3–4.0) | 20.5 | 70.5 | 9.1 |
| Calcium, mg/dl | 9.65 (8.9–10.1) | 44 | 9.2 (7.0–10.3) | 29.5 | 59.1 | 11.4 |
| iPTH, $\mu$l eq/ml | 22 (undetectable to 40) | 12 | 74.8 (9–240) | 83.3 | 16.7 | 0 |
| **URINE** | | | | | | |
| Calcium. mg/24 hrs | 133 (<263) | 30 | 89.6 (3.4–220) | 23.3 | 76.7 | 0 |
| Phosphorus, mg/24 hrs | 1001 (590–1742) | 26 | 678.8 (358–1167) | 23.1 | 76.9 | 0 |
| %TRP | 87 (>80%) | 7 | 74.9 (36–91) | 14.3 | 71.4 | 14.3 |

Patient population: mean age 55.7 yrs.
Out of 44 patients:
10 patients had had previous gastrectomy;
 3 patients were on anticonvulsant medication;
 1 patient had milk intolerance.
Other causes were sprue, colitis, malabsorption, and unknown.

3. Eventually the osteoblasts stop laying down matrix and dedifferentiate, and the osteoid does not thicken further but remains unmineralized and inactive. The third phase therefore is of the appearance of unmineralized osteoid not in the process of bone formation, generally called inactive osteoid.

4. Osteoblasts form elsewhere on the bone surface and lay down osteoid which also fails to mineralize, increases in thickness, and then becomes inactive. The fourth phase then is one of an increase in the length of bone surface covered by wide osteoid borders. This phase continues until more and more of the bone is covered by unmineralized osteoid. The accumulation of unmineralized osteoid tends to prevent osteoclastic bone resorption and the osteoid builds up both by being deposited and by a failure of removal by normal osteoclastic remodeling. In chronic osteomalacia this can lead to "osteosclerosis," a dense appearance on x-ray which is explained by the increase in bone matrix which absorbs x-rays significantly more effectively than the adjacent soft tissue (Fig. 22–1). Phase 4 is almost always accompanied by biochemical and often by radiological manifestations of osteomalacia.

If osteomalacia has existed for some time, and particularly if the incidences of mineralization failure have been intermittent, the osteoid may become partially

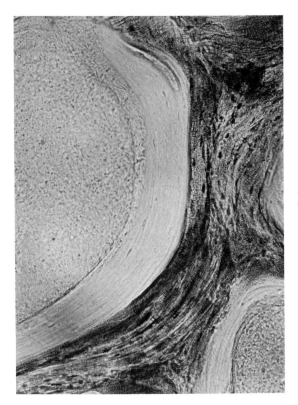

**Figure 22–8** A mineralized section of bone, unstained, showing a border of osteoid which is of increased width and lacks a mineralization front between it and the bone surface (magnification x 160).

mineralized. However, there seems to be a period of time in which calcium and phosphorus can be deposited in the matrix, followed by a period which may last for perhaps many years, when the matrix becomes unmineralizable. This property results in areas of bone, generally related to the microanatomy of the osteones, which are incompletely mineralized and which appear as dark zones in the microradiographs. If an individual has had osteomalacia that has been corrected, and if normal mineralization is taking place, areas of incomplete bone mineralization may still be seen (Fig. 22–9). The patient can then be described as being presently normal but as having experienced a previous episode of osteomalacia.

**Etiology.** Since osteomalacia most frequently represents an exaggerated form of calcium lack, which in a milder form will cause osteoporosis, it is to be expected that there will be a number of factors that cause both diseases. This will present as osteoporosis, as yet uncomplicated by osteomalacia, or as osteomalacia with underlying osteoporosis. Of the various causes for rickets or osteomalacia, most can be related to vitamin D deficiency or to an abnormality of metabolism of this hormone (Table 22–2). A smaller group consists of the osteomalacic individuals who lack sufficient phosphorus for bone mineralization. It should be stressed, as is evident by omission in Table 22–2, that calcium deficiency is not a cause of osteomalacia.[1] In the presence of adequate vitamin D, increased absorption of calcium from the intestine in the presence of a low calcium intake and parathyroid hormone induced bone resorption may result in osteoporosis but will not progress to clinically evident osteomalacia.

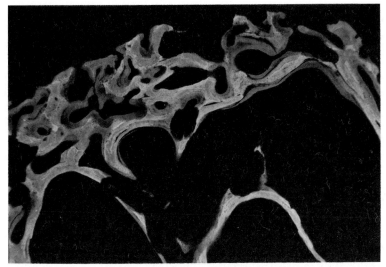

**Figure 22–9** Microradiograph from the rib of an adult female with nutritional osteomalacia which has been cured by a correct diet. There are areas of low density within the bone conforming to the orientation of the bone, which represent the bone laid down at the time of an excessively low calcium intake, and subsequent failure of mineralization (magnification x 75).

Vitamin D deficiency is rare in the United States because vitamin D supplements are added to a large variety of commonly used foods, such as milk, some cereals, bread, and so on. Americans on the whole tend to expose themselves to sunshine, a tanned skin indicating wealth or a recent holiday. In other parts of the world, vitamin D is not usually added to food, deficient diets are common (China,

**Table 22–2** ETIOLOGY OF RICKETS OR OSTEOMALACIA

**Lack of calcium for mineralization**
1. VITAMIN D DEFICIENCY
   (a) dietary deficiency
       vegetarians; low vitamin D intake
       lactase deficient with no vitamin D supplement
   (b) environmental vitamin D deficiency
       excessive protection from the sun
           social customs (excessive clothing)
           "allergy" to sunlight
   (c) man-made
       gastrectomy: steatorrhea and lack of vitamin D
       phenobarbitone administration
           abnormal 25-OH vitamin D metabolism
   (d) disease
       severe liver disease: no 25-OH vitamin D
       severe renal disease or no kidneys: no $1–25(OH)_2$ vitamin D
       malabsorption: idiopathic steatorrhea, non-tropical sprue

**Lack of phosphorus for mineralization**
   (a) "phosphate diabetes"
   (b) adult onset hypophosphatemic osteomalacia, tumor associated osteomalacia
   (c) phosphate binding agents causing dietary phosphate depletion
   (d) severe hyperparathyroidism, as in renal failure (causing a low serum phosphorus)

Japan), sunlight is scarce or tangential (Scotland, Finland), or a tanned skin or exposure of skin is a social stigma of low class (Spain, Bedouin Arabs). Table 22–3 illustrates the large variety of ways in which vitamin D deficiency can occur in normal people, expressed as levels of the first metabolite, 25-OH-vitamin D. The data on the submariners suggest that vitamin D storage is not as effective as was originally supposed and that deficiency can develop relatively rapidly, while the Asian immigrants in Glasgow and Birmingham illustrate a new and relatively large population of persons with vitamin D deficiency.[5, 6, 7, 8] These persons had high alkaline phosphatase, low urine calcium, and low serum vitamin D.[5] The bone biopsies showed increased amounts of osteoid. The predominantly vegetarian diet, the relative lack of sunshine, and the high phytate intake have all been blamed for the vitamin deficiency.

Removal of dietary phytates will cause an improvement in the biochemical signs of osteomalacia;[6] however, nutritional and dietary vitamin D deficiency has been described in poor persons living in north Indian slums.[9] Symptoms are found almost exclusively in women, and the osteomalacia is apparently the result of a combination of the social custom of confining themselves to their houses and protecting their skin from sunlight with excessive clothing. If all cases of vitamin D deficiency were to be reviewed, the single factor of lack of exposure of the skin to sunlight, frequently due to covering the body almost completely with clothing, would appear to be the most important element. The presence of phytates alone cannot be blamed, although they may be the precipitating factor in some populations.[8] The same etiology explains the vitamin D deficiency in geriatric patients who do not consume vitamin D–supplemented food. Their exposure to sunlight is minimal, and vitamin D levels are consequently low. Chalmers and his co-workers reported a series of 34 women and three men presenting with osteomalacia.[4] All the men and 16 of the women had had total or partial gastrectomies, which probably accentuated the vitamin D deficiency. Nevertheless, elderly persons, otherwise in good health, are prone to develop osteomalacia as a result of lack of this essential hormone.

A vegetarian diet and, in the United States, lactase deficiency and dislike of dairy products may produce osteomalacia if associated with environmental vitamin D deficiency;[1] however, such an etiology is rare, although, when more obvious causes of deficiency have failed to explain the cause of the bone disease, such an etiology is worth exploring and the disease is generally easily remedied.

Table 22–3   SERUM 25-OH VITAMIN D LEVELS IN
VITAMIN D DEFICIENCY

| Group of Persons | 25-OH Vitamin D (ng/dl, mean ± SE) |
| --- | --- |
| Submariners – 2 month patrol, n = 7 | 7.9 ± 1.2 |
| Asians living in England, n = 1; | undetectable |
| Asians living in Glasgow, n = 24; | 3.3 ± 0.4 |
| Asians living in country near Glasgow, n = 24; | 5.9 ± 0.8 |
| Geriatric patients as they entered Middlesex Hospital, n = 21 | 4.9 ± 1.0 |
| Normals from London and Glasgow, n = 51 | 12.1 ± 0.8 |

Data from Preece et al.[5]

Gastrectomy as a cause of osteomalacia is controversial. Probably the majority of patients with a total or partial gastrectomy develop only osteoporosis and rarely osteomalacia. However, osteomalacia can be a complication, and it has been reported to occur in as many as 25 per cent of patients. Vitamin D is a fat soluble vitamin and is therefore lost in the feces if there is significant steatorrhea. Vitamin D loss also occurs in cases of non-tropical sprue and in patients with pancreatitis and biliary disease because of the disruption in fat metabolism and absorption in these diseases.

Phenobarbitone administration for the treatment of epilepsy is a more recently documented cause of both osteoporosis and osteomalacia. Early studies in rats suggested an abnormality of vitamin D metabolism resulting from an effect of barbiturates on liver microsomes and therefore on the hydroxylation of vitamin D. Recent evidence suggests that there is a partial failure of the first hydroxylation step, and patients treated with dilantin or phenobarbitone have high vitamin $D_3$ or $D_2$ levels but inappropriately low 25-OH vitamin D levels (Table 22–4).

Since the liver and kidney are the organs which convert vitamin D to the active hormone, it is obvious that disease of both these organs will affect the production of the hormone. Because of the feedback machanisms of vitamin D, severe liver disease and nephrectomy are necessary to produce significant vitamin D deficiency that will result in bone abnormalities or symptoms.

**Treatment.**   The treatment of any vitamin D deficient bone disease rests on the correct diagnosis. If the osteomalacia is caused by dietary lack of vitamin D, a normal diet containing vitamin D will correct the disease.[1] If a defect in vitamin D metabolism is established, administration of the appropriate metabolite will be successful; i.e., $1-25(OH)_2$ vitamin D (or its more easily available $1 \alpha$ 25-OH analogue) will be successful in the treatment of anephric patients. In some instances, even when a metabolite abnormality has been documented, as in Dilantin-treated epileptic patients, vitamin $D_3$ will be successful, since a proportion of the vitamin will be hydroxylated and the feedback mechanisms will assure maximum effectiveness of the 25-OH form that is produced.[10]

In patients who are vitamin D deficient because of malabsorption due to sprue or gastrectomy, treatment with oral vitamin $D_3$ will not be successful. The simple solution is to administer vitamin $D_2$ by exposing the patients to ultraviolet light, artificial where necessary, sunlight where this is available.

Appropriate vitamin D treatment will "cure" osteomalacia, often rapidly and dramatically. If osteomalacic osteosclerosis is present, then complete mineralization of the osteoid may take a long time, since chronic osteomalacia will frequently

**Table 22–4**   VITAMIN D LEVELS IN THE PLASMA OF NORMAL CHILDREN, CHILDREN TREATED WITH ANTICONVULSANT DRUGS, AND CHILDREN WITH LIVER DISEASE (values mean ± SD)

| | No. of Subjects | Age in Years | Cholecalciferol (CC) ng/ml | 25 OH CC ng/ml | Ratio CC:25-OHCC |
|---|---|---|---|---|---|
| CONTROLS | 15 | 3–12 | 13.2 ± 6.7 | 31.4 ± 17.5 | 2.8 ± 1.5 |
| DILANTIN TREATED | 25 | 3–16 | 55.7 ± 30.3 | 34.1 ± 23.8 | 0.6 ± 0.3 |
| LIVER DISEASE | 5 | children | 18.1 ± 13.2 | 10.4 ± 6.9 | 0.7 ± 0.2 |

From Glorieux, et al.[10]

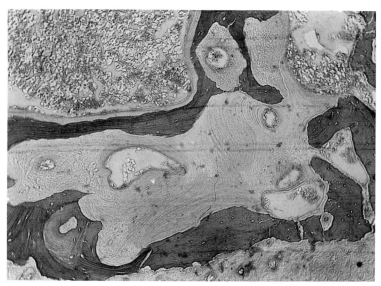

**Figure 22–10** Stained, mineralized section of bone showing the small fraction of dark-staining mineralized bone and a large proportion of pale unmineralized matrix. It is evident that successful mineralization of this matrix will result in restoration of a large volume of bone which will probably result in symptomatic relief of bone pain (magnification x 100).

result in large volumes of unmineralized matrix (Fig. 22–10). This will require large quantities of calcium and phosphorus to be deposited in it before the mineralization of the osteoid is normal or before biochemical responses are normal. Successful treatment of the osteosclerotic osteomalacia should result in approximately normal amounts of bone. However, if, as is most often the situation in the United States, the osteomalacia is complicated by previous osteoporosis, the patient will then be osteoporotic and will have to be treated for this disease subsequently. On the other hand, any patient with "osteoporosis" who is "cured" with vitamin D most certainly has osteomalacia as the predominant disease.

## REFERENCES

1. Stanbury, S. W.: Osteomalacia. J. Clin. Endocrinol. Metab., *1*:239–266, 1972.
2. Bloom, W., Nalbandov, A. V., and Bloom, M. A.: Parathyroid enlargement in laying hens on a calcium-deficient diet. Clin. Orthop., *17*:206–209, 1960.
3. Chalmers, J.: Osteomalacia. J. R. Coll. Surg. Edinb., *13*:255–275, 1968.
4. Chalmers, J., Conacher, W. D. H., Gardner, D. L., and Scott, P. J.: Osteomalacia—a common disease in elderly women. J. Bone Joint Surg., *49B*:403–423, 1967.
5. Preece, M. A., Tomlinson, S., Ribot, C. A., Pietrek, J., Korn, H. T., Davies, D. M., Ford, J. A., Dunnigan, M. G., and O'Riordan, J. L. H.: Studies of vitamin D deficiency in man. Q. J. Med. (new series), *44*:575–589, 1975.
6. Ford, J. A., Colhoun, E. M., McIntosh, W. B., and Dunnigan, M. G.: Biochemical response of late rickets and osteomalacia to a chupatty-free diet. Br. Med. J., *3*:446–447, 1972.
7. Ford, J. A., Colhoun, E. M., McIntosh, W. B., and Dunnigan, M. G.: Rickets and osteomalacia in the Glasgow Pakistani community, 1961–1971. Br. Med. J., *2*:677–680, 1972.
8. Swan, C. H. J., and Cooke, W. T.: Nutritional osteomalacia in immigrants in an urban community. Lancet, *2*:456–459, 1971.
9. Vaishnava, H., and Rizvi, S. N. A.: Vitamin-D deficiency osteomalacia in Asians (letter to the Editor). Lancet, *2*:621–622, 1973.
10. Glorieux, F. H., Delvin, E. E., and Dussault, M.: Evaluation of liver hydroxylation of vitamin D by simultaneous measurement of circulating cholecalciferol (CC) and 25-hydroxycholecalciferol (25-HCC). Trans. Orthop. Res. Soc., *1*:123, 1976 (abstract).

# Chapter Twenty-Three

# UNUSUAL FORMS
# OF OSTEOMALACIA

Eight other forms of osteomalacia are occasionally encountered which do not fall under the previous heading of the more common form of this disease, and which have distinct features which allow them to be classified separately.

## FIBROGENESIS IMPERFECTA OSSIUM (FIO)

This bone disorder was first described by Baker in 1956, and only four cases have been reported since.[1, 2] The patients described have been between 60 and 70 years old and include four men and one woman. The biochemical findings are generally unremarkable. The x-ray is abnormal but in no clearly distinct way and has been most frequently described as Paget's disease. The bone biopsy, however, appears to be distinctly different from both Paget's disease of bone and from any other form of osteomalacia. In fact, it has been questioned whether fibrogenesis imperfecta ossium should be classified as osteomalacia. However, unmineralized matrix is present, Therefore, at least morphologically, it falls under the heading of osteomalacia.

Bone biopsies demonstrate wide osteoid borders which lack the birefringence of normally deposited collagen (Fig. 23–1). Unlike Paget's disease, the arrangement of the osteones is normal and regular. The lack of birefringence is explained by a disordered arrangement of the collagen fibrils. The disease appears to be acquired, since previously healthy adults develop the disease fairly late in life, and the bone biopsy shows abnormal bone lying on top of normal bone.

The disease appears to be one of a defect in matrix production, in some ways not different from the changes produced by lathyrism. There is a greater solubility of collagen in both FIO and lathyrism, although in lathyrism, skin and other connective tissue collagen appear to be affected, while in FIO only the bone is abnormal. The lack of mineralization appears to be secondary to the matrix defect.

Treatment with vitamin D, and with A.T. 10 has been tried in three patients and appears to be only partially effective; symptomatic improvement may represent the natural history of the disease, about which little is known.

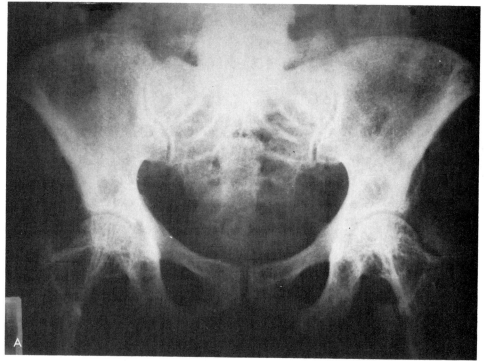

**Figure 23–1**  (a) Radiograph of the pelvis of a 66-year-old female patient with fibrogenesis imperfecta ossium. There is symmetrical involvement of the pelvis and femurs characterized by coarse trabeculation.

*Legend continued on opposite page*

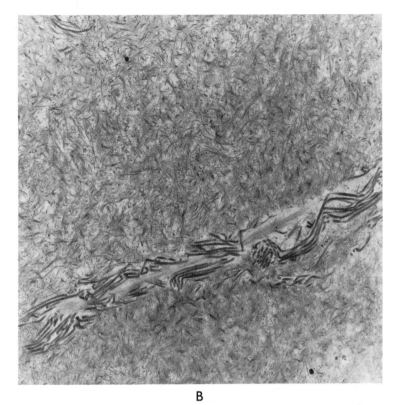

B

**Figure 23–1** *Continued* (b) Electron microscopic appearance of the collagen in the same patient as Figure 23–1(a), showing a narrow band of normal collagen fibrils with adjacent abnormal collagen fibrils which lack the cross-banding and orientation of the normal collagen (magnification x 18,900). (From Swan, C. H. J., Shah, K., Brewer, D. B., and Cooke, W. T.: Fibrogenesis imperfecta ossium. Quart. J. Med., *45*:233–253, 1976. By permission of Oxford University Press.)

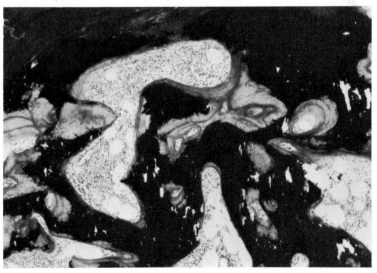

C

**Figure 23–1** *Continued* (c) von Kossa stained section of mineralized bone section from the pubic ramus from the same patient as Figure 23–1(a). The trabeculae are thickened and there are many areas of undemineralized, pale-staining osteoid within the normally mineralized matrix. Such areas do not show birefringence with polarized light (magnification x 64). (Material courtesy of Dr. W. T. Cooke.)

## "AXIAL OSTEOMALACIA"

Three males between the ages of 60 and 75, complaining of spine or rib pain, presented with radiological evidence of a coarse trabecular appearance in the spine, pelvis, and ribs.[3] No biochemical abnormalities or pseudofractures were associated with the radiological findings, and, like fibrogenesis imperfecta ossium, the classification depended on the finding of osteomalacia in the bone biopsy. The coarsened trabeculae were likened to the x-ray appearance of Paget's disease, as in the cases of fibrogenesis imperfecta ossium. However, the description is also reminiscent of fluorosis, as is the increase in osteoid border width. The appearance of the coarsened trabeculae in the spine, pelvis, and some ribs is particularly reminiscent of fluorosis. No history of fluoride exposure was reported, however, and no attention apparently was given to mild fluorosis as an alternative diagnosis to a description of what may or may not be a new disease. Neither was the presence or absence of osteoid established in cortical bone, where it would be unlikely to show radiographically but, if present, would make the name of the disorder inappropriate. In the original report by Frame and co-workers[3] in 1961, abnormalities of serum calcium, phosphorus, and alkaline phosphatase were not associated with the disease, which distinguishes it from more advanced, generalized osteomalacia.

## DIPHOSPHONATE-INDUCED OSTEOMALACIA

Disphosphonates are deposited in bone matrix and prevent mineralization of new bone. As for fibrogenesis imperfecta ossium and axial osteomalacia, the use of the term osteomalacia depends on the finding of excessive amounts of osteoid tissue in the bone biopsy rather than the characteristic symptoms of osteomalacia in the patient. Although the serum alkaline phosphatase is high, calcium and phosphorus are not low, but rather elevated. As in FIO and "axial osteomalacia," the osteomalacia cannot be explained on the basis of lack of calcium or phosphorus; a normal matrix in which mineralization is almost totally prevented is the basic defect in diphosphonate-induced osteomalacia. It is reversible when diphosphonates are withdrawn and mineralization of the osteoid occurs in an apparently normal fashion. However, 100 times the normal dose of vitamin D or calcium fails to reverse the abnormality if diphosphonate administration is continued. (For further discussion see Chapter Twenty-Eight, Osteoporosis, discussion under Treatment.)

## VITAMIN D–DEPENDENT HYPOCALCEMIC RICKETS

Vitamin D–dependent rickets appears to be a different entity from vitamin D–deficient rickets. The former disorder is inherited as an autosomal recessive and, unlike hypophosphatemic rickets, responds well to large doses of vitamin D.

**Clinical, Radiological and Biochemical Abnormalities.** Hypocalcemia and mild hypophosphatemia with elevated alkaline phosphatase are the biochemical features of the disease, and there may be a negative calcium balance. Radiographically, the bone lesions are characteristic of rickets and show widened spaces between the epiphysis and metaphysis. Patients present with growth failure and with signs of tetany accompanied by muscular weakness and often with positive Trousseau and

Chvostek signs. There may also be poor enamel development. Serum parathyroid levels are raised in untreated patients, presumably a response to the hypocalcemia.

Although large doses of vitamin $D_2$ or $D_3$ are necessary to cause healing of the rickets, smaller doses of 25-OH-$D_3$ are effective. Even more effective is 1–25-$(OH)_2D_3$ ($1\alpha$, 25-$(OH)_2D_3$ has been the precise metabolite used); the abnormality can be corrected using 200 to 900 times less than the dose of 25-OH-$D_3$ required to produce the same results.[4] It is reasonable to conclude therefore that the metabolic aberration is a failure of the second hydroxylation of vitamin D to 1,25-$(OH)_2$ vitamin D in the kidney. The evidence points to a genetic defect in 25-hydroxycholecalciferol-1-hydroxylase.

**Treatment.** $1\alpha$, 25-$(OH)_2D_3$ is the treatment of choice, since the block to hydroxylation of 25-OH $D_3$ in the kidney is bypassed by providing the active metabolite. This causes increased calcium absorption and a positive calcium balance; serum phosphorus and calcium both rise, the calcium because of the direct effect of the vitamin D metabolite, and the phosphorus because of a decrease in secondary hyperparathyroidism, since serum parathyroid hormone levels decrease to normal levels.

## HYPOPHOSPHATEMIC RICKETS OR OSTEOMALACIA

**Radiological and Biochemical Findings.** Failure of mineralization as a result of a lack of phosphorus is an infrequent cause of bone disease. Of the various causes, vitamin D–resistant rickets is probably the most common. It is a sex-linked dominant trait with variable penetrance, occurring more frequently in males than females. It may be severe in children but often becomes less so as the individual becomes older. The x-ray appearance is like that of vitamin D–deficient rickets except that thin bones (osteoporosis) less frequently accompany the osteomalacia, for obvious reasons.

The outstanding biochemical abnormality is the low serum phosphorus, which is caused by a failure of reabsorption of phosphorus in the kidney and a resulting low %TRP. In some patients calcium infusion has resulted in a partial rise in serum phosphorus, which suggests that the parathyroids may be responsible for at least part of the phosphaturia. Hyperplastic parathyroids have also been reported, which tends to favor this as a mechanism. However, parathyroid hormone immunoassay studies show that this hormone is only elevated in some patients. It is possible that only in some do the parathyroids complicate the phosphate loss; however, it is also possible that the phosphate diuretic hormone that Dent described as being a part, both functionally and structurally, of parathyroid hormone plays a role in this disease.[5] A fraction of parathyroid hormone that is responsible for the renal phosphaturic effect and not recognized by immunoassay may be being secreted, and this would account for all the features of this disease—the low serum phosphorus and consequent mineralization defect—while the high ionized calcium would explain any tendency for extraskeletal ossification.

The hypophosphatemia also causes a failure of growth of the individual. This may, at times, mask the severity of the disease and also explain why the symptoms tend to decrease in adulthood.

**Morphology.** A large volume of unmineralized osteoid, accompanied by the microradiographic appearance of mineralization defects, is almost pathognomonic of vitamin D–resistant rickets. Since the disease is hereditary, all the bone is affected to some degree, in contrast to adult onset osteomalacia. Perhaps the most characteristic feature is the lack of mineral around the osteocytes, suggesting a failure of mineralization which persists despite more complete mineralization in the surrounding bone (Fig. 23–2). Failure of osteoclastic resorption of osteoid will often lead to osteomalacic osteosclerosis; however, where mineralized bone lies on the marrow or periosteal surface of the bone, osteoclasts can usually be found in abundance.

**Treatment.**    Phosphate, administered by infusion or orally, will cause temporary increases in serum phosphate and improvement in the rickets. However, the bone disease is generally severe, and there may be half or more of the skeleton which lacks mineral. If relatively normal serum phosphate levels can be maintained, then the serum calcium will tend to fall; in fact, aggressive treatment with phosphate infusions may precipitate hypocalcemic tetany. For this reason vitamin D and calcium supplements are often used in conjunction with the phosphate supplements. Careful measurements of serum calcium, as well as serum phosphorus, are therefore necessary. It is obvious from Figure 22–10 that treatment must be continued for a long time before the radiological, symptomatic, and biochemical findings become normal. The amount of unmineralized osteoid in the entire skeleton may be equivalent to two thirds of the total skeletal matrix complement. This amount of osteoid would require approximately 500 g of calcium and an equivalent amount of phosphorus. Even with a positive calcium balance of 300 mg per day, three years or more would be necessary to produce a normal skeleton under these circumstances.

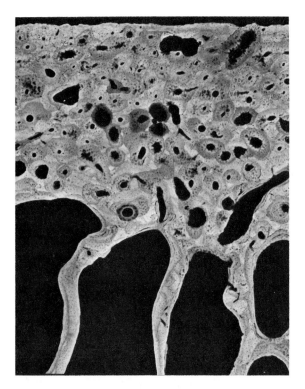

**Figure 23–2** Microradiograph of cortical bone from an individual with Vitamin D–resistant rickets. Around many of the osteocytes are areas of low mineral density indicating a failure of mineralization (magnification x 18).

## ADULT ONSET HYPOPHOSPHATEMIC OSTEOMALACIA

If it is accepted that in vitamin D–resistant rickets the primary defect is one of increased renal excretion of phosphate, then adult hypophosphatemic osteomalacia is similar except that it is not hereditary; it appears spontaneously in adult life and has been associated with a tumor that may either be in bone or be extraskeletal.

**Clinical and Biochemical Findings.** The youngest patient to be reported with this condition was the original 17-year-old girl described by Prader and associates in 1959;[6] other patients have been adults. The patients present with a remarkable degree of bone pain and muscle weakness, particularly in light of the frequently mild changes seen radiologically. In fact, in the three patients who are reported in Table 23–1, a suggestion of hysteria had been documented at some time or other. The most consistent and, in fact, the only biochemical abnormalities are the low serum phosphate, which is frequently 1.0 mg/dl, and the low %TRP (Table 23–1). Since the serum calcium is normal and the serum phosphate low, the ionized calcium is presumably high and the undetectable value for serum parathyroid hormone in one patient is not surprising. However, the parathyroid hormone value is important in that it exonerates the parathyroids as being the cause of the increased renal secretion of phosphate and proves that the glands are responding appropriately to the ionized calcium. The high ionized calcium may in fact explain the severe pain that is a feature of the disease; free calcium plays a major role in nerve conduction.

Perhaps the most striking feature is the finding of a tumor in these patients which, if successfully removed, results in complete remission of the disease and a return to normal of the biochemical abnormalities.[7] The serum phosphate may in fact be somewhat high in the initial stages of recovery, presumably because parathyroid hormone secretion has been suppressed and the gland takes some time to return to normal function. The %TRP returns to normal, as does urine phosphorus, and serum parathyroid hormone rises to detectable, normal levels.

**Table 23–1** BIOCHEMICAL AND BONE MORPHOLOGICAL PARAMETERS IN ADULT HYPOPHOSPHATEMIC OSTEOMALACIA

| | Patient 1 (38 yr. ♂) | Patient 2 (30 yr. ♂) | Patient 3 (47 yr. ♀) | Normal Range |
|---|---|---|---|---|
| SERUM Ca mg/dl | 9.4 (10.0)* | 9.8 (9.7)* | 9.3 | 8.9 to 10.1 mg/dl |
| SERUM P mg/dl | 1.3 (4.7)* | 1.2 (4.0)* | 1.4 | 2.5 to 4.5 mg/dl |
| SERUM iPTH μl eq/ml | — | Undetectable (normal) | — | up to 40 μl eq/ml with a normal Ca |
| TRP% | 23 (81)* | 46 (86)* | — | >80 |
| OSTEOID WIDTH microns | 35.0 | 33.5 (13.2)* | 26.4 | 15 (10–20) microns |

( )* Values after removal of the tumor.

**Morphology.** The majority of the bone in the bone tissue which has been examined appears to be normal, as would be expected in a disease that presents most often in adulthood. However, the width of unmineralized osteoid is clearly increased (Fig. 23–3). The tumors that have been removed have been found in the femur, the ribs, or in the soft tissues of the leg (groin and behind the knee). They have been described as sclerosing hemangiomas or granulomas and may contain bone. If undemineralized tumor tissue is evaluated for osteomalacia, the tumor is found to have the same osteomalacic appearance with wide osteoid borders as is seen in the bone biopsies.[7]

**Etiology.** The disease is rare; nine cases with associated tumors have been reported in the literature, although at least twice as many instances of acquired adult osteomalacia have been described in which no associated tumor could be found. However, the tumors may be small (one or two centimeters or less in size) and it is not impossible that all acquired hypophosphatemia is associated with a tumor, and that the tumor is not peripheral or superficial and therefore is not found. From the theoretical point of view, the finding of tumors in approximately one third of all cases of acquired hypophosphatemia must be more than a coincidence and strongly suggests that a tumor is present in all instances of this disease and is the cause of the disease.

Although the amino acid sequence of the substance contained in or secreted by the tumor has not been established, it is presumed that the tissue makes a hormone that increases the renal excretion of phosphate. The hormone may be similar in structure to the fraction of parathyroid hormone that increases the renal excretion of phosphorus.

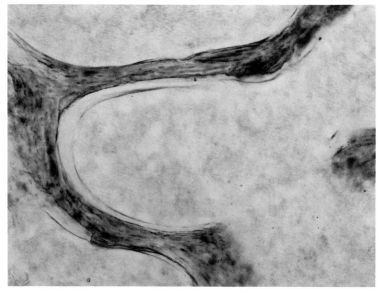

**Figure 23–3** Unstained, mineralized section from a patient with adult onset hypophosphatemic rickets. The translucent border of osteoid is of increased thickness, the osteoid covers a large proportion of the bone surface and there is no mineralization front between the matrix and the mineralized bone (magnification x 64).

## PHOSPHATE BINDING AGENTS

A small number of otherwise normal persons have been reported to have taken large doses of aluminum hydroxide, generally as an antacid. In the instances where osteomalacia has developed, the intake clearly has been many times above the prescribed therapeutic dose.[8] Such individuals present with all the signs and symptoms of osteomalacia. Hypophosphatemia is usually marked, and, presumably, in the presence of a normal total serum calcium, the ionized calcium is high. As a consequence, parathyroid gland activity is suppressed, and the urinary calcium is high. Reduction in the ingestion of phosphate binding agents is a successful remedy.

Phosphate binding agents are also used for the treatment of the hyperphosphatemia of renal failure to compensate for the inability of the kidneys to secrete appropriate amounts of this ion. Hypophosphatemia has been known to develop in such patients but generally for only short periods, since there is a strong metabolic tendency toward hyperphosphatemia operating at all times.

## HYPOPHOSPHATEMIA IN HYPERPARATHYROIDISM

There have been a number of reports of clinically evident osteomalacia in patients with hyperparathyroidism. Stanbury has summarized these recently, and it is perhaps more than a coincidence that the reports are from Europe rather than from the United States.[9] In Europe vitamin D deficiency is relatively common.

**Clinical and Biochemical Features.** The patients present with the symptoms and radiological signs of osteomalacia, while the biochemical findings indicate mildly elevated or even normal or low serum calcium levels and serum phosphorus values are usually depressed. Alkaline phosphatase is high and the urinary calcium normal or low. These biochemical values may vary from time to time in any one individual, which suggests that perhaps hypercalcemic hyperparathyroidism develops into hypocalcemic hyperparathyroidism as a result of the low serum phosphate which causes osteomalacia. It is at this stage that the urinary calcium may be very low, probably as a result of the failure of the skeleton to release mineral into the serum.

**Etiology and Treatment.** The presentation is at first difficult to distinguish from vitamin D–deficiency osteomalacia except that vitamin D administration results in hypercalcemia, even when the dose of vitamin D is moderate. Stanbury has suggested that the syndrome is, in fact, vitamin D–deficiency osteomalacia with associated secondary hyperparathyroidism, which after a long period of time develops into an "autonomous" hyperparathyroidism. The absence of consistent hypercalcemia can be explained by the presence of unmineralized osteoid and the consequent inability of the parathyroid hormone, even at increased levels, to release calcium from a skeleton "sealed" by so much osteoid.

**Morphology.** The morphology appears to be a mixture of osteomalacia and hyperparathyroidism.[9] There are brown tumors and fibrous connective tissue replacement of the marrow spaces, which is characteristic of hypercalcemia hyperparathyroidism. Non-symptomatic osteomalacia, evident only on bone biopsy by an increase in width of osteoid borders, is frequently found as in the more classical instances of hyperparathyroidism. In mild forms the presence of a low serum

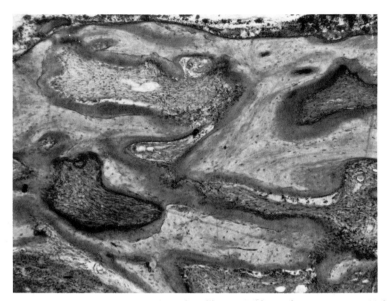

**Figure 23–4**  Stained, mineralized section of an iliac crest biopsy from a 69-year-old female with primary hyperparathyroidism who developed osteitis fibrosa, hypercalcemia, and bone loss, followed by normo- and hypocalcemia and a gross increase in osteoid (darkly stained), which is thicker and increased in amount to the point that almost no mineralized bone surface is available for osteoclastic resorption (magnification x 80).

phosphorus (secondary to the action of the hormone on the renal excretion of phosphate) accompanied by a minimally elevated serum calcium level results in the failure of mineralization. In more severe, chronic forms, the microradiographic and histological pictures are of extensive bone loss, fibrosis, osteoclasts, and a large proportion of surface covered by inactive osteoid (Fig. 23–4).

**Treatment.**  Vitamin D administration is not only useful diagnostically but also should correct the bone disease by decreasing the osteomalacia. It is also possible that a period of hypercalcemia will result in suppression of the hyperparathyroidism, and the feedback response will return to normal.

## REFERENCES

1. Baker, S. I.: Fibrogenesis imperfecta ossium: a generalized disease of bone characterized by defective formation of the collagen fibres of the bone matrix. J. Bone Joint Surg., *38B*:378–417, 1956.
2. Swan, C. H. J., and Cooke, W. T.: Fibrogenesis imperfecta ossium. Excerpta Medica, International Congress Series No. *270*:465–468, 1973.
3. Frame, B., Frost, H. M., Ormond, R. S., Hunter, R. B.: Atypical osteomalacia involving the axial skeleton. Ann. Intern. Med., *55*:632–639, 1961.
4. Fraser, D., Hooh, S. W., Kind, H. P., Holick, M. F., Tanaka, Y., and DeLuca, H. F.: Pathogenesis of hereditary vitamin D-dependent rickets. N. Engl. J. Med., *289*:817–822, 1973.
5. Dent, C. E.: Some problems of hyperparathyroidism. Br. Med. J., *2*:1495–1500, 1962.
6. Prader, A., Illig, R., Uehlinger, E., et al.: Pachitis infolge Knochentumors. Helv. Paediat. Acta, *14*:554–565, 1959.
7. Salassa, R. M., Jowsey, J., and Arnaud, C. D.: Hypophosphatemic osteomalacia associated with "nonendocrine" tumors. N. Engl. J. Med., *283*:65–70, 1970.
8. Dent, C. E., and Winter, C. S.: Osteomalacia due to phosphate depletion from excessive aluminium hydroxide ingestion. Br. Med. J., *1*:551–552, 1974.
9. Stanbury, S. W.: Osteomalacia. J. Clin. Endocrinol. Metab., *1*:239–266, 1972.

# Chapter Twenty-Four

# THYROID BONE DISEASE

## HYPOTHYROIDISM

Bone disease that causes pain and discomfort is not generally a feature of hypothyroidism; however, there are profound alterations of bone remodeling and a clearly impaired ability to respond to fluctuations in serum calcium. In animal studies, complete thyroidectomy with the parathyroids left intact resulted in a reduction of bone formation and resorption to values near zero (Table 24–1).[1] Parallel with the reduction in bone turnover and responsible for the impaired ability to maintain normal serum calcium levels is a decreased response to exogenous parathyroid hormone. In these studies both bone remodeling and the response to parathyroid hormone were completely restored with thyroxine (Table 24–1). It can be concluded therefore that calcitonin plays no role in either the bone or calcium homeostasis changes induced by thyroidectomy. Williams and co-workers came to the same conclusion in a group of thyroxine-replaced thyroidectomized patients.[2] The data in adult man and animals at first glance appear to be contradictory to the report of Hirsch and Munson, who found that significant hypercalcemia occurred in calcium-loaded rats who had been thyroidectomized.[3] Since the thyroidectomy was performed only five minutes before the calcium load was given, the animals could not have become physiologically hypothyroid, and the lack of precise control of the hypercalcemia at short times may be explained in terms of calcitonin.

The decrease in resorption of bone seen in hypothyroidism is also reflected in the decreased hydroxyproline and low radiocalcium kinetic values found in this disorder.[4, 5] Bone biopsies in hypothyroid patients, as in thyroidectomized animals, also show a decrease in bone resorption and bone formation, an alteration in bone turnover that can be expected to cause little change in the skeleton or any symptom related to its role in the support of the body.[6] Presumably, thyroxine deficiency results in a decreased metabolic activity of bone cells as well as of other cells in the body, and the low turnover of bone in hypothyroidism reflects only a generalized effect of this hormone on cell activity.

## HYPERTHYROIDISM

In contrast to hypothyroidism, hyperthyroidism, or thyrotoxicosis, may present with bone symptoms and osteoporosis. Thyroidectomized animals given

Table 24–1  SERUM AND BONE MORPHOLOGY CHANGES IN
HYPER- AND HYPOTHYROID DOGS (mean ± SD)

| Group n = 6 | Serum Ca mg % | Serum Thyroxine g/100 ml | Bone Form % Surface | Bone Resp. % Surface | Serum Ca % Increase c̄ PTH |
|---|---|---|---|---|---|
| Control | 9.8 ± .08 | 1.1 ± 0.6 | 3.30 | 3.63 | 11.3 ± 1.7 |
| Hypothyroid | 10.1 ± .07 | 0.2 ± 0.2 | 0.02 | 0.24 | 3.7 ± 1.2 |
| Thyroxine replaced (0.3 mg thyroxine) | 9.8 ± .06 | 1.3 ± 0.6 | 2.98 | 2.76 | 15.6 ± 1.3 |
| Hyperthyroid (5 mg thyroxine) | 10.1 ± .10 | 10.4 ± 3.8 | 11.70 | 9.11 | 22.4 ± 2.3 |

From Jowsey and Detenbeck.[1]

excess thyroxine have elevated levels of both resorption and formation and an exaggerated response to exogenous parathyroid hormone administration. They also demonstrate an increase in the capability to control fluctuations in serum calcium, either hypo- or hypercalcemia (Table 24–1).[1]

Kinetic analysis and bone biopsies in human beings mirror the findings in animals. Thyroxine appears to stimulate the activity of the osteoclasts and osteoblasts, just as lack of the hormone diminishes it (Table 24–2). The effect appears to be direct, since thyroxine administration will affect calcium and bone in the absence of both parathyroid hormone and cortisone. The osteoclast appears to be somewhat more sensitive to the hormone than the osteoblast, so bone resorption predominates in this disease, and bone is lost in the majority of cases. The morphology is not unlike that of osteoporosis, except that formation is almost always elevated rather than being only occasionally so. Because resorption exceeds formation, the bone becomes porous (Fig. 24–1). The porosity can be seen radiologically as a loss of trabeculae and a tunneling within the cortex.[8] It is of interest that the subperiosteal resorption of cortical bone, which is characteristic of hyperparathyroidism, is not seen in hyperthyroidism, although "osteitis fibrosa" has been reported at least in trabecular bone.[9] Resorptive activity by the periosteum seems to be a finding in states of increased parathyroid hormone alone, as noted in Chapter Twenty-Seven, Hyperparathyroidism.

As a consequence of the elevated osteoblastic bone formation level, there is an increase in the amount of osteoid. In earlier reports this finding had led to the suggestion that patients with hyperthyroidism have osteomalacia.[10] However, neither of the morphological criteria of osteomalacia, increased width of osteoid or the

Table 24–2  BONE TURNOVER IN HYPERTHYROIDISM (mean ± SD)

| | No. of Subjects | Bone Formation (% surface) | Bone Resorption (% surface) | Osteoid Width (microns) |
|---|---|---|---|---|
| Controls, age 25–50 | 26 | 2.0 ± 1.1 | 3.5 ± 0.9 | 16.1 ± 2.4 |
| Hyperthyroid, age 25–53 | 8 | 5.0 ± 3.3 | 10.2 ± 1.7 | 13.5 |

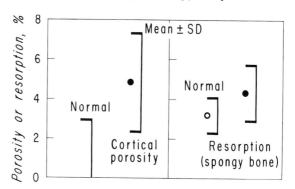

**Figure 24–1** Cortical porosity and trabecular bone resorption in patients with hyperthyroidism compared with age-matched normals. (Redrawn from Bianchi et al.[7])

presence of inactive osteoid, occurs, and the abundant osteoid merely reflects increased bone tissue deposition; the osteoid is of normal width and is always associated with osteoblasts.[11] The increased ability of the skeleton to respond to calcium depletion and calcium loads can probably also be explained on this basis. An increased number of bone cells are already differentiated and available to respond to hormonal stimulation.

Patients with hyperthyroidism tend to have high serum calcium and phosphorus levels. Adams reports a group of ten hyperthyroid patients with a mean serum calcium of 9.7 mg/dl, compared with a normal of 9.3 mg/dl; similarly serum phosphorus was high (4.0 mg/dl, compared with 3.2 for euthyroid controls) although serum calcium and phosphorus were above normal in only one out of the ten patients.[11] The raised serum phosphorus may be the cause of the decreased calcium absorption found in hyperthyroid patients, since elevated phosphorus will impair the renal hydroxylation of 25-OH vitamin D to 1–25 vitamin D.

Since serum albumin is low normal, ionized calcium is raised and produces a relative hypoparathyroidism, which may be the cause of the raised serum phosphorus. The mild hypoparathyroidism may also account for the hypercalciuria associated with hyperthyroidism, since diminished parathyroid gland secretion would result in low tubular reabsorption of calcium.

A less explicable relationship appears to exist between hyperthyroidism and hyperparathyroidism in that several patients with hyperthyroidism have coexisting hyperparathyroidism, and vice versa. The incidence of hyperthyroidism is higher in hyperparathyroid patients than in the general population.[12]

### REFERENCES

1. Jowsey, J., and Detenbeck, L. C.: The importance of thyroid hormones to bone metabolism and calcium homeostasis. Endocrinology, 85:87–95, 1969.
2. Williams, G. A., Martinez, N. J., Bowser, E. N., and Henderson, W. J.: The importance of calcitonin in adult human physiology. Excerpta Medica International Congress, No. 270:, pp. 644–647, 1973.
3. Hirsch, P. F., and Munson, P. L.: Importance of the thyroid gland in the prevention of hypercalcemia in rats. Endocrinology, 79:655–658, 1966.
4. Heaney, R. P., and Whedon, G. D.: Radiocalcium studies of bone formation rate in human metabolic bone disease. J. Clin. Endocrinol. Metab., 18:1246–1267, 1958.
5. Kivirikko, K. I., Laitinen, O., and Lamberg, B. A.: Value of urine and serum hydroxyproline in the diagnosis of thyroid disease. J. Clin. Endocrinol. Metab., 25:1347–1352, 1965.

6. Jowsey, J., and Simons, G. W.: Normocalcemia in relation to cortisone secretion. Nature, *217*: 1277–1278, 1968.

7. Bianchi, G. S., Meunier, P., Courpron, P., Edouard, C., Bernard, J., and Vignon, G.: Le retentissement osseux des hyperthyroidies. Rev. Rhum. Mal. Osteoartic., *39*:19–32, 1972.

8. Meema, H. E., and Schatz, D. L.: Simple radiologic demonstration of cortisone bone loss in thyrotoxicosis. Radiology, *97*:9–15, 1970.

9. Follis, R. H., Jr.: Skeletal changes associated with hyperthyroidism. Johns Hopkins Med. J., *92*:405–421, 1953.

10. Clerkin, E. P., Haas, H. G., Mintz, D. H., Meloni, C. R., and Canary, J. J.: Osteomalacia in thyrotoxicosis. Metabolism, *13*:161–171, 1964.

11. Adams, P. H., Jowsey, J., Kelly, P. J., Riggs, B. L., Kinney, V. R., and Jones, J. D.: Effects of hyperthyroidism on bone and mineral metabolism in man. Q. J. Med., *36*:1–15, 1967.

12. Calcium metabolism and bone in hyperthyroidism. Lancet (editorial), *2*:1300–1301, 1970.

# Chapter Twenty-Five

# ACROMEGALY

**Clinical and Radiological Findings.** If epiphyseal growth has ceased, the manifestations of acromegaly are minimal and may be non-symptomatic. However, there is generally increased weight and height even in late onset acromegaly and almost always an increase in hand volume (Fig. 25–1).[1] Despite the increase in size of the skeleton, a decreased bone mass is commonly associated with the disease. Paradoxically, recent experimental studies have suggested the use of growth hormone in the treatment of osteoporosis;[2] the discrepancy can be resolved simply by realizing that growth of the skeleton is a different phenomenon from increasing bone mass, which is only accomplished in an adult by raising the level of bone formation. The radiological and morphological findings in acromegaly as well as the failure of growth hormone to alter the bone loss in osteoporosis fit with this concept of the action of growth hormone on the skeleton.

Symptoms such as headaches and visual field defects and abnormal perimetry are, in fact, more frequent findings in acromegalic patients than are hypercalcemia or hypercalciuria.[1] The symptoms can be related in the most part to abnormalities of bone growth. The total mass of bone appears to be normal or low, both by quantitative roentgenography of the ulna using the multi sampling technique of Doyle[3] and by total body neutron activation analysis.[4] In the latter study, 40 per cent of patients demonstrated below normal values for the percentage of calcium in the body. Since these were calculated as calcium-to-potassium ratios, and therefore included a correction for body size, it can be assumed that 60 per cent have not only normal values for bone mass but also normal values in relation to lean body mass, the remainder being comparable to a matched osteoporotic group (Table 25–1).[4] A similar percentage (40 per cent) of patients lies in the relative osteoporotic range using the Singh Index, with 60 per cent in the normal range. Bone densitometry, using the Cameron-Sorenson densitometer, indicated that the same group of acromegalic patients had a higher than normal bone mass than average. Aloia, using uncorrected values, also reported an increase in total body calcium which was marked in some patients.[4] Both techniques reflect the increase in size of the patients rather than indicating any abnormality in bone density.

**Morphology.** Bone biopsies have been taken from both ribs, which contain predominantly cortical bone, and also from the iliac crest, which contains a mixture of the two (Table 25–2) (Fig. 25–2). The data suggested an increase in resorption in trabecular bone, but to a lesser extent in cortical bone. The latter may appear contradictory at first until it is appreciated that external periosteal bone remodeling is not included in the technique used, quantitative microradiography.

219

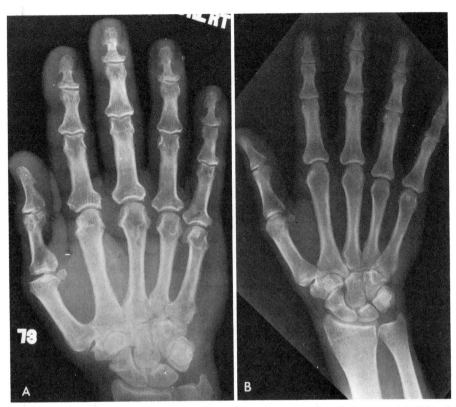

**Figure 25–1** X-rays of the hand of a patient with acromegaly (a) and of a normal individual (b). The generalized increase in size, both in length of the bones and in width is evident in (a). The bone also appears somewhat porotic.

Both bone formation and resorption correlate with growth hormone (r=0.754 and v=0.562, respectively), so it is reasonable to assume a stimulation of bone remodeling by growth hormone; there is no alteration in serum parathyroid hormone in acromegalic patients. However, both growth hormone and bone remodeling are closely related to serum phosphorus levels, and this has been demonstrated to be important in the control of both formation and resorption activity in bone. It is possible, though perhaps less probable, that the remodeling of bone is secondarily related to growth hormone, rather than primarily related.

**Table 25–1**  TOTAL BODY CALCIUM IN NORMALS AND
ACROMEGALIC PATIENTS (mean ± SD)

| | |
|---|---|
| Acromegalics, grams calcium | $1199 \pm 258.4$ |
| % calcium (grams) | $110 \pm 10.8$ |
| Acromegalic females, grams calcium | 978 |
| Osteoporotic females, grams calcium | 645 |
| Normal females, grams calcium | 748 |
| Normal males, grams calcium | $1093 \pm 148.7$ |

$$\left( \% \text{ calcium} = \frac{\text{predicted Ca}}{\text{observed Ca}} \times 100; \text{ where predicted Ca} = 0.203 \times \text{height in meters}^3 \right)$$

From Aloia et al.[4]

**Table 25-2**  BONE TURNOVER IN ACROMEGALY

|  | Bone Formation %* | Bone Resorption % |
|---|---|---|
| | (mean ± SD) | |
| RIB | | |
| normal | 2.5 ± 1.7 | 4.5 ± 1.9 |
| acromegaly | 7.6 ± 5.8 | 6.5 ± 6.3 |
| ILIAC CREST | | |
| normal | 2.1 ± 1.5 | 3.7 ± 1.3 |
| acromegaly | 2.1 ± 1.1 | 10.6 ± 4.0 |

* Bone formation was not evaluated on the periosteal surface, and the values are therefore an underestimate by the amount of new bone which occurs periosteally and accounts for increase in size of the bone.

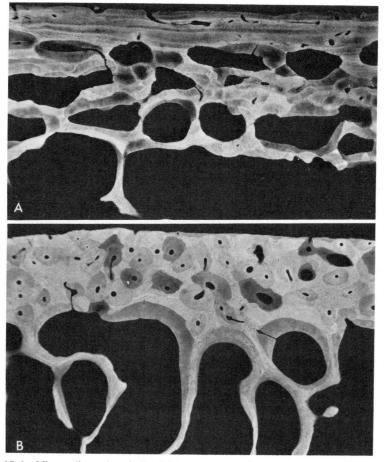

**Figure 25-2**  Microradiographs of rib of (a) an acromegalic patient, 32-year-old male and (b) a normal person, 33 years old. The acromegalic specimen shows increased porosity in the cortex and new periosteal bone formation (magnification x 30) (From Jowsey, J., and Gordan, G.: Bone turnover and osteoporosis. In Bourne, G. H. (ed.): The Biochemistry and Physiology of Bone, 2nd edition, vol. III. New York, Academic Press, 1971, pp. 201–238.)

**Table 25-3** THE EFFECTS OF GROWTH HORMONE ON
TOTAL SKELETAL MASS IN OSTEOPOROSIS (mean ± SD)

| | Low Dose, 6 mos. | | High Dose, 12 mos. | |
|---|---|---|---|---|
| | BEFORE | AFTER | BEFORE | AFTER |
| Calcium, g | 640 ± 104 | 643 ± 90 | 661 ± 84 | 638 ± 104 |
| Potassium, g | 70.5 ± 16.2 | 71.9 ± 16.6 | 76.8 ± 12.6 | 77.6 ± 13.3 |
| Skeletal Ca accretion, g/24 hrs* | 0 mos. | | 12 mos. | |
| | 0.407 ± 0.057 | | 0.506 ± 0.073 | |
| | (control 0.418 ± 0.037) | | | |

From Aloia et al.[6]
*[47]Ca tracer kinetic method.

The remodeling of bone differs from the bone turnover increase seen in hyperthyroidism and cannot be attributed to any abnormality of thyroid function, despite the suggestion that excessive growth hormone production may be a stimulus for aberrations in thyroid function.[5]

In acromegaly there is new bone deposition in the same areas which respond by growth in an immature person or animal, the physis and the periosteum, resulting in an increase in bone length and size. In other bone disorders of increased bone turnover, such as hyperthyroidism or hyperparathyroidism, the periosteal dimensions do not alter; in fact, in no bone disorder is periosteal size uniformly increased, although melorheostosis and Paget's disease may result in patchy, localized increase in bone size.

Growth hormone administration may therefore be expected to cause an increase in size of the whole skeleton, but at the expense of endosteal and trabecular loss of bone; osteoporosis will result because the amount of bone, normal for a normal person, will be inadequate for a large person. It is therefore not reasonable to expect improved bone density in osteoporotic patients treated with growth hormone. Aloia and colleagues, in a group of eight patients treated with growth hormone, showed that there was no change in total body calcium, although kinetic studies indicated increased calcium accretion (Table 25-3). Treatment with somatomedin would parallel the experience with growth hormone and also be contraindicated in the treatment of osteoporosis.[7]

**Treatment.** Acromegaly is frequently benign, especially in adult onset forms, which probably explains the severity of the disease that is often seen when patients eventually seek medical aid. It is also a treatable disease, although relief of symptoms is often not achieved.[1]

## REFERENCES

1. Kanis, J. A., Gillingham, F. J., Harris, P., Horn, D. B., Hunter, W. M., Redpath, A. T., and Strong, J. A.: Clinical and laboratory study of acromegaly: assessment before and one year after treatment. Q. J. Med., *43*:409–431, 1974.
2. Harris, W. H., and Heaney, R. P.: Effect of growth hormone on skeletal mass in adult dogs. Nature, *223*:403–404, 1969.

3. Doyle, F. H.: Radiologic assessment of endocrine effects on bone. Radiol. Clin. North Am., 5:289–302, 1967.
4. Aloia, J. F., Roginsky, S., Jowsey, J., Dombrowski, C. S., Shukla, K. K., and Cohn, S. H.: Skeletal metabolism and body composition in acromegaly. J. Clin. Endocrinol. Metab., 35:543–551, 1972.
5. Mukhtar, E., Wilkinson, R., Alexander, L., Appleton, D., and Hall, R.: Thyroid function in acromegaly. Lancet, 2:279–283, 1971.
6. Aloia, J. F., Zanzi, I., Ellis, K., Jowsey, J., Roginsky, M., Wallach, S., and Cohn, S. H.: Effects of growth hormone in osteoporosis. J. Clin. Endocrinol. Metab., 43:992–999, 1976.
7. Bomboy, J. D., Jr., and Salmon, W. D., Jr.: Somatomedin. Clin. Orthop., 108:228–240, 1975.

# Chapter Twenty-Six

# HYPERCORTISONISM

**Clinical Presentation.** Historically, bilateral adrenal cortical hyperplasia and oversecretion of corticosteroids have formed the classic description of hypercortisonism or Cushing's disease; the symptoms are now well recognized, and the disease can generally be treated successfully. By far the larger number of individuals with bone disease as a result of glucocorticoid excess have been receiving cortisone as rheumatoid patients, for asthma, for some kind of allergy, or as a part of treatment for a kidney transplant. Both in Cushing's disease and in patients treated with high doses of steroids the clinical features are obesity, hirsutism, and, frequently, purple striae on the abdomen. In children, sexual development and body height are retarded. Osteoporosis, with vertebral fractures, is common.[1]

In patients with rheumatoid arthritis, one should keep in mind both the average age of the rheumatoid patient and the possibility that the severity of the arthritis will result in a certain degree of disuse, which tend to produce bone loss independently from the steroid treatment. The involvement of the skeleton is controversial; McConkey and his co-workers found a change in radiological evidence of osteoporosis from only 28 per cent to 32 per cent in a normal, age-matched group of rheumatoid patients receiving steroids at doses of 2.5 to 20 mg of prednisone daily.[2] Strangely, in the same study, the incidence of vertebral fractures rose from 0 to 8 per cent, suggesting an increase in severity, if not in radiological evidence, of bone disease. Since there is a clear relationship between the dose of steroids and the development of significant or symptomatic bone disease, McConkey's group suggested that at doses of approximately 10 mg, old age was the predisposing factor in the development of osteoporosis, rather than chronic steroid administration.[2] Also, 10 mg or less is generally not expected to cause the rapid development of osteoporosis in a young individual.

**Morphology.** There is no doubt that in rats, rabbits, and people large doses of corticosteroids cause bone loss (Fig. 26–1). The cellular abnormalities depend on the duration of the cortisone excess as well as dose. In relatively recent hypercortisonism, bone formation is reduced and bone resorption is elevated. (Table 26–1).[3] Frost and co-workers, using osteoid borders as a reflection of bone formation, also showed remarkably diminished bone formation (Fig. 26–2).[4] The initial increased resorption and decreased formation explain the often rapid onset of symptomatic or radiological bone changes in this disorder. As in chronic osteoporosis, in long-term hypercortisonism the skeleton appears to reach an altered state in which the major cause of the bone loss ceases and bone resorption stops. In treated Cushing's disease or intermittent steroid treatment, bone cell function returns to normal. Intermittent treatment has been compared with daily treatment and, in animals, the

224

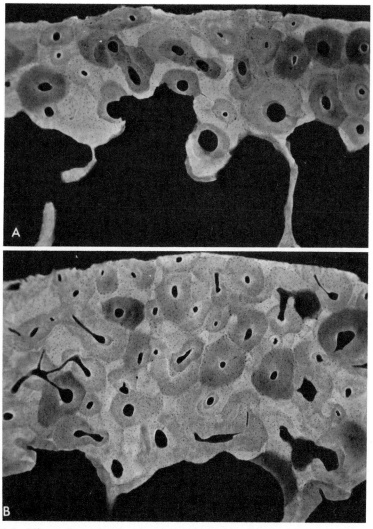

**Figure 26–1** Microradiographs of cross-section of the external cortex of the rib of (a), a 49-year-old female with hypercortisonism, compared with a 49-year-old female (b). The loss of endosteal bone and resulting decrease in cortical thickness is evident (magnification × 50). (From Jowsey, J., and Gordan, G.: Bone turnover and osteoporosis. *In* Bourne, E. H. (Ed.): The Biochemistry and Physiology of Bone, 2nd ed. Vol. III. New York, Academic Press, 1971. pp. 201–238.)

difference is striking.[5] Also, in children or in adults on intermittent treatment, there appears to be an opportunity for recovery of the skeleton to normal or an initial failure to develop the skeletal changes of hypercortisonism, respectively (Table 26–2).[6] In adult hypercortisonism the process stops but is irreversible without treatment.[7]

The suppression of bone formation is doubtless the result of the general depressive effect of corticosteroids on the fibroblastic-inflammatory cell process, which includes the fibroblast-derived osteoblasts. The effect on accelerated bone resorption is less definite. Corticosteroids inhibit the endsorption of calcium in the ileum and, in fact, may have a general effect on absorption in the intestine merely by depressing cell action. Evidence that parathyroid hormone is stimulated by cor-

**Table 26–1**  BONE TURNOVER IN HYPERCORTISONISM ($\bar{x} \pm SD$)

|  | Bone Formation, % | Bone Resorption, % |
| --- | --- | --- |
| Hypercortisonism | $0.13 \pm 0.17$ | $14.9 \pm 6.67$ |
| Age-matched normals | $2.04 \pm 1.32$ | $3.71 \pm 1.33$ |

From Jowsey and Riggs.[3]

tisone secondary to any hypocalcemic effect is unconvincing, since serum iPTH is not increased in steroid treated patients (Table 26–3). Nevertheless, hypercalciuria and a negative calcium balance are common; the effect of corticosteroids on bone resorption is probably therefore direct. It may be that adrenal cortical hormones are responsible to some degree for maintaining the serum calcium and therefore have a primary effect on osteoclasis and stimulate osteoclast activity directly in order to maintain normocalcemia.

**Treatment.**  Recovery takes place in the growing individual after adrenalectomy or cessation of steroid treatment.[6] The irreversibility of the bone disorder in the adult is the result of the low bone-forming activity present in persons over the age of 21. Obviously, alternate day treatment, reduction of dose to 10 mg per day or less, or complete withdrawal are preferable forms of treatment, but, in many instances, it is not possible, and steroid administration must continue to control the primary disease, often for many years. In such a patient or in an adult with steroid-induced osteoporosis, treatment of the bone disease is now achievable. Increased bone mass, and therefore "recovery," require a significant level of osteoblastic activity; stimulation of osteoblasts can be achieved by fluoride. A fluoride-calcium regime, similar to that for postmenopausal osteoporosis, appears promising. The levels of fluoride used must be relatively high, since steroids appear to cause malabsorption of fluoride (Table 26–4), as they do of calcium. This form of treatment, used concomitantly with steroid therapy, will prevent the development of osteoporosis; if osteoporosis has already developed, it should restore the skeletal mass toward normal and prevent further fracture.

Bone Formation With
Cortisone Administration
(from Frost)

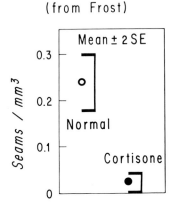

**Figure 26–2**  Bone formation reflected in osteoid "seams" (borders) both are clearly decreased in patients receiving steroids. (Drawn from Frost and Villanueva.[4])

**Table 26-2**   EFFECT OF EVERYDAY AND ALTERNATE DAY STEROID
ADMINISTRATION IN ADULT RABBITS ($\bar{x} \pm$ SD)

|  | Control | Everyday | Alternate Day |
|---|---|---|---|
| $^{45}$Ca uptake in whole femur (counts/s per mg) | 1.95 ± 0.12 | 0.73 ± 1.10* | 2.00 ± 0.14 |
| Cortical thickness, tibial diaphysis (microns) | 440 ± 17 | 346 ± 35* | 434 ± 36 |

From Sheagren et al.[5]
*Significantly (p. < 0.05) different from either corresponding alternate-day group or control group.

**Table 26-3**

|  | Serum Parathyroid Hormone, $\mu$l eq/ml (mean ± SD) |
|---|---|
| Untreated subjects (n = 19) | 30.7 ± 11.2 |
| Steroid treated subjects (n = 20) | 30.0 ± 19.8 N.S. |

**Table 26-4**   SERUM FLUORIDE LEVELS IN PERSONS ON OR NOT ON
STEROID TREATMENT.

|  | Serum Fluoride, $\mu$MF (mean ± SD) |
|---|---|
| (A) Patients on time-release fluoride (50 mg/day); not on steroids (n = 16) | 6.7 ± 3.2 |
| (B) Patients receiving time-release fluoride (50 mg/day); on steroids (n = 11) | 3.1* ± 2.3 |
| (C) Patients on fluoride; (75 mg/day); receiving steroids (n = 11) | 12.0** ± 2.2 |

*Significance of difference between A and B, p < .005.
**Significance of difference between B and C, p < .001.
*Note:*The rise in serum fluoride in group (C) is partly the result of the increase in dose (33 per cent), but it is mainly due to the more easily absorbable form of sodium fluoride compared with the time-release capsule form.

It is important to realize that the serum level of fluoride is directly related to the amount of new bone and levels below 7.0 to 10.0 $\mu$M are not associated with significant increases in bone formation.

## ADRENAL CONTROL OF SERUM CALCIUM

If the adrenals are removed the serum calcium rises. In adrenalectomized patients with Cushing's disease, the replacement with normal levels of steroids prevents this from being evident unless an interval occurs between adrenalectomy and steroid replacement therapy. The first, most obvious, conclusion drawn from the development of the hypercalcemia was that corticosteroids tend to lower serum calcium and antagonize the effect of parathyroid hormone. This theory has been reported and until recently was the current concept to explain the hypercalcemia.[8]

**Table 26–5**  LEVELS OF SERUM CALCIUM IN ADRENALECTOMIZED DOGS*

| Day | Thyroidectomized | Parathyroidectomized |
|---|---|---|
| | (percentage of change in serum calcium) | |
| 0 | 109 | 109 |
| 1–10 | 113 | 159 |
| 11–20 | 119 | 229 |
| 21–32 | 121 | dead |

*From Jowsey and Simons.[9]

However, later work in animals showed that adrenalectomy followed by parathyroidectomy results in a further rise in serum calcium and in dramatic hypercalcemia, the levels of serum calcium rising to the lethal range in experimental animals.[9]

On reflection, it is obvious that the calciostat mechanism of the parathyroids would itself tend to suppress hypercalcemia resulting from adrenalectomy, so that removal of both the adrenals and parathyroids might be expected to result in excessive—in fact, mortal—hypercalcemia. That the adrenals control high serum calcium levels is more reasonable when it is considered that they derive from the fifth ultimobranchial pouch and may have a calcitonin-like action. There is good evidence that the adrenals do, in fact, secrete a substance which is structurally very like calcitonin;[10] considering the mild or non-existent hypercalcemia that develops with calcitonin deficiency, and the clinical and experimental evidence of marked hypercalcemia after adrenalectomy, it is probable that the adrenals have a real physiological role in the control of serum calcium levels, while calcitonin remains a residual part of the fifth ultimobranchial gland with only a minor and transient function in man. It appears that the calcium which produces the hypercalcemia is derived from the bone, since thyroidectomy, which reduces bone cell activity to low levels, decreases the hypercalcemic effect of adrenalectomy (Table 26–5). Steroids appear to play a role both in bone cell regulation and in the control of serum calcium levels.

## *REFERENCES*

1. McArthur, R. G., Cloutier, M. D., Hayles, A. B., and Sprague, R. G.: Cushing's disease in children: findings in 13 cases. Mayo Clin. Proc., 47:318–326, 1972.
2. McConkey, B., Fraser, G. M., and Bligh, A. S.: Osteoporosis and purpura in rheumatoid disease: prevalence and relation to treatment with corticosteroids. Q. J. Med., new series. 31:419–427, 1962.
3. Jowsey, J., and Riggs, B. L.: Bone formation in hypercortisonism. Acta Endocrinol., 63:21–28, 1970.
4. Frost, H. M., and Villanueva, A. R.: Human osteoblastic activity. Part III: The effect of cortisone on lamellar osteoblastic activity. Henry Ford Hosp. Med. Bull., 9:97–99, 1961.
5. Sheagren, J. N., Jowsey, J., Bird, D. C., Gurton, M. E., and Jacobs, J. B.: Effect on bone growth of daily versus alternate-day corticosteroid administration: an experimental study. J. Lab. Clin. Med., 89:120–130, 1977.
6. Skeels, R. F.: Reversibility of osteoporosis in Cushing's disease: case report. J. Clin. Endocrinol. Metab., 18:61–64, 1958.
7. Aloia, J. F., Roginsky, M., Ellis, K., Shukla, K., and Cohn, S.: Skeletal metabolism and body composition in Cushing's syndrome. J. Clin. Endocrinol. Metab., 39:981–985, 1974.
8. Eliel, L. P., Thomsen, C., and Chanes, R.: Antagonism between parathyroid extract and adrenal cortical steroids in man. J. Clin. Endocrinol. Metab., 25:457–464, 1965.
9. Jowsey, J., and Simons, G. W.: Normocalcemia in relation to cortisone secretion. Nature, 217:1277–1278, 1968.
10. Kaplan, E. L., Peskin, G. W., and Arnaud, C. D.: Nonsteroid, calcitonin-like factor from the adrenal gland. Surgery, 66:167–174, 1969.

# Chapter Twenty-Seven

# HYPERPARATHYROIDISM

## HYPERCALCEMIA OR "PRIMARY" HYPERPARATHYROIDISM

In the discussion on parathyroid hormone it was pointed out that the parathyroid glands had two functions; the first is to recognize the numerical value of the ionized calcium in the blood (the calciostat), and the second is to alter the rate of secretion of the hormone in response to fluctuations above and below that value. The first function results in what are accepted as normal serum calcium levels, since they occur in normal people, while the second results in the maintenance of this level. It has also been shown that each individual tends to maintain a characteristic serum calcium level within relatively narrow boundaries, so that the "normal range" of serum calcium values in any hospital laboratory will include a collection of values, some of which may be high or low for any particular person, compared with the average laboratory value.

With these points in mind, Fuller Albright's definition of hyperparathyroidism remains the most accurate and meaningful. He defined what is usually referred to as "primary" hyperparathyroidism in terms of the serum calcium level.[1] "The disease," he states, "is the result of more parathyroid hormone being secreted than is necessary for the maintenance of a normal serum calcium." In terms of the comments made above, this means that hyperparathyroidism is a disease of the serum calcium setting or the calciostat, and that the ability to respond to fluctuations around this calcium level, however abnormal, is frequently unimpaired. This is born out by serial measurements of serum calcium levels over many years in patients with hypercalcemia who have been diagnosed as having "primary" hyperparathyroidism and whose hypercalcemia remains relatively constant, although above normal.

**Clinical and Biochemical Abnormalities.** In the early and mid-1900s the diagnosis of hyperparathyroidism was dependent on bone disease and fractures, and the disease was always associated with osteitis fibrosa cystica, that is, massive loss of bone, replacement of marrow by fibrous connective tissue, and the occurence of cysts in the bone. Albright recognized the relationship between hypercalcemia and hyperparathyroidism, and since then symptoms related to hypercalcemia have most frequently led to the diagnosis of this disease.[1] The symptoms include a general malaise, loss of appetite, nausea, vomiting and polydipsia. There may be muscular weakness, sometimes personality changes, and eventually drowsiness and coma. There is a close association between hyperparathyroidism and the presence of recurrent renal stones, and also an association with pancreatitis (Table 27–1).[2, 3]

229

However, only from 1 to 20 per cent of patients with renal stones have hyper-parathyroidism. The stones are predominately calcium phosphate; it has been suggested that they develop as a result of a high urine calcium and phosphorus load and a tendency to alkalinity.[4] The high urine calcium and phosphorus and the alkalinity result from increased resorption of mineralized bone.

The disease is approximately twice as common in females as in males, and it can be familial,[4] although in such instances it may be part of a multiglandular syndrome.[2] Diagnostic tests consist of a serum calcium determination, which, by the more commonly accepted definition of the disease, is always high (Table 27–2). The %TRP is frequently low because of the effect of parathyroid hormone on the renal absorption of this ion. As a result, the serum phosphate may be low. Howev-er, phosphate is continually being released from bone, and hypophosphatemia is only found in approximately 30 per cent of patients. Serum immunoreactive parathyroid hormone is often above normal; when compared with the serum calci-um, it is found to be inappropriately high, following Albright's original definition of this disease. However, serum immunoreactive parathyroid hormone levels may be within the normal range in a significant number of patients;[5] also, the assay system used can give different results depending on the antibody used. Antibodies directed against the C-terminal of the parathyroid hormone may completely differentiate pa-tients with hyperparathyroidism (HPT) from those without, while the N-terminal assay will show no such discrimination but rather almost complete overlap between the two groups.[6,7]

**Radiological Abnormalities.** In recent years, because the diagnosis has come to depend on the presence of hypercalcemia, overt radiological changes have only been seen in approximately one third of patients who eventually have a confirmed parathyroid gland abnormality. When x-ray evidence of the disease is present it is characterized by thin cortices, which, in more severe disease, have ragged, indis-tinct endosteal and periosteal margins (Fig. 27–1). This may progress in the termi-nal digits to almost complete erosion of the bone. Trabeculae are more evident, largely because of loss of intermediate trabeculae and the transformation of the en-dosteal cortical bone into trabecular bone. In flat bones, the cortical erosion and trabecular loss results in a mottled appearance, often seen in the skull. Cysts may appear, either singly or in numbers, frequently in the cortices of the long bones and in the jaws; these are similar to giant cell tumors and, since they are lytic, may lead to fractures through that area. Loss of the lamina dura is frequently found (Fig. 27–2); however, disappearance of this narrow band of cortex around the teeth

Table 27–1  ASSOCIATED FINDINGS IN PATIENTS WITH
HYPERPARATHYROIDISM

|  | Percentage of Patients Involved | |
|  | Purnell et al. | Louw et al. |
| --- | --- | --- |
| RENAL LITHIASIS | 51 | 56 |
| NEPHROCALCINOSIS | 5 | (all had renal lithiasis) |
| RENAL IMPAIRMENT (GFR < 60 ml/min) | 8 | 2 |
| PEPTIC ULCER | 9 | 4 |
| PANCREATITIS | 2 | 4 |
| RADIOLOGICAL EVIDENCE OF BONE DISEASE | 41 | — |

From Purnell et al.[2]; from Louw et al.[3]

Table 27–2  DEGREE OF ABNORMALITY IN A RANDOM SELECTION OF
32 PATIENTS WITH PRIMARY HYPERPARATHYROIDISM AND
SURGICALLY PROVEN ADENOMAS

| Serum Values | | % of Patients | Range of Values |
|---|---|---|---|
| Ca, mg/dl | >10.1 | 97 | 10.0–14.8 |
| P, mg/dl | <2.5 | 30 | 3.4–1.7 |
| Alk. phos, IU | >60 | 47 | 28–211 |
| iPTH, μl eq/ml | >40 | 81 | 23–720 |

is seen in many diseases of bone loss and is therefore not considered to be very helpful as a diagnostic tool in hyperparathyroidism.

Extraskeletal mineralization of soft tissues may also occur, particularly in the kidney and the peripheral blood vessels (Fig. 27–3). Mineral deposits in particular can be easily seen in the cornea as band keratopathy, while mineral deposits in cartilage, joint capsules, and tendons may give rise to joint discomfort and inflammation.

**Bone Morphology.**  As in other bone disorders, the radiological appearance in hyperparathyroidism reflects not only the severity of the disease but also the duration of the disease. On the other hand, the bone biopsy tends to represent mainly the present status of the bone disorder, particularly if bone cell counts are used. Bone biopsy is also a more sensitive method for evaluation of an abnormality, with the result that, although a minority of patients with confirmed hyperparathyroidism have x-ray evidence of bone disease, all bone biopsies demonstrate abnormalities

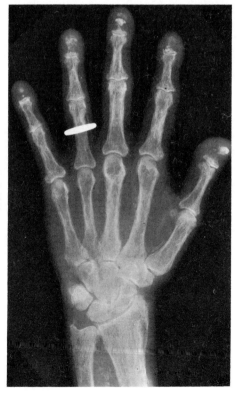

**Figure 27–1**  X-ray of the hand of a patient with hypercalcemic hyperparathyroidism. There has been erosion of the cortices of the phalanges, both on the endosteal and periosteal surfaces and almost complete loss of the terminal phalanges.

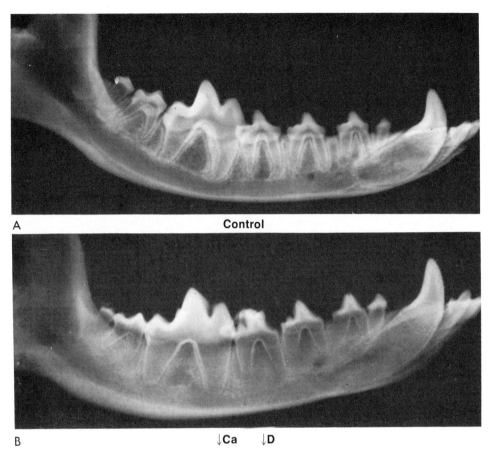

A                                     **Control**

B                              ↓Ca    ↓D

**Figure 27–2**  X-ray of the jaws of two young dogs, (a) on a normal calcium and vitamin D diet and (b) on a diet deficient in both calcium and vitamin D. The loss of the cortex that normally envelops the tooth roots can be seen in (b), as well as the decrease in trabeculae between the teeth.

(Fig. 27–4). The most consistently abnormal change is an increase in the number of osteoclasts and bone resorption.[8, 9, 10, 11, 12] The osteoclast numbers and bone resorption values are related positively to the amount of hormone in the blood. Although values are numerically different depending on the techniques used and the bone sample that is evaluated, the general conclusions are that bone resorption is increased three- to four-fold and bone formation is also elevated in many individuals (Table 27–3). The values in Table 27–3 are average values, and it would be more correct to say that resorption is increased above normal in all patients, while formation is increased above normal only in one third of the patients (Fig. 27–4). It is perhaps relevant to recall that in osteoporosis bone formation may be above normal in a number of patients, if untreated and only ambulatory patients comprise the group analyzed; bone formation may be above the normal range in up to one fourth of patients. Since bone resorption is high in osteoporosis, the changes are similar to those seen in hyperparathyroidism, though quantitatively less.

It must be pointed out, however, that there are differences between osteoporosis and hyperparathyroidism that appear to be more than a matter of degree. Biochemically, hypercalcemia is the most distinctive feature of hyperparathyroidism, in the chronic state generally associated with an adenoma of the parathyroid gland.

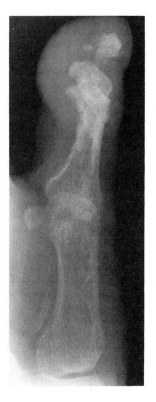

**Figure 27–3** X-ray to demonstrate the extraskeletal mineralization which has taken place in the vessels in the soft tissue of the hand (enlargement of Figure 27–1).

Radiologically, subperiosteal erosion is found in about one-third of the patients with hyperparathyroidism and this is reflected in the appearance of increased porosity in the outer third of the cortex (Fig. 27–5). In osteoporosis the outer third of the cortex appears to remain intact, hypercalcemia does not occur, and hyperplasia rather than parathyroid adenomata is found when this gland is examined.

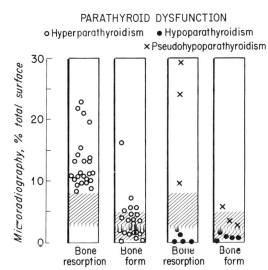

**Figure 27–4** Bone resorption and bone formation surfaces in iliac crest bone biopsies in patients with hyperparathyroidism, hypoparathyroidism and pseudohypoparathyroidism. Only one third of the patients with primary hyperparathyroidism showed radiological evidence of the disease, although all had abnormally high bone resorption values. (Hatched areas represent normal values.)

**Table 27-3**   BONE MORPHOLOGY IN PATIENTS WITH
HYPERPARATHYROIDISM

| | Controls | Primary Hyperparathyroidism |
|---|---|---|
| BONE RESORPTION | | |
| *(Jowsey, 1968)[8] | 3.1 ± 0.3 | 14.1 ± 1.2 |
| *†(Meunier et al., 1971)[9] | 2.4 ± 0.4 | 9.0 ± 4.9 |
| *(Riggs et al., 1965)[10] | 4.3 ± 0.4 | 13.8 ± 1.0 |
| ††**(Wilde et al., 1973)[11] | 0.5 ± 0.3 | 1.2 ± 0.8 |
| **(Jowsey, 1974)[12] | 3.6 ± 1.1 | 13.3 ± 5.7 |
| | | |
| BONE FORMATION | | |
| *(Jowsey, 1968)[8] | 1.7 ± 0.2 | 3.1 ± 0.4 |
| *†(Meunier et al., 1971)[9] | – | – |
| *(Riggs et al., 1965)[10] | 2.1 ± 0.8 | 4.1 ± 1.2 |
| ††**(Wilde et al., 1973)[11] | 0.04 ± 0.01 | 0.2 ± 0.2 |
| **(Jowsey, 1974)[12] | 2.4 ± 1.3 | 3.1 ± 2.2 |

*mean ± SE
**mean ± SD
†trabecular bone only⎫
††cortical rib bone    ⎬ all others are trabecular and cortical bone of iliac crest.

Other bone morphological findings in hypercalcemic hyperparathyroidism are those of an increase in osteocyte size, the presence of fibrous connective tissue, and occasionally mild morphological osteomalacia.

Increase in size of the osteocyte lacunae has been suggested as being an exclusive finding in hyperparathyroidism.[9] It appears that parathyroid hormone will affect the osteocytes, which then resorb the bone surrounding them, a process termed osteocytic osteolysis. In normal individuals, Meunier and colleagues found osteocyte dimensions of 48.3 ± SD 4.8 $\mu^2$, while in hyperparathyroidism the average size increased to 68.3 ± SD 9.5 $\mu^2$, which was a significantly higher value.[9] This size did not increase in secondary hyperparathyroidism, in which vastly increased levels of circulating parathyroid hormone are found, suggesting that the osteolytic response of osteocytes is limited. On the other hand, the osteoclastic response to increased levels of the hormone appears to be linear.[7, 13] The resorption of bone in hyperparathyroidism is therefore mainly the responsibility of the osteoclasts rather than osteocytes, although the latter clearly respond to raised hormone levels. (See also Chapter Ten, Bone Cells, section under "The Osteocyte.")

In a small number of cases (10 per cent), small foci of irregular holes may appear, suggesting that osteocytic osteolysis may very occasionally, in discrete areas, agglomerate into tiny resorption cavities (Fig. 27-6). It is possible that such foci become the brown tumors that are a feature of this bone disorder.

The presence of fibrous connective tissue is a common feature of bone histology in early instances of hyperparathyroidism which present with bone disease; this has led to the use of the term osteitis fibrosa for this disease (Fig. 27-7). Until more sophisticated quantitative methods became available, the presence or absence of fibrosis was taken as proof of the presence or absence of hyperparathyroidism.[12] However, as already mentioned, quantitation of osteoclasts has shown that resorption is increased in all bone biopsies from patients with proven

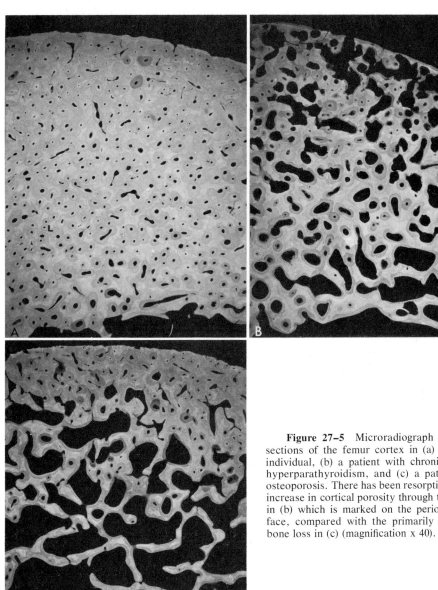

**Figure 27–5** Microradiograph of cross-sections of the femur cortex in (a) a normal individual, (b) a patient with chronic, severe hyperparathyroidism, and (c) a patient with osteoporosis. There has been resorption and an increase in cortical porosity through the cortex in (b) which is marked on the periosteal surface, compared with the primarily endosteal bone loss in (c) (magnification x 40).

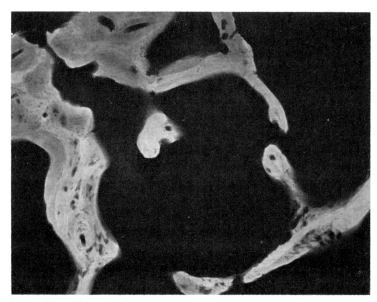

**Figure 27–6**  Microradiograph of trabecular bone from a patient with hyperparathyroidism. Some of the osteocyte lacunae are enlarged and in a few areas appear to have become confluent (magnification x 64).

hyperparathyroidism, and that only in the severely affected patients is there any fibrosis.

The increase in width of osteoid tissue, found in some instances of primary hyperparathyroidism, is perhaps surprising to find in a disease characterized by hypercalcemia. However, in the minimally affected cases that currently form the majority of patients diagnosed with the disease, the serum calcium may be only slightly above normal and the serum phosphate reduced, with a resulting low calcium-phosphorus product in the blood and therefore a failure of mineralization.[8] This may be one of the few instances in which the calcium-phosphorus product has physiological significance. The width of osteoid is usually only very minimally increased; in one study of biopsies from hyperparathyroid patients the values for osteoid thickness rose from a mean of 17.7 ± SE 0.4 in normal age-matched people to 22.0 ± SE 1.2.[8] Clinical or radiological signs of osteomalacia are not associated with the bone biopsy findings. In an occasional patient with chronic hyperparathyroidism, the hypophosphatemia has existed for a long time and caused significant failure of mineralization and a consequent increase in the surface of bone covered by unmineralized and inactive osteoid. The eventual result is a decrease in serum calcium to levels which are within the normal range, despite continued high values for iPTH and a biopsy which resembles osteomalacia. (See Chapter Twenty-three, Unusual Forms of Osteomalacia, section under "Hypophosphatemia in Hyperparathyroidism.")

Albright suggested that hyperparathyroidism could be associated with a history of low calcium intake.[1] The low calcium intake or any other stimulus for hypocalcemia, such as vitamin D deficiency, would tend to lower the serum calcium level and stimulate the parathyroid glands. At first, generalized hyperplasia would develop; however, if one gland responded more actively, there would be a tendency for the remaining glands to become atrophic and the hyperplastic gland to

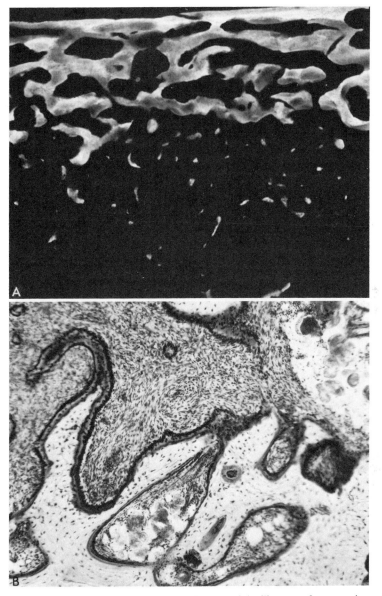

**Figure 27–7**  (a) Microradiograph of the external cortex of the iliac crest from a patient with severe, chronic hyperparathyroidism showing both extensive bone loss and a high turnover level. (b) A stained undemineralized bone section from the same patient demonstrating the extensive fibrosis and high cellular activity of the biopsy (magnification (a) x 20, (b) x 64).

develop into an adenoma. Evidence for a mixture of hyperplastic and adenomatous glands has been demonstrated a number of times.[14] A previous hypocalcemic stimulus has also been documented in patients with hyperparathyroidism, and patients with documented hypocalcemia have been shown to develop autonomous glands.[12, 15]

It is possible therefore that all instances of "primary" hyperparathyroidism are, in fact, cases of secondary hyperparathyroidism that have developed into the "tertiary" form. There are further morphological data to suggest that this is so. In microradiographs of bone from patients with primary hyperparathyroidism, patches of hypomineralized bone appear which indicate an episode of incomplete minerali-zation of bone (Fig. 27–8). The involved zone is almost invariably in an area of old, mature bone distant from the bone-soft tissue surface. In a group of 20 patients with hyperparathyroidism, 80 per cent showed clear evidence of this defect and provided the data to support Albright's original hypothesis as to the origin of the disease.[8] A period of hypocalcemia sufficient to produce a mineralization defect and to alter parathyroid gland function may never be associated with any clinical symp-toms, and it is unlikely that all instances of "primary" hyperparathyroidism can be documented as being associated with a hypocalcemic period or with symptoms that cause an individual to seek medical advice. However, enough examples exist that, with the morphological evidence from the microradiographs, there is evidence that "primary" hyperparathyroidism represents a disorder which began with hypocal-cemia and ended with secretion of the hormone from the parathyroids at a higher than normal calciostat setting for the serum calcium value. It would probably be more accurate to refer to the disease as hypercalcemic hyperparathyroidism; this has the advantage of not inferring a cause and of describing the most consistent fea-ture of the disease.

**Treatment.**   One of the more serious complications, as indicated in Table 27–1, is the development of renal stones. These consist most commonly of calcium phosphate and oxalate and are found in the kidney tissue, the ureter, or the bladder. In hyperparathyroidism the majority of the stones formed contain a preponderance of phosphate, suggesting that an increase in the renal excretion of this ion may be related to the composition of the stone and may be the result of a high calcium-phosphorus product. This is not to say that this is why most renal calculi are of cal-cium phosphate, since only an average of 7 per cent of stone-formers have hyper-parathyroidism. A decrease in calcium intake, with or without calcium-binding agents such as cellulose phosphate, or a high fluid intake are usual forms of treat-

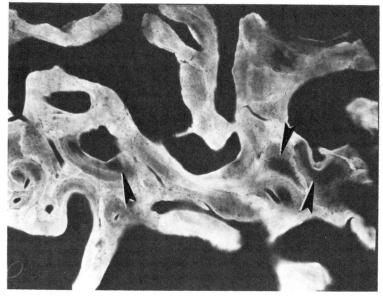

**Figure 27–8**   Microradiograph of part of a biopsy of the iliac crest of a patient with hypercalcemic hyperparathyroidism. There are areas of increased density indicating hypomineralization deep within the bone tissue ➤ (magnification x 64).

ment for recurrent renal lithiasis. A high phosphate intake and infusions have also been used; the former lowers the urinary calcium, and decreases the incidence of stone formation, but it may also cause bone disease.

Hypercalcemia, which results in soft tissue calcification, is probably the factor of most concern in hyperparathyroidism. If this is persistently high, parathyroidectomy is the reasonable course, part of one normal gland being left in situ to take over the role of calcium homeostasis. However, a number of patients may have only minimal hypercalcemia which may remain stable for many years without surgical intervention.

## SECONDARY HYPERPARATHYROIDISM

The parathyroids function all the time in normal individuals, decreasing and increasing the excretion of the hormone as serum calcium levels rise and fall. If the serum calcium decreases excessively, parathyroid hormone levels rise, and, when they reach levels above the normal range, secondary hyperparathyroidism is established.

**Biochemical and Radiological Features.**   Because most of the causes of secondary hyperparathyroidism are the result of calcium "deficiency," generally associated with vitamin D abnormalities, a mild hypocalcemia often occurs, and in chronic secondary hyperparathyroidism the serum phosphorus may also be low. Both the low calcium and low phosphorus will tend to result in a failure of bone mineralization and the development of increased amounts of osteoid tissue; consequently, the parathyroids will become less and less able to maintain a normal serum calcium, and the levels of the hormone will rise to heights that far exceed those seen in primary hyperparathyroidism. Alkaline phosphatase may be high, although the vitamin D status will influence this parameter as well as the degree of hypocalcemia. In Europe and other areas where vitamin D is not added to food, borderline vitamin D deficiency is relatively common, so that any further calcium deficiency will rapidly result in osteomalacia. In the United States and countries where vitamin D is adequate or more than adequate, hypocalcemia does not develop to such a degree, and osteomalacia is a rare accompaniment of the bone loss. The most severe forms of secondary hyperparathyroidism are seen in renal failure, which is associated with hyperphosphatemia and consequently a decrease in the production of $1,25\text{-}(OH)_2$ vitamin D.

The radiological appearance is very like that of hypercalcemic ("primary") hyperparathyroidism, but it is more exaggerated. There are sub-periosteal erosion, osteopenia, and ectopic mineralization, and fractures may occur. Because diagnosis is not possible in the early stages of the disease (as in the early diagnosis of hypercalcemic hyperparathyroidism by hypercalcemia), and because the disease often has a rapidly progressive course, treatment is frequently more difficult.

**Bone Morphology.**   In secondary hyperparathyroidism increased bone resorption is, not surprisingly, the most striking finding. Osteoclasts are abundant and there is generally a marked increase in fibrous connective tissue. Osteoblasts are generally also increased in number and, with the osteoclasts and fibrosis, are often located somewhat patchily on the bone surface (Fig. 27–9). Compared with hypercalcemic hyperparathyroidism, the cellular activity and abnormality of the bone tissue is more pronounced. This is particularly true of the degree of osteopenia (Fig. 27–10).

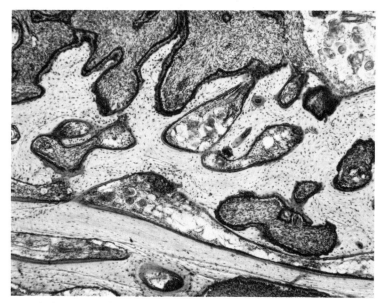

**Figure 27-9**  Stained, undemineralized section. There are areas of fibrosis above with active osteoblasts lining the bone surface, and some areas of osteoclasts. The areas of the bone which are not fibrotic
are almost always devoid of bone cells (magnification x 40).

When vitamin D intake is low, osteomalacia is a striking feature of the bone
tissue; in the few areas of mineralized bone which abut onto a soft tissue surface,
an osteoclast can almost always be found. It is the protective coating of osteoid
that prevents effective parathyroid function in the osteomalacic form of the disease,
not the absence of vitamin D or any synergism between parathyroid hormone and
vitamin D. Because of the layer of osteoid that inhibits osteoclastic bone resorption
in osteomalacic renal osteodystrophy, the total amount of mineralized or partially
mineralized bone may be greater than normal, and the x-ray may demonstrate osteosclerosis. However, in secondary hyperparathyroidism which develops in the
presence of adequate or more than adequate vitamin D intake, calcium absorption
is high, osteomalacia generally does not occur, and the bone tissue demonstrates
severe osteoporosis.

**Etiology.**  There are a number of instances in which vitamin D deficiency
causes secondary hyperparathyroidism, and, as mentioned above, cases are found
most frequently in northern Europe.[16] In the United States, by far the most
frequent cause of secondary hyperparathyroidism is renal failure. The culprit is the
phosphorus which is retained in the body rather than excreted by the kidney. Since
gastrointestinal phosphorus absorption is not significantly decreased in renal failure, impaired renal function results in an accumulation of phosphorus and a raised
serum phosphate level, which lowers the ionized calcium, although total serum calcium may be normal. Slatopolsky has shown elegantly that the early stages of
parathyroid hormone stimulation and the development of bone disease occur at the
first stages of renal failure. He has also shown that oral phosphorus deprivation to
maintain serum phosphorus at normal levels will prevent the development of secondary hyperparathyroidism.[17] This procedure is being used in the control of renal
osteodystrophy in man by using phosphate binding agents rather than oral phosphate restriction.

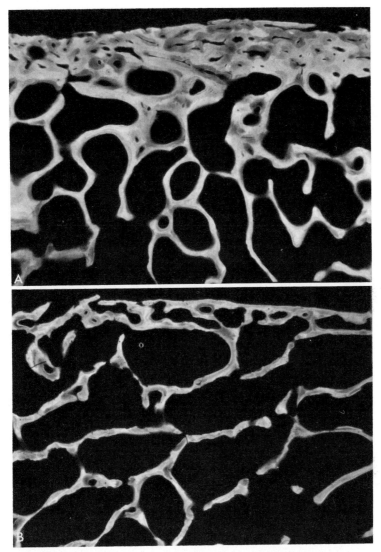

**Figure 27–10**  Microradiographs of the iliac crest of (a) a patient with hypercalcemic hyperpara-thyroidism and (b) a patient with secondary hyperparathyroidism. There has been more extensive bone loss in (b); there is also evidence of osteocytic osteolysis. The serum iPTH level in (a) was 160 $\mu$l eq/ml and in (b) was 600 $\mu$l eq/ml (magnification x 20).

For some time it has been recognized that decreased calcium absorption com-pounds the problems of secondary hyperparathyroidism associated with elevated serum phosphorus. The elevated serum phosphorus will cause a decrease in the hydroxylation of 25–(OH) vitamin D to the dihydroxy form that is essential for cal-cium absorption in the gut. It may, at first inspection, be puzzling why, at a time when calcium is deficient, the mechanism of vitamin D metabolism acts to prevent calcium entry through the intestine. However, a high calcium and phosphorus prod-uct in the blood will cause extraskeletal mineralization, which may have serious consequences in terms of vessel and kidney mineralization and result in further im-pairment of renal function. Many of the relations between vitamin D and parathyroid hormone, and an important function of parathyroid hormone alone, act to prevent the development of a high calcium-to-phosphorus ratio in the body, which may be more deleterious than bone loss or the development of unmineralized osteoid.

**Treatment.**  Secondary hyperparathyroidism caused by calcium deficiency or vitamin D deficiency can be corrected by supplemental calcium and vitamin D. If vitamin D deficiency is the result of gastrectomy, a useful form of therapy is ultraviolet light treatment—sunlight, if this is available, or irradiation from a sunlamp if natural sunshine is not available, as in some parts of northern Europe.[4]

Table 27–4  BIOCHEMICAL CHANGES IN UREMIC PATIENTS
AFTER TREATMENT WITH 1,25-(OH)$_2$D$_3$

| | 1,25-(OH)$_2$D$_3$ | | Serum Ca (mg/dl) | | Serum P (mg/dl) | | Serum iPTH (ng/ml) | |
| --- | --- | --- | --- | --- | --- | --- | --- | --- |
| PATIENT | DOSE ($\mu$g/day) | DURA-TION (wk) | CONTROL | RX | CONTROL | RX | CONTROL | RX |
| 1 | 0.28 | 8 | 7.3 | 8.6 | 4.1 | 4.8 | 1.40 | 1.20 |
| 2 | 0.28 | 8 | 8.5 | 9.4 | 3.8 | 2.9 | 0.57 | <0.18 |
| 3 | 0.28 | 8 | 8.6 | 9.1 | 5.6 | 6.0 | 1.30 | 0.24 |
| 4 | 0.28 | 8 | 6.9 | 8.7 | 5.5 | 2.9 | 4.70 | 0.61 |
| 5 | 0.28 | 10 | 8.2 | 8.8 | 5.4 | 5.6 | 0.46 | 0.57 |
| 6 | 0.14 | 2 | 11.2 | 13.3 | 6.3 | 5.2 | 5.30 | – |
| 7 | 0.14 | 17 | 10.2 | 10.8 | 4.4 | 4.3 | 2.40 | 0.52 |
| 8 | 0.14 | 14 | 10.0 | 10.5 | 4.8 | 5.9 | 1.80 | 0.89 |
| 9 | 0.14 | 8 | 6.2 | 6.8 | 5.5 | 3.7 | 1.20 | 0.95 |
| | | mean | 8.6 | 9.6* | 5.0 | 4.6 | 2.1 | 0.6* |
| | | SD | 1.7 | 1.8 | 0.8 | 1.2 | 1.7 | 0.4 |

From Brickman et al.[18]
*Significantly different from pretreatment values.

Table 27–5  BONE CHANGES IN UREMIC PATIENTS
AFTER TREATMENT WITH 1,25-(OH)$_2$D$_3$

| | Resorption % | | Osteoid Width, ($\bar{x} \pm$ SD) | |
| --- | --- | --- | --- | --- |
| Patients | CONTROL | RX | CONTROL | RX |
| 1 | 8.3 | 4.0 | 17.4 ± 6.0 | 12.8 ± 2.3 |
| 2 | 13.9 | 7.3 | 14.7 ± 5.6 | 11.8 ± 5.9 |
| 3 | 11.4 | 5.0 | 10.5 ± 2.6 | 12.1 ± 1.9 |
| 4 | 12.7 | 4.4 | 19.7 | 13.5 |
| 5 | 13.6 | 15.0 | 21.8 ± 6.2 | 23.3 ± 11.0 |
| 6 | 9.1 | 2.9 | 19.0 ± 5.8 | 15.3 ± 2.7 |
| 7 | 7.4 | 7.0 | 12.3 | 9.0 |
| 8 | 3.0 | 2.9 | 18.8 | 17.7 |
| Mean | 9.9 | 6.1* | 16.8 | 14.4* |
| SD | 3.7 | 4.0 | 3.9 | 4.4 |

From Brickman et al.[18]
*Significantly different from pretreatment values.

If the secondary hyperparathyroidism is the result of renal failure, 25-$(OH)_2$ vitamin D would successfully treat the bone disease in most instances (Tables 27–4, 27–5).[18] Renal transplant or dialysis remain the usual forms of treatment for anephric patients at the present time.

## TUMORAL CALCINOSIS

Tumoral calcinosis is a relatively uncommon disease which appears to have a familial incidence. The majority of reported cases have occurred in Negroes; when familial, they have all occurred in siblings and are not found in more than one generation in a particular family, suggesting an autosomal recessive mode of inheritance. As in hypoparathyroidism and renal failure, the state is associated with hyperphosphatemia; however, the serum calcium is normal or elevated, so that a high calcium-to-phosphorus product is present in most cases (Table 27–6).[19, 20]

The x-ray appearance is of a mineralized mass of lobulated material with occasional cystic areas (Fig. 27–11). The lesions are almost invariably associated with joints, although they are not attached to bone or skin and are usually freely movable within the tissue. The lesion consists of a connective tissue stroma that is filled with calcium-phosphate deposits that can be washed out. The "tumor" therefore does not usually resemble bone or a tumor but rather ectopic mineralization localized to certain regions and associated with a loose collagen matrix. Some small areas of cartilage and osteoid have been seen, and occasional cystic areas were filled with multinucleate giant cells.

Treatment consists of surgical excision, which is usually followed by recurrence of the mineralized mass. One older patient has been treated with a low cal-

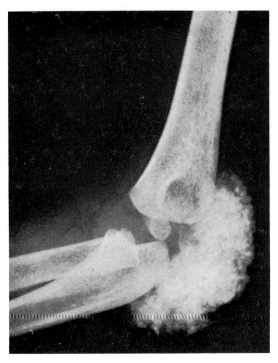

**Figure 27–11** Radiograph of a four-year-old Negro boy with tumoral calcinosis occurring at the elbow joint. The calcific deposit is extraskeletal and appears to consist of large granules of dense material. (From Baldursson et al.[19])

Table 27–6  SERUM CHEMISTRY VALUES IN TUMORAL CALCINOSIS

| Age (yr) | Sex | Ca (mg/100 ml) | P (mg/100 ml) | Alkaline Phosphatase, KA |
|---|---|---|---|---|
| 4 | M | 9.3–10.0 | 7.1– 9.8 | 8.7 |
| 4 | M | 9.4–12.2 | 7.0–11.5 | 9.6 |
| 4 | M | 11.6 | 7.7 | normal |
| 6 | F | 8.7–12.5 | 6.2–10.0 | 12.0 |
| 14 | M | 9.7 | 4.6 | 26.5 |
| 46 | M | 9.5 | 4.5– 5.8 | 35.0 |

From Baldursson et al.;[19] Slavin et al.;[20] Mozaffarian et al.[21]

cium and phosphorus diet and phosphorus depletion using aluminum antacid phosphate binding agents.[21] The phosphorus depletion resulted in negative calcium and phosphorus balance, and a regression of the calcific deposits occurred after one and one-half years of therapy.

## HYPOPARATHYROIDISM

**Clinical and Biochemical Features.**  Absence of parathyroid function most commonly occurs as a result of thyroid surgery for hyperthyroidism. It may be transient, as when the blood supply is reversibly damaged, or it may be permanent. The percentage of patients who become hypoparathyroid in this manner varies from 0 to 50 per cent of patients undergoing thyroidectomy, the percentage depending on the investigator and the test used for discovery of the hypoparathyroidism. Both "surgical" and idiopathic hypoparathyroidism may be tolerated for some years in adults with no symptoms, although the serum calcium will be below normal and the serum phosphorus high. For example, Vlietstra reported a 45-year-old male who developed classical hypoparathyroid symptoms and responded to parathyroid extract, four years after gastric surgery.[22] Pregnancy has also been a cause of uncovering hypoparathyroid symptoms. Presumably a certain degree of hypocalcemia can be tolerated unless an extra calcium stress is placed on the individual. Hypoparathyroidism may also be caused by radioiodine treatment of hyperthyroidism, but such instances are rare. Idiopathic hypoparathyroidism is also rare, but, in contrast to the surgically induced disease, it more frequently leads to symptoms, since it occurs in growing individuals.

The same symptoms and biochemical changes are present in the idiopathic and the adult onset disease; there are hypocalcemia and hyperphosphatemia as a result of lack of parathyroid hormone effect on the bone and the kidney, respectively. The response to exogenous parathyroid hormone is generally excessive, both in terms of urinary phosphorus excretion and cyclic AMP excretion. Consistent hyperphosphatemia may cause soft tissue calcification, and cataract formation. Diagnosis of the disease is generally simple, based on the findings above, which exclude pseudohypoparathyroidism. Calcium deprivation by phytate, cellulose phosphate, or EDTA will uncover nonsymptomatic individuals, as will calcium stress of most kinds, and tetany will develop. The fall in serum calcium, which does not occur in parathyroid intact patients, is accompanied by a slower fall than normal in urinary calcium, reflecting the inability of the skeleton to give up calcium to the blood.[23]

**Bone Morphology.** The two major findings on biopsy of patients with absent parathyroids are the presence of increased amounts of osteoid tissue and, in idiopathic hypoparathyroidism, a lack of bone remodeling. The osteoid shows a slight increase in thickness and, perhaps more significantly, the bone demonstrates a large percentage of surface covered by unmineralized matrix. The layer of osteoid effectively seals off the bone and may prevent a normal response to parathyroid hormone. Bone formation and bone resorption are decreased significantly; resorption falls to below the normal range and formation falls to values below one standard deviation from normal.[8] It may well be that the decrease in both formation and resorption is the explanation for the appearance of the radiological features in young individuals affected with the disease, in contrast to adults. The majority of adults appear normal radiologically and no abnormality should be expected if the disease is adult in onset, since the bone remodeling essentially stops and the skeleton remains unperturbed. The term "hyper-hypoparathyroidism" has been invented to describe a clinical picture in children which is identical to hypoparathyroidism except for the appearance of some radiological changes which resemble hyperparathyroidism, that is, metaphyseal rarefaction and uneven periosteal cortices in the phalanges.[24] It is possible, even highly probable, that these changes are the result of a failure of bone formation and the presence of osteoid, which of course would not appear on an x-ray. The lack of clear signs of rickets in young hypoparathyroid patients probably also depends on the decrease in bone formation and also, presumably, on the cartilage growth in the epiphyses that accompanies the lowered resorption.

**Treatment.** Vitamin D and calcium are generally successful in the treatment of these patients, resulting in a rise in absorption of dietary calcium and consequently of serum calcium. Serum phosphorus will often decrease, as the normal serum calcium permits mineralization of new bone, which requires phosphorus. Hypercalcemia may develop and cause transient renal failure, apparently irrespective of the dose of vitamin D.[25] The hypercalcemic response may well reflect the amount of unmineralized osteoid, in that large accumulations of osteoid will require and accumulate large amounts of calcium, while smaller amounts will be rapidly mineralized and a rise in serum calcium will follow. The opposite may also occur; a patient may appear to be resistant to doses of vitamin D which would normally produce and maintain normal serum calcium levels.[26] Such vitamin D resistance appears to occur in younger patients and again may reflect the bone morphology. A 10 to 16 year old person with idiopathic disease may well have kilograms of unmineralized osteoid that need mineralization and that continue to need mineralizing as growth continues and new matrix is formed, although perhaps at a decreased rate. If the vitamin D therapy is successful as far as mineralization of new bone is concerned, a fall in serum phosphorus may occur and mineralization will then cease and hypercalcemia and renal failure may develop. The patient will then appear to hyper-respond to normal doses of vitamin D.

It is evident therefore that both the calcium and phosphorus levels in the serum need careful monitoring in the treatment of this disease and that a bone biopsy, to evaluate the amount of unmineralized skeleton, can be helpful.

A final and rare cause of "hypoparathyroidism," which is expressed as hypocalcemia and hyperphosphatemia, may appear as the result of magnesium deficiency.[27] Large doses of calcium and vitamin D will fail to alter the hypocalcemia and hyperphosphatemia. In such instances magnesium will restore the ability of the parathyroid glands to respond to the hypocalcemia, and vitamin D and calcium supplements will only be necessary as long as the bone contains excessive amounts of unmineralized matrix. (See also Chapter Four, Magnesium, section under "Action of Magnesium.")

## PSEUDOHYPOPARATHYROIDISM

Pseudohypoparathyroidism is a congenital condition that resembles hypoparathyroidism biochemically, with hypocalcemia and hyperphosphatemia; subcutaneous mineralization is also common, and short stature and bilateral shortening of the metacarpals (generally the fourth) and metatarsals may occur. A clear distinction between pseudohypoparathyroidism and hypoparathyroidism can be made in that parathyroid extract does not produce a rise in serum calcium, nor is there a rise in urinary cyclic AMP. The disease appears to be the result of a lack of response by the kidney to parathyroid hormone, and consequently a lack of phosphaturic response and possibly a renal leak of calcium, although this is confused by the very low serum calcium values and consequent decreased filtered load, which would tend to mask any hypercalciuria.

It has now been established that there is no end-organ defect in bone and no abnormality of the parathyroid glands. Indeed, most cases in which gland histology has been reported describe hyperplasia, and bone biopsies show increased bone resorption.[24] However, since osteoid surface is increased because of the hypocalcemia, the parathyroid-bone response is no doubt impaired to some extent. Removal of the parathyroids results in a further fall of serum calcium, substantiating a responsiveness of the bone to the hormone.

Pseudo-pseudohypoparathyroidism is similar radiologically to pseudohypoparathyroidism; however, the serum chemistries are normal, as is the renal adenyl cyclase response to parathyroid hormone. Subcutaneous mineralization and cataracts are common, which suggests that the disorder may be a pseudohypoparathyroidism which has a developed normal adenyl cyclase response in the kidney, and the patient is therefore normal biochemically but has still the stigmata of the previous episode of pseudohypoparathyroidism.

Treatment has been the administration of vitamin D in an attempt to raise the serum calcium to normal. It has recently been suggested that 25-(OH) vitamin D is more effective, and even more effective is 1,25-(OH)$_2$ vitamin D.[28] This is somewhat to be expected, since it is known that the dihydroxy form of the vitamin D is the active hormone in calcium absorption. It was suggested by Kooh and colleagues that both hypoparathyroidism and pseudohypoparathyroidism are diseases of lack of conversion to 1,25-(OH) vitamin D. However, the evidence is tenuous, and the thesis requires further studies.

## *REFERENCES*

1. Albright, F.: A page out of the history of hyperparathyroidism. J. Clin. Endocrinol., *8*:637–657, 1948.
2. Purnell, D. C., Smith, L. H., Scholz, D. A., Elveback, L. R., and Arnaud, C. D.: Primary hyperparathyroidism: a prospective clinical study. Am. J. Med., *50*:670–678, 1971.
3. Louw, J. H., and Joffe, S. N.: Hyperparathyroidism. S. Afr. Med. J., *48*:343–346, 1974.

4. Nordin, B. E. C.: Metabolic Bone and Stone Disease. Baltimore, Williams and Wilkins, 1973.

5. Potts, J. T., Murray, T. M., Peacock, M., Niall, H. D., Tregar, G. W., Keutmann, H. T., Powell, D., and Deftos, L. J.: Parathyroid hormone: sequence, synthesis, immunoassay studies. Am. J. Med., *50*:639–649, 1971.

6. Fischer, J. A., Binswanger, U., and Dietrick, F. M.: Human parathyroid hormone—immunological characterization of antibodies against a glandular extract and the synthetic amino-terminal fragments 1–12 and 1–34 and their use in the determination of immunoreactive hormone in human sera. J. Clin. Invest., *54*:1382–1394, 1974.

7. Arnaud, C. D., Goldsmith, R. S., Bordier, P. J., Sizemore, G. W., Larsen, J. A., and Gilkinson, J.: Influence of immunoheterogeneity of circulating parathyroid hormone on results of radioimmunoassays of serum in man. Am. J. Med., *56*:785–793, 1974.

8. Jowsey, J.: Bone in parathyroid disorders in man. Excerpta Medica. International Congress Series No. *159*:137–151, 1968.

9. Meunier, P., Bernard, J., and Vignon, G.: Le mesure de l'élargissement périostéocytaire appliquée au diagnostic des hyperparathyroidies. Pathol. Biol., *19*:371–378, 1971.

10. Riggs, B. L., Kelly, P. J., Jowsey, J., and Keating, F. R., Jr: Skeletal alterations in hyperparathyroidism: determination of bone formation, resorption and morphologic changes by microradiography. J. Clin. Endocrinol. Metab., *25*:777–783, 1965.

11. Wilde, C. D., Jaworski, Z. F., Villanueva, A. R., and Frost, H. M.: Quantitative histological measurements of bone turnover in primary hyperparathyroidism. Calcif. Tissue Res., *12*:137–142, 1973.

12. Jowsey, J.: Bone histology and hyperparathyroidism. Clin. Endocrinol. Metab., *3*:267–284, 1974.

13. Jowsey, J.: Microradiography. A morphologic approach to quantitating bone turnover. Excerpta Medica, International Congress Series No. *270*:114–123, 1973.

14. Roth, S. I.: Recent advances in parathyroid gland pathology. Am. J. Med., *50*:612–622, 1971.

15. Sherwood, L. M., Lundberg, W. B., Jr., Targovnik, J. H., Rodman, J. S., and Seyfer, A.: Synthesis and secretion of parathyroid hormone in vitro. Am. J. Med., *50*:658–669, 1971.

16. Stanbury, S. W.: Osteomalacia. Clin. Endocrinol. Metab., *1*:239–266, 1972.

17. Slatopolsky, E., Caglar, S., Pennell, J. P., Taggart, D. D., Canterbury, J. M., Reiss, E., and Bricker, N. S.: On the pathogenesis of hyperparathyroidism in chronic experimental renal insufficiency in the dog. J. Clin. Invest., *50*:492–499, 1971.

18. Brickman, A. S., Sherrard, D. J., Jowsey, J., Singer, F. R., Baylink, D. J., Maloney, N., Massry, S. G., Norman, A. W., and Coburn, J. W.: 1,25-Dihydroxycholecalciferol: Effect on skeletal lesions and plasma parathyroid hormone levels in uremic osteodystrophy. Arch. Intern. Med., *134*:883–888, 1974.

19. Baldursson, H., Evans, E. B., Dodge, W. F., and Jackson, W. T.: Tumoral calcinosis with hyperphosphatemia: a report of a family with incidence in four siblings. J. Bone Joint Surg., *51A*:913–925, 1969.

20. Slavin, G., Klenerman, L., Darby, A., and Bansal, S.: Tumoral calcinosis in England. Br. Med. J., *1*:147–149, 1973.

21. Mozaffarian, G., Lafferty, F. W., and Pearson, O. H.: Treatment of tumoral calcinosis with phosphorus deprivation. Ann. Intern. Med., *77*:741–745, 1972.

22. Vlietstra, R. E.: Idiopathic hypoparathyroidism following gastric surgery. N. Z. Med. J., *78*:113–114, 1973.

23. Parfitt, A. M.: Effect of cellulose phosphate on calcium and magnesium homeostasis: studies in normal subjects and patients with latent hypoparathyroidism. Clin. Sci. Mol. Med., *49*:83–90, 1975.

24. Costello, J. M., and Dent, C. E.: Hypo-hyperparathyroidism. Arch. Dis. Child., *38*:397–407, 1963.

25. Hossain, M.: Vitamin-D intoxication during treatment of hypoparathyroidism. Lancet, *1*:1149–1151, 1970.

26. Chertow, B. S., Plymate, S. R., and Becker, F. O.: Vitamin-D-resistant idiopathic hypoparathyroidism. Arch. Intern. Med., *133*:838–840, 1974.

27. Rösler, A., and Rabinowitz, D.: Magnesium-induced reversal of vitamin-D resistance in hypoparathyroidism. Lancet, *1*:803–805, 1973.

28. Kooh, S. W., Fraser, D., DeLuca, H. F., Holick, M. F., Belsey, R. E., Clark, M. B., and Murray, T. M.: Treatment of hypoparathyroidism and pseudohypoparathyroidism with metabolites of vitamin D; evidence for impaired conversion of 25-hydroxy-vitamin D to 1α, 25-dihydroxyvitamin D. N. Engl. J. Med., *293*:840–844, 1975.

# Chapter Twenty-Eight

# OSTEOPOROSIS: JUVENILE

## INTRODUCTION

The definition of osteoporosis has remained a clinical one, based on symptoms such as back pain and on radiological evidence of fractures. The most common fracture site is the spine. Such patients are generally seen by endocrinologists, and the spinal fracture is treated with the use of a brace or corset; patients with femoral neck and Colles' fractures, on the other hand, usually arrive at an Orthopedic Department for surgical treatment of the fracture. Possibly for this reason, osteoporosis expressed as a spinal fracture is more frequently treated than when the disease is associated with a femoral neck or Colles' fracture, although the relationship between these fractures and osteoporosis is well recognized. For example, if loss of height resulting from vertebral collapse is measured using the ratio of sitting height to standing height, then those individuals with a decreased rump-to-head height have more femoral neck fractures (Table 28–1).[1] Similarly, if the metacarpal cortical thickness compared with the total diameter is measured in women with Colles' fractures, the majority of values fall below the normal mean and a significant number below the normal range of control cortical thickness-to-total diameter ratios.[2]

It has been stated that the areas of the skeleton most subject to fracture are those composed mainly of trabecular bone, and osteoporosis has been called a disease of trabecular bone. However, close investigation of this premise suggests that the site of fracture depends on biomechanical factors rather than on the proportion of trabecular bone. For example, the lumbar and thoracic vertebrae are more frequently the first to suffer fracture, compared with the cervical vertebrae, presumably because more weight is born by lower vertebrae. The femur neck is an area particularly prone to fracture because of its angular relationship to the vertical load applied to this area in a biped. The high incidence of Colles' fractures depends on the manner of the fall; when a person slips or trips, and puts out a hand to "save" himself, the wrist bears the first impact of the fall. In comparison, the distal end of the tibia contains a proportion of trabecular bone equal to or above that of the femoral neck, and yet it is very rarely a site for pathological fracture, presumably because the biomechanical forces predispose to fracture to a lesser degree.

Because stress plays an important role in the fracture, and because the existence of a fracture is part of the definition of the disease, it is obvious that the

248

**Table 28–1**  FREQUENCY OF FRACTURES IN RELATION TO HEIGHT LOSS
(mean ± SD)

|  | Control | Fracture Femoral Neck** | Fracture Upper Limb** |
|---|---|---|---|
| Number of patients | 32 | 93 | 21 |
| Age (years) | 66.7 ± 13.0 | 69.4 ± 12.7 | 68.9 ± 12.8 |
| Weight (kilograms) | 66.4 ± 14.1 | 57.1* ± 10.3 | 66.9 ± 9.2 |
| Ratio $\frac{\text{head and trunk height}}{\text{total height}}$ | 0.524 ± 0.023 | 0.505. ± 0.023 | 0.528 ± 0.026 |

From Nilsson.[1]
*Significantly different from control, $P < 0.001$
**Pathological fractures
***Traumatic fractures

degree of bone loss that predisposes to cause the fracture exists in individuals both with and without the disease; two individuals may have lost the same amount of bone, yet one may have a fracture, and therefore be an osteoporotic patient, while the other is "normal." Many attempts have been made to define the disease more physiologically by measuring the amount of bone loss using such techniques as bone densitometry or metacarpal cortical thickness. However, these methods measure absolute bone mass rather than appropriate mass, that is, mass related to body weight and height. Even the Singh Index, which does measure bone loss and therefore evaluates how much bone any individual has in relationship to how much is normal for that individual, is not the ultimate answer, partly because it is not a truly quantitative method, but mainly because of the question of what degree of bone loss should be treated. Is it best to treat individuals when they first show signs of bone loss on x-ray or by the Singh Index, or should the patient only be treated when a fracture occurs and symptoms are present? The question is largely answered by the fact that patients with osteoporosis and no fracture seldom seek medical aid; only annual examinations which include a Singh Index would separate such individuals from those with normal amounts of bone. Since preventive therapy is often preferable, there is much on the positive side to be said for this manner of medical care. However, the vast majority of osteoporotic patients become "visible" medically only after a fracture has occurred.

Although this point will be made later when treatment is considered, it is essential to realize that because the diagnosis of osteoporosis still rests on the presence of a fracture, bone mass must be decreased and an increase toward normal must be induced before the fracture incidence can be expected to decrease. An osteoporotic patient with a fracture will continue to have fractures if left untreated for osteoporosis or if given preventive treatment only.

It is also important to realize how much bone has been lost in an osteoporotic patient. The iliac crest has been shown to be relatively representative of the skeleton as a whole, and measurements of cortical and trabecular bone in this area show that 50 to 70 per cent of bone has been lost by the time a fracture occurs (Fig. 28–1). This is a large percentage, and it far exceeds the loss of muscle mass seen with increasing age. It reflects the constant need for calcium necessary to maintain calcium homeostasis, which is not supplied by dietary intake but which comes from mineralized bone tissue. Other etiological factors are associated with this calcium homeostatic function of the skeleton that no doubt contribute to the bone loss.

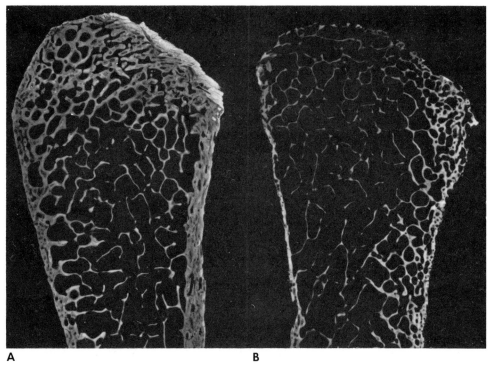

**A**                                                                    **B**

**Figure 28–1**   Microradiographs of iliac crest specimens from (a) normal individual aged 50 and (b) an osteoporotic individual aged 50. There has been a generalized loss of mineralized tissue; however it is important to notice the considerable loss of bone seen in the internal and external cortices of the osteoporotic bone sample (magnification x 6).

In relation to considerations of etiological factors it must be mentioned that some data have suggested that osteoporosis is a result of senescence rather than a disease that affects only a certain proportion of the population.[3] The former view is based on the somewhat uniform loss of bone with age that occurs in the majority of men and women and that is avoided only by a small percentage of people (see section under "Etiology"). Unfortunately, the majority of data overwhelms the minority, and, indeed, there appears to be a "generalized" loss of bone with increasing age. However, to try to explain a hormonally controlled homeostatic phenomenon, which has been relatively well described and documented with data, by as obscure a term as "senescence" is not enlightening. It is also obvious from the following discussion of etiological factors that the longer an etiological factor affects bone, the more bone will be lost, and therefore that older individuals should be expected to have less bone.

## JUVENILE OSTEOPOROSIS

This is considered a relatively rare disease, and, compared with postmenopausal or senile osteoporosis, it is certainly uncommon. It may be more common, however, if kyphosis is taken as a possible indication of the disease, as well as the more classic cases described by Dent and Friedman.[4] Their comprehensive report includes six patients; later reports of sporadic cases and a collection of seven patients indicate an age of onset of symptoms between six and 13 years of age.[5, 6] More males than females (11:7) seem affected, but the difference may be in the tendency for boys to be more active and strenuous than girls at this age and therefore be at greater risk for fracture.

**Radiological Features.** The fractures occur as the result of relatively minor accidents, and a spinal x-ray shows anterior wedging or fracture of the vertebral bodies and loss of height in all cases (Fig. 28–2). Careful examination of the biochemical findings and the clinical histories has failed to reveal any abnormality or to provide any explanation for the loss of bone and development of fractures. The exception was a tendency for high urine calcium values in some patients accompanied by increased levels of urinary hydroxyproline.[4, 5] Malabsorption of calcium is also a feature of some patients.[4] The characteristics are identical to those of post-menopausal or senile osteoporosis except for the age of symptoms and the regression of the disease that seems to occur at the end of the growth spurt. Görgényi's review of 19 cases indicates the same characteristics.[6]

In the 20 reported cases considered here, ten sustained fractures of the lower extremities because of the manner of the fall, and only later were they found to have associated vertebral fractures. Of the remaining ten, six fell in such a way that vertebral fractures resulted, while only a minority of the group as a whole had

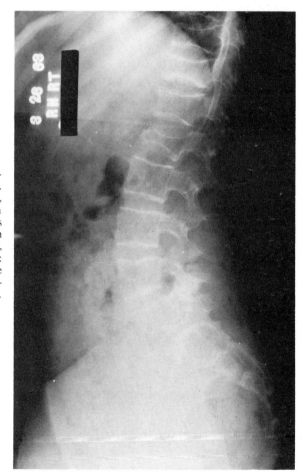

**Figure 28–2** X-ray of a 12-year-old patient with juvenile osteoporosis. A number of vertebrae show height loss, while a clear fracture has taken place in one. The remainder show thin cortices and translucent-appearing bodies. (From Cloutier, M. D., Hayles, A. B., Riggs, B. L., Jowsey, J. and Bickel, W. H.: Juvenile osteoporosis. Report of a case including a description of some metabolic and microradiographic studies. Pediatrics, 40:649–655, 1967.)

primary symptoms of low back pain and spinal fracture apparently unrelated to any recorded trauma. This suggests that any child of six to 15 years of age who sustains a fracture without very reasonable cause should have a spinal x-ray and a Singh Index evaluation. It also suggests that the incidence of the classical form of juvenile osteoporosis is not as rare as is generally supposed.

### Scheuermann's Kyphosis

Anterior wedging of the vertebrae is most probably the cause of Scheuermann's kyphosis. As in juvenile osteoporosis, it is most frequent in the early teens and bears a telling resemblance to the kyphosis of the post-menopausal osteoporotic female. The question of whether Scheuermann's kyphosis is a form of juvenile osteoporosis has been recently examined; on the basis of finding abnormally low Singh Indices in all but one of these patients, it was felt that this syndrome was indeed a form of the disease.[7] Like the better-recognized forms, it also tends to be self-limiting; that is, with conservative treatment, by maturity there is generally a normal appearance, both externally and by radiography.

**Etiology.** The only abnormality reported in juvenile osteoporosis, including Scheuermann's kyphosis, has been malabsorption of calcium on a normal calcium intake[4] or a low dietary calcium intake.[6] Possibly the age is the most significant factor in that, in the presence of either calcium malabsorption or a somewhat low dietary calcium intake, the ages of eight to 13 represent a time when calcium requirements are high. These ages are not necessarily those at which the skeletal growth *rate* is greatest, but, more importantly, they are ages at which the number of grams of calcium added to the skeleton per month or year is highest. A dietary intake of 1 gram of calcium may be adequate at age six; at age 12, however, in order to remain in the degree of positive calcium balance necessary to accrete bone at a normal rate, the necessary dietary calcium intake is significantly higher. Lack of any aspect of osteomalacia suggests that vitamin D lack or abnormal metabolism of this hormone is unlikely, since at this age some sign of a failure of correct mineralization of bone would be expected, at least in some instances. The opposite, in fact, is the case (see below).

**Bone Morphology.** A total of 12 patients with Scheuermann's kyphosis and seven with juvenile osteoporosis have had bone biopsies, and the common finding is one of increased bone resorption.[5, 7] Two other reports of single cases state that osteoblasts are diminished; however, these were non-quantitative results,[6, 8] while in two other additional cases in which bone biopsies were taken, increased bone destruction was the predominant finding.[9] The result is a decreased amount of bone tissue seen in both the cortex and the trabeculae (Figs. 28–3, 28–4) (Table 28–2). No biopsy showed the presence of increased amounts of osteoid or any indication of osteomalacia; indeed, osteoid border widths were decreased in the majority (six out of seven), probably as a consequence of the high serum calcium and phosphorus (Fig. 28–5). One report suggested that serum immunoreactive parathyroid hormone may be inappropriately elevated in relation to the serum calcium in comparison with normal children of that age.[5] This finding would be consistent with the evolving picture of normocalcemic hyperparathyroidism that is evident from the pathology and high urinary hydroxyproline, but the measurement was only made in one case and must remain tentative.

Table 28–2  BONE REMODELING IN OSTEOPOROSIS IN
YOUNG INDIVIDUALS (mean ± SD)

|                                    | Formation, % | Resorption, % |
| ---------------------------------- | ------------ | ------------- |
| Scheuermann's kyphosis*            | 6.5 ± 2.5    | 8.1 ± 4.6     |
| Idiopathic juvenile osteoporosis** | 7.1 ± 2.4    | 18.8 ± 1.7    |
| Controls (5–19 years old)          | 6.2 ± 3.3    | 7.0 ± 1.0     |

*From Bradford et al.[7] These cases include some in whom the active phase of the bone disorder had "burned out."
**From Jowsey and Johnson.[5]

**Treatment.**  On the basis of finding calcium malabsorption, Dent treated his patients with dihydrotachysterol, although vitamin $D_2$ would presumably have been equally effective.[4] Mild vitamin D deficiency has been documented in some populations in England, and the calcium malabsorption may be merely a reflection of a vitamin D deficiency at a time of increased calcium requirement. In the cases reported from the United States no treatment was given, mainly because of the tendency for urine calcium values to be high, causing apprehension therefore about using either vitamin D or calcium supplements. However, the low calcium intake

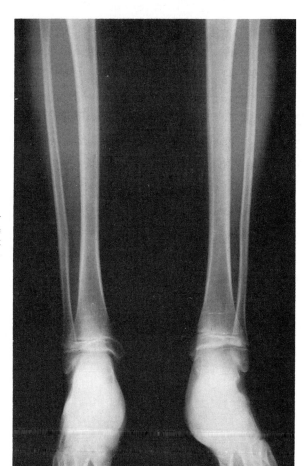

**Figure 28–3**  X-ray of the lower extremities of a patient with juvenile osteoporosis. The cortices are thin, but the bones are of normal external dimensions, unlike osteogenesis imperfecta, and there is no evidence of rickets.

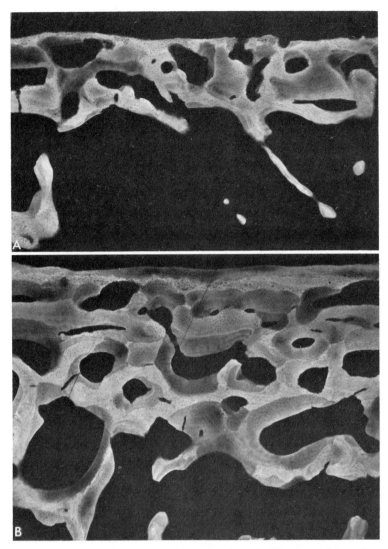

**Figure 28–4**  Microradiograph of the external cortex from the iliac crest of (a) a 13-year-old male with juvenile osteoporosis and (b) a normal male of the same age. In the osteoporotic sample the cortex is narrow and more porous than in the normal; the number of secondary haversian systems and the amount of bone remodeling, however, seem normal, unlike osteogenesis imperfecta (magnification x 40).

that was found in a number of the patients with Scheuermann's kyphosis would indicate that at least in these patients calcium supplements should be given to maintain a 1 gram calcium intake. Vitamin D status should also be estimated and any deficiency corrected. A somewhat restricted phosphorus intake was suggested as a form of treatment in cases which showed no tendency to spontaneous remission.[5]

The clinical presentation in juvenile osteoporosis, the x-ray findings, and the pathology all support a close similarity between this syndrome in children and the adult form of the disease. However, the etiology and the treatment differ, mainly because increase in bone mass is possible because of the normal high bone formation rate in children and because inactivity and estrogen deficiency are not features of the etiology. Therefore, lowering of the bone resorption level to normal or below normal, without any stimulation of formation, should result in recovery.

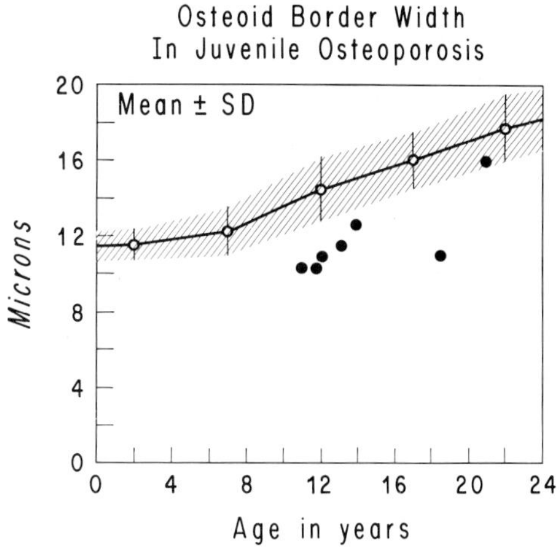

Osteoid Border Width
In Juvenile Osteoporosis

**Figure 28–5**  Osteoid border widths in seven patients with juvenile osteoporosis. The lower than normal values exclude any osteomalacic form of bone disease. (From Jowsey and Johnson.[5])

## REFERENCES

1. Nilsson, B. E.: Spinal osteoporosis and femoral neck fracture. Clin. Orthop., *68*:93–95, 1970.
2. Nordin, B. E. C.: Metabolic Bone and Stone Disease. Baltimore, The Williams and Wilkins Company, 1973.
3. Newton-John, H. F., and Morgan, D. B.: Osteoporosis: disease or senescence? Lancet, *1*:232–233, 1968.
4. Dent, C. E., and Friedman, M.: Idiopathic juvenile osteoporosis. Q. J. Med. new series, *34*:177–210, 1965.
5. Jowsey, J., and Johnson, K. A.: Juvenile osteoporosis: bone findings in seven patients. J. Pediatr., *81*:511–517, 1972.
6. Görgényi, Á.: Idiopathic juvenile osteoporosis: report of a case and review of the literature. Acta Pediat., Acad. Sci. Hung., *10*:315–321, 1969.
7. Bradford, D. S., Brown, D. M., Moe, J. H., Winter, R. B., and Jowsey, J.: Scheuermann's kyphosis: a form of juvenile osteoporosis? Clin. Orthop., *118*:10–15, 1976.
8. Gooding, C. A., and Ball, J. H.: Idiopathic juvenile osteoporosis. Radiology, *93*:1349–1350, 1969.
9. Berglund, G., and Lindquist, B.: Osteopenia in adolescence. Clin. Orthop., *17*:259–264, 1960.

# Chapter Twenty-Nine

# OSTEOPOROSIS: IDIOPATHIC, POST-MENOPAUSAL, AND SENILE

Patients who fall into the category of idiopathic, post-menopausal, or senile osteoporosis distinguish themselves from the previous group of juvenile osteoporotic patients by age. The implications in the three names also somewhat subdivide this group into the idiopathic, who are between 20 and 45, the post-menopausal, who are women who have had oophorectomy or have become post-menopausal naturally, and the senile group, which includes all older men and also women who have been taking estrogens in physiological amounts post-menopausally. It is perhaps obvious that these groups overlap to some extent and that the nomenclature is descriptive of the individuals rather than explanatory of their disease, with the possible exception of post-menopausal women in whom estrogen deficiency plays a clear role in their bone loss.

**Radiologic Features.** The most common osteoporotic patient is the post-menopausal woman with fractures of the spine. The fractures may be symmetrical but more frequently consist of collapse of the anterior part of the vertebral body (Fig. 29–1). This leads eventually to both height loss and dorsal kyphosis, which can be of such a degree that the anterior rib cage may eventually rest on the iliac crest, with associated anterior folds of the skin. In very severe spinal osteoporosis the respiratory cage may be so collapsed and the volume decreased to the point that respiratory failure is a cause of death. The common patient with osteoporosis generally experiences a sharp pain associated with some activity such as lifting, which is frequently related to a fracture of a vertebral body. The fracture heals normally and the pain generally disappears. The history is not the same as that of the patient who complains of backache. Nordin and associates analyzed the relative vertebral density of a group of 152 female volunteers and found the incidence of backache was equal in those with low and high vertebral density values.[1, 2] The history in a patient with backache also tends to be accompanied by complaint of a chronic dull pain not associated with any particular event, although possibly with a deformity of the spine severe enough to cause "mechanical" chronic discomfort.

The incidence of vertebral fractures becomes significant in women at age 45 and is at least four times as common in women as in men. After age 65 the inci-

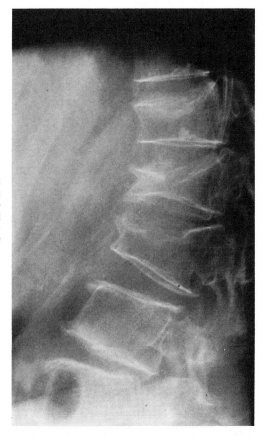

**Figure 29–1** X-ray of the spine of a patient with post-menopausal osteoporosis. There is some deformity of all the vertebrae, plus a "pencilling" of the cortices. Three of the vertebral bodies show fracture or collapse, which has decreased the anterior height and would inevitably lead to kyphosis.

dence climbs steeply, as does the incidence of femoral neck fracture (Fig. 29–2).[3, 4, 5] The fractures are generally associated radiologically with a generalized translucency of the spine and loss of intercortical density as a result of the disappearance of trabeculae. As a result of the loss of trabeculae and endosteal bone there is an accentuation of the remaining cortical bone, which gives the x-ray of the bones a pencilled appearance. This is in contrast to the mushy, diffuse appearance of intercortical bone in osteomalacia, presumably owing to the presence of thick borders of osteoid on the remaining trabeculae within the cortex and the thickening of the cortex, also by osteoid.

Fractures of the femoral neck are also related to osteoporosis, and these are more common (2.4 times more common) in women than in men.[4, 6] Femoral neck fractures occur more frequently in patients with other fractures associated with osteoporosis, such as Colles' or vertebral fractures; in studies in which histological measurements of bone mass have been made, histological osteoporosis is associated with femoral neck fractures.[4, 7] Just as one vertebral fracture is frequently followed by a second and third, so a femoral neck fracture may be followed by a fracture on the contralateral side. Stewart found that 27 out of 388 patients returned with a fracture of the contralateral side.[6] The average age of the patients at the time of admission for their first fracture was 73 years (±2 SE 4.9), an age which obviously included a number of 80-year-old individuals in whom the fracture was not a surprising phenomenon; however approximately 22 per cent of these persons were less than 65 years old. In the group returning with a second fracture, all on the

Fracture Rate In Females In Relation To Age

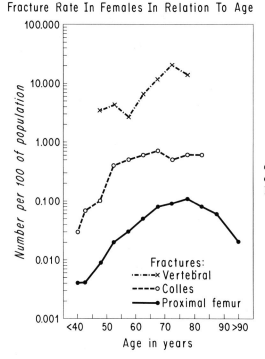

**Figure 29–2** Vertebral fractures appear early and are more frequent than either Colles' or femoral fractures. (Redrawn from Smith and Rizek,[3] Alfram,[4] and Bauer.[5])

contralateral side, the interval between the first and second fracture varied greatly, from patients who returned the same year to those who returned after seventeen or eighteen years (mean $3.8 \pm 2$ SE 1.9 years). The short interval in some could be attributed, at least in part, to the period of immobilization that occurred after the first fracture and caused accelerated bone loss.

**Bone Morphology.** In response to lack of stress or some type of calcium deficiency, such as a chronic low calcium intake compared with phosphorus, or a vitamin D deficiency, or because of accentuated parathyroid hormone action on bone caused by the absence of estrogens, bone resorption is higher than bone formation and results in a net loss of bone in osteoporosis. Resorption tends to be higher than formation in normal, (that is, non-osteoporotic) individuals also, but the bone resorption values in such a group tend to be only moderately elevated (two-fold) above formation compared with the three- or four-fold increases in patients with osteoporosis (Table 29–1). Albright, in 1948, suggested that osteoporosis was the result of a failure of bone formation; this was based on experimental studies in pigeons in which estrogens produce a laying down of new bone. However, this

**Table 29–1** BONE TURNOVER IN OSTEOPOROSIS (mean ± SD)

|  | Age | N | Formation % | Resorption % |
|---|---|---|---|---|
| NORMALS | 20–44 | 37 | 2.3 ± 1.3 | 4.0 ± 1.4 |
|  | 45–75 | 58 | 2.0 ± 1.4 | 3.9 ± 1.4 |
| OSTEOPOROTICS | 20–44 | 12 | 2.9 ± 1.7 | 8.9 ± 3.5 |
|  | 45–75 | 143 | 2.6 ± 1.7 | 10.5 ± 5.1 |

bone is intermedullary bone, formed of highly cellular trabeculae, and is both rapidly formed and rapidly resorbed in response to the deposition of the eggshell on the egg.[8] Nevertheless, impressed by this response to estrogens (which later studies proved to be true only in egg-laying birds), and well aware of the preponderance of estrogen-deficient women who develop osteoporosis, Albright suggested that osteoporosis is the result of a failure of new bone formation. This thesis obviously failed to account for osteoporosis in pre-menopausal women and in children, and it also failed to explain osteoporosis in men. More recent work has shown that osteoporosis is the result of an absolute increase in bone resorption, while bone formation is normal.[9]

Different values and sometimes different conclusions are reached and appear to be conflicting until the data are carefully examined. The majority of bone morphology is carried out on trabecular bone alone, which appears to cease to form bone and later ceases to resorb bone with increasing age. The age of the patient in whom the measurement is made is therefore of importance if only trabecular bone is studied. In a group of eleven younger osteoporotic individuals (mean age 37), the majority falling into the idiopathic group, Bordier and colleagues showed that while resorption was increased compared with normal, bone formation tended to be low; the decrease in formation was not significantly less than normal, because the variation in the percentage of bone formation among his group of patients was high (0.7–6.1 per cent) (Table 29–2).[10] The technique used was of osteoid associated with osteoblasts as a measure of formation and of the surface covered by osteoclasts to evaluate resorption, but only trabecular bone was analyzed. Again using only trabecular bone (from the iliac crest), Schenk studied an elderly population (mean age 73) and found that osteoblasts were diminished and that bone resorption had fallen to normal levels.[11] It is possible that cell counts in the two studies cannot be related to bone loss, since in both studies the formation exceeded resorption by 700 per cent in normals and by 300 per cent in the osteoporotic group. This would mean that both normal and, to a slightly lesser extent, osteoporotic individuals must be gaining bone mass if equal cell counts were taken to imply equal bone deposition and removal rates.

The majority of bone loss takes place on the endosteal cortical and intracortical bone (Fig. 29–3). If the entire specimen of the iliac crest, including the cortex, is examined, then resorption is found to exceed formation. In addition, the majority of bone-forming sites appear to be in the cortex, and, in osteoporosis, the number and extent of these areas are not different from those of normal individuals who have suffered acute deaths.

An important point to be made regarding the histological analysis of bone biopsies is that bed rest will rapidly reduce bone formation. Any patient who is studied in a hospital environment with more than normal amounts of bed-rest will show a

**Table 29–2** BONE REMODELING IN ADULT OSTEOPOROSIS (11 PATIENTS)
(values are mean ± SD)

| Group | Age in yrs. | Hydroxyproline (mg/24 hrs.) | Active Surface % Resorption | % Formation |
|---|---|---|---|---|
| Normals | — | 25.0 ± 5 | 0.59 ± 0.52 | 4.5 ± 2.0 |
| Osteoporotic patients | 36.5 ± 7.5 | 50.2 ± 14 | 0.95 ± 0.86 | 2.4 ± 1.56 |

From Bordier et al.[10]

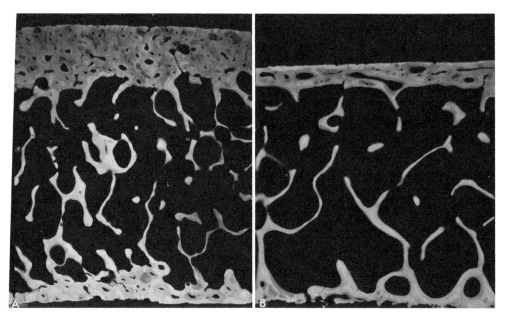

**Figure 29–3** Microradiographs of iliac crests of (a) normal 43-year-old female and (b) a 51-year-old patient with osteoporosis. Cortical thicknesses have decreased markedly, and there has been some loss of trabecular bone (magnification x 16).

fall in this parameter at as short an interval as one day (see section under "Physical Activity"). In addition, a number of relatively common forms of "therapy" for osteoporosis, including calcium and estrogen supplements, will cause a fall in bone formation.

The relationship between the presence of a cell and the relative number of cells, either an osteoclast or an osteoblast, does not imply equal rates. (See also Chapter Seventeen, Morphology, section under "Histology.") This has already been mentioned in studies in osteoporosis with respect to the puzzling numerical values of Bordier and Schenk, where the osteoblasts outnumber osteoclasts significantly in populations who are known to be losing bone. It is evident therefore that osteoclasts work harder per cell than osteoblasts. Indeed, in histological studies directed toward this point, osteoclasts have been measured as having bone resorption rates of up to seven times those of osteoblasts. The rates have also been found to be increased in bone-losing diseases compared with rates in normal states. Therefore, any form of cell count or surface measurement must be taken as such and not be interpreted in terms of addition or removal of bone tissue. If changes in bone mass or cancellous bone volume are also determined, the histological data can be further interpreted to some extent, at least in terms of activity. In any event, observation of bone cells and other biopsy methods are the only way to evaluate bone turnover and are therefore essential, despite their shortcomings.

A final point, which has been documented in the earlier discussion on cortical and trabecular bone, is that cortical bone contributes the majority of tissue to the homeostatic mechanism that involves bone loss. Although trabecular bone has a higher turnover rate because of the high surface-to-volume ratio, and because it disappears more rapidly at early ages (between 20 and 45), the amount of mineral it contributes to the serum is relatively small in absolute terms. Therefore, although measurements of trabecular bone will demonstrate the most sensitive and rapidly measurable changes in bone mass, it is in cortical bone, almost exclusively after age 45, where most bone resorption is occurring and the absolute loss is higher, although the percentage values may be low.

## ETIOLOGY

It is clear that in many instances of bone loss or osteopenia, hormone excess or some single factor such as immobilization is responsible for the skeletal abnormality. In the disease called osteoporosis (often incorrectly "primary" osteoporosis), a single etiological factor is often hard to single out as being the most important. It is evident that in post-menopausal women estrogen deficiency plays a role, since the incidence of the disease is common in this group, and the disease occurs at a relatively early age in women with surgical menopause. However, it is probably most accurate to say that a number of different causes together produce the bone loss seen in the typical patient with this disease. Some factors can be ruled out by history or by laboratory tests, but there remain a number of factors in each patient that can usually be considered contributory. Of these, in the United States, lack of activity and a poor dietary calcium-to-phosphorus ratio are probably the most important, combined with the fact that a larger percentage of people in the United States, particularly women, live longer than in other countries, such as India or Africa, and therefore have a greater chance to acquire the disease.

Secondary osteoporosis, that is, osteopenia with a known causative abnormality, is less common than so-called "primary" osteoporosis. Secondary osteoporosis has been described under the various headings of hyperthyroidism, hyperparathyroidism, and hypercortisonism, to name a few. Primary osteoporosis is distinguished from the secondary form in two ways. First, the abnormality of bone in "primary" osteoporosis is frequently associated with a homeostatic response to a necessity for maintaining serum calcium levels; for example, osteoporosis in a chronic, severe alcoholic might well be called secondary alcoholic osteoporosis (as steroid-induced osteoporosis is called hypercortisone osteoporosis). However, the term primary is used because an exact and single cause of the disease is unknown, although it can generally be related to a response by the body to calcium and probably also to vitamin D deficiency, while in secondary osteoporosis, such as steroid-induced osteoporosis or hyperthyroidism, for instance, the bone loss is generally the result of unrequired (by the bone or serum calcium) increases of corticosteroids and thyroxine, respectively. The second, perhaps less distinguishing feature, is that the cause of bone loss in primary osteoporosis is multifactorial.

**Immobilization**   The most sensitive measure of the effect of immobilization on bone is the rise in serum ionized calcium, particularly if a fracture is present or if the individual is less than 20 years of age. Total serum calcium is not always measured in immobilized patients, and ionized calcium is rarely monitored.[12] In fact, severe symptoms such as nausea, incoherence and dehydration, may be the first signs of hypercalcemia. These findings suggest a serum calcium determination may be of value in immobilized patients. In the report by Winters and co-workers[13] the symptoms of hypercalcemia were accompanied by a total serum calcium of 16.0 mg per 100 ml. In general, however, immobilization will cause a rise in serum calcium, rather than frank hypercalcaemia, with the exception of Paget's disease of bone. Furthermore, symptomatic hypercalcemia in immobilized patients is almost exclusively found in adolescents with fractures where the values may be of concern because of the possibility of impairment of renal function, which has indeed been found to be a complication.[14] However, non-symptomatic hypercalcemia is found in the majority of immobilized patients, with fractures or without; there is a rise in the ionized serum calcium to above normal, although the total serum calcium may remain normal. The elevated ionized calcium is usually associated with hypercalciuria, a secondary effect of the rise in serum calcium (Table 29-3). Presumably the immobilization alone will cause release of calcium into the blood and initiate a rise in both serum calcium (total and ionized) and phosphorus. The ionized calcium will suppress parathyroid hormone secretion, which will then result in a lowering of the renal absorption of calcium and an increase in renal excretion, as reflected in the hypercalciuria.[14] There is generally no renal calculus formation, and, since the ionized calcium is infrequently measured, the phenomenon is often unrecognized; it may be clinically unimportant except that it illustrates the severe upset in calcium homeostasis produced by immobilization which may result in significant bone loss. Nevertheless, an additional secondary effect of the raised ionized serum calcium and the consequently suppressed parathyroid hormone is a tendency for the serum phosphate to be higher than normal, and there is an increased possibility of extraskeletal mineralization. In a short-term study in five immobilized male patients, the ionized calcium rose from 4.9 to 5.2 mg per dl, and the serum parathyroid hormone after twelve days had fallen from 1.08 to 0.65 ng per ml.[15] This would suggest a major effect of serum pH or some factor present in an immobilized individual, which increases the effectiveness of parathyroid hormone–induced bone resorption. Although bone resorption values and parathyroid hormone are generally related, there are a number of bone abnormalities in which this relationship does not hold; immobilization, either local or total body immobilization, is an example. Other examples include estrogen-replaced post-menopausal women and the bone diseases, such as multiple myeloma and hypercortisonism, in which the parathyroids appear not to be implicated.

Some of the increased urinary calcium is doubtless the result of an increase in the filtered load of calcium. Through renal elimination alone, not including fecal excretion, the loss may be up to or above 400 mg per 24 hours,[16] producing a negative calcium balance of 300 mg per day which over a six-month period would reflect a 20 per cent loss of the skeleton. This is considerable and correlates well with the loss of skeletal mass measured directly by balance studies and quantitative roentgenography in normal, immobilized patients. (See Chapter Thirteen, Bone Density Measurements, section under "Quantitative Radiography.")

**Table 29–3**

|  | Total Serum Ca (mg/dl) | Ionized Serum Ca (mg/dl) | Urine Ca mg/24 hrs |
|---|---|---|---|
| NORMALS |  |  |  |
| Control | 8.9 | 4.8 | 128 |
| Bed rest | 9.2 | 5.2 | 252 |
| FRACTURE PATIENTS |  |  |  |
| With bed rest | 9.3 | 5.3 | 364 |

From Heath et al.[12]

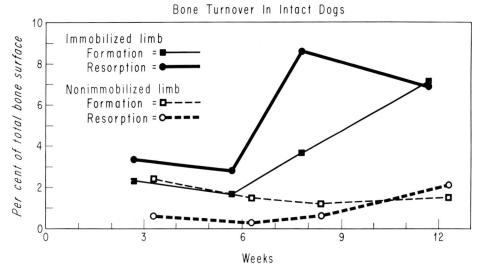

**Figure 29–4** Changes in bone resorption and formation in immobilization. One hind-limb of an adult dog has been immobilized by a plaster cast. Bone remodeling values measured at zero, six, eight and 12 weeks show the marked rise in resorption, which is followed by a delayed rise in formation.

There is a rapid decrease in bone formation followed by a gradual increase in bone resorption.[17] Later, bone formation is increased and bone resorption levels off and then tends to return to normal (Fig. 29–4). The relative effectiveness of the two processes appears to depend on the presence or absence of stress. If the person, or even just the limb itself, continues to be immobilized and weightless, resorption predominates and the bone loses mass, although at a decreasing rate. If stress is resumed, then bone formation increases, calcium balance becomes less negative, and bone mass increases.[12, 18]

The loss of bone therefore is directly related to use; an immobilized limb will show a decrease, while the rest of the skeleton will remain normal. If the whole body is immobilized, then the bone loss is generalized. From this it is evident that the loss is dependent on the lack of stress rather than on a general systemic hormonal alteration. The implication is not that hormones are uninvolved, rather the reverse, since removal of the parathyroids will essentially prevent the development of the bone loss (Table 29–4).[15, 19] The implication is that there is an increased sensitivity of the bone tissue to normal or even lowered circulating levels of parathy-

**Table 29–4** FRACTIONAL CHANGES IN REMODELING OF IMMOBILIZED AND NON-IMMOBILIZED LIMBS IN ADULT DOGS

| Group | No. of Weeks | Formation % | Resorption % |
|---|---|---|---|
| Intact | 2 | −0.5 | + 5.0 |
|  | 6 | +0.5 | +10.0 |
|  | 8 | +3.4 | +14.0 |
|  | 12 | +5.0 | + 5.0 |
| Parathyroidectomized | 2–12 | +1.4 | −1.6 |
| Thyroidectomized | 6–12 | −0.8 | +0.05 |
| Thyroparathyroidectomized | 2–12 | −0.3 | −4.0 |

From Burkhart and Jowsey.[19]

roid hormone, resulting possibly from the localized fall in pH due to the disuse and related hemodynamic changes.

The relationship between disuse osteoporosis and transient osteoporosis of the lower extremities is obscure. Lower extremities (foot, knee, and hip) are usually affected and the condition is painful. Resolution of the condition generally follows with no treatment, in contrast to patients with reflex dystrophy, a similar entity, but one generally associated with a history of injury.[20, 21] Since bone necrosis has been seen on biopsy, it is possible that this form of localized osteoporosis represents a response to avascularity and death of tissue secondary to impairment of blood supply. The history of symptoms and repair would not be in conflict with this suggestion.

When "immobilization" osteoporosis is carefully examined, it is apparent that the correct terminology should be "lack of weight-bearing and changing stress" osteoporosis. In strictly immobilized volunteers neither horizontal stress nor pressure resulted in a return toward normal of the bone, which had decreased approximately 20 per cent in mass after 130 days.[22] Only weight-bearing ambulation is effective in restoring bone mass. Lack of gravity also results in a negative calcium balance, and the loss per month is similar to that produced by bed immobilization.[23] As in the studies by Lockwood, rigorous exercise in a non-gravity atmosphere did not succeed in preventing the loss, again pointing out the importance of weight-bearing in the maintenance of skeletal mass. It is also perhaps relevant not only to document the type of stress necessary to evoke an increase in bone mass, but also to come to some conclusion about the length of time for which the stress should be applied. A normal person in a 16-hour day must probably spend 25 per cent of that time in weight-bearing movement in order not to lose bone mass. It is therefore reasonable to plan at least four hours per day of ambulatory exercise in any rehabilitation program in order to stimulate bone formation significantly. It may seem unnecessary to point this out; however, as with the possible hypercalcemia of the immobilized adolescent which seems to be frequently ignored, immobilized patients are often treated with woefully inadequate exercise programs which cannot even be expected to halt, let alone reverse, the bone loss of bed rest.

**Physical Activity**  The mechanism whereby increased load results in an increase in bone mass is unknown, but, as with immobilization osteoporosis, it is probably in the field of piezoelectricity.[24] The bone response is no more unusual than muscle or skin response to increased activity or pressure; examples might include the bulging muscles of the professional weightlifter, the phenomenon of "weaver's bottom," or the skin calluses of the manual laborer. In bone, the phenomenon becomes important not only because of the contribution of disuse or inactivity to bone loss, and therefore to an increased fracture incidence, but also because of the use of exercise in increasing bone mass as a treatment for osteoporosis. It is relevant to document the effect of exercise or stress on bone mass changes; however, the most significant point is the amount of exercise required to make measurable changes in the bone.

Any increase in stress is normally associated with hypertrophy of both muscle and bone. In fact, a bone mass and muscle mass correlation has been demonstrated in man (Fig. 29–5).[25] This relationship was also observed in the studies of Smith and Saville, who devised the ingenious, albeit unkind, device of depriving growing rats of their two front legs;[26] the rats therefore used their hind legs entirely for locomotion, in a manner similar to the desert rat. The body weight of this group

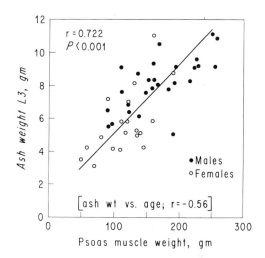

**Figure 29-5** The relationship between bone mass in a single vertebra and the weight of the psoas muscle. The muscle mass has been taken as a measure of activity. (Redrawn from Doyle et al.[25])

was initially less than controls because of loss of the forelimbs. However, after a few days body weight rose to normal and above. At the same time stress on the hind limbs increased, femur weight increased. Femur weight and volume in the bipeds was greater than in controls, although a perhaps surprising finding was that the cross-sectional area remained the same in the two groups, as did the slope of stress (weight per unit volume) against femur calcium over volume; however, the intercept in the bipeds was greater by a factor of nearly two, suggesting that the bone was better arranged to withstand stress. It is possible that the bending test which provided the stress data favored a femur grown under bipedal conditions; nevertheless, the increase is impressive (Table 29-5). It is likely that the increase in breaking strength is related to stress alone rather than to altered posture, since symmetrical loading, as in lambs wearing lead coats, or excessive but normal ambulation, as well as excessive exercise in normal rats all lead to increased bone and muscle volume.[27, 28, 29]

Studies in Malmö and Stockholm, Sweden, have rightly emphasized the type and duration of exercise necessary. Perhaps fortuitously in the animal studies, large stresses were applied (the rats ran more than a mile and the lambs' jackets weighed 40 per cent of their body weight). In man, also, large stresses are necessary before

**Table 29-5**   INCREASE IN BREAKING STRESS IN BIPEDAL
AND NORMAL RATS

|  | Control | Bipedal | Units |
|---|---|---|---|
| FEMUR BREAKING STRESS AT 300 gms BODY WT | 1.9 | 2.8 | kg/cm$^2$ × 10$^{-3}$ |
| FEMUR BREAKING STRESS AT A BONE DENSITY OF 1.25 mg/cm$^3$ | 0.7 | 1.7 | kg/cm$^2$ × 10$^{-3}$ |

From Smith and Saville.[26]

any significant alterations in bone mass are seen. Employing the bone mineral densitometer, but using the distal femur rather than the radius, a significant difference was found between professional athletes and non-athletes and also between those who exercised and those who had no exercise program (Table 29–6).[28] When the athletes were separated into groups by the load on the lower limb, it was evident that the effect on bone density was mainly the result of weight-bearing movement; for example, swimmers tended to have a relatively normal bone density, although they also tended to be younger than the weightlifters and throwers, with whom they were compared, which may to some extent explain the data.[28] As can be seen from Table 29–6, this study supported the idea that exercise programs are effective in increasing "bone density." However, the subjects were all young, about 22 years old, which may explain the discrepancy between this conclusion and the evidence for a lack of effect seen by the Stockholm group.[29] The subjects were normal volunteers, aged about 53, who were in a three-month exercise program, possibly too short a time to elicit a response. However, long-distance runners formed the "athletes" in this study, and they were 55 years old. Their bone density was significantly greater, on an average 13 per cent in the seven different sites measured. This figure was somewhat lower than the 30 per cent difference seen between the young athletes and non-exercisers reported from Malmö.[28]

Stress will clearly increase bone mass; it appears that the effect can be elicited in both young and older individuals and that relatively large amounts of stress must be applied; however these lie within the realm of rigorous exercise programs. Weight-bearing ambulation appears to be the form of stress that is effective, recalling the experience of Hulley's group, in which ambulation reversed the bone loss of immobilization but horizontal exercises did not.[18] Exercise will therefore tend to result in a dense skeleton that is more resistant to fracture, and long-term exercise will maintain skeletal mass.

The practical problems that arise in the use of this information for the treatment of osteoporosis are two-fold. In an individual who has fractures, any increase in stress is liable to cause further fractures, and if the patient is "bed-ridden" then an effective exercise program is essentially impossible. Probably the most significant factor is the impracticality of making people change their way of life. A large number of women in the 1970's play bridge, watch television, and "visit," while a large number of men, once they arrive at "the office," are sedentary all day except for the short walk to the sedentary automobile. In comparison with the amount of effort required to function 60 years ago (no cars, no washing machines, etc.), the everyday expenditure of energy is significantly less now, quite apart from the average amount of energy required to do the average job, which is true for both males and females. It is probably not possible to make people change the way of

**Table 29–6**   EFFECT OF EXERCISE ON BONE DENSITY IN MAN

|  | Bone Density (g/cc) | Age (yrs) | Weight (kg) |
|---|---|---|---|
| ATHLETES | 0.25 ± 0.05 | 22.3 ± 4.1 | 90.3 ± 26.3 |
| CONTROLS, EXERCISING | 0.21 ± 0.03 | 22.5 ± 5.1 | 69.8 ± 10.7 |
| CONTROLS, NOT EXERCISING | 0.17 ± 0.04 | 22.8 ± 5.2 | 68.5 ± 9.2 |

From Nilsson and Westlin.[28]

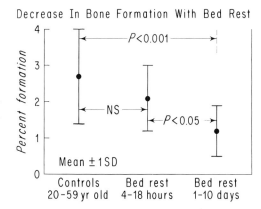

**Figure 29–6** Bone formation, measured by the technique of microradiography, in the iliac crest of normal individuals who died suddenly (controls) or were at bed-rest, immobilized, or died after a 1 to 10-day-period of coma after an accident. The decrease occurs rapidly and becomes marked after ten days.

life they have chosen, and, except for the few who have taken up jogging or physical activity programs, there are a large majority of people whose level of activity insures that they will lose bone mass.

The mechanism of action of stress on bone is through an increase in bone formation. Lack of stress, such as in bed rest or immobilization, will cause profound decreases in bone formation in a short time (Fig. 29–6). Continuous exertion has not been studied in terms of bone turnover, but the net effect is one of increased bone mass. To return to the question of how much exercise is significant, it is relevant that active occupations involving physical labor over an eight-hour day appear to result in a retention of bone, compared with the loss that occurs in sedentary workers (Table 29–7). The bone density values derived from videodensitometry were divided into two groups: those that fell above (group 1) and those that fell below (group 2) the mean regression line in all normal men between the ages of 40 and 75. The occupations of the group 1 men were of the laboring type, requiring heavy work, while those that fell below the mean normal level had sedentary employment. While it is evident that osteoporosis frequently has a multifactorial etiology, any sedentary occupation should be suspected as contributory, particularly when associated with a sedentary hobby. Exercise is unreasonable to recommend in the therapy of most severely osteoporotic individuals; however, it is certainly worthwhile and effective wherever possible, and it is undoubtedly useful in prevention of the disease.

**Table 29–7** BONE DENSITY IN NORMAL INDIVIDUALS WITH DIFFERENT OCCUPATIONS

| | Age in yrs | Number | % Bone | Occupations |
|---|---|---|---|---|
| GROUP 1 | | | | |
| Above mean value | 64.0 | 12 | 80.8 | farmers (4), carpenter, laborers (2), elevator operator, furniture mover, custodian, cleaner, roadworker |
| GROUP 2 | | | | |
| Below mean value | 52.3 | 15 | 61.1 | college professor, insurance agent, supplies supervisor, state hospital patients (2), alcoholics (3), disabled railroad switchman, bookkeeper, office secretary (2), unknown (3) |

Related to the importance of exercise and stress is the impression that emerges frequently from encounters with patients suffering from osteoporosis — such individuals are frequently small and light. This impression has been translated into quantitative values by Saville, who carefully compared body weight in randomly selected individuals with and without osteoporosis. He found that the great proportion of osteoporotic individuals weighed less than those with no symptoms. It is uncommon for women over 140 pounds to have osteoporosis, while it is a frequent finding in women who are less than 140 pounds (Fig. 29–7).[30] Increased stress because of increased body weight may constitute a factor through the piezoelectric effect. A second factor which may play a role, since increased body weight is largely represented by increased fat, is the storage of estrogens in fatty tissue and a greater estrogen effect on bone resorption, presuming that this hormone is not only stored but released from body fat. High body weight perhaps should not be encouraged; however, body weight will play a part in the etiology of bone loss.

**Genetics.**   It has been suggested that there is a uniform loss of bone with increasing age in both men and women and in all races.[31] The different amount of bone in different individuals and the non-uniformity of fractures in, for example, men and women has been accounted for by the difference in the amount of bone at the age of skeletal maturity, that is at age 20. There certainly are data to support the latter, and clear variations in bone mass have been demonstrated in young adults by methods as variable as the Cameron-Sorenson densitometer, metacarpal cortical thickness, and total body neutron activation analysis. However, variables in the rate of bone loss have also been documented which suggest that bone loss is not an inevitable accompaniment of old age, but for a number of reasons is avoided by a significant number of persons.

One of the major difficulties of assessing rates of bone loss is the necessity of using longitudinal studies in which the same individuals are studied over a significant period of time, rather than using cross-sectional studies and comparing groups of people of different ages. The latter studies are based on two assumptions: first, that all the individuals were once the same and therefore that any decreased mass is a reflection of rates of loss; secondly, that the year of birth makes no difference to rate of loss. It has already been seen in the discussion on the increase in bone

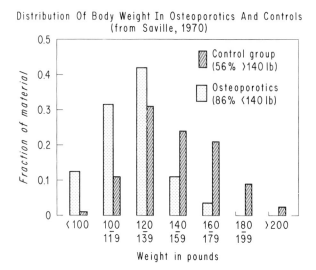

**Figure 29–7** Body weight in a random group of women, with and without osteoporosis. The majority of osteoporotic women weigh less than 140 lbs., whereas osteoporosis is uncommon in women who weigh more than 160 lbs. (Redrawn from Saville.[30])

size with age that the increase in periosteal size in older individuals does not represent increase in the external diameter with age, but rather the fact that in 1900 men and women had larger external diameters to their bones to begin with at the age of skeletal maturity. Although it is unlikely that porosity was increased in individuals born longer ago, it is a possibility to be considered. Neither assumption is necessary in a longitudinal study. In 1956 and again in 1967 a total of 123 men and women were studied by Adams and his colleagues.[32] These persons were a random selection of people living in the Vale of Glamorgan in Wales; careful measurements were made of the metacarpal cortical thickness, and serum calcium, phosphorus, and alkaline phosphatase were also measured. Spinal x-rays were made, and body height and weight were also recorded. Although there was an overall loss of bone in both men and women over the 11-year period, a significant group of both sexes did not show any bone loss (Fig. 29–8). Singh Index measurements on older persons also support the concept that a small proportion of both sexes, particularly men, do not lose bone with increasing age, since they still have a Singh Index of VII at the age of 70 (Fig. 29–9).[33] Therefore, although the majority of both men and women lose bone as they grow older, this is not a universal event.

A true genetic effect on bone mass has been found in a study on monozygotic and dizygotic twins. If genetic constitution is important, then the bone mass differences in monozygotic or genetically identical twins should be small, while those in genetically different twins should differ as a reflection of any differences in environment or food habits.[34] The variance in both children and adults supports a genetic trait, in that these values are small in the monozygotes and greater in the dizygotes (Table 29–8). The variances are a factor of four different in the juveniles and only a factor of two in the adults, suggesting that environmental differences tend to make the monozygous pairs drift further apart with time.

BLACK VERSUS WHITE.   Probably the best known and most clearly documented bone mass differences that indicate a genetic difference are those between white and black races. As early as 1965 it was shown that the incidence of hip fracture was far greater in whites than blacks (Table 29–9).[35] There was no evidence of a geographic, age, or economic difference to explain the data, and the numbers for the percentage of patients with hip fractures, varying from 6 per cent in black men to 44 per cent in white women, are compelling. The explanation appears to be

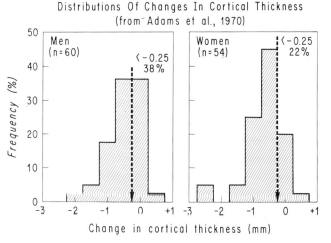

**Figure 29–8**  The change in the metacarpal thickness at an 11-year interval. A significant percentage of both men and women have not lost bone over this period of time. (Redrawn from Adams et al.[32])

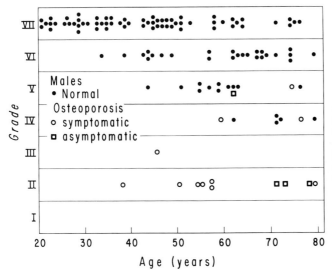

**Figure 29–9** The Singh Index in normal and osteoporotic males in relation to age. A number of men over the age of 70 have an Index of VII, indicating that they have not lost appreciable amounts of bone with age. (From Singh et al.[33])

**Table 29–8   VARIANCE OF INTERPAIR DIFFERENCES**

|  | Bone Mass | Bone Width |
|  | gm²/cm² | cm |
|---|---|---|
| JUVENILE TWINS |  |  |
| monozygotic | 0.0013 | 0.0021 |
| dizygotic | 0.0052 | 0.0091 |
| ADULT TWINS |  |  |
| monozygotic | 0.0069 | 0.0057 |
| dizygotic | 0.0137 | 0.0104 |

From Smith et al.[34]

**Table 29–9   PROXIMAL FEMUR FRACTURES IN PERSONS OVER AGE 65 ADMITTED TO THE JEFFERSON DAVIS HOSPITAL, HOUSTON**

|  | Average Age (yrs.) | % Total Admissions | % Total Hip Fractures |
|---|---|---|---|
| BLACK MEN | 76 | 27.1 | 6.3 |
| BLACK WOMEN | 79 | 18.7 | 14.4 |
| WHITE MEN | 78 | 32.5 | 35.1 |
| WHITE WOMEN | 78 | 21.7 | 44.2 |

From Moldawer et al.[35]

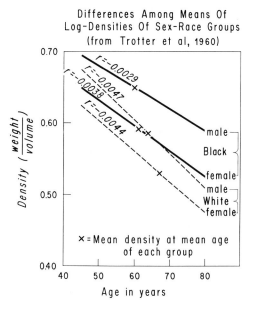

**Figure 29–10** Regression lines of bone density in black and white males and females. Black males and females have a higher bone mass at age 40 and lose it at a slower rate than white males and females. (Drawn from Trotter et al.[36])

that blacks reach skeletal maturity with a greater bone mass than whites, and similarly males of either race have a higher skeletal mass at maturity than females.[36] In addition, blacks lose bone less rapidly than whites of either sex (Fig. 29–10). The bone loss differences are not the result of any periosteal new bone growth, since this has been shown not to occur.[37] It must be the consequence of endosteal and intercortical bone resorption and, of course to a lesser extent, the loss of bone trabeculae. It seems only reasonable at this time to ascribe the differences to a genetic factor, since other known racial factors would tend to push the data in the opposite direction; these include the decreased vitamin D absorption by black skin and the increase in lactose deficiency in blacks compared with whites.

Three impressions emerge frequently from clinical encounters with patients presenting with symptoms of osteoporosis. The first is that the patients are frequently small and thin, while the second is that they are predominantly white rather than black. The third, and perhaps most obvious, is that they are women rather than men. In other words, the most common osteoporotic patient is a white, lightweight woman. The prevalence of this type as a patient can be explained to some extent and contributes to our knowledge of the etiology of the disease.

**Protein Deficiency.** Protein lack can occur as a result of starvation and will result in metabolic acidosis. Bone will be resorbed in abnormally high quantities as a buffer in the renal excretion of the hydrogen ions.[38] However, in the United States, chronic starvation is not a common cause of bone disease, and, with the exception of severe weight-loss programs, this is an unusual form of induced bone abnormality and has probably never resulted in clinically recognizable skeletal disease.

Protein deficiency, however, is a recognized cause of bone disease. In protein deficiency which occurs soon after birth and onwards, the body weight and skeletal age are always less than normal, suggesting a failure in anabolism rather than exaggerated catabolism as a cause of the bone immaturity and osteoporosis. This is also suggested by experimental studies; in an investigation in monkeys, lack of matrix deposition and a decreased endochondral bone formation were both features of a protein deficient diet.[39] There is less bone than normal in addition to the decreased skeletal age; cortical thickness is decreased and the trabeculae also appear subjectively less.[40]

Only occasionally in the United States, but not uncommonly in other countries where starvation levels of food intake occur, protein deficiency presents clinically with the full picture of kwashiorkor. Frequently the syndrome results from a high-carbohydrate intake, unaccompanied by adequate protein. Kwashiorkor includes the clinical presentations of irritability, generalized edema, and often characteristic hair changes, particularly noticeable in black-haired people. In addition, there is retarded skeletal maturity and a general failure to thrive. The protein deficiency that results in kwashiorkor is rare but not unknown in the United States. In common with many of the instances of kwashiorkor in Africa, where it is more frequent, it is now most often related to poor nutritional education. In the instances that are documented most frequently in Africa, the disease results from a diet consisting of only one staple food (e.g., mealies or matooke) which contains very little protein but adequate calories, while in the United States the instances of kwashiorkor result from a cereal diet supplemented often with fruit and vitamins but with inadequate protein.[41] The most serious complications are not bone disease but failure to thrive, and the condition is readily reversed by a normal diet. In Africa and some instances in the United States, the infant with kwashiorkor may present with rickets if the calcium intake as well as the protein intake is low, and the patients may have rib fractures and muscle weakness.[40, 41] Milk added to the diet will provide not only protein but also calcium and should reverse all symptoms readily.

**Calcium and Vitamin D Deficiency.**   Epidemiological studies of dietary calcium intake and the incidence of osteoporosis have been suggestive but not conclusive. Using metacarpal cortical thickness as a measure of bone loss, Nordin found a marked decrease with age in Japan, where calcium intake is low and phosphorus intake high, compared with the bone loss in Finland where calcium intake is high.[42] However, in all epidemiological studies, there are many factors operating in any one population and the role of calcium deficiency is not always easy to establish as an important etiological factor.

If dietary calcium intake is compared between normal and osteoporotic individuals, the same conflict appears. Riggs and associates reported, in a group of 166 osteoporotic individuals, that the calcium intake was lower; in a sub-group of 35 of this population 46 per cent had a lower intestinal absorption, using $^{47}$Ca tracer methods, than age- and calcium-intake-matched controls.[43] This could be the result of differences in vitamin D intake, although of the patients who were receiving vitamin D supplements at a low level (<1000 IU per day), five out of nine of them were in the group who malabsorbed calcium.[44] In countries other than the United States, insufficient vitamin D is a common factor in the etiology of the disease, especially in areas such as the north of England and Scotland, where sunlight exposure is low and skin exposure to sunlight is minimal. Osteomalacia is often mixed with the osteoporosis in such a population. Other studies have measured calcium intake in people of different ages, and dietary intake appears to decrease significantly with age as a result of the change in dietary habits.[45] The latter data would be relevant only in that more older persons have osteoporosis than those in the younger age groups. Avioli has reported a general decrease in absorption with age, which, added to the declining calcium intake, would result in approximately 50 per cent less calcium being available in people over 50 compared with those below 20 years of age.[46] The data are supported by the almost universally observed negative calcium balance seen in older individuals, which appeared in the report by Avioli to be reflected in a similar degree of decreased absorption of calcium in older people whether or not they had osteoporosis. The problem of distinguishing between people losing bone at an increased rate, some of whom have incurred enough trauma to cause a fracture and to be classified as osteoporotic, and some of whom have lost equal amounts of bone but have no fracture, is again a problem here. In addition, Avioli's study was carried out with all patients on a low calcium intake, which could suggest that fracture patients are as unable to adapt to a low calcium diet as are non-fracture patients.

An etiological factor that is possibly important in northern parts of any continent is the variation in sunlight exposure. Contrary to previously held views, it is evident that vitamin D stores begin to be depleted after only a few weeks. Asian immigrants to the north of Britain show a 50 per cent depletion in two months.[47] In Glasgow, the mean monthly hours of sunshine vary from a low of 28 in January to a high of 179 in June. Metacarpal mineral content measurements in surgically postmenopausal women between 31 and 58 showed a loss in the winter and a gain in the summer; this change was followed by a minor cyclical variation in the serum phosphorus from high values in the summer to low values in the winter and would be consistent with a fall in parathyroid activity in response to a higher vitamin D level (Fig. 29–11).[48] It is possible that the population which develops osteoporosis

**Figure 29–11**  There is a close relationship between the metacarpal cortical bone thickness and the hours of sunshine. The rise in serum phosphorus is also greatest in the high sunshine period. (Drawn from Aitkin et al.[48])

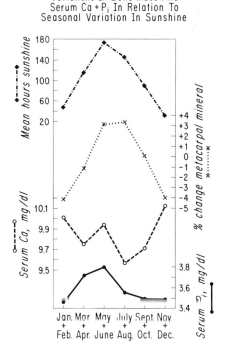

Variations In Bone Mass And Serum Ca + P$_i$ In Relation To Seasonal Variation In Sunshine

**Table 29–10** CAUSES OF INADEQUATE CALCIUM INTAKE (Into the Blood)

Inadequate calcium in the diet
Lactase deficiency
Vitamin D deficiency, dietary or environmental
Abnormality of vitamin D metabolism
Sprue
Gastrectomy
Dilantin therapy
Chronic alcoholism
Acidosis

with vertebral fractures are those who fail to replace the bone they lost in the winter with new bone during the summer.

Some specific causes of calcium malabsorption which function alone or in combination are apparent in small groups of individuals. These include the agents listed in Table 29–10. In 1965 Saville showed that the bone mass, measured by weighing defatted bone biopsies of the iliac crest, was reduced in young (<45 years old), chronic alcoholics.[49] This was found to be true in both men and women, and the decrease was on the order of 30 per cent compared with age- and sex-matched non-alcoholics. Although dietary intake is certainly a factor, the information is significant. In experimental animals, 20 per cent ethanol supplied in drinking water was found to reduce the absorption of calcium. Using $^{45}Ca$ transport in everted gut-sacs, Krawitt showed that the effect was not dependent on inhibition of 1,25-$(OH)_2$ vitamin $D_3$ but appeared to be the result of an interference in the transfer of calcium from the microvilli to intracellular sites (Table 29–11).[50] This is likely, since vitamin 25-$(OH)D_3$ is also unable to reverse the alcohol depressive effect on calcium absorption, so presumably the effect does not depend on the presence of liver or kidney disease.

Although the alcohol content in the experimental study was high, and presumably the group of patients studied by Saville also consumed large volumes of alcohol, the effect of alcohol on calcium absorption can be considered to make a contribution to the absorption of calcium in adult individuals who are more than "social drinkers."

Sprue, malabsorption, and gastrectomy will all cause loss of both calcium and vitamin D, while treatment for epilepsy with barbiturates will interfere with vitamin D metabolism. Lactase deficiency is considered in the next section.

Pregnancy and heparin administration have been implicated in the development of osteoporosis, but the data are somewhat inconclusive.

Since calcium deficiency of some kind, most frequently associated with an abnormality of vitamin D, appears to be associated with osteoporosis, calcium sup-

**Table 29–11** THE EFFECT OF ETHANOL ON CALCIUM ABSORPTION IN THE RAT WITH AND WITHOUT ACTIVE VITAMIN D
(Mean ± SE, 7–10 animals in each group)

|  | Control (Pair Fed) | ETOH | ETOH + 1,25$(OH)_2D_3$ |
|---|---|---|---|
| $^{45}Ca$ S/M ratio | 7.5 ± .8 | 4.6 ± .4 | 4.2 ± .6 |

From Krawitt.[50]

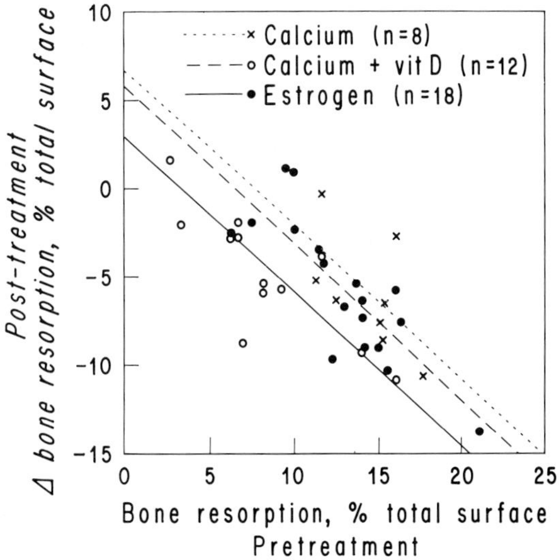

**Figure 29–12** Changes in bone resorption on three different treatment regimes. There is no significant difference between the three forms of treatment. (From: Riggs et al.[51])

plements have been used in an attempt to treat this disease. In a one-year study calcium (2 grams), calcium (1.5 to 2 grams) and vitamin D and estrogen treatment in osteoporotic women have been compared. The effects on bone resorption were similar with all three forms of treatment (Fig. 29–12).[51] The decrease in resorption was accompanied by a fall in serum parathyroid levels from $28 \pm 3$ to $23.2 \pm 2$ (mean $\pm$ SD, $\mu l$ eq/ml), which was significant at $p<0.05$. Calcium infusion has also been used to treat patients with osteoporosis on a basis similar to the use of oral calcium supplements; a rise in serum calcium should depress parathyroid hormone and result in a fall in bone resorption. As with oral supplements of calcium, calcium infusion also decreased resorption. Values fell to normal from the high levels found before treatment ($p=<0.001$); no change occurred in bone formation (Table 29–12).[52]

It should be recalled that a decrease in resorption of bone with no increase in formation will not result in increased bone mass. Indeed, if resorption, though decreased, continues to exceed formation, bone loss may continue, although at a reduced rate. Videodensitometry of patients before and after oral calcium and vitamin D showed no change ($27.3 \pm 3.3$ to $26.5 \pm 2.5$) (mean $\pm$ SE, porosity per

**Table 29–12** THE EFFECT OF CALCIUM INFUSIONS ON BONE REMODELING IN RIB AND ILIAC CREST ($n = 12$)

| | Before Treatment | | After Treatment | | Age- and Sex-Matched Controls | |
|---|---|---|---|---|---|---|
| | % BF | % BR | % BF | % BR | % BF | % BR |
| RIB | | | | | | |
| Mean | 2.7 | 10.7 | 5.1 | 5.2 | 2.8 | 4.6 |
| SD | 2.0 | 3.5 | 2.5 | 2.2 | 1.9 | 2.1 |
| ILIAC CREST | | | | | | |
| Mean | 1.6 | 7.8 | 2.2 | 4.9 | 3.6 | 6.6 |
| SD | 1.3 | 2.4 | 2.3 | 2.1 | 2.0 | 1.5 |

From Jowsey et al.[52]

cent) over a 12-month period. Using total body neutron activation analysis, a continued loss was noted in five osteoporotic patients treated by calcium infusion over a 13- to 22-month period.[53] Calcium supplements, or the more elaborate and tedious calcium infusion techniques, may be used preventatively but will not reverse the disease.

The lack of any added advantage of vitamin D supplements with calcium has suggested that vitamin D is not useful in the treatment of osteoporosis. Treatment with 1,25-(OH)$_2$ vitamin D may prove useful if a deficiency of this hormone is established in osteoporotic subjects. A study in a small number of patients using 1$\alpha$-hydroxy vitamin D has been reported, showing a decrease in bone resorption in four out of the six patients.[54] However, the data are confusing, since four out of the six patients had osteomalacia, rather than osteoporosis uncomplicated by increased amounts of osteoid. Also, one gram of supplemental calcium constituted part of the treatment, and it has already been mentioned that calcium alone is effective in reducing resorption. Further studies on osteoporotic patients given vitamin D metabolites alone are necessary to settle the question of the possible therapeutic effectiveness of this metabolite.

On the other hand, in states of vitamin D deficiency, which are common in the north of England and Scotland and which may be seasonally significant in the northern United States, vitamin D can be expected to cause an increase in mineralized bone mass and possibly clinical improvement. In fact, a patient who improves with vitamin D treatment almost certainly had osteomalacia, not osteoporosis, as the primary clinical problem.

A secondary cause of calcium loss may be acidosis. The skeleton forms a buffer for the ingestion of a large amount of acid and bone is lost to compensate for the acid intake. Increased acid intake occurs with a high fat diet (ketogenic acidosis), ammonium chloride, or an acid ash diet which can result from a high protein intake. The increased amounts of calcium found in the urine are significant (Table 29–13).[55] With severe acid loading, blood and urine pH may also fall, while blood bicarbonate increases. Acidosis is an uncommon form of calcium deficiency (in terms of loss exceeding intake) but occurs in diabetes and may be significant in patients ingesting large amounts of salicylates. Chronic renal disease also causes acidosis as the damaged kidney is unable to excrete hydrogen ions. Acidosis may result from ureterosigmoidostomy, since the intestinal mucosa reabsorbs chloride which has already been filtered by the kidney and is destined for urinary excretion.

Gonick and colleagues reported three patients with renal tubular acidosis who were in strong negative calcium balance and had high parathyroid hormone levels.[56] Both the calcium balance and the serum parathyroid hormone returned toward normal after alkali therapy, with the exception of one patient whose serum parathyroid hormone levels tended to remain elevated until a subtotal parathyroidectomy was

**Table 29–13**  CHANGES IN URINARY CALCIUM IN ADULTS (20–80 years old), IN RESPONSE TO ACIDOSIS

|          | Ketogenic | Ammonium Chloride | Acid Ash |
|----------|-----------|-------------------|----------|
| CONTROL  | 4.2       | 24.1              | 29.1     |
| ACIDOTIC | 90.0      | 133.6             | 101.2    |

From Knapp.[55]
The values represent urine calcium as a percent of calcium intake.

performed. This and other studies have implicated the parathyroids in the development of bone disease in acidosis. The bone disease has been described as osteomalacia caused by the tendency to hypercalciuria, which produces a lowering of the serum calcium and secondary hyperparathyroidism. It is also possible that bone resorption is increased because of increased effectiveness of normal parathyroid hormone levels in an acid environment. A similar mechanism was suggested for the bone loss of immobilization. (See section under "Immobilization," page 261.)

**Lactase Deficiency.** Lactase deficiency causes lactose intolerance, which results in gastric discomfort and diarrhea after ingestion of milk or dairy products. People with lactase deficiency therefore avoid calcium-containing foods and are on a voluntary low calcium intake. The incidence of lactase deficiency, in a series reported by Birge and co-workers, was approximately 50 per cent in a group of patients presenting with osteoporosis.[57] The diagnosis was made on the basis of a lactose tolerance test; in those in whom this test was below normal the dietary calcium intake was low (Fig. 29–13). In a series of 100 patients seen at the Mayo Clinic who had symptomatic osteoporosis, 38 per cent were reported in the routine dietary history as being habitual non-milk drinkers. The dietary history of this latter group of patients at the time they entered the study was deceptive, since the majority of the non-milk drinkers had been told by their local physician to start drinking milk when they first presented with back pain. In a normal population, in comparison with an osteoporotic and therefore older group, lactase deficiency is, perhaps surprisingly, widespread; the prevalence varies in different populations and geographical areas (Table 29–14). In Scandinavians, lactose intolerance is rare, while in Orientals and Africans it is high. It is tempting to speculate that the prevalence of the deficiency is related to the habitual diet, which in Norway, Finland, Sweden, and Switzerland contains a large amount of cheese and milk products, while Asians and Africans produce and drink very little milk, probably partly because of the difficulties of storage.[58] Where races are mixed in one geographical area, the amount of milk con-

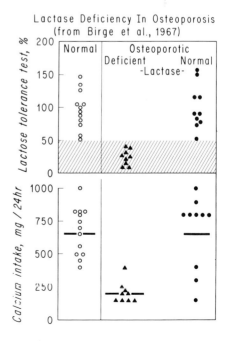

**Figure 29–13**   Nine out of nineteen patients with osteoporosis proved to be lactase deficient compared with normals. This group also had a low habitual calcium intake. (Redrawn from Birge et al.[57])

Table 29–14

| Population | Locale | Abnormal Lactose Tolerance Test | Abnormal Lactose Assay |
|---|---|---|---|
| Eskimo | Greenland | 88 | — |
| Chinese, Japanese, Korean | Minnesota and Maryland (USA) | 100 | 100 |
| Japanese | Japan | — | 92 |
| African Bantu | Uganda and Rhodesia | 95 | 95 |
| American Negro | Maryland (USA) | 72 | 70 |
| Israeli Jewish | Israel | 61 | — |
| Finnish | Finland | 18 | — |
| Danish | Denmark | 2 | — |
| Swiss | Switzerland | — | 6 |
| White American | Minnesota and Maryland (USA) | 10 | 10 |
| White American | Illinois (USA) | — | 19 |
| White Australian | Australia | 16 | — |

From Gastroenterology.[58]

sumed continues to vary, although not to the extent seen when the group was in its country of origin. For example, in two studies, one in Boston and one in South Carolina, whites were reported to drink twice as much milk as the blacks living in the same place.[58] Lactose intolerance in Japanese and Chinese does not change when these individuals migrate to the United States, nor does it change in American-born Orientals. This is most likely to be the result of dietary habit rather than a genetic factor.

There appears to be a difference in the incidence of lactose intolerance (the habitual non-milk drinker) and the incidence of lactase deficiency. Some people who cannot drink milk have normal lactase levels, and, in these people, lactose or a gradually increasing milk intake will produce tolerance. Experimentally, an increase of lactase and increased tolerance to a high lactose diet can be induced by feeding lactose to previously lactose-intolerant animals whose habitual intake was low in lactose.[59] In human beings small amounts of lactose (up to 100 mg) can be ingested, either in water or as milk in intolerant subjects without significant discomfort.[60] The addition of small increments of milk to the diet of non-milk drinkers, therefore, seems a reasonable approach to assuming an adequate calcium intake. The lactose should be tolerated and induction of lactase should follow after a significant period of time. Since the only alternative way of increasing dietary calcium is by supplements in the form of chemicals, milk supplements would seem preferable. However, milk also contains phosphorus. (See next section.) The relationship between intake and tolerance is also stressed by the studies in infants who, irrespective of race, are all tolerant and absorbed lactose. Only after the age of one or two years does the intolerance develop, presumably as milk ingestion ceases, since it develops in nearly all who do not drink milk subsequent to weaning but does not develop in those who continue to drink milk.[61]

In the United States, Asians and, to a lesser extent, American blacks would be likely to have a low calcium intake as a result of lactose intolerance. American Indians also have a high incidence of intolerance and, like the Asians and blacks, this is associated with a habitual low milk intake.[61] Lactase deficiency[57] and the percentage of non-milk drinkers among osteoporotic patients was higher (37 and 50 per cent), compared with the incidence of lactase deficiency in a similar group of non-osteoporotic individuals (10 to 19 per cent). This would suggest that this defect and, consequently, the dietary calcium intake are lower in osteoporotic patients, and that lactase deficiency is possibly an important etiological factor in osteoporosis. A dietary history and a test for lactase deficiency would provide useful information in the evaluation of an osteoporotic patient. The latter can be relatively complex; an evaluation of symptoms after a 150 gram load of lactose appears to give reliable data simply, although physiological response to milk ingestion results in a wide range of responses.[60]

**Phosphate Excess.**   The causal relationship between calcium deficiency and osteoporosis may appear unclear; it is not the absolute amount of this element but rather the ratio between it and the phosphorus intake that is critical in the effect on bone. Whenever the ionized calcium is decreased, as it is when serum phosphorus rises after phosphorus ingestion, parathyroid hormone is stimulated and increased osteoclastic activity results. Although there are some species differences, the data all lead to the same conclusion—that a calcium-to-phosphorus ratio of less than one will cause bone loss.

Early reports had suggested that a low calcium, high phosphorus intake leads to osteogenesis imperfecta. However, it was hard to explain an inherited disease of bone being produced in a normal animal by dietary means, and later studies in a number of species established the bone abnormality produced by such a dietary imbalance as osteoporosis.[62, 63, 64] A number of investigators have concerned themselves with altering the calcium-to-phosphorus ratio; however, one of the most telling studies involved adult rabbits given a high calcium and phosphorus intake compared with a group in which the amounts of the two elements were similar to that in man (Table 29–15). It is evident from this table that the ratio of calcium to phosphorus of less than one leads to osteoporosis irrespective of the absolute

Table 29–15   DAILY CALCIUM AND PHOSPHORUS INTAKE IN EXPERIMENTAL RABBITS AND MAN

| | Ca Intake, mg | Phosphorus Intake, mg | Ca:P | Bone Status |
|---|---|---|---|---|
| GROUP 1 (RABBITS) | | | | |
| Control | 1125 | 662 | 1.7 | Normal |
| High P | 1125 | 2047 | 0.6 | Osteoporotic |
| | | | | |
| GROUP 2 (RABBITS) | | | | |
| Control | 90 | 84 | 1.1 | Normal |
| High P | 90 | 208 | 0.4 | Osteoporotic |
| OSTEOPOROTIC PATIENTS | | | | |
| (n = 152) | 864 ± 39*† | 1325 ± 473* | 0.6 ± 0.12* | |

*Values are mean ± SD.
†Includes those taking milk for medical reasons.

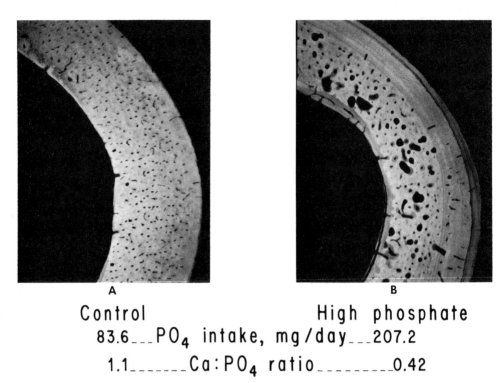

A                                                    B

Control                              High phosphate
83.6___PO$_4$ intake, mg/day___207.2
1.1_____Ca:PO$_4$ ratio_____0.42

**Figure 29–14** Microradiographs of cortical bone of adult rabbits fed (a) a calcium-to-phosphorus ratio of 1.1 and (b) a calcium-to-phosphorus ratio of 0.42. There is an increase in porosity of the cortex in the animals fed the low ratio diet (magnification x 20). (From Jowsey, J.: Osteoporosis: its nature and the role of diet. Postgrad. Med., *60*:75–79, 1976.)

amounts of the two elements. The osteoporosis is seen in the bone in the form of an increased porosity in the cortex and in a loss of trabeculae and endosteal bone (Fig. 29–14). Perhaps the most important point is that the group 1 control animals received 662 mg per day of phosphorus and did not develop osteoporosis, while the group 2 osteoporotic animals received only 208 mg of phosphorus per day and yet developed the disease, emphasizing that it is the ratio of the two elements, not the absolute amounts of either, that is important. The group of osteoporotic patients (Table 29–15) can be seen to fall into the category of a low calcium-to-phosphorus ratio that caused osteoporosis in the experimental animals. Of these patients, 37 per cent had been non-milk drinkers most of their lives, but, at the time their dietary history was taken, they were ingesting one to three glasses of milk daily under their physician's advice. This would make the calcium value higher than their "normal" intake. Despite this fact, 47 per cent of these patients were ingesting less than 500 mg of calcium daily (mean intake of this group was 363 mg calcium per day). It is therefore highly probable, since a ratio of calcium to phosphorus of about 0:5 invariably produces bone loss in animals, that in adult man a similar imbalance between the two elements leads to bone loss.

The mechanism by which the bone loss takes place involves the parathyroids. This has been shown in experimental animals and in man. In normal animals the values rose during a high phosphate intake period by a factor of two to three (Table 29–16). In both these long-term studies, the rise in serum parathyroid hormone was

**Table 29–16**  PARATHYROID GLAND ACTIVITY IN ADULT ANIMALS
ON A HIGH PHOSPHORUS INTAKE

| Group | Number | Parathyroid Value | |
|---|---|---|---|
| | | (BEFORE HIGH P DIET) | (AFTER HIGH P DIET) |
| Adult cats | 12* | 2.9 ± 0.6 | 6.5 ± 2.0 |
| time | | 0 | 5–13 months |
| Adult dogs | 6** | 55.3 ± 14.1 | 142 ± 53.2 |
| time | | 0 | 5 months |

Values are mean ± SD.
*A/B index from Jowsey et al.[64]
**iPTH μl eq/ml from Jowsey et al.[65]

accompanied by a decline in serum phosphorus and no change in serum calcium. In adult man the data support the concept that a high phosphate intake stimulates parathyroid activity. Short-term studies in adult dogs and in man were directed toward the immediate postprandial changes in serum values. In the dogs, serum phosphorus rose and ionized calcium declined maximally at four hours and six hours, respectively. In man, the rise and fall of parathyroid hormone occurred at shorter intervals (Fig. 29–15). This may be a species difference or it may be because the dogs had been fed the high phosphorus diet for six weeks, while the human volunteers were only studied after a single oral load of phosphorus.[66] That the rise in parathyroid hormone was dependent on the rise in serum phosphate was shown by a concomitant calcium infusion which prevented the rise in serum phosphate and the subsequent rise in serum parathyroid hormone (Fig. 25–15). The

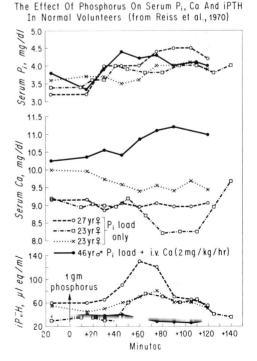

The Effect Of Phosphorus On Serum $P_i$, Ca And iPTH
In Normal Volunteers (from Reiss et al., 1970)

**Figure 29–15**  The rise in serum $P_i$ causes a fall in calcium which stimulates parathyroid hormone release: Only if the fall in calcium is prevented as by intravenous calcium infusion does the serum parathyroid hormone level remain unchanged. (Drawn from Reiss et al.[66])

serum calcium in the volunteer rose to values of about 11.2 mg per dl, which would result in a calcium-to-phosphorus product of 45. Such a value would lead to calcium phosphate precipitation in soft tissues. In a later study, the postprandial changes in calcium and phosphorus were studied after two weeks of phosphate supplementation, and it was found that the serum calcium fell rather than rose as it did in unsupplemented controls after both noon and evening meals, while serum phosphorus was consistently increased during the day (Fig. 29–16).[67] The higher-than-normal fasting morning phosphorus suggested that sustained periods of phosphate supplementation produce an effect that is maintained for longer times than after a one-day postprandial load of phosphorus.

One of the most consistent changes after phosphate supplements is the decrease in urinary calcium and increased body retention of calcium, leading to the concept that the positive calcium balance represented an increase in mineralized bone mass. In both animal experiments (Table 29–15) the calcium content of soft tissues was measured, and it appears that the retained calcium is deposited not only in bone but also in soft tissues. In different species, various tissue have a tendency to retain specifically more of the calcium in the form of calcium phosphate salt. In the rabbit the aorta is the tissue most prone to mineralization, while the kidney mineralizes to a lesser extent (Fig. 29–17).[68] In the dog the kidney retained more than other tissues (Fig. 29–18).[69] The studies so far mentioned occurred without the production of a rise in serum calcium. In earlier work, Spaulding and Walser showed that phosphate fed to rats that had been made hypercalcemic with vitamin D caused fatal calcification of heart and kidney tissue.[70] The soft tissue mineralization was considered to be associated with both hypercalcemia and hyperphosphatemia; indeed, fatal consequences have resulted in a hypercalcemic individual who was treated with intravenous phosphate infusions. In general, however, intravenous or oral phosphate is an effective treatment for severe hypercalcemia when it is continued for one or two days only. While soft tissue calcium deposition is to be expected in hypercalcemic individuals given phosphate, the animal studies in rabbits and dogs demonstrated that deposition of calcium and phosphate will occur in the soft tissues in the absence of hypercalcemia.

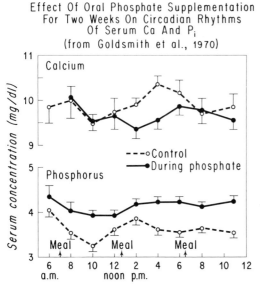

Effect Of Oral Phosphate Supplementation For Two Weeks On Circadian Rhythms Of Serum Ca And $P_i$ (from Goldsmith et al., 1970)

**Figure 29–16** Changes in serum calcium and phosphorus values after two weeks of phosphorus supplementation in patients with metabolic bone disease. (Redrawn from Goldsmith et al.[67])

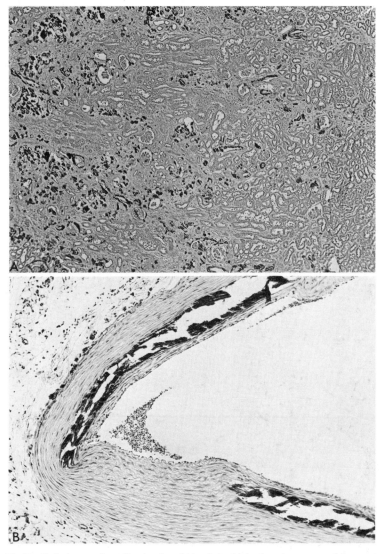

**Figure 29-17**    Soft tissue mineralization in rabbits fed a high phosphorus-to-calcium ratio (Group 1, Table 29-15). The von Kossa stain shows mineral in the glomeruli of the kidney cortex (a) and in the intima of the aorta (b). In none of the animals were calcium deposits visible on autopsy (magnification (a) x 30 and (b) x 75). (From Jowsey and Balasubramaniam.[68])

A parallel situation exists in renal failure, in which hyperphosphatemia results from the inability of the kidney to excrete phosphate despite the presence of secondary hyperparathyroidism. Soft tissue mineralization is a well-known complication of this disease; corneal and skin mineralization are the most common; gastric mucosa, alveolar septae, and the media and intima of the blood vessels are also areas where mineral is deposited. Phosphate deprivation, under experimental conditions such that the serum phosphorus remains constant despite a reduction in the glomerular filtration rate, results in no change in serum parathyroid hormone.[71] In patients with renal failure the hyperphosphatemia has usually developed before the patient becomes ill. Secondary hyperparathyroidism develops because of the fall in

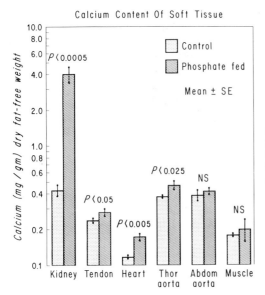

Figure 29–18  The calcium content of soft tissues after five months of phosphate supplementation. All tissues in the phosphate supplemented animals retained more calcium than the control animals. (Drawn from Laflamme and Jowsey.[68])

ionized calcium, and, as in the animal studies, there is bone loss. In the United States renal failure is nearly always a disease of rapidly developing bone loss and osteopenia, while in areas where vitamin D is not as prevalent osteomalacia may complicate the bone picture.

The original premise that the reduction in urinary calcium reflected an increase in mineralized bone mass has therefore no support. Neither, of course, has the suggestion that phosphate should be useful in the treatment of fracture healing or metabolic bone disease. If phosphate is given as a supplement during fracture healing, the healed portion of the bone is porous, and the normal remodeling that occurs around a fracture site demonstrates more extensive remodeling and more holes (Figure 29–19). The effect of phosphate supplements on metabolic bone disease has been studied in only a few patients. The results reflected the data derived from the animal studies. The patients studied had osteoporosis, and the raised bone resorption values increased further after three to four months of one gram of supplemental phosphate per day. Serum parathyroid hormone rose in four out of the six patients, and the urinary calcium fell, as was to be expected. The TRP% fell, no doubt as a result of both the increase in parathyroid hormone and the increased renal load of phosphate (Table 29–17). Bone mass also decreased in these patients.[72]

In immobilized volunteers who were given phosphorus supplements during the first or second half of a 30-week period of bed rest, the bone loss of disuse was unaffected by the addition of phosphate (Fig. 29–20).[17] Although immobilization osteoporosis is a different entity from the more common metabolic osteoporosis, this study again stressed the lack of an effect of phosphorus in preventing or increasing bone mass.

It is evident that the majority of data shows clearly that phosphate ingestion results in temporary and eventually sustained elevation in serum phosphate, which causes a decreased ionized calcium and stimulation of parathyroid hormone. It is also evident that the average calcium-to-phosphorus ratio in the normal person's diet is less than half and that bone loss must result from this imbalance.

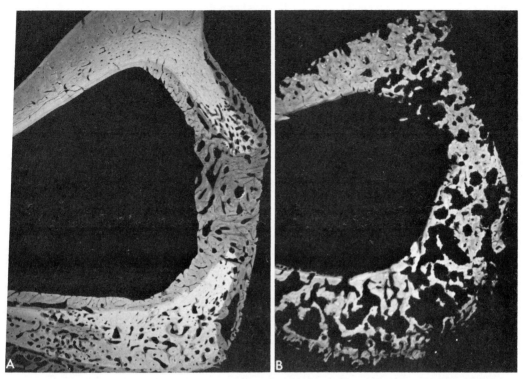

**Figure 29–19** Microradiographs of the proximal tibia of two rabbits, eight weeks after a 2 mm defect has been produced in the anterior tubercle. (a) The control rabbit has been fed a 1.1 calcium ratio and the defect, appearing as an area of incompletely mineralized bone, is relatively solid, although some holes show in both the new bone and the adjacent cortex; (b) a rabbit from the same litter receiving the same amount of calcium but an additional 1.4 gms of phosphorus. There has been a considerable increase in porosity both in the fracture area and the adjacent bone (magnification x 12).

**Table 29–17** SIGNIFICANT CHANGES IN BIOCHEMICAL AND BONE FINDINGS AFTER ORAL PHOSPHATE THERAPY IN SIX PATIENTS WITH OSTEOPOROSIS (mean ± SD)

|  | Before Treatment | After Treatment |
|---|---|---|
| SERUM |  |  |
| Phosphorus, mg/dl | 3.8 ± 0.4 | 3.5 ± 0.3* |
| iPTH. $\mu$l eq/ml | 17.3 ± 6.0 | 22.3 ± 10.6 |
| URINE |  |  |
| Calcium, mg/24 hrs | 123 ± 44.1 | 68 ± 37.8** |
| Phosphorus, mg/24 hrs | 722 ± 201.3 | 1418 ± 167.4** |
| TRP % | 73.5 ± 7.6 | 62.2 ± 4.5*** |
| BONE |  |  |
| Resorption, % surface | 11.0 ± 2.7 | 17.2 ± 4.1† |

*p < .05
**p < .001
***p < .005
†p < .01

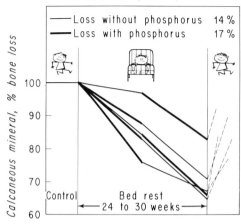

Figure 29–20  Quantitative radiography measurements of the os calcis in normal young adults given phosphate supplements or no phosphate supplements during a 30-week period of bed rest. Phosphorus supplements fail to arrest the progress of osteoporosis, despite reduced urinary calcium excretion. (Drawn from Hully et al.[17])

From both the animal and human studies it is to be expected that parathyroid hormone levels should be higher in elderly individuals whose calcium intake is low and whose absorption also tends to be decreased. This has been documented in a study in normal and osteoporotic individuals from age 20 to 80.[73] In this series 15 per cent of osteoporotic patients showed a higher-than-normal level of parathyroid hormone using the GP-1M antibody (Fig. 29-21), which is assumed to measure the circulating hormone, rather than the secreted form measured by CH-14M. Later data have shown that 12 per cent of osteoporotic patients have values above the normal range and yet have normal serum calcium levels. The basic problem is that it is highly likely that the majority of men and women over the age of 50 have "osteoporosis" but have not yet sustained the fracture that will place them in the category of osteoporosis. Similar data have been reported from Johannesburg in elderly individuals, both with and without pigmented skin (Table 29-18).[74]

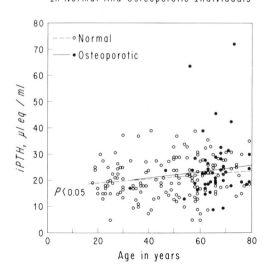

Figure 29-21. Serum immunoreactive PTH in non-osteoporotic and osteoporotic individuals.

**Table 29–18**  BIOCHEMICAL FINDINGS IN BLACK, INDIAN, AND
WHITE ELDERLY FEMALE SUBJECTS (mean ± 2 SE)

| Group | No. | Age (years) | Serum Calcium (mg/dl) | Serum Phosphorus (mg/dl) | Serum Alk P'tase KA Units | Serum PTH (pg/ml) |
|-------|-----|-------------|------------------------|---------------------------|----------------------------|--------------------|
| Black | 21 | 74 ± 4 | 9.4 ± 0.2 | 3.1 ± 0.2 | 6.2 ± 0.6 | 553 ± 80 |
| Indian | 19 | 67 ± 2 | 9.7 ± 0.4 | 3.0 ± 0.4 | 5.7 ± 1.2 | 446 ± 23 |
| White | 20 | 73 ± 4 | 9.8 ± 0.2 | 3.4 ± 0.2 | 7.3 ± 1.0 | 483 ± 42 |

(Control PTH range 25–400 pg/ml)
From Joffee et al.[74]

Four further reports suggest that osteoporotic patients have parathyroid hormone levels above normal. Fujita and his colleagues measured parathyroid hormone in eleven patients with postmenopausal osteoporosis and vertebral fractures.[75] Age- and sex-matched normals were used as controls and they found a significant difference ($p=0.01$), although, as expected, there was overlap between the two groups. They further found a relationship between the lumbar score and a second assay for parathyroid hormone, indicating that the severity of the disease was related to higher levels of the hormone (Fig. 29–22). Berlyne compared young individuals (19 years) with older, osteoporotic individuals (77 years) and found that there was a ten-fold increase in parathyroid hormone is his osteoporotic population.[77] By using young individuals as controls he avoided the complication of including in his controls individuals with osteoporosis but no vertebral fractures, and so obtained a greater distinction between normal and osteoporotic patients. The older age group showed some indication of impaired renal function, which was considered to account for an unpredictable proportion of the increase in serum parathyroid hormone. Two other reports consider osteoporosis as a disease of normocalcemic hyperparathyroidism. Gallagher and co-workers reported ten postmenopausal women with evidence of hyperparathyroidism and raised serum parathyroid hormone levels, eight of whom had normal serum calcium levels.[77] Teitelbaum and associates studied 16 post-menopausal women, six of whom had

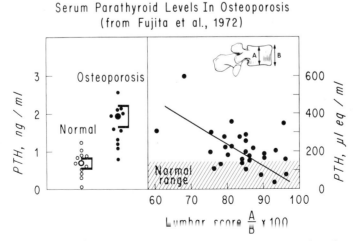

**Figure 29–22**  Serum parathyroid hormone levels in normal and osteoporotic patients, and the relationship between lumbar score and the serum parathyroid hormone. (Redrawn from Fujita et al.[75])

serum parathyroid hormone levels above normal and high bone resorption values, but all of whom were normocalcemic.[78]

In view of the earlier finding of phosphate supplements in animals and the two-to-one ratio of phosphorus to calcium in the normal human diet, it is not unexpected to find increased bone loss and raised parathyroid hormone levels in patients with osteoporosis. It may well be that in those patients in whom a high phosphate intake plays a major role in the etiology of their disease, the syndrome is normocalcemic hyperparathyroidism.

Phosphate excess probably rarely exists as a single etiological factor in the development of osteoporosis. However, a report of an epidemiological study carried out on Eskimos, who subsist mainly on seal and walrus meat and fat, suggested that the high phosphate intake is perhaps the primary factor that causes the bone loss.[79, 80] That diet was of major importance was suggested by the early loss of mineral, which started at age 20, in comparison with an age-matched Wisconsin population in whom the bone loss was not apparent until age 55 in women and age 65 in men (Fig. 29–23).

Although the role of the parathyroids in the development of osteoporosis has not been uncontrovertibly established, the evidence is strong that phosphate ingestion results in a homeostatic response by the parathyroids; in all individuals with a calcium-to-phosphorus ratio of less than unity this response will lead to bone loss and contribute to osteoporosis.

Phosphate excess and the consequent transient increases in serum phosphate must be carefully separated from phosphate depletion. Lack of phosphate to a point that causes biochemical abnormalities and bone disease is rare. The three instances, all themselves relatively uncommon, are adult onset hypophosphatemic os-

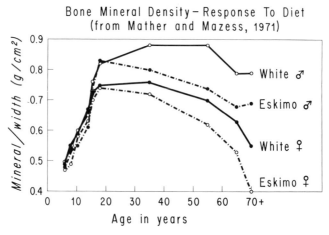

**Figure 29–23** Bone mass changes measured by bone densitometry in North Point Barrow Eskimos (primarily meat-eaters) and in normal Wisconsin volunteers (omnivores). There is a decline in bone mass in all groups, but the decrease starts at maturity in the Eskimos, rather than after age 50 as in the Wisconsin population. (Drawn from Mather and Mazess.[79])

teomalacia, vitamin D-resistant rickets, and the excessive use of phosphate binding agents. (See Chapter Twenty-three, pages 205–214.) Hypophosphatemia appears to result in decreased bone formation as well as a failure of mineralization; there is no doubt that in such instances increased dietary phosphate intake until normophosphatemia is achieved, if this is possible, is the treatment of choice.

**Hormone Deficiency.**   It is impossible to avoid realizing that the majority of osteoporotic patients are post-menopausal women, and to suspect therefore that estrogen deficiency is related in some way to the development of the disease. Nordin and his colleagues in 1966 examined 152 volunteers randomly selected from visitors to a Glasgow hospital. A number of tests were used to evaluate osteoporosis, including the metacarpal and femoral shaft cortical index and the vertebral index of the third lumbar vertebra. The series ranged in age from 19 to 83 years, and the density measurements all showed a significant negative regression with age. The regression of these same parameters against the years since menopause, in general, showed slightly lower correlation coefficients, which would suggest that age is the predominant factor in bone loss. However, if cortical bone is evaluated using the femoral index, a fall from 0.57 to 0.51 ($p=<0.01$) occurs 15 years after the menopause, at approximately age 60.[1] It has already been shown that cortical bone contributes most significantly in the older age groups, and presumably this finding is a reflection of that point.

In later work, loss of bone measured by the metacarpal cortical thickness was related to age and menopause; it was again apparent that age was the predominant factor in the decrease in mass. However, if younger women with pre-menopausal bilateral oophorectomy were examined, then lack of estrogens appeared to contribute significantly to the bone loss. Biochemical changes also occurred, in that the serum and urinary calcium rose, as did urinary hydroxyproline.[78] These data suggested that increased bone resorption results from estrogen deficiency, which produces a significant loss of bone over and above that resulting from age-related loss. Serum and urinary calcium fall to normal with estrogen therapy, confirming earlier work, which included the relationship between estrogen therapy and parathyroid hormone secretion.[81] In the latter report the fall in serum calcium was associated with both a rise in serum immunoreactive parathyroid hormone and a fall in bone resorption, measured by microradiography (Fig. 29–24). This led to the conclusion that estrogens form a protective barrier between the bone and the osteoclast-stimulating properties of parathyroid hormone. The effect appears to be a direct one of the hormone on bone, since it can be elicited in tissue culture.[82]

The same effect can be produced in patients with hypercalcemic hyperparathyroidism; as a result of estrogen administration serum calcium and urinary calcium both fall, presumably as a reflection of the inhibition of bone resorption.[78]

Just as young adults who have had an oophorectomy develop osteoporosis prematurely, so patients with Turner's syndrome or hypogonadism develop osteoporosis well before the expected age;[83] roentgenographic evidence is related to the lack of development of secondary sexual characteristics, which becomes evident usually at 10 to 13 years of age. As in adult post-menopausal osteoporosis, the serum calcium and phosphorus levels are normal, as are most other biochemical parameters.[83] In a study of eight patients with Turner's syndrome or congenital estrogen deficiency, the Singh Index was II or III in five patients, thus placing them in the category of osteoporosis, at least by this criterion. All normal individuals of this age have a Singh Index of VII. Bone remodeling values indicated normal

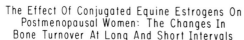

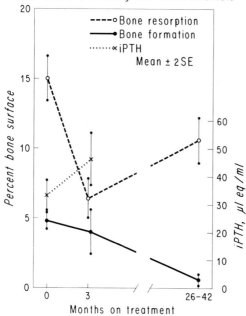

Figure 29-24  Decrease in bone resorption and formation with estrogen treatment in postmenopausal women with osteoporosis. (Redrawn from Riggs et al.[81])

formation and increased resorption, as in adult estrogen deficient osteoporosis (Table 29–19). Parathyroid hormone levels were normal, which substantiated the dietary calcium and vitamin D histories in these patients, which also were normal.

The effect of estrogens on the bone in both osteoporotic and hyperparathyroid individuals explains the perhaps now historic work of estrogen replacement therapy in post-menopausal women by Henneman and Wallach (Table 29–20).[84] This study showed that hormone treatment in osteoporotic women who had already fractured several vertebrae, as indicated by height loss, prevented further loss of height. It also showed that in women treated for post-menopausal symptoms, but who were without osteoporosis, the hormone treatment prevented fracture and height loss. Estrogen replacement after the menopause has been used extensively since and has been shown to halt or slow the progress of bone loss compared with untreated estrogen-deficient women (Table 29–21). The variations in bone mass changes were large in each group, but the results are similar to previous studies by Meema's group.[85]

It is necessary to point out that all the data on the estrogen treatment of post-menopausal women, as well as the information derived from osteoporotic individuals with fractures treated with estrogens, have failed to show any increase in bone mass but merely a cessation or slowing down of bone loss (Fig. 29–25).

Table 29–19  BONE REMODELING IN TURNER'S SYNDROME (mean ± SD)

|  | Age in yrs. | Number | % Formation | % Resorption |
|---|---|---|---|---|
| Patients with Turner's Syndrome | 9–19 | 8 | 5.4 ± 1.7 | 9.2 ± 1.8 |
| Controls | 9–19 | 28 | 5.4 ± 2.8 | 6.1 ± 1.6 |

**Table 29–20**  HEIGHT LOSS IN POST-MENOPAUSAL WOMEN, WITH AND WITHOUT OSTEOPOROSIS, WITH AND WITHOUT HORMONE THERAPY
(Mean ± 2 SE)

|  | No. | Post-menopausal Years Before Estrogen Treatment | Height Loss (inches) | Years of Estrogen Treatment | Further Height Loss (inches) |
|---|---|---|---|---|---|
| POST-MENOPAUSAL OSTEOPOROTICS | 16 | 15.3 ± 3.6 | 2.3 ± 0.6 | 6.2 ± 2.2 | 0.3 ± 0.2 |
| POST-MENOPAUSAL WITHOUT OSTEOPOROSIS | 23 | 2.0 ± 1.6 | 0 | 11.7 ± 2.8 | 0 |

From Henneman and Wallach.[84]

**Table 29–21**  BONE MINERAL MASS IN POST-MENOPAUSAL WOMEN, UNTREATED OR TREATED WITH EQUINE-CONJUGATED ESTROGENS. BONE MINERAL MASS, mg/cm²

|  | Surgical Oophorectomy | | Natural Menopause | |
|---|---|---|---|---|
|  | UNTREATED | TREATED | UNTREATED | TREATED |
| Number | 26 | 23 | 27 | 6 |
| Years of study | 6 | 6½ | 6 | 5½ |
| Initial value | 629.8 | 664.9 | 632.4 | 407.8 |
| Change | −49.0 | +12.8 | −39.9 | +45.8 |
| Significance | <.05 | NS | <.05 | <.05 |

From Meema et al.[85] (Figures derived from radiological measurements of the radius.)

**Figure 29–25**  Bone densitometry, using $^{125}I$ radiation of the second phalanx of the third digit of the left hand, in postmenopausal women treated and untreated with estrogens. $\mu_B$ represent radiation absorption corrected for bone thickness derived from a lateral view of the same phalanx. Estrogen treatment decreases the bone loss seen in the untreated patients. (From Davis et al.[86])

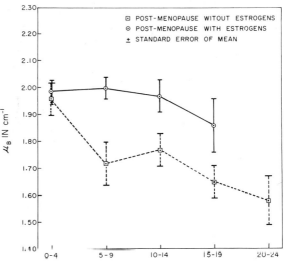

$\hat{\mu}$ TOTAL BONE VS NUMBER OF YEARS POST MENOPAUSE  (NORMAL FEMALES)

□ POST-MENOPAUSE WITOUT ESTROGENS
⊙ POST-MENOPAUSE WITH ESTROGENS
± STANDARD ERROR OF MEAN

$\mu_B$ IN cm$^{-1}$

NUMBER OF YEARS POST-MENOPAUSE

The effect of estrogens in estrogen-deficiency is to repress resorption, which then tends to rise slightly toward the untreated level after one year; long-term treatment causes a fall in bone formation. It may be expected that the early response may be good, but the long term effect, though still present, is small since the difference between formation and resorption is large.

The general opinion by both physicians and orthopedic surgeons who are faced with the problem of how to treat post-menopausal or senile osteoporosis supports this view. Hormones, both estrogens and androgens, have little beneficial effect, and these patients tend to return with further fractures, although possibly less frequently than if left entirely untreated.

## *REFERENCES*

1. Nordin, B. E. C., MacGregor, J., and Smith, D. A.: The incidence of osteoporosis in normal women: its relation to age and the menopause. Q. J. Med. (new series), *35*:25–38, 1966.
2. Nordin, B. E. C.: Metabolic Bone and Stone Disease. Baltimore, The Williams and Wilkins Company, 1973.
3. Smith, R. W., Jr., and Rizek, J.: Epidemiologic studies of osteoporosis in women of Puerto Rico and Southeastern Michigan with special reference to age, race, national origin and to other related or associated findings. Clin. Orthop., *45*:31–48, 1966.
4. Alfram, P.: An epidemiologic study of cervical and trochanteric fractures of the femur in an urban population. Acta Orthop. Scand., *65*:1–109, 1964.
5. Bauer, G. C. H.: Epidemiology of fractures. *In* Barzel, U. S. (Ed.): Osteoporosis. New York, Grune & Stratton, 1970, pp. 153–163.
6. Stewart, I. M.: Fracture of neck of femur. Br. Med. J., *2*:922–924, 1957.
7. Stevens, J., and Abrani, G.: Osteoporosis in patients with femoral neck fractures. J. Bone Joint Surg., *46B*:24–27, 1964.
8. Albright, F., and Reifenstein, E. C.: The Parathyroid Glands and Metabolic Bone Disease. Baltimore, Williams and Wilkins Company, 1948, pp. 145–197.
9. Jowsey, J.: Quantitative microradiography: a new approach in the evaluation of metabolic bone disease. Am. J. Med., *40*:485–491, 1966.
10. Bordier, Ph. J., Miravet, L., and Hioco, D.: Young adult osteoporosis. Clin. Endocrinol. Metab., *2*:277–292, 1973.
11. Schenk, R. K., Attila, D. J., and Merz, W. A.: Bone cell counts. Excerpta Medica, International Congress Series, No. *270*:103–113, 1973.
12. Heath, H., III, Earll, J. M., Schaaf, M., Piechocki, J. T., and Li, T.: Serum ionized calcium during bed rest in fracture patients and normal men. Metabolism, *21*:633–640, 1972.
13. Winters, J. L., Kleinschmidt, A. G., Jr., Frensilli, J. J., and Sutton, M.: Hypercalcemia complicating immobilization in the treatment of fractures (a case report). J. Bone Joint Surg., *48A*:1182–1184, 1966.
14. Lawrence, G. D., Loeffler, R. G., Martin, L. G., and Connor, T. B.: Immobilization hypercalcemia. J. Bone Joint Surg., *55A*:87–94, 1973.
15. Heath, H., III, Schaaf, H. L., Wray, J. M. M., and Earll, J. M.: Parathyroid activity and immobilization-induced changes in calcium metabolism. Excerpta Medica, International Congress Series No. *270*:257–260, 1973.
16. Millard, F. J. C., Nassim, J. R., and Woollen, J. W.: Urinary calcium excretion after immobilization and spinal fusion in adolescents. Arch. Dis. Child., *45*:399–403, 1970.
17. Minaire, P., Meunier, P., Edouard, C., Bernard, J., Courpron, P., and Bourret, J.: Quantitative histological data on disuse osteoporosis. Calcif. Tissue Res., *17*:57–73, 1974.
18. Hulley, S. B., Vogel, J. M., Donaldson, C. L., Bayers, J. H., Friedman, R. J., and Rosen, S. N.: The effect of supplemental oral phosphate on the bone mineral changes during prolonged bed rest. J. Clin. Invest., *50*:2506–2518, 1971.
19. Burkhart, J. M., and Jowsey, J.: Parathyroid and thyroid hormones in the development of immobilization osteoporosis. Endocrinology, *81*:1053–1062, 1967.
20. Swezey, R. L.: Transient osteoporosis of the hip, foot and knee. Arthritis Rheum., *13*:858–868, 1970.
21. Langloh, N. D., Hunder, G. G., Riggs, B. L., and Kelly, P. J.: Transient painful osteoporosis of the lower extremities. J. Bone Joint Surg., *55A*:1188–1196, 1973.

22. Lockwood, D. R., Lammert, J. E., Vogel, J. M., and Hulley, S. B.: Bone mineral loss during bedrest. Excerpta Medica, International Congress Series No. 270:261–265, 1973.
23. Mack, P. B., and LaChance, P. L.: Effects of recumbency and space flight on bone density. Am. J. Clin. Nutr., 20:1194–1205, 1967.
24. Becker, R. O., and Murray, D. G.: A method for producing a cellular dedifferentiation by means of very small electrical currents. Trans. N. Y. Acad. Sci., Series 2, 29:606–615, 1967.
25. Doyle, F., Brown, J., and LaChance, C.: Relation between bone mass and muscle weight. Lancet, 1:391–393, 1970.
26. Smith, R. E., and Saville, P. D.: Bone breaking stress as a function of weight bearing in bipedal rats. Am. J. Phys. Anthropol., 25:159–164, 1966.
27. Tulloh, N. M., and Romberg, B.: An effect of gravity on bone development in lambs. Nature, 200:438–439, 1963.
28. Nilsson, B. E., and Westlin, N. E.: Bone density in athletes. Clin. Orthop., 77:179–182, 1971.
29. Dalen, N., and Olsson, K. E.: Bone mineral content and physical activity. Acta Orthop. Scand., 45:170–174, 1974.
30. Saville, P. D.: Observations on 80 women with osteoporotic spine fractures. In Barzel, U. S. (Ed.): Osteoporosis. New York, Grune & Stratton, 1970, pp. 38–46.
31. Morgan, D. B., and Newton-John, H. F.: Bone loss and senescence. Gerontologia 15:140–154, 1969.
32. Adams, P., Davies, G. T., and Sweetnam, P.: Osteoporosis and the effects of aging on bone mass in elderly men and women. Q. J. Med. (new series) 39:601–615, 1970.
33. Singh, M., Riggs, B. L., Beabout, J. W., and Jowsey, J.: Femoral trabecular-pattern index for evaluation of spinal osteoporosis. Ann. Intern. Med., 77:63–67, 1972.
34. Smith, D. M., Nance, W. E., Kang, K. W., Christian, J. C., and Johnston, C. C., Jr.: Genetic factors in determining bone mass. J. Clin. Invest., 52:2800–2808, 1973.
35. Moldawer, M., Zimmerman, S. J., and Collins, L. C.: Incidence of osteoporosis in elderly whites and elderly Negroes. JAMA, 194:117–120, 1965.
36. Trotter, M., Broman, G. E., and Peterson, R. R.: Densities of bone of white and Negro skeletons. J. Bone Joint Surg., 42A:50–58, 1960.
37. Trotter, M., Peterson, R. R., and Wette, R.: The secular trend in the diameter of the femur of American whites and Negroes. Am. J. Phys. Anthropol. ns., 28:65–73, 1968.
38. Lemann, J. Jr., Litzow, J. R., and Lennon, E. J.: Studies of the mechanism by which chronic metabolic acidosis augments urinary calcium excretion in man. J. Clin. Invest., 46:1318–1328, 1967.
39. Jha, G. J., Deo, M. G., and Ramalingaswami, V.: Bone growth in protein deficiency. Am. J. Pathol., 53:1111–1121, 1968.
40. Adams, P., and Berridge, F. D.: Effects of Kwashiorkor on cortical and trabecular bone. Arch. Dis. Child., 44:705–709, 1969.
41. Lozoff, B., and Fanaroff, A. A.: Kwashiorkor in Cleveland, Am. J. Dis. Child., 129:710–711, 1975.
42. Nordin, B. E. C.: International patterns of osteoporosis. Clin. Orthop., 45:17–30, 1966.
43. Riggs, B. L., Kelly, P. J., Kinney, V. R., Scholz, D. A., and Bianco, A. J., Jr.: Calcium deficiency and osteoporosis. J. Bone Joint Surg., 49A:915–924, 1967.
44. Gallagher, J. C., Riggs, B. L., Eisman, J., Arnaud, S., and DeLuca, H.: Impaired intestinal calcium absorption in postmenopausal osteoporosis: possible role of vitamin D metabolites and PTH (abstract). Clin., Res., 24:360A, 1976.
45. Odland, L. M., Mason, R. L., and Alexeff, A. I.: Bone density and dietary findings of 409 Tennessee subjects. II. Dietary considerations. Am. J. Clin. Nutr., 25:908–911, 1972.
46. Avioli, L. V., McDonald, J. E., and Lee, S. W.: The influence of age on the intestinal absorption of $^{47}$Ca in women and its relation to $^{47}$Ca absorption in postmenopausal osteoporosis. J. Clin. Invest., 44:1960–1967, 1965.
47. Preece, M. A., Tomlinson, S., Ribot, C. A., Pietrek, J., Korn, H. T., Davies, D. M., Ford, J. A., Dunnigan, M. G., and O'Riordan, J. L. H.: Studies of vitamin D deficiency in man. Q. J. Med. (new series) 44:575–589, 1975.
48. Aitken, J. M., Gordon, S., Anderson, J. B., Hart, D. M., Lindsay, R., Horton, P. W., Smith, C. B., Smith, D. A., and Shimmins, J.: Seasonal variations in calcium and phosphorus homeostasis in man. Excerpta Medica, International Congress Series No. 270:80–84, 1973.
49. Saville, P. D.: Changes in bone mass with age and alcoholism. J. Bone Joint Surg., 47A:492–499, 1965.
50. Krawitt, E. L., Sampson, H. W., and Katagiri, C. A.: Effect of 1,25-dihydroxycholecalciferol on ethanol mediated suppression of calcium absorption. Calcif. Tissue Res., 18:119–124, 1975.
51. Riggs, B. L., Jowsey, J., Kelly, P. J., Hoffman, D. L., and Arnaud, C. D.: Effects of oral therapy with calcium and vitamin D in primary osteoporosis. J. Clin Endocrinol. Metab., 42:1139–1144, 1965.
52. Jowsey, J., Hoye, R. C., Pak, C. Y. C., and Bartter, F, C.: The treatment of osteoporosis with calcium infusions: evaluation of bone biopsies. Am. J. Med., 47:17–22, 1969.

53. Chesnut, C. H., III, Nelp, W. B., Denney, J. D., and Sherrard, D. J.: Measurement of total body calcium (bone mass) by neutron activation analysis: applicability to bone-wasting disease. Excerpta Medica, International Congress Series No. 270:50–54, 1973.

54. Lund, B., Kjaer, I., Friis, T., Hjorth, L., Reimann, I., Andersen, R. B., and Sorensen, O. H.: Treatment of osteoporosis of ageing with 1 α-hydroxycholecalciferol. Lancet, 2:1168–1171, 1975.

55. Knapp, E. L.: Factors influencing the urinary excretion of calcium. I. In normal persons. J. Clin. Invest., 26:182–202, 1947.

56. Gonick, H. C., Lee, D. B. N., Drinkard, J. P., and Coulson, W. C.: Interrelationship of acidosis, calcium balance, serum parathormone concentration, and bone morphology in type I renal tubular acidosis (RTA). Excerpta Medica, International Congress Series No. 270:403–406, 1973.

57. Birge, S. J., Keutmann, H. T., Cuatrecasas, P., and Whedon, G. D.: Osteoporosis, intestinal lactase deficiency and low dietary calcium intake. N. Engl. J. Med., 276:445–448, 1967.

58. Editorial: Lactose intolerance and milk drinking habits. Gastroenterology, 60:605–609, 1971.

59. Wen, C., Antonowicz, I., Tovar, E., McGandy, R. B., and Gershoff, S. N.: Lactose feeding in lactose-intolerant monkeys. Am. J. Clin. Nutr., 26:1224–1228, 1973.

60. Stephenson, L. S., and Latham, M. C.: Lactose intolerance and milk consumption: the relation of tolerance to symptoms. Am. J. Clin. Nutr., 27:296–303, 1974.

61. Bose, D. P., and Welsh, J. D.: Lactose malabsorption in Oklahoma Indians. Am. J. Clin. Nutr., 26:1320–1322, 1973.

62. Krook, L., Barrett, R. B., Usui, K., and Wolke, R. E.: Nutritional secondary hyperparathyroidism in the cat. Cornell Vet., 53:224–240, 1963.

63. Sie, T. L., Draper, H. H., and Bell, R. R.: Hypocalcemia, hyperparathyroidism and bone resorption in rats induced by dietary phosphate. J. Nutr., 104:1195–1201, 1974.

64. Jowsey, J., and Raisz, L. G.: Experimental osteoporosis and parathyroid activity. Endocrinol., 82:384–396, 1968.

65. Jowsey, J., Reiss, E., and Canterbury, J. M.: Long-term effect of high phosphate intake on parathyroid hormone levels and bone metabolism. Acta Orthop. Scand., 45:801–808, 1974.

66. Reiss, E., Canterbury, J. M., Bercovitz, M. A., and Kaplan, E. L.: The role of phosphate in the secretion of parathyroid hormone in man. J. Clin. Invest., 49:2146–2149, 1970.

67. Goldsmith, R. S., Richards, R., Dube, W. J., Hulley, S. B., Holdsworth, D., and Ingbar, S. H.: Metabolic effects and mechanism of action of phosphate supplements. In Hioco, D. J. (Ed.): Phosphate et Métabolisme Phosphocalcique Régulation Normale et Aspects Physiopathologiques: Symposium International. Paris, Laboratories Sandoz. 1972.

68. Jowsey, J., and Balasubramaniam, P.: Effect of phosphate supplements on soft-tissue calcification and bone turnover. Clin. Sci., 42:289–299, 1972.

69. Laflamme, G. H., and Jowsey, J.: Bone and soft-tissue changes with oral phosphate supplements. J. Clin. Invest., 51:2834–2840, 1972.

70. Spaulding, S. W., and Walser, M.: Treatment of experimental hypercalcemia with oral phosphate. J. Clin. Endocrinol., 31:531–538, 1970.

71. Slatopolsky, E., and Bricker, N. S.: The role of phosphorus restriction in the prevention of secondary hyperparathyroidism in chronic renal disease. Kidney Int., 4:141–145, 1973.

72. Goldsmith, R. S., Jowsey, J., Dube, W. J., Riggs, B. L., Arnaud, C. D., and Kelly, P. J.: Effects of phosphorus supplementation on serum parathyroid hormone and bone morphology in osteoporosis. J. Clin. Endocrinol. Metab., 43:523–532, 1976.

73. Riggs, B. L., Arnaud, C. D., Jowsey, J., Goldsmith, R. S., and Kelly, P. J.: Parathyroid function in primary osteoporosis. J. Clin. Invest., 52:181–184, 1973.

74. Joffe, B. I., Seftel, H. C., Goldberg, R. C., Bersohn, I., and Hackeng, W. H. L.: Metabolic bone disease in the elderly. S. Afr. Med. J., 49:965–966, 1975.

75. Fujita, T., Orimo, H., Okano, K., and Yoshikawa, M.: Clinical application of parathyroid hormone radioimmunoassay. Excerpta Medica, International Congress Series No. 270:274–280, 1973.

76. Berlyne, G. M., Ben-Ari, J., Galinsky, D., Hirsch, M., Kushelevsky, A., and Shainkin, R.: The etiology of osteoporosis: the role of parathyroid hormone. JAMA, 229:1904–1905, 1974.

77. Gallagher, J. C., Bulusu, L., and Nordin, B. E. C.: Oestrogenic hormones and bone resorption. Excerpta Medica, International Congress Series No. 270:266–273, 1973.

78. Teitelbaum, S. L., Rosenberg, E. M., Richardson, C. A., and Avioli, L. V.: Histological studies of bone from normocalcemic postmenopausal osteoporotic patients with increased circulating parathyroid hormone. J. Clin. Endocrinol., 42:537–543, 1976.

79. Mather, W. E., and Mazess, R. B.: Bone mineral content of the Eskimos of Point Hope and Barrow: preliminary report. A.E.C. Progress Report, C00-1422-103, 1971.

80. Mazess, R. B., and Mather, W.: Bone mineral content of North Alaskan Eskimos. Am. J. Clin. Nutr. 27:916–925, 1974.

81. Riggs, B. L., Jowsey, J., Goldsmith, R. S., Kelly, P. J., Hoffman, D. L., and Arnaud, C. D.: Short- and long-term effects of estrogen and synthetic anabolic hormone in postmenopausal osteoporosis. J. Clin. Invest., *51*:1659–1663, 1972.
82. Atkins, D., Zanelli, J. M., Peacock, M., and Nordin, B. E. C.: The effect of oestrogens on the response of bone to PTH in vitro. J. Endocrinol., *54*:107–117, 1972.
83. Brown, D. M., Jowsey, J., and Bradford, D. S.: Osteoporosis in ovarian dysgenesis. J. Pediatr., *84*:816–820, 1974.
84. Henneman, P. H., and Wallach, S.: The use of androgens and estrogens and their metabolic effects: a review of the prolonged use of estrogens and androgens in postmenopausal and senile osteoporosis. Arch. Intern. Med., *100*:715–723, 1957.
85. Meema, S., Bunker, M. L., and Meema, H. E.: Preventive effect of estrogen or postmenopausal bone loss. Arch. Intern. Med., *135*:1436–1440, 1975.
86. Davis, M. E., Lanzl, L. H., and Cox, A. B.: The detection, prevention and retardation of menopausal osteoporosis. In Barzel, U. S. (Ed.): Osteoporosis. New York, Grune & Stratton, 1970, pp. 140–149.

# Chapter Thirty

# THE TREATMENT
# OF OSTEOPOROSIS

## INTRODUCTION

The treatment of osteoporosis, for a long time a matter of controversy, has met with little success until the last few years. Part of the problem is that the majority of metabolic bone diseases are treated successfully by reversing the cause of the disease; for example, hypercalcemic hyperparathyroidism is treated by removal of the parathyroids; vitamin D deficiency osteomalacia is corrected by administration of vitamin D. Although numerous etiological factors have been described as contributing to osteoporosis, it has already been pointed out that a number of these factors generally operate in any one person to produce the disease. It is also true to say that the majority of the etiological factors are difficult to reverse; it is hard to make elderly people change their way of life in order to increase exercise levels significantly. Without taking calcium supplements in the form of a pill, it is practically impossible to achieve the recommended dietary calcium-to-phosphorus intake with a ratio of one.

In the discussions on etiology, causative factors of osteoporosis were considered and also discussed in terms of treatment. These included the factors listed in Table 30–1. Their effect on the status of the bone disorder is also summarized in this table, and it is evident that none of what might be termed the physiological forms of therapy will reverse the bone loss; although the mineralized bone may disappear at a decreasing rate, the individual will remain fracture-prone and will continue to experience the clinical symptoms of osteoporosis.

A number of substances have been studied which are not implicated in the etiology of osteoporosis. These include the diphosphonates, calcitonin, growth hormone, and fluoride.

## THE DIPHOSPHONATES

The diphosphonates are synthetic pyrophosphates which have the ability to prevent the growth of hydroxyapatite crystals. They are used in industry to prevent the deposition of boiler-scale in hot water systems. In human beings it was

296

**Table 30-1**   OSTEOPOROSIS

| Etiology | Treatment | Result |
|---|---|---|
| ESTROGENS DEFICIENCY<br>post-menopausal<br>surgical oophorectomy<br>Turner's syndrome | Hormone replacement | Partial halting of bone loss |
| HIGH PHOSPHORUS-TO-CALCIUM INTAKE<br>high phosphorus diet<br>calcium deficient diet<br>lactase deficiency | Calcium supplements | Partial halting of bone loss |
| INACTIVITY<br>immobilization<br>lack of exercise | Activity (generally impractical in elderly people) | Halting of bone loss or increase in bone mass |
| VITAMIN D DEFICIENCY | Vitamin D | Halting of bone loss |

felt that they would coat mature hydroxyapatite crystals and prevent resorption of bone. In early studies in growing rats, immobilization osteoporosis was prevented, to a small extent, by administration of either EHDP (disodium ethane-1-hydroxy-1, 1-diphosphonate) or $Cl_2MDP$ (disodium dichloromethane diphosphonate).[1] The difference between untreated rats and those given the maximal dose (5.0 mg P/kg/day) was only about 5 per cent, although this was significant (p = <.05). Both compounds result in the development of osteomalacia; the effect of decreased bone loss may be the result of an inhibition of osteoclastic activity by the unmineralized osteoid. Since the animals grew 20 per cent, bone remodeling at the metaphyses and epiphyses was extensive enough to insure that all bone in these areas was largely covered by osteoid tissue, which would prevent removal of mineralized tissue as well as add to the total weight of the limb.

In studies in humans, adult patients with osteoporosis were treated for three months with doses of EHDP that varied from 4.5 to 20.0 mg/kg/day, with similar results; bone biopsies showed broad osteoid borders (Fig. 30–1). Bone resorption did not change significantly; however, above 4.5 mg/kg/day bone formation fell to very low values.[2] The most consistent change was the development of hyperphosphatemia, which continued in three of the four patients even at a dose of 4.5 mg/kg/day. This was accompanied by elevated serum calcium values. The rise in serum phosphorus caused a fall in ionized calcium and a rise in serum parathyroid hormone. The elevated calcium and phosphorus are of concern because of their potential effect on soft tissue mineralization. Diphosphonates will therefore produce morphological and, eventually, clinical osteomalacia, while the bone resorption, bone mass, or serum parathyroid hormone values do not encourage, but rather discourage, its use in the treatment of osteoporosis.

The diphosphonates may be useful in the treatment of myositis ossificans. Seventy patients with myositis ossificans progressiva have been treated with 10 to 20 mg of EHDP/kg/day. Approximately 50 per cent of the patients improved, and the others were stabilized on treatment.[3] Somewhat better results were obtained in the treatment of calcinosis in which the mineral (not bone) deposits were decreased in 12 out of 18 patients.

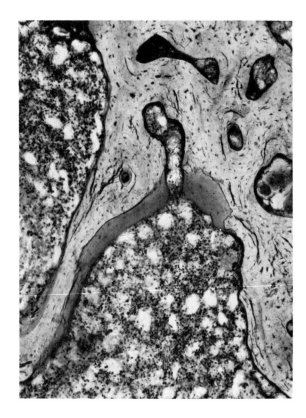

**Figure 30–1** Stained, undemineralized section of bone from a 67-year-old female patient with osteoporosis, treated for three months with an average of 14 mg/kg/day of EHDP. The wide osteoid border, which is more deeply stained, lacks a mineralization front and is not associated with an osteoblastic layer (magnification x 100).

## CALCITONIN

In Chapter Seven most of the information regarding the effect of calcitonin on bone was discussed. Because of the rapid (5 minutes) hyperphosphatemia that develops after calcitonin administration to calcitonin-depleted animals, it appears that the action of the hormone is to transfer phosphorus out of the cell and into the serum, thus energy-depleting the cell.[4] For this reason calcitonin has appeared to be effective in the treatment of Paget's disease of bone when the cells are extraordinarily active and have high energy requirements. The results of the use of this hormone in osteoporosis are unclear. There appears to be a consistent increase in the urine calcium, a tendency toward a negative calcium balance, and, in most studies, a decrease in serum calcium to the point that calcitonin has been used for the treatment of hypercalcemia. Serum phosphate is also decreased, and the effect appears to be independent of parathyroid hormone, since both the hypophosphatemia and hypocalcemia occur in the parathyroidectomized state.[5] The decrease is chronic, and it is obviously an expression of the increased renal excretion of these ions and therefore does not conflict with the previously noticed acute hyperphosphatemic effect in depleted animals, which has essentially disappeared by one hour.

Bone histological measurements made on biopsies of patients with osteoporosis treated with calcitonin are variable but, on the whole, show either no effect on bone loss or else a tendency toward an acceleration of loss (Table 30–2).[6, 7, 8] In addition bone densitometry measurements in patients with medullary carcinoma of the thyroid and chronic high serum calcitonin measurements fail to reveal any evi-

**Table 30-2** THE EFFECT OF PORCINE CALCITONIN OR BONE REMODELING
AND PARATHYROID HORMONE IN FIVE POST-MENOPAUSAL WOMEN
FOR ONE TO FOUR MONTHS*
(Mean ± SD)

|  | Before Treatment | After Treatment |  |
| --- | --- | --- | --- |
| Bone resorption % surface | 11.9 ± 2.7 | 14.8 ± 5.2 | NS |
| Bone formation % surface | 2.2 ± 1.1 | 1.7 ± 1.1 | NS |
| Serum parathyroid hormone $\mu$l eq/ml | 19.6 ± 6.3 | 32.8 ± 5.3 | <.025 |

From Jowsey et al.[6]

dence of osteosclerosis. This may be because the hypocalcemic effect of the hormone, which is presumably secreted spontaneously in large amounts by the C-cells of the thyroid, up to 100 times normal, causes hypocalcemia and therefore secondary hyperparathyroidism. It is relevant that, in the patients studied by Jowsey and associates, the two patients treated for only one month with increasing amounts of calcium (100 to 500 $\mu$g/day) showed a steady fall in serum calcium from 10.2 to 9.4 and from 9.9 to 9.3, while the patients treated with 200 $\mu$g/day for three and four months showed no fall in serum calcium but a three-fold increase in serum parathyroid hormone. This represents an average increase of 18 $\mu$l eq/ml compared with the 6 $\mu$l eq/ml rise seen at one month.[6] Since parathyroid hyperplasia is the more characteristic pathologic process seen in medullary carcinoma of the thyroid gland, a response to hypocalcemia is further suggested. The increased parathyroid hormone possibly counteracts any tendency for lowered bone resorption that might occur in this disease with calcitonin alone, just as in osteoporotic patients treated with the hormone.

Thyroidectomized patients with thyroxine replacement, but with no calcitonin, should develop osteoporosis if calcitonin has a real function in depressing bone resorption. However, no association between calcitonin deficiency and osteoporosis has been observed.

In adult man and probably in children, with the possible exception of neonates, calcitonin appears to be a hormone inherited from earlier forms of life in which it was essential, as in the salmon migrating from high to low calcium environments. Its lack of effectiveness in the control of hypercalcemia is illustrated by the many instances of hypercalcemia, and its lack of use in the treatment of osteoporosis is demonstrated by a lack of any consistency in the results obtained and by the majority of studies which show no effect on bone loss.

## GROWTH HORMONE

Since the majority of patients with osteoporosis are over 45 years of age and of normal height, skeletal growth may be considered far removed from both the etiology and treatment of osteoporosis. In the discussion of acromegaly it became evident that the increased skeletal growth in this disorder is a different entity from the increased bone mass required for the successful treatment of osteoporosis. Further-more, decreased bone density and occasional vertebral fractures occur in acro-megalic patients.

Growth hormone has been administered to a limited number of osteoporotic patients (see Chapter Twenty-five, Acromegaly), and no effect has been seen that can be interpreted as positive in terms of successful treatment; the only visible change has been an increase in new bone deposited periosteally at the expense of increased cortical porosity and loss of bone endosteally.[9]

## FLUORIDE AND CALCIUM

Many studies have been documented in which fluoride, known to cause os-teosclerosis in areas of endemic fluorosis, has been administered to osteoporotic patients. In some, fluoride alone was given and caused the stimulation of bone for-mation expected, but the failure to mineralize the bone, and an accompanying fall in serum calcium resulting from the excessive amount of new matrix, caused os-teomalacia and secondary hyperparathyroidism, the latter resulting in accelerated bone loss.[10] Vitamin D added to the regime resulted in no particular improvement when given in physiological amounts (400 to 800 IU/day). Similarly, patients on adequate vitamin D to whom fluoride was administered in relatively large doses (88 to 100 mg sodium fluoride daily) resulted in no change except for a decrease in urinary calcium excretion.[11] The latter was probably an expression of a stimulation of parathyroid gland activity.

Experimentally it has been shown that the osteoblastic activity induced by fluoride results in new matrix, which will be mineralized if adequate calcium is avail-able and, perhaps obviously, if vitamin D deficiency is not present. Animals fed fluoride developed mild osteomalacia and secondary hyperparathyroidism, while, on the same amount of fluoride, with a high calcium supplement, neither os-teomalacia nor any evidence of increased parathyroid hormone developed.[12] In man similar results have been reported, and, while in some respects the data appear con-fusing, careful examination has shown that studies that appear ineffective involved either fluoride alone, fluoride and inadequate amounts of calcium, or inadequate amounts of both. When sufficient fluoride and calcium are given, new bone, which is well mineralized, is formed and bone mass increases.[13] Fluoride and calcium, ad-ministered in appropriate amounts, will produce significant volumes of new bone in a reasonable time. For example, a 25 per cent increase in bone in one year will require approximately 75 mg per day of sodium fluoride (equivalent to about 38 mg of fluoride ion), accompanied by 3.4 grams per day of calcium carbonate (which is equivalent to about 1.3 grams of elemental calcium). The bone will be hyper-mineralized compared with pre-treatment bone, and it may contain small areas around the osteocytes of low mineral density (Fig. 30–2). Vitamin D is apparently an unnecessary adjunct to the calcium-fluoride treatment. Radiological evidence of increased bone mass is also apparent (Fig. 30–3). Double radioisotope densi-tometry studies also confirm the efficacy of fluoride and calcium.[14] A mean increase of 21 per cent in bone mass in the lumbar vertebra was seen in nine patients stud-ied by this method; the values increased from 2.85 to 3.43 in units of bone mineral content, which are equivalent to grams of hydroxyapatite mineral per cm of bone.

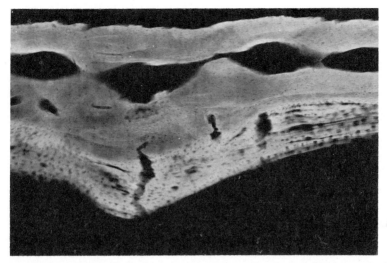

**Figure 30–2**   Microradiograph of the cortex of the iliac crest of an individual treated with fluoride and calcium. The new bone has been laid down endosteally and can be distinguished from the pre-treatment bone by its relative high mineral density and "large" osteocyte lacunae. It is evident that in this sample the bone volume has been increased approximately two-fold (magnification x 40).

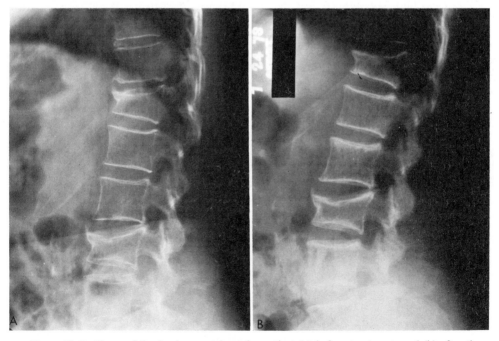

**Figure 30–3**   X-ray of the lumbar vertebra of a patient (a) before treatment, and (b) after three years of treatment with fluoride and calcium. Note the appearance of vertical trabeculae and thickening of the cortices. Some horizontal trabeculae also appear post-treatment. (From Jowsey, J.: Osteoporosis: its etiology and treatment. Sandoz Medical Services Dept. Sandoz Pharmaceuticals, Division of Sandoz (Canada) Ltd., Dorval, Que.)

The original report in which calcium and fluoride were shown to result in a radiological increase in bone mass was that of Cohen and colleagues, who studied patients with multiple myeloma. They administered 50 to 75 mg of sodium fluoride per day, accompanied by 540 mg of elemental calcium as a supplement.[15] Androgens were also given, and, although some of the effect may have been ascribed to the hormone, later studies showed that hormone therapy is an unnecessary adjunct to the fluoride and calcium.[13] The study by Cohen and co-workers is of additional interest because it showed that, in a group of 13 osteoporotic patients, only the two who received additional calcium showed increased bone mass radiologically. The most recent investigations would suggest that the 540 mg calcium supplement used in the study was inadequate; indeed, despite the strong positive calcium balance, the marked radiological density increases, and the gross thickening of trabeculae seen on biopsy, in Cohen's study the bone was poorly mineralized in some instances, although x-ray diffraction indicated increased crystallinity of the hydroxyapatite. A more recent study has confirmed Cohen's work in patients with multiple myeloma; using 100 mg of sodium fluoride and 4 grams of calcium carbonate per day, bone mass increased, compared with a placebo-treated group, despite continued intermittent melphalan and prednisone therapy (Fig. 30–4). The patients treated with steroid alone did not form bone and continued to lose bone; after one year a 10 per cent decrease in bone mass was evident, using videodensitometry. In the patients receiving fluoride–calcium therapy in addition to steroids, bone formation was increased and bone resorption decreased to almost normal levels; bone mass increased by an average of 11 per cent. Presumably, the fluoride increased the osteoblastic activity, as in osteoporosis, while the calcium, in addition to allowing mineralization of new bone, depressed parathyroid hormone activity.

Having established that a combination of fluoride and calcium will increase bone mass in osteoporosis and in the osteopenia of multiple myeloma, the question arises as to whether the bone is stronger and if fractures will stop. The latter question will require many years of investigation in patients who have been treated and many attempts to derive accurate incidences of fracture rates. However, the question concerning the strength of fluoride-induced new bone has been studied by Franke and co-workers in two normal individuals who had industrial fluorosis.[17] Compared with the normal bone, cylinders of cortical bone from the two fluorotic individuals showed a diminution in the resistance to pressure, a slight loss of elasticity, but no decrease in breaking strength; in addition, the whole lumbar vertebral

BONE TURNOVER IN MYELOMA

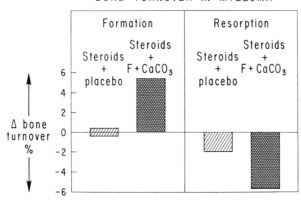

**Figure 30–4** The change in bone turnover in patients with multiple myeloma treated with steroids and placebo, or steroids and fluoride and calcium. The fluoride-calcium treatment increased bone formation and decreased bone resorption.

body showed a three-fold increase in breaking strength, reflecting the increase in bone mass.

A final point is related to fluoride and its effect on dental caries. The fluoride ion replaces the hydroxyl ion in both enamel and hydroxyapatite, and improves the crystallinity of the crystals. Fluoridation of water is associated with a reduction in caries because the enamel is resistant to attack by the bacteria that cause the defect. In vitro, fluoride-substituted hydroxyapatite is more resistant to solution than apatite containing no fluoride. However, a resistance to resorption is not the mechanism by which fluoride is effective in osteoporosis. It is the stimulation of osteoblastic activity and the potential, with calcium, of increasing bone mass that results in the success of this combination therapy. Drinking fluoridated water, unless it contains large amounts of fluoride and is accompanied by calcium supplements, will not alter the course of osteoporosis, and may, in fact, cause osteomalacia if the concentration of fluoride in the water is high enough.

## CONCLUSIONS

The field covered by mineral metabolism and metabolic bone disease is enormous, and there are omissions in this book which include such subjects as genetically heritable disorders, biomechanics of bone, joint diseases, and so forth. However, it is obvious that the scope of any book must be limited. The present volume has been concerned with the understanding of bone tissue and the abnormalities of this tissue as they occur in metabolic bone disease and in some disorders that are not truly metabolic, such as Paget's disease of bone, but that often appear in an orthopedic practice as well as in a general medical practice.

Some subjects are not dealt with in particular detail; however, the references are specifically chosen to fill in any deficiency in the depth to which a subject is discussed.

In the end, all that can be said is that it is hoped that this book proves to be helpful and instructive and that it provides a useful reference for those interested in bone disease, particularly for orthopedists, for whom the volume has been primarily written.

## *REFERENCES*

1. Michael, W. R., King, W. R., and Francis, M. D.: Effectiveness of diphosphonates in preventing "osteoporosis" of disuse in the rat. Clin. Orthop., 78:271–276, 1971.
2. Jowsey, J., Riggs, B. L., Kelly, P. J., Hoffman, D. L., and Bordier, Ph.: The treatment of osteoporosis with disodium ethane-1-hydroxy-1, 1-diphosphonate. J. Lab. Clin. Med., 78:574, 584, 1971.
3. Geho, W. B., and Whiteside, J. A.: Experience with disodium etidronate in diseases of ectopic calcification. Excerpta Medica, International Congress Series No. 270:506–511, 1973.
4. Jowsey, J., and Detenbeck, L. C.: Importance of thyroid hormones in bone metabolism and calcium homeostasis. Endocrinology, 85:87–95, 1969.
5. Munson, P. L., Hirsch, P. F., Brewer, H. B., Reisfeld, R. A., Cooper, C. W., Wästhed, A. B., Orimo, H., and Potts, J. R., Jr.: Thyrocalcitonin. Recent Progr. Horm. Res., 24:589–650, 1968.
6. Jowsey, J., Riggs, B. L., Goldsmith, R. S., Kelly, P. J., and Arnaud, C. D.; Effects of prolonged administration of porcine calcitonin in postmenopausal osteoporosis. J. Clin. Endocrinol. Metab., 33:752–758, 1971.
7. Melick, R. A., Martin, T. J., and Storey, E,: Use of porcine calcitonin in osteoporosis. Aust. N. Z. J. Med., 3:285–289, 1973.

8. Lockwood, D. R., Lammert, J. E., Vogel, J. M., and Hulley, S. B.: Bone mineral loss during bedrest. Excerpta Medica, International Congress Series No. *270*:261–265, 1973.
9. Aloia, J. F., Zanzi, I., Ellis, K., Jowsey, J., Roginsky, M., Wallach, S., and Cohn, S. H.: Effects of growth hormone in osteoporosis. J. Clin. Endocrinol. Metab., *43*:992–999, 1976.
10. Jowsey, J., Schenk, R. K., and Reutter, F. W.: Some results of the effect of fluoride on bone tissue in osteoporosis. J. Clin. Endocrinol. Metab., *28*:869–874, 1968.
11. Spencer, H., Lewin, I., Osis, D., and Samachson, J.: Studies of fluoride and calcium metabolism in patients with osteoporosis. Am. J. Med., *49*:814–822, 1970.
12. Burkhart, J. M., and Jowsey, J.: Effect of variations in calcium intake on the skeleton of fluoride-fed kittens. J. Lab. Clin. Med., *72*:943–950., 1968.
13. Jowsey, J., Riggs, B. L., Kelly, P. J., and Hoffman, D. L.: Effect of combined therapy with sodium fluoride, vitamin D and calcium in osteoporosis. Am. J. Med., *53*:43–49, 1972.
14. Hansson, T., and Roos, B.: Effect of combined therapy with sodium fluoride, calcium, and vitamin D on the lumbar spine in osteoporosis. Am. J. Roentgenol. Radium Ther. Nucl. Med., *126*:1294–1296, 1976.
15. Cohen, P., Nichols, G., Jr., and Banks, H. H.: Fluoride treatment of bone rarefaction in multiple myeloma and osteoporosis. Clin. Orthop., *64*:221–249, 1969.
16. Kyle, R. A., Jowsey, J., Kelly, P. J., and Taves, D. R.: Multiple-myeloma bone disease: the comparative effect of sodium fluoride and calcium carbonate or placebo. N. Engl. J. Med., *293*:1334–1338, 1975.
17. Franke, J., Runge, H., Grau, P., Fengler, F., Wanka, C., and Rempel, H.: Physical properties of fluorosis bone. Acta Orthop. Scand., *47*:20–27, 1976.

# Index

Page numbers in *italics* refer to illustrations; (t) indicates a table.

Acidosis, effect of, on urinary calcium, 276(t)
Acromegaly, 219–223
  bone turnover in, 221(t)
  clinical and radiological findings, 219
  microradiographic appearance in, *221*
  morphology of, 219
  radiologic appearance in, *220*
  total body calcium in 220(t)
  treatment of, 222
Adenyl cyclase mechanism, possible effect of
  magnesium on, 22
Adrenalectomy, effect of, on serum calcium,
  228(t)
Aequonin luminescent reaction, with calcium, 9
Alkaline phosphatase, in serum. See *Serum
  alkaline phosphatase.*
  levels of, abnormalities in, causes of, 17, 17(t)
  measurement of, 16
Anticonvulsant therapy, 100, *101*, 203, 203(t),
  274, 274(t)
Atomic absorption spectrophotometry
  for measurement of calcium, 7
  for measurement of magnesium, 20
  for measurement of phosphorus, 14
Autoradiography, 127–137
  principles and method of, 127, *129*
  quantitative, 128
  uses of, 131
    localization of element by, 131, *131*
    localization of labeled compound by, 131,
      *132*
    metabolism of bone, 132, *133*
"Axial osteomalacia," 208


Biopsy, of bone, 138
  sites of, *139*
Blue sclera, associated with osteogenesis imperfecta, 186
Bone(s), and mineral, metabolism of, and
  calcium–phosphorus ratio, 89
  as source of calcium, 4
  biopsy of, 138

Bone(s) (*Continued*)
  calcium–phosphorus ratio in different types of,
    154, 154(t)
  cancellous, anatomy of, 42
  changes in, in hyperthyroidism, *217*
  cortical, anatomy of, 42
    and trabecular, changes in, with age, 44,
      44(t)
      in skeleton, percentage of, 44, 44(t)
      loss of, 45, 45(t)
        with age, 43, *43*
      surface-area ratio and volume of, 43(t)
    lamellar arrangement in, 79, *82*
    thickness of, measurement of, 102
  disease of, associated with bone loss, 163
    Paget's disease of, 163–171
  effect of calcitonin on, 38, 39(t)
  effect of daily calcium and phosphorus intake
    on, 279(t)
  erosion of, by myeloma cells, 76
  evaluation of, autoradiography in, 127
    bone growth markers for, 124–126
    chemical determinations of, 157
    electron microscopy, technique for, 147
    electron probe, technique for, 153
    microradiography in, 142
    morphology of, 138–156
    neutron activation analysis of, 119
    radioisotope methods of, 115–123
      importance of vascular supply in, 117
    techniques for, 87
  formation of, and resorption, use of micro-
    radiography in quantitating, 145
    by osteoblast, 62
    rate of, in dogs, 74(t)
  haversian, arrangement of, 79, *79*
    lamellae in, 79, *80*
  kinetic analysis of, 117, *118*
  lamellar, 78, *79*
  lamellar non-haversian, *62, 79, 79, 81*
  loss of. See *Bone loss.*
  measurement of, by photon absorption
    methods, 108, *108*
    by x-ray, imperfections in, 104
    technique for, 104

Bone(s) (*Continued*)
  metabolism of, relationship to calcium balance,
    90
  mineral content of, measurement of, 109, *111*
  mineral density of, in animals, 147(t)
  mineralization of, 53
    current studies of, 54
    early studies of, 53
    electron-dense granules and, 54, *55*
  morphology of, major considerations in, 145
  non-lamellar, 78
  radium-burdened, 134, *134*, 135(t)
  remodeling of, by osteoclasts, 74
  remodeling rate, 135(t)
    effect of calcium infusions on, 275(t)
    stimuli for, 42
  resorption of, and formation of, correlation of,
      139(t)
    by mast cells, 74
    by osteoclasts, 73
    in various treatment regimes, *275*
    rate of, in dogs, 74
  structure of, 41–47. See also *Skeleton.*
  tissues of. See *Bone tissue(s).*
  trabecular, and cortical, formation of, 64(t)
    measurement of, Singh Index for, 97
  woven, 78, *80*
Bone cells, 58–77
  osteoblasts, 59, *59*
  osteoclasts, *59, 69*
  osteocytes, 64, *65, 67*
  osteoprogenitor, *59*
  progenitor, location of, 58
  types of, differences in, 149(t)
Bone density, effect of exercise on, 266, 266(t)
  effect of occupation on, 267(t)
  genetics, effect on, *271*
  increased, causes of, 184
  loss of, with age, *98*
  measurement of, mass and volume deter-
      minations of, 96
    techniques for, 96
    wax or plastic coating with, 96
  millet seed displacement method of, 96
  osteoporosis and, *27*
Bone disease, protein deficiency and, 271
Bone growth, markers of, 124–126
  alizarin, 124
  chloro-s-triazines, 124
  microradiographic and tetracycline data
      concerning, 126(t)
Bone loss, associated with bone disease, 163
  calcium deficiency and, 272
  effect of exercise and compression on, 106,
    *106*
  effect of gastrectomy on, 103
  in immobilization, 263, 284
  insufficient calcium-to-phosphorus ratio and,
    284, *286*
  mechanism of, role of parathyroids in, 280,
    281(t), *281*
  race and, 271
  vitamin D deficiency and, 272
  with age, *97*
Bone mass, and race, 269
  and sex, 269, 269(t)
  effect of calcium intake on, 105(t)

Bone mass (*Continued*)
  effect of exercise on, 264, *265*
  effect of genetics on, 269
  effect of immobilization on, 111, *112*
  in post-menopausal osteoporosis, 290, *291*
  in twins, 270(t)
  mineralized, and calcium balance, 282
Bone mineral, 53
  concentration of, glycosaminoglycan-to-
    collagen ratio and, 78
  formation of, 53
  loss of, and hypocalcemia, *27*
  structure of, 53
  trace elements in, 55, 56(t)
Bone size, increase in, causes of, 46
    measurement of, 46, 47(t)
    with age, 46
Bone tissue(s), 48–57
  appearance of, 78
  composition of, 48(t)
  morphology of, 138–156
  types of, 78–86, *79*
Bone tumor(s), associated with Paget's disease
    of bone, 171
Bone turnover rate, data on, 135
  definition of, 132
  method of determining, 132
Brush border, role of, in function of osteoclasts,
    72

Calciostat, 26
  primary hyperparathyroidism and, 26
Calcitonin, biological activity of, 39
  C-cells of thyroid gland and, 35, *35*
  effects of, hypocalcemic, 37
    on bone, 38, 39(t)
    on serum phosphate, 38, 38(t)
  metabolism, 35–40
  role of, in control of serum calcium, 36
    in lowering serum phosphorus, 11
  secondary hyperparathyroidism and, 37
  secretion of, and hypocalcemia, in animals, *36*
  serum calcium levels and, 37, 37(t)
  sources of, 36
  use of, in treatment of osteoporosis, 298
    in treatment of Paget's disease of bone, 170
Calcium, absorption of, effect of ethanol on,
      274(t)
  factors influencing, 4
  influence of parathyroid hormone on, 28.
    See also *Calcium absorption.*
  sites of, 4
  aequonin luminescent reaction with, 9
  and fluoride, use of, in treatment of osteo-
    porosis, 300, *301, 302*
  and hyperparathyroidism, 236
  and phosphorus, dietary intake of, history of,
    87
    ratio between, in relation to bone and
      mineral metabolism, 89
  concentrations of, in water, fish, and man,
    3(t)
  dietary intake of, decrease in, with age, 88, *88*
  dietary sources of, variations in, 87
  exchange of, in bone, 135, 136(t)
  excretion of, by urine, rate of, 5

Calcium (*Continued*)
  homeostasis of, 4
    as function of osteocytes, 66
    role of diet in, 4
    role of kidney in, 5
  in serum. See *Serum calcium.*
  infusions of, effect of, on bone remodeling, 275, 275(t)
  intake of, and phosphorus, effect of, on bone, 87, 89, 279(t)
    inadequate, causes of, 274, 274(t)
    ionized, carbon dioxide in, loss of, prevention of, 7
      measurement of, 6
      frog heart method of, 7
      variations in, 8
    methods of storage of, 8(t)
  malabsorption of, 91
  measurement of, in urine, feces, and food, 91
  metabolism of, 3–10
  minimum daily requirement of, 5
  recommended daily intake of, 89
  role of, in body functioning, 3
    in conversion of prothrombin to thrombin, 4
  skeleton as source of, 41
  sources of, 3, 4, 41
Calcium absorption, effect of age on, 94
  in gut, measurement of, 93
  measurement of, technique for, variations in, 94
  role of calcium deficiency in, 93
  site of, 93
Calcium balance, measurements of, 87–95
  mineralized bone mass and, 282
  relationship to bone metabolism, 90
  studies of, 87, 90
    conditions for insuring accuracy of, 91
    data obtained from, reliability of, 92
    shortcomings of, 92
    technique and interpretation of, 90
    variables considered in, 90
Calcium deficiency, bone loss and, 272
  role of, in calcium absorption, 93
Calcium intake, effect of, on bone mass, 105, 105(t)
Calcium levels, depressed, effects of, 4
Calcium–phosphorus product, 14
  soft tissue mineralization and, 15
Calcium–phosphorus ratio, osteoporosis and, 280, 281(t)
  in different types of bone, 154(t)
Cameron–Sorenson method, for bone measurement, 108, *108, 110, 111*
  body size and, 109
  imperfections in, 109
  in fracture and non-fracture patients, *110*
  variations of, 112
Carbon dioxide, in ionized calcium, loss of, prevention of, 7
  measurement of, 7
Cell(s), myeloma, 76
  of bone. See *Bone cells.*
Cell cycles, equation expressing, 130
Cement line, of secondary haversian systems, 82, *83*
Collagen, formation of, 51
  in osteoid, 50
  production of, by osteoblast, 61

Colles' fracture, 248, 257, *258*
Compression, effect of, on bone loss, 106, *106*
Cortical thickness, measurement of, to distinguish normal from abnormal bone, 102, *102*
Corticosteroids, administration of, and bone formation, 224, *226*
Cushing's disease, 94, 224

Dehydration, as cause of abnormal serum protein levels, 6
Dental caries, effect of fluoride on, 303
Diet, as source of calcium and phosphorus, 89
  calcium–phosphorus ratio in, 90
  role of, in control of phosphorus, 11
Diphosphonates, use of, in treatment of osteoporosis, 296, *298*
Diphosphonate-induced osteomalacia, 208, 297
Disodium dichlormethane diphosphonate ($Cl_2MDP$), use of, in treatment of osteoporosis, 297, *298*
Disodium ethane–1–hydroxy–1,1–diphosphonate (EHDP), use of, in treatment of osteoporosis, 297, *298*
Dual photon absorptiometry, 111, *112*
Duodenectomy, as cause of vitamin D deficiency, 34

Electron microscopy, use of, in evaluation of bone, 147, *148*
Electron probe, for evaluation of bone, technique for, 153
Engelmann's disease, 182, *182*
Estrogen therapy, in post-menopausal women, bone mineral mass in, 291(t), *291*
  bone turnover in, 290, *290*
Ethanol, effect of, on calcium absorption, 274, 274(t)
Ethylenediamine tetra-acetic acid (EDTA), in measurement of serum calcium, 6
  used as food additive, 89
Exercise, effect of, on bone density, 266
  on bone loss, 106, *106*
  on bone mass, 264

Feces, calcium in, measurement of, 91
Femoral trabecular index. See *Singh index.*
Fibrogenesis imperfecta ossium (FIO), 205
  electron microscopic appearance of, *207*
  radiographic appearance of, *206*
Fish, calcium concentration in, 3(t)
Fluoride, and calcium, use of, in treatment of osteoporosis, 300, *301, 302*
  effect of, on dental caries, 303
  use of, in treatment of osteogenesis imperfecta, 190
Fluorine–18, 115
Fracture(s), femur, proximal, in persons over 65, 270(t)
  frequency of, in relation to height loss, 249(t)
  of femoral neck, and osteoporosis, 257

Fracture(s) (*Continued*)
  role of, in diagnosing metabolic bone disease, 163
Frog heart, in measurement of ionized calcium, 7

Gastrectomy, as cause of osteomalacia, 203
  effect of, on bone loss, 103, *103*
Glycosaminoglycans, production of, by osteoblast, 61
Glycosaminoglycan–collagen ratio and, bone mineral, 78
Glyoxal bis (2–hydroxyavil) (GBHA), in measurement of serum calcium, 7
Growth hormone, administration of, in acromegaly, 222
  use of, in treatment of osteoporosis, 299, 299(t)

Hand, bones of, quantitative radiography of, technique for, 104
Haversian systems, primary, 79, *79*
  distinguished from secondary, 80, *82*
  remodeling of, 83
  secondary, 79, *79*
    cement line of, 82, *83*
Heparin, administration of, and pregnancy, 274
Histology, of bone, procedure for, 140, *141, 142*
Hormone deficiency, and osteoporosis, 289, *290*
Howship's lacunae, 71, *72*
Hydroxyapatite, 53, 56(t)
  in normal osteoporotics, *27*
Hydroxyproline, in bone, 51
  in osteogenesis imperfecta, 187
  in osteoporosis, 259(t), 289
  in urine, 51, 52
  measurement of, 52
Hypercalcemia, 213, 229, 238, *238*, 239, 261, 282
Hypercortisonism, 224–228
  clinical presentation of, 224
  microradiographic appearance of, *225*
  morphology of, 224
  treatment of, 226
Hyperparathyroidism, 229–247
  Albright's definition of, 229
  associated findings in, 230(t)
  bone formation and bone resorption in, 233
  bone loss in, *237*
  bone morphology in, 231, 239, *240*
  calcium intake and, 236
  chronic, severe, microradiographic appearance of, *235*
  clinical and biochemical abnormalities in, 229
  "conventional," microradiographic appearance of, *178*
  hyperplasia and, 23, *24*
  hypophosphatemia in, 213, *214*
  microradiographic appearance of trabecular bone in, *236*
  osteoporosis and, similarities and differences in, 232
  osteosclerotic, 176, *177*
    biochemical changes in, 179(t)
  primary, 229
    calciostat and, 26

Hyperparathyroidism (*Continued*)
  radiologic abnormalities in, 230
  radiologic appearance of, *231, 232, 233*
  secondary, 239
    calcitonin and, 37
    effect of, on osteocytes, 66, *67*
    etiology of, 240
    microradiographic appearance in, *240, 241*
    treatment of, 242
  subperiosteal erosion and, 233, *235*
  treatment of, 238
Hyperphosphatemia, prevention of, by parathyroid hormone, 28
Hyperplasia, hyperparathyroidism and, 23, *24*
Hyperthyroidism, 215
  and serum and bone morphology changes in, 216(t)
  bone changes in, *217*
  bone turnover in, 217(t)
Hypocalcemia, hyperparathyroidism and, 213, 238, 239, *241*
  hyperphosphatemia and, 245
  hypocalcemia and, 245
  hypoparathyroidism and, 244
  loss of bone mineral and, *27*
  magnesium depletion and, 21
Hypoparathyroidism, bone morphology in, 245
  clinical and biochemical features of, 243, 243(t)
  magnesium depletion and, 21, 245
  osteocytes in, 68
  pregnancy and, 244
  radiographic appearance of, *244*
  treatment of, 245
Hypophosphatasia, 179, *179, 180*
  symptoms of, 177
Hypophosphatemia, in hyperparathyroidism, 213, *214*
Hypothyroidism, 215

Iliac crest, anterior, site for bone biopsy, 138
Isotope, ways of entering bone, 118, *119*

Jejunectomy, as cause of vitamin D deficiency, 34

Kidney, production of vitamin D in, 33
  role of, in calcium homeostasis, 5
Kinetic analysis, of bone, 117, *118*
Kwashiorkor, 272

Lactase, deficiency in, and osteoporosis, 277, *277*
Lactose, intolerance to, 278, 278(t)
Lacunae, Howship's, 71, *72, 145*
  of osteocytes, *68*
    and osteocytic osteolysis, distinction between, 67, *67*
Liver, role of, in degradation of parathyroid hormone, 29

Magnesium, adenyl cyclase mechanism and, 22
  depletion of, bone morphology in, 22, 22(t)
    causes of, 20
    hypocalcemia and, 20, 21
    hypoparathyroidism and, 21
    in chickens, 21(t), 22
    in dogs, 20(t), 21(t), 22
  homeostasis of, 19
  in bone, 19
  in serum. See *Serum magnesium.*
  influence of, on parathyroid hormone, 19
  measurement of, 20
  metabolism of, 19–22
  role of, in body functioning, 19
Magnesium deficiency, associated with hypopara-
    thyroidism, 245
  bone morphology in, 22(t)
  effect on osteoid width, 21(t)
  microradiographic appearance of, 21
Man, calcium concentration in, 3(t)
Mast cells, increase in number of, causes of, 74
  resorption of bone by, 74
Mast cell disease, 74, 75
Melorheostosis, microradiographic and x-ray
    appearance of, 181, 181
  symptoms of, 180
Microradiography, use of, in evaluation of
    mineral density, 142
    in quantitating bone formation and re-
      sorption, 144, 145, 146
    tetracycline and, 126(t)
Milkman pseudofractures, 196
Millet seed, displacement of, as method of bone
    density measurement, 96
Mineral density, evaluation of, by microradiog-
    raphy, 143
Mineral exchange, in bone, 135, 136(t)
Mineralization, of bone, 53–55
Mineralization front, electron probe analysis
    of, 154
Mithramycin, in treatment of Paget's disease, 171
Morphology, of bone, 138–156
    major considerations in studying, 146
Myeloma, osteopenia, treatment of, 302
  bone turnover in, 302
  osteoporosis and, 76


Neutron activation analysis, 119
  technique for, 120
Non-serum calcium, 9
Normocalcemia, maintenance of, as function of
    osteocytes, 66


Organ and tissue culture, 157–160
Organ culture, 158
Os calcis, quantitative radiography of, tech-
    nique for, 104, 105, 106, 286
Osteitis fibrosa, 229, 234, 235
Osteoblast(s), covering osteoid border, 63
  features of, 59, 59
  formation of bone by, 62
  in secondary hyperparathyroidism, 239, 240
  lamellar pattern of, 61, 62

Osteoblast(s) (*Continued*)
  nucleus–cytoplasmic ratio of, 60
  on bone matrix surface, 60
  production of collagen by, 61
  production of glycosaminoglycans by, 61
  ratio of, to osteoclasts, 73
  structure of, 60
Osteoclast(s), bone resorption by, 73
  brush border of, 72
  formation of, 69
  function of, 71, 74
  growth and dedifferentiation of, 71
  location of, 71, 72
  nuclei in, 69, 70
  ratio of, to osteoblasts, 73
  structure of, 69, 70
Osteocyte(s)
  effect of physiologic stimulation on, 66, 67
  electron microscopic appearance of, 148
  formation of, 64, 65
  function of, 65, 66
  in rickets and hypoparathyroidism, 68, 69
  mineral density of, 68
  physiologic role of, 66
  responses of, to parathyroid hormone, 28
  size of, 65
Osteogenesis imperfecta, 186–191
  bone morphological findings in, 190(t)
  clinical, radiological, and biochemical findings,
    186
  malignant, radiographic appearance of, 187
  microradiographic appearance of, 189
  morphology of, 188
  radiographic appearance of, 188
  symptoms of, 186
  treatment of, 190
Osteoid, appearance of, 48, 49
  collagen in, 50
  composition of, 48
  definition of, 48
  matrix, 48, 50, 55
Osteoid borders, measurement of, 63, 64, 64
  method for demonstrating, 62, 63
  number of, effect of age on, 64
  osteoblasts and, 63
  width change, with age, 50
Osteoid tissue, volume of, 51
    measurement of, 49
Osteomalacia, biochemical features of, 197, 199(t)
  bone morphology in, 198, 200, 204
  clinical presentation of, 195
  comparison with osteoporosis, 195
  development of, 193, 194
  etiology of, 200, 201(t)
  gastrectomy as cause of, 203
  hypophosphatemic, adult onset, clinical and
      biochemical findings in, 211, 211(t)
    morphology and etiology of, 212
  in children (rickets), 192–204
  nutritional factors in, 201
  radiographic appearance of, 193
  stages in the development of, 198
  treatment of, 203
  unusual forms of, 205 214
Osteopetrosis, 172–185
  etiology of, 172
  microradiographic appearance of, 173, 175

Osteopetrosis (*Continued*)
  morphology, 174, *175*
  radiologic appearance of, 172, *173, 174*
  treatment of, 176
Osteopoikilosis, 182
Osteoporosis, as result of senescence, 250, *250*
  body weight and, 268, *268*
  bone turnover in, 258(t), 259(t)
  calcium absorption in, 92
  calcium–phosphorus ratio and, 279, 280(t)
  cells in, 75
  development of, 193, *194*
  differentiated from normal, use of Singh Index
    in, 112
  effect of immobilization on, 261, 262(t), *263,*
    263(t)
  effect of oral phosphate therapy on, 285(t), *286*
  effect of vitamin D administration on, 276
  etiology of, 261, 297(t)
  exposure to sunlight and, 273, 273(t)
  femoral neck fractures and, 257
  height loss in, with hormone therapy, 291(t)
  hormone deficiency and, 289, *290*, 297(t)
    estrogen treatment in, 290, *290*
  hyperparathyroidism and, similarities and
    differences in, 232, *235*
  idiopathic, post-menopausal and senile, 256–
    296
  "immobilization," 261–264
  juvenile, 248–255
    and adult, 254
    bone remodeling in, 253(t)
    definition and symptoms of, 248
    diagnosis of, 249
    external cortex in, comparison with normal,
      254
    osteoid border width in, *255*
    radiologic features of, 251, *251, 253*
    Singh Index in, 249
  lactase deficiency and, 277, *277*
  microradiographic appearance of, *235, 250,*
    260
  osteomalacia and, relation to rickets, 192
  parathyroid hormone levels in, *286, 287*, 288
  physical activity and, 264
  post-menopausal, bone loss in, 259, 259(t), *260*
    bone morphology in, 258
    bone turnover in, *290*
    radiologic features of, 256, *257*
  Singh Index and, 99, 100, *100*
  treatment of, 296–304
    calcitonin in, 298
    diphosphonates in, 296, 297(t)
    fluoride and calcium in, 300, *301, 302*
    growth hormone in, 299, 299(t)
  Turner's syndrome and, 289, 290, *291*
Osteosclerosis, in hyperparathyroidism, 176


Pachyostosis, 183, *183*
  appearance of bone in, *183, 184*
Paget's disease of bone, 163–171
  diagnosis of, 167
  frequency of bone tumors with, 171
  history of, 164
  hypercortisonism and, 224

Paget's disease of bone (*Continued*)
  hyperparathyroidism and, 229, *235*, 239, 241
  hypophosphatasia and, 249, *250, 260,* 261,
    297(t)
  microradiographic appearance of, lytic phase,
    *168*
    sclerotic phase, 168
  morphologic features of, 166, *167*
  radiographic appearance of, *165, 166*
  treatment of, 169
    calcitonin used in, 170
Paragon stain, 140, 144
Parathyroid gland(s), and thyroid, as sources of
  calcitonin, 36
  functions of, 25
  role of, in bone loss, 279, 281(t), *281*
  secretion of parathyroid hormone by, 25
  serum calcium levels and, 26, 27
Parathyroid hormone, amino acid sequence of,
  23
  assays of, 24
  biological activity of, 29
  calcium absorption and, 28
  degradation of, by liver, 29
  half-life of, in blood, 29
  in osteoporotic patients, 286–288
  increased levels of, causes of, 25, 25(t)
    in serum, 28
  influence of magnesium on, 19
  maintenance of serum calcium by, role of
    osteoclasts in, 74
  metabolism of, 23–30
  osteoclastic bone resorption and, 28
  responses of osteocytes to, 28
  role of, in body functioning, 23, 28
    in lowering serum phosphorus, 11
    in prevention of hyperphosphatemia, 28
Phosphate, effect of calcitonin on, 38, 38(t)
  excess of, 279–289
    as factor in osteoporosis, 288
Phosphate binding agents, 213
Phosphorus, calcium and, dietary intake of,
    history of, 87
    ratio between, in relation to bone and
      mineral metabolism, 89
  control of, role of diet in, 11
  daily intake of, and effect of calcium on bone,
    279(t)
  dietary sources of, variations in, 88
  effect of, on serum calcium, 282, *282, 284*
  in blood and serum, distribution of, 12(t)
  in serum. See *Serum phosphorus.*
  metabolism of, 11–15
  renal excretion of, 11
  role of, in body functioning, 11
Phosphorus–calcium ratio, insufficient, and
    bone loss, 279, *280,* 284
  soft tissue mineralization and, *283, 284*
Photon absorption, for bone measurement, tech-
    nique for, 108, *108, 110, 111*
Physical activity, and osteoporosis, 264
Polyphosphate, mechanism of uptake of, 117
Pregnancy, and osteoporosis, 274
  and hypoparathyroidism, 244
Progenitor cell(s), 58, 59
  location of, 58
Proline. See *Hydroxyproline.*

Protein deficiency, and bone disease, 271
Prothrombin, conversion of, to thrombin, role of calcium in, 4
Pseudohypoparathyroidism, *236,* 246

Radioisotope methods, of bone evaluation, 115–119
Remodeling, of secondary haversian systems, 83
Renal stones, as complication of hyperparathyroidism, 230(t), 238, *238*
Rickets, 192–204
  hypophosphatemic, morphology of, 209, 210
    radiological and biochemical findings in, 209
    treatment of, 210
  osteocytes in, 68, *69*
  radiographic appearance of, *196*
  relation to osteoporosis and osteomalacia, 192
  symptoms of, 192
  vitamin D-dependent hypocalcemic, 208
    treatment of, 209
  vitamin D-resistant, microradiographic appearance of, *210*

Scanning electron microscopy (SEM), 149, *150, 151, 152*
Scheuermann's kyphosis, 252
  Singh Index and, 100, *101*
SEM. See *Scanning electron microscopy.*
Serum alkaline phosphatase, in adults and children, normal values for, 16(t), 17, *17*
Serum calcium, adrenal control of, 227
  bone density and, *9*
  effect of adrenalectomy on, 228(t)
  forms of, 5
  levels of, effect of age on, 26(t)
    in males and females, *8*
    parathyroid glands and, 26, 27
  maintenance of, under control of parathyroid hormone, role of osteoclasts in, 74
  measurement of, ethylenediamine tetra-acetic acid in, 6
    glyoxal bis (2–hydroxyavil) in, 7
    methods for, 6
  partition of, 6(t), 20(t)
  role of calcitonin in control of, 36, *36*
  role of parathyroid gland in, 25, 25(t), 26
  serum phosphorus and, in man and animals, 13(t)
Serum fluoride, levels of, and steroid treatment, 227(t)
Serum magnesium, 20(t)
  measurement of, 20
Serum parathyroid, levels of, in osteoporosis, *287*
Serum phosphate, elevated, stimulation of parathyroid hormone by, 285, *286*
Serum phosphorus, 12
  distribution of, 12
  effect of, on mineral metabolism, 12
  levels of, effect of age on, *14*
    in children and adults, *12*
    in men and women, comparison of, 13
    in normal and disease states, 13(t)

Serum phosphorus (*Continued*)
  lowering of, by parathyroid hormone and calcitonin, 11
  measurement of, methods of, 14
  serum calcium and, comparison of, 12
    in man and animals, 13(t)
Serum protein, levels of, abnormal, dehydration as cause of, 6
Singh Index, 97–102
  anticonvulsant therapy and, 100, *101*
  basis of, 97
  grading patterns in, 99, *99*
  in differentiating osteoporosis from normal, 112
  in separating osteoporotic from normal individuals, 100
  osteoporosis and, 99, *100, 249, 270*
  Scheuermann's kyphosis and, 100, *101*
  skeleton size and, 100
Skeleton, as source of calcium, 3, 41
  cortical and trabecular bone in, percentage of, 44, 44(t)
  role of, in calcium supply, 4
[85]Sr-Strontium, 115
Steroids, administration of, effect of, 224–227
  in myeloma, 302, *302*
Stress, breaking, in rats, 264, 265(t)
  in fluorotic bone, 302
Sunlight, exposure to, elevated levels of vitamin D and, 32, 201, 202(t), 272
  osteoporosis and, 273, *273*

[99m]Tc-Technetium, use of, in detecting bone abnormalities, 116, *116*
Tetracycline, use of, as bone growth marker, 124, 125, *125*
Thrombin, conversion of prothrombin to, role of calcium in, 4
Thyroid bone disease, 215–217
Tissue culture, 159
Total body calcium measurements, 120, 122, 220(t)
Total body neutron activation analysis (TBNAA), 120(t), 121, 121(t), *122*
Trace elements, in bone mineral, 55, 56(t)
Tumoral calcinosis, 242
  radiographic appearance of, 242, *244*
Turner's syndrome, and osteoporosis, 289, 290, *291*

Ulna, x-ray measurement of, technique for, 107
Urinary calcium, changes in, in response to acidosis, 276(t)
  mineralized bone mass and, lack of correlation between, 284, *285*
Urine, as means of calcium excretion, 5
  calcium in, measurement of, 91

Vascular supply, importance of, in radioisotope methods of bone evaluation, 117
Vesicles, matrix, 54, *55*

Videodensitometry, advantages of, 107
  technique for, 107
  use of, in quantitating bone mineral, 144
Vitamin D, administration of, effect of, in osteo-
    porosis, 276
  biological activity of, 32
  deficiency of, as cause of secondary hyperpara-
    thyroidism, 240
    bone loss and, 272
    causes of, 34
  lack of, in osteomalacia, 201
  levels of, 32, 32(t)
    in different populations, 202, 202(t)
  metabolism of, 31–34
    geographical differences and, 33
    role of calcium in, 33

Vitamin D (*Continued*)
  production of, in kidney, 33(t)
  role of, in calcium absorption, 5
  sources of, 31
    environmental adaptation to, 31
  use of, in treatment of secondary hyper-
    parathyroidism, 242(t), 243(t)
Vitamin D-dependent hypocalcemic rickets, 208
Vitamin D metabolites, transport of, 32
Volkmann's canal, connecting secondary
  haversian systems, 83
von Kossa stain, use of, in bone histology, 48,
  140

Ward's triangle, 98
Water, calcium concentration in, 3(t)

# Understand Your Diabetes
## and Live a Healthy Life

**Recommended by The Canadian Diabetes Association**

# Understand Your Diabetes
## and Live a Healthy Life

**Diabetes Day-Care Unit – Hôtel-Dieu, Montreal**

**New Edition 2008**
**(Translation of the 6th French Edition)**

**Bibliothèque et Archives nationales du Québec and Library and Archives Canada cataloguing in publication**

Main entry under title :

Understand your diabetes and live a healthy life
New ed. 2008.
Translation of: Connaître son diabète pour mieux vivre.
ISBN 978-2-922260-26-7

1. Diabetes - Popular works. 2. Diabetics - Health and hygiene. 3. Diabetes - Diet therapy. I. Mircescu, Hortensia, 1969-  . II. CHUM. Pavillon Hôtel-Dieu. Unité de jour de diabète.

RC660.4.C6613 2008          616.4'62   C2008-941303-2

Legal deposit : 3rd quarter
Bibliothèque nationale du Québec, 2008
National Library of Canada, 2008

The publication of this work was made possible thanks to an unrestricted educational grant from sanofi-aventis.

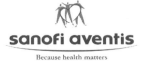

sanofi aventis
Because health matters

**Editor:**
Chantal Benhamron
**Graphic Design and Layout:**
Rogers Business and Professional Publishing group

Printed in Canada

# Preface

This publication is offered as a support for people who have recently been diagnosed with diabetes and for those who are taking the steps required to live an active and productive life as persons with diabetes. Diabetes is challenging, there is no doubt about it, and this is particularly true now, as new medications, technologies and informations are transforming our understanding of how Canadians can better care for themselves as they manage and treat their condition. Knowledge is the first and most important step.

This New edition 2008 of *Understand Your Diabetes and Live a Healthy Life* is an excellent resource. The information it contains is aimed at assisting people with diabetes in adopting healthy lifestyles and maintaining glucose levels that will delay and/or prevent both short- and long-term complications. Our mission at the Canadian Diabetes Association is to promote the health of Canadians through diabetes research, education, service and advocacy, and we recognize the importance of resources such as this publication as part of a support network for people with diabetes. On behalf of the Association, I applaud the authors' efforts in developing this new edition of *Understand Your Diabetes and Live a Healthy Life*.

**Karen Philp**
*Vice-President*
*Public Policy and Government Relations*
*Canadian Diabetes Association*

## From the same publisher*

Dr. Michael McCormack and Dr. Fred Saad
*Understanding Prostate Cancer* (2008)

Dr. Michael McCormack and Dr. Fred Saad
*Diagnosis and Management of Prostatic Diseases* (2006)

Dr. André-H. Dandavino et al.
*The Family Guide to Symptoms*, 2nd edition (2003)

Dr. Michael McCormack
*Male Sexual Health* (2003)

Dr. André-H. Dandavino et al.
*The Family Guide to Health Problems* (2000)

Dr. Jacques Boulay
*Bilingual Guide to Medical Abbreviations*, 3rd edition (1998)

* All the above titles are also available in French.

# Foreword

Here is another edition of *Understand Your Diabetes and Live a Healthy Life*.

Diabetes has a long history. The Ancient Greeks used the term *dia-baino*, which means "to pass through", to describe people who urinated as soon as they took a drink. Thankfully, our understanding of diabetes, its causes, diagnosis, complications, treatment and prevention has never stopped evolving. It is now possible to prevent or delay the onset of type 2 diabetes through healthy living and certain medications.

It is very important for people with diabetes or at risk of developing the disease to be aware of new discoveries and approaches. This type of knowledge can help them change their lifestyles and make it easier to take control of this chronic disease, which is rapidly increasing in occurrence.

We hope that this book will be a valuable source of information for the population in general. More specifically, we hope that it can motivate people with diabetes to achieve a better understanding of themselves in relation to the disease and learn how to improve their treatment in order to get the most out of life.

CHUM–Hôtel-Dieu Diabetes Day-Care Unit Team

# Acknowledgments

We would like to thank the members of the Division of Endocrinology-Metabolism and Nutrition of the CHUM-Hôtel-Dieu for their contribution, and to Ms. Susanne Bordeleau for her work as coordinator.

We would also like to express our gratitude to the following health professionals for their revisions, comments, and suggestions:

- Marc Aras, Director of Communications, Diabetes Québec
- Andrée Gagné, dietician, Diabetes Québec
- Julie Lalancette, dietician, Hôpital Charles-LeMoyne
- Carole Lavoie, Ph.D., professor, Department of Human Kinetics, Université du Québec à Trois-Rivières
- Catherine Noulard, dietician, CHUM
- Thérèse Surprenant, dietician, CHUM
- Julie St-Jean, dietician, Diabetes Québec
- Louise Tremblay, nurse and M.Ed., Diabetes Québec

# List of Authors

This book has been re-edited by the multidisciplinary team of the Centre hospitalier de l'Université de Montréal, Hôtel-Dieu, namely:

- o Françoise Desrochers, graduate nurse
- o Lyne Gauthier, pharmacist
- o Michelle Messier, dietician
- o Hortensia Mircescu, endocrinologist
- o Charles Tourigny, psychologist

We would also like to acknowledge the work done by the authors who contributed to previous editions:

- o Nathalie Beaulieu, dietician
- o Jean-Louis Chiasson, endocrinologist
- o Julie Demers, pharmacist
- o Micheline Fecteau-Côté, dietician
- o Sylvie Fournier, pharmacist
- o Christiane Gobeil, dietician
- o Nicole Hamel, pharmacist
- o Lise Lussier, psychologist
- o Caroline Rivest, pharmacist
- o Danièle Tremblay, psychologist
- o Francis Viguié, psychologist

# Objectives of This Book

This book has the following objectives:

## General objective

To help people with diabetes achieve optimal control of their health so that they may improve their well-being and reduce the risk of developing complications of diabetes.

## Specific objectives

To provide tools to people with diabetes to help them improve their habits, maintain normal blood glucose levels, and enable them to:

1) acquire general knowledge about diabetes;
2) adapt their diet to their diabetes and their various activities;
3) take into account the effects of stress and physical exercise on the management of their disease;
4) recognize the complications caused by poorly controlled blood glucose levels;
5) take effective steps when complications do occur;
6) recognize situations that require emergency intervention;
7) understand the treatments (such as drugs and insulin) that are used to treat diabetes and its complications;
8) understand the adjustments necessary in special situations (for example, while exercising or on trips);
9) understand the importance of good foot care and general hygiene;
10) correctly operate blood glucose measurement and insulin delivery devices;
11) use community resources, when needed;
12) adopt a positive attitude and management strategies to take better control of their health.

# Table of Contents

**1**   General Information about Diabetes    17

**2**   Hyperglycemia    23

**3**   Hypoglycemia and Glucagon    27

**4**   Self-monitoring:
Blood Glucose and Glycosylated Hemoglobin (A1C)    39

**5**   Measuring Ketone Bodies    53

**6**   Eating Well    57

**7**   How to Recognize Carbohydrates    65

**8**   Fats: Making the Right Choices    75

**9**   How to Read Food Labels    85

**10**   Preparing Meals    93

**11**   Special Situations:
- Eating in Restaurants    97
- Delayed Meals    98
- Alcohol    99
- Minor Illnesses    102
- Planning a Trip    104

**12**   Oral Antidiabetic Drugs    113

**13**   Over-the-counter Drugs    123

**14**   Insulins    129

**15**    Preparation and Injection of Insulin                                        139

**16**    Insulin Injection: Injection Site Rotation                                  149

**17**    Storage of Insulin                                                          153

**18**    Insulin Dose Adjustment                                                     159

**19**    The Insulin Pump: Another Treatment Option                                  171

**20**    Physical Activity                                                           181

**21**    Hyperglycemic Emergencies:
          Diabetic Acidosis and the Hyperosmolar State                               191

**22**    Chronic Complications                                                       197

**23**    Foot Care and General Hygiene                                               205

**24**    Living with Diabetes                                                        215

**25**    Managing Daily Stress                                                       223

**26**    The Motivation to Change                                                    231

**27**    Sex and Family Planning                                                     237

**28**    Community Resources                                                         243

**29**    Research: What the Future Holds                                             269

**30**    Diabetes Follow-up Tools                                                    277

Appendice                                                                            285

# General Information about Diabetes

1. **What is diabetes?**

   Diabetes is a disease characterized by a lack of insulin and/or impaired insulin action, which causes an **elevation of blood glucose** (blood sugar) to levels above normal.

2. **How many Canadians are affected by diabetes?**

   About **2.5 million Canadians** (8% of the population) have diabetes, but nearly 40% of these people remain undiagnosed and unaware of their condition. It is anticipated that the number of cases will have doubled by 2025, making diabetes the **disease of the 21st century.**

   Engendering increasingly significant costs, currently estimated to be close to $13 billion per year, diabetes is a growing societal problem, which must be battled on all fronts.

3. **What are the criteria of a diagnosis of diabetes?**

   The diagnosis of diabetes is based on the following laboratory results from tests performed on venous blood:

   1) **fasting blood glucose** equal to or above 7.0 mmol/L;
   2) **random blood glucose** equal to or above 11.1 mmol/L;
   3) **oral glucose tolerance test (OGTT)**, with a blood glucose level equal to or above 11.1 mmol/L two hours after the consumption of 75 g of glucose.

   If there are no symptoms, however, a medical diagnosis of diabetes requires that an abnormal result on one of these tests be confirmed by repeating any one of the tests on a different day.

**4.   What is normal blood glucose?**

Blood glucose is considered normal when it remains steady **between 4 mmol/L and 6 mmol/L before meals, and between 5 mmol/L and 8 mmol/L one to two hours after meals.**

**5.   What blood glucose levels are targeted in the treatment of diabetes?**

The **target glucose levels** for most people with diabetes should be between 4 mmol/L and 7 mmol/L before meals, and between 5 mmol/L and 10 mmol/L one or two hours after meals. In cases where there is no risk of hypoglycemia, however, **normal glucose levels** should be targeted, that is, between 4 mmol/L and 6 mmol/L before meals and between 5 mmol/L and 8 mmol/L one or two hours after meals.

**6.   Why is it important to achieve a normal or target blood glucose level?**

The closer blood glucose is to normal, the more a person with diabetes will:
1)   feel **fit**, and
2)   **lower the risk** of long-term complications associated with diabetes.

**7.   Why do blood glucose levels increase in a person with diabetes?**

Blood glucose rises because of a **lack of insulin**, which can be caused by reduced insulin secretion, decreased insulin action, or a combination of the two. When there is **insufficient insulin** or insulin action to cause glucose to enter the cells, glucose levels in the blood increase. This is called **hyperglycemia.**

**8.   What is insulin?**

Insulin is a hormone produced by the **pancreas**, an organ located in the abdomen, behind the stomach.

Insulin is like a **key that opens the door and lets glucose enter the cells**, which in turn lowers blood glucose levels.

**9. How does the body use glucose?**

Glucose is a vital **energy source** for the body's cells, much as gasoline is an important fuel for cars.

**10. Where does excess glucose in the blood of a person with diabetes come from?**

Excess glucose in the blood comes from two main sources:
1) foods containing **carbohydrates in meals and snacks;**
2) the **liver**, which produces glucose, when it makes too much.

**11. What are the characteristics of type 1 diabetes?**

Type 1 diabetes is typically characterized by the following features:
1) a **total lack of insulin;**
2) the appearance of the disease **around puberty** or in early adulthood (**usually before age 40**)
3) **weight loss;**
4) the need for treatment with **insulin injections**.

**12. What are the characteristics of type 2 diabetes?**

Type 2 diabetes is typically characterized by the following features:
1) **insulin resistance**, where the insulin produced becomes less effective;
2) **insufficient insulin production;**
3) appearance of the disease **after age 40** (although in certain populations at risk, it is becoming increasingly frequent in younger people);
4) **excess weight;**
5) significant family history;
6) treatment through lifestyle modification (dietary program, increased physical activity) **alone** or in combination with **oral antidiabetic drugs. In some cases, insulin injections are necessary**.

**13. Are some people predisposed to diabetes?**

Yes. Susceptibility to diabetes is inherited genetically.

## 14. Are there factors that can trigger diabetes in people who are predisposed to the disease?

Yes, there are a number of external (i.e. non genetic) factors that can trigger the disease in those with a predisposition.

Certain viral infections, for example, can precipitate type 1 diabetes in people who are predisposed. As for type 2 diabetes, two major factors play roles in its development: excess weight and lack of physical activity. Physical or physiological stress, such as heart attacks, strokes, or infections, can also trigger the development of diabetes, especially type 2, in predisposed individuals. It can also be brought on by psychological stressors, such as the loss of a loved one. Certain drugs, such high doses of cortisone or antipsychotics, can also be triggers.

## 15. Can some diseases cause diabetes?

Yes, certain diseases can cause diabetes. Cystic fibrosis and pancreatitis (inflammation of the pancreas) can destroy the pancreas, bringing on the disease. Other conditions, such as gestational diabetes, polycystic ovary syndrome, schizophrenia and certain types of muscular dystrophy also increase the risk of developing type 2 diabetes.

## 16. Are there tests to identify people who are predisposed to developing type 2 diabetes?

There are tests to identify people with an elevated risk of developing the disease.

A fasting blood glucose level above 6 mmol/L but below 7 mmol/L is considered an **abnormal fasting blood glucose level**; this phenomenon is called **impaired fasting blood glucose (IFG)**. An oral glucose tolerance test, which involves drinking a beverage containing 75 g of glucose on an empty stomach, can indicate **impaired glucose tolerance (IGT)** if blood glucose is measured anywhere between 7.8 mmol/L and 11.0 mmol/L two hours after the test.

These two conditions—**impaired fasting blood glucose and impaired glucose tolerance**—are considered pre-diabetic states and indicate an elevated risk of developing the disease.

Reactive hypoglycemia (below-normal blood glucose, usually three to four hours after a meal containing carbohydrates) is sometimes the first sign of type 2 diabetes.

### 17. Is it possible to prevent or slow down the development of diabetes in pre-diabetic people?

Yes. It has been shown that weight loss and physical activity can decrease the risk of developing type 2 diabetes by over 50% in people who are glucose intolerant. Certain medications (metformin, acarbose, thiazolidinediones) have also been shown to be effective, decreasing the risk of developing diabetes in subjects with impaired glucose tolerance by over 30%.

### 18. How can a person with diabetes achieve and maintain a target or normal blood glucose level?

To control their disease, people with diabetes have to take responsibility for it. The following guidelines can help:
1)  acknowledge and accept the condition;
2)  eat healthy food;
3)  lose weight, if necessary;
4)  be physically active;
5)  measure **blood glucose** regularly;
6)  take oral antidiabetic **drugs** and/or insulin as prescribed;
7)  learn to **manage** stress;
8)  stay well **informed** about diabetes.

o As the person with diabetes, you are the one person best equipped to manage it—along with the help and support of your doctor and other health care professionals.

o Diabetes is a chronic disease; it cannot be cured, but it can be controlled.

o You have done nothing to bring on your diabetes, and you have nothing to feel guilty about.

o The closer you keep your blood glucose to normal, the better you will feel.

o The more you learn about diabetes, the better able you will be to take responsibility for your condition.

# Hyperglycemia

**1.   What is hyperglycemia?**

Hyperglycemia occurs when **blood glucose rises above target levels** (above 7mmol/L before meals and 10 mmol/L one or two hours after meals).

**2.   How do people with diabetes develop hyperglycemia?**

People with diabetes develop hyperglycemia when there is an **insufficient amount of insulin in the blood to handle the amount of glucose being released into the bloodstream.**

**3.   What are the symptoms of hyperglycemia?**

When blood glucose rises above a certain threshold, the following symptoms can appear:

1)   **increase in the volume of urine and the frequency of urination;**
2)   intense **thirst**;
3)   dry **mouth**;
4)   excessive **hunger**;
5)   involuntary **weight loss.**

Hyperglycemia can also cause the following symptoms:

6)   **blurred vision**;
7)   **infections**, especially of the genital organs and bladder;
8)   **sores or wounds** that do not heal;
9)   **fatigue**;
10)  **drowsiness**,
11)  **irritability.**

### 4. What are the main causes of hyperglycemia?

The main causes of hyperglycemia are:

1) over-consumption of **foods** containing carbohydrates;
2) **a decrease in physical activity**;
3) **incorrect dosage of** antidiabetic drugs (insulin or pills);
4) an **infection** or other medical conditions, such as a heart attack, that impair the secretion/action of insulin;
5) poor **stress** management;
6) taking certain **medications** (for example, cortisone);
7) uncorrected **nocturnal hypoglycemia** (low blood sugar) followed by a hyperglycemic rebound in the morning.

### 5. What should a person with diabetes do when hyperglycemia is suspected?

When hyperglycemia is suspected, blood glucose must be measured to confirm.

**If hyperglycemia is confirmed, the following steps are necessary:**

1) **people with type 1 diabetes must check for ketone bodies** if blood glucose is higher than 14 mmol/L. Reagent strips (Ketostix®) are used to measure the level of ketone bodies in the urine, and a meter (such as the Precision Xtra®) is used to measure the level of ketone bodies in a blood sample taken from the fingertip;
2) **drink plenty of water** to avoid dehydration (250 mL of water per hour, unless contraindicated);
3) identify the cause of the hyperglycemia;
4) correct the cause if possible;
5) continue eating (including carbohydrates) and follow the prescribed treatment (oral antidiabetic drugs or insulin);
6) call the doctor if the situation does not correct itself;
7) call the doctor or go to the emergency room if:
   - blood glucose rises above 20 mmol/L;
   - liquids taken orally cannot be retained because of nausea and vomiting;
   - the level of ketone bodies in the urine is moderate (4 mmol/L) to large (16 mmol/L); or
   - the level of ketone bodies in a blood sample taken from the fingertip is above 3 mmol/L.

6.  **What are the long-term complications of hyperglycemia?**

    In the long term, hyperglycemia can cause complications affecting the eyes, kidneys, nerves, heart and blood vessels.

# Hypoglycemia and Glucagon

1. **What is hypoglycemia?**

   Hypoglycemia is a **drop in blood glucose levels below normal** (below 4 mmol/L).

2. **Why does a person with diabetes develop hypoglycemia?**

   A person with diabetes develops hypoglycemia when there is **too much insulin in the blood in relation to the amount of glucose entering the circulation**.

3. **Who is susceptible to hypoglycemia?**

   People **who inject insulin or who take medications that stimulate the pancreas to produce more insulin can develop hypoglycemia**. Such medications include chlorpropamide (Apo®-Chlorpropamide), tolbutamide (Apo®-Tolbutamide), glyburide (Diaβeta®, Euglucon®), gliclazide (Diamicron® and Diamicron® MR), glimepiride (Amaryl®), repaglinide (GlucoNorm®) and nateglinide (Starlix®).

4. **What are the symptoms of hypoglycemia?**

   The body has two types of warning systems. The first causes symptoms with **rapid onset**, brought on by the secretion of adrenalin.

When hypoglycemia develops **rapidly**, it can cause the following symptoms:
1) **tremors or shakes**;
2) **palpitations**;
3) **sweating**;
4) **anxiety**;
5) **acute hunger**;
6) **pallor**;
7) **nightmares and restless sleep, if the hypoglycemia occurs during sleep**;
8) waking with a **headache** and **rebound hyperglycemia in the morning** following uncorrected nocturnal hypoglycemia during the previous night's sleep.

The second warning system creates less perceptible symptoms with **slower onset**. These symptoms are caused by a shortage of glucose being transported to the brain.

When hypoglycemia occurs **slowly**, the symptoms are more subtle:
1) **numbness or tingling around the mouth**;
2) **yawning**;
3) **fatigue or weakness**;
4) **the urge to sleep**;
5) **mood swings**;
6) **aggressiveness**;
7) **dizziness**;
8) **blurred vision**;
9) **unsteady gait, poor coordination**;
10) **difficulty pronouncing words**;
11) **confusion**.

## 5. Does hypoglycemia always cause these symptoms?

No. The symptoms of hypoglycemia vary from one person to another and can change over time. In some cases people with diabetes develop asymptomatic hypoglycemia, especially if blood glucose decreases slowly or the person has had diabetes for many years and no longer easily senses the hypoglycemia – a situation called hypoglycemia unawareness. The more frequent the hypoglycemia, the more likely it is that warning symptoms will appear later on and the correction of the problem will be delayed.

## 6.  What are the causes of hypoglycemia?

The most common causes of hypoglycemia can be broken down into four categories:

1)  **food**
    o  skipping a snack or a meal;
    o  delaying a meal;
    o  insufficient consumption of foods containing carbohydrates;
    o  an error in measuring the carbohydrate content of food;
    o  inability to keep food down or rapid loss (vomiting, diarrhea);
    o  drinking alcohol (this can lead to hypoglycemia as long as 16 hours after consumption);
    o  fasting while taking antidiabetic medications;
    o  gastroparesis (delayed emptying of the contents of the stomach);
2)  **physical activity**
    o  physical activity without adjusting the intake of food or medication;
3)  **antidiabetic drugs**
    o  incorrect (excessive) dosage of antidiabetic drugs or insulin;
    o  overcorrection of elevated blood glucose by the injection of an excessive dose of insulin;
    o  failure to adjust to a lower dosage, despite glucose levels frequently lower than 4 mmol/L;
    o  improper timing of antidiabetic drug doses.

## 7.  What should people with diabetes do if hypoglycemia is suspected?

If a person with diabetes suspects the onset of hypoglycemia, he or she **must not go to sleep** and assume that the blood glucose level will correct itself. Rather, the person must:

1)  **measure blood glucose;**
2)  **eat food with 15 g of rapidly absorbed carbohydrates.** Glucose or sucrose in pill or liquid form is the best option;
3)  **wait 15 minutes;**
4)  **measure blood glucose again**; if hypoglycemia is still present, **consume an additional 15 g of carbohydrates.**

If the hypoglycemia is corrected but the next meal is over an hour away, have a snack containing 15 g of carbohydrates and a protein source (e.g., 300 mL of milk or 7 soda crackers and cheese or fruit and cheese)

**Note: Do not overtreat hypoglycemia as one risks getting hyperglycemia.**

If the person with diabetes is **unable to administer his or her own treatment**:
1) measure his or her blood glucose level, if possible;
2) give the person food containing **20 g of carbohydrates** (if person able to swallow);
3) repeat after 15 minutes, giving the person food with 15 g of carbohydrates if blood glucose remains lower than 4 mmol/L.

Examples of foods with **15 g of carbohydrates**:
**1st choice (rapidly absorbed)**
- o 3 tablets of Glucose BD® (1 tablet = 5 g of carbohydrates)
- o 4 tables of Dex4® (1 tablet = 4 g of carbohydrates)
- o 5 tablets of Dextrosol® (1 tablet = 3 g of carbohydrates)
- o 7 tablets of Glucosol® (1 tablet = 2.25 g of carbohydrates)
- o 125 mL (½ cup) of regular (not diet) soft drink (pop) or fruit beverage
- o 5 mL (3 tsp or 3 packets) of sugar dissolved in water
- o 15 mL (3 tsp) of honey, jam or syrup
- o Insta-Glucose® (1 tube = 24 g of carbohydrates; take the equivalent of 15 g)

**2nd choice (slower absorption)**
- o 125 mL (½ cup) of fruit juice without added sugar
- o 300 mL (1¼ cups) of milk
- o 200 mL (1 single-serving size carton) of milk with 2 Social Tea biscuits
- o 4 Social Tea biscuits
- o 7 soda crackers
- o 1 dried fruit bar (for example, "Fruit To Go")
- o 1 small apple or 1/2 banana or 2 kiwis or 2 dates, etc.

Examples of quickly absorbed foods containing **20 g of carbohydrates**:
- o 4 tablets of Glucose BD® (1 tablet = 5 g of carbohydrates)
- o 5 tablets of Dex4® (1 tablet = 4 g of carbohydrates)
- o 7 tablets of Dextrosol® (1 tablet = 3 g of carbohydrates)
- o 9 tablets of Glucosol® (1 tablet = 2.25 g of carbohydrates)
- o 175 mL (3/4 cup) of regular soft drink (not diet) or fruit beverage
- o 20 mL (4 tsp) or 4 packets of sugar dissolved in water
- o 20 mL (4 tsp) of honey, jam or syrup
- o Insta-Glucose (1 tube = 24 g of carbohydrates; take the equivalent of 20 g)

**8.  Why is it important to treat hypoglycemia immediately?**

Hypoglycemia must be treated **immediately**; if left uncorrected, hypoglycemia can lead to loss of consciousness, coma and sometimes convulsions. There is no such thing as "minor hypoglycemia".

**9.  Does uncorrected hypoglycemia always lead to coma?**

No, uncorrected hypoglycemia does not necessarily lead to coma. The body attempts to defend itself from hypoglycemia by secreting hormones such as glucagon and adrenalin, which can elevate blood glucose and correct hypoglycemia. If there is too much insulin in the blood, however, these efforts might not be sufficient to correct hypoglycemia and prevent coma.

**10.  How can hypoglycemia be avoided?**

The following precautions are usually effective in avoiding hypoglycemia:
1)  measure blood glucose regularly;
2)  keep regular mealtime hours and include foods containing carbohydrates;
3)  check blood glucose before undertaking any physical activity and consume carbohydrates as necessary (*see chapter 20 on physical activity*);
4)  avoid consuming alcohol on an empty stomach;
5)  check blood glucose around 2 a.m., if necessary because one suspects nocturnal hypoglycemia;
6)  take antidiabetic drugs as prescribed, following the recommended dosage and timetable.

Note: People with type 1 diabetes are advised to periodically check blood glucose around 2 a.m. A snack containing at least 15 g of carbohydrates and a protein source is also recommended before turning in for the night if blood glucose is below 7 mmol/L at bedtime.

**11.  What safety measures should be taken by people with diabetes who are at risk for hypoglycemia?**

People with diabetes at risk for hypoglycemia must:
1)  always have at least **two 15 g servings of carbohydrates within reach**;
2)  wear a diabetic ID **bracelet** or **pendant**;

3) **inform** family, friends and colleagues that they have diabetes and tell them about the symptoms of hypoglycemia and the way to deal with it;

4) if they take insulin, always have **glucagon** within reach at home, at work or when travelling. A friend or relative must learn how to inject the glucagon in the event of a hypoglycemic coma.

## 12. What should be done if a person with diabetes has fallen into a hypoglycemic coma?

If a person with diabetes is unconscious or in a hypoglycemic coma, another person must immediately:

- inject him or her with glucagon, if available; if not,
- call for an ambulance by dialling 911.

**Never try to feed sugary foods to an unconscious person. Food can be inhaled into the lungs instead of being swallowed into the stomach.**

## 13. What is glucagon?

Glucagon is a hormone produced by the pancreas to elevate blood glucose. In the event of a hypoglycemic coma, glucagon must be injected by another person to correct the hypoglycemia.

A glucagon injection first-aid kit should always be on hand; it can be stored at room temperature. Check the expiry date periodically.

Here are the steps to follow in the event of a hypoglycemic coma:

1) lay the person on his or her side (glucagon can occasionally cause nausea and vomiting);

2) remove the plastic cap from the bottle of glucagon;

3) remove the needle sheath and inject the entire contents of the syringe into the bottle of glucagon. Do not remove the plastic stop ring from the syringe. Remove the syringe from the bottle;

4) gently shake the bottle until the glucagon powder is completely dissolved in the solvent;

5) draw up all of the solution from the vial using the same syringe;

6) inject the contents of the syringe (1 mg) subcutaneously (under the skin) or intramuscularly. The person should awaken within 15 minutes. There is no risk of overdose. A doctor may recommend a half dose for children who weigh less than 20 kg (44 lbs);

7) give the person some food as soon as he or she is awake and able to swallow. Provide a substantial snack containing 45 g of carbohydrates and a protein source (e.g., orange juice and a meat sandwich or crackers and cheese);

8) inform the person's doctor of the incident so that treatment can be evaluated and possibly adjusted. A visit to the emergency room may still be necessary to follow-up on the correction of the hypoglycemia.

If the person with diabetes does not regain consciousness within 15 to 20 minutes after the glucagon injection, ensure that he or she is brought to the emergency room immediately.

## 14. What are the recommendations for people with diabetes who are at risk for nocturnal hypoglycemia but live alone?

People with diabetes who live alone may be apprehensive of experiencing nocturnal hypoglycemia. It should be remembered, however, that hypoglycemia rarely persists for extended periods of time. In a crisis situation, the body reacts by raising the blood glucose level using sugar stored in the liver. Nevertheless, the situation is stressful. In addition to taking preventive measures to avoid a crisis, a person with diabetes should also have a social network in place to ensure his or her safety in case of prolonged hypoglycemia. Here are some suggestions:

1) ask a friend or relative to telephone every morning;

2) ask the mailman to deliver the mail in person;

3) agree on a code system with a neighbour (for example, one curtain open or closed upon waking);

4) use a personal response telephone service with a two-way voice communication system such as Philips Lifeline: 514-735-2101 or 1 877 423-9700.

It is a good idea to leave a house key with a friend or relative who can help if necessary.

## 15. Can symptoms of hypoglycemia occur when blood glucose is normal?

Yes, there are two situations in which a person with diabetes can have symptoms of hypoglycemia when blood glucose is normal:

1) When hyperglycemia has existed for some time, using antidiabetic medications to normalize blood glucose levels too quickly can trigger symptoms of hypoglycemia sometimes lasting several days. To avoid this unpleasant feeling, it may be necessary to slow down the treatment so that blood sugar can decrease more gradually. The ultimate goal is always to regain a normal blood glucose level.

2) When blood glucose is quite elevated and then quickly drops to a normal level, symptoms of hypoglycemia may appear and then fade quickly. Therefore, if hypoglycemia is suspected, blood glucose levels must be tested to avoid treating a false case of hypoglycemia, which could cause the hyperglycemia to recur.

o  The symptoms or signs of hypoglycemia do not always occur simultaneously.

o  The symptoms of hypoglycemia can differ from one from person to person.

o  Symptoms and discomforts can change over time. When a person has had diabetes for 10 to 20 years, he or she may no longer experience the symptoms of hypoglycemia (neuropathy).

o  The symptoms of hypoglycemia can be masked by certain medications, such as beta-blockers.

o  The symptoms of hypoglycemia may be absent if the person suffers from repeated episodes  hypoglycemia unawareness.

o  Certain signs and symptoms of hypoglycemia are difficult to assess. Glucose levels should therefore be confirmed with a glucose meter to avoid making unnecessary correction.

o  Hypoglycemia should be corrected immediately, following the recommended steps, to ensure that there is no damage to the brain. It should be remembered that hypoglycemia, no matter how severe or mild, must always be taken seriously.

## RECOMMENDATIONS FOR THE TREATMENT OF HYPOGLYCEMIA FOR PEOPLE WITH DIABETES

↓

### Test blood glucose immediately

↓

### If blood glucose is lower than 4.0 mmol/L

1. If no assistance is required for treatment, take 15 g of carbohydrates in one of the appropriate forms:

**1st choice (absorbed quickly)**
- o  3 tablets of Glucose BD® (1 tablet = 5 g of carbohydrates)
- o  4 tablets of Dex4® (1 tablet = 4 g of carbohydrates)
- o  5 tablets of Dextrosol® (1 tablet = 3 g of carbohydrates)
- o  7 tablets of Glucosol® (1 tablet = 2.25 g of carbohydrates)
- o  125 mL (½ cup) of regular soft drink or fruit beverage
- o  15 mL (3 tsp. or 3 packets) of sugar dissolved in water
- o  15 mL (3 tsp.) of honey, jam or syrup
- o  Insta-Glucose® (1 tube = 24 g of carbohydrates, take the equivalent of 15 g)

**2nd choice (absorbed more slowly)**
- o  125 mL (½ cup) fruit juice without added sugar
- o  300 mL (1 ¼ cup) of milk
- o  200 mL (1 single-serving carton) of milk plus 2 dry Social Tea biscuits
- o  4 dry Social Tea biscuits
- o  7 soda crackers
- o  1 dry fruit bar (for example, "Fruit to go")
- o  1 small apple, ½ banana, 2 kiwis, or 2 dates, etc.

2. If the person is conscious but needs assistance for treatment, give him or her 20 g of carbohydrates in the appropriate form:
- o  4 tablets of Glucose BD® (1 tablet = 5 g of carbohydrates)
- o  5 tablets of Dex4® (1 tablet = 4 g of carbohydrates)
- o  7 tablets of Dextrosol® (1 tablet = 3 g of carbohydrates)
- o  9 tablets of Glucosol® (1 tablet = 2.25 g of carbohydrates)

- 175 mL (¾ cup) of regular soft drink or fruit beverage
- 20 mL (4 tsp. or 4 packets) of sugar dissolved in water
- 20 mL (4 tsp.) of honey, jam or syrup
- Insta-Glucose® (1 tube = 24 g of carbohydrates; take the equivalent of 20 g)

↓

**Wait 15 minutes and test blood glucose again**

↓

**If blood glucose is still below 4.0 mmol/L,
have another 15 g of carbohydrates**

↓

**Wait 15 minutes, and repeat treatment as needed**

↓

**When blood glucose reaches or exceeds 4.0 mmol/L**

↓

**Meal (or snack) expected within one hour or less**

↓                   ↓

**Yes**                      **No**

**Have the meal or snack as planned**     **Have a snack containing 15 g of
carbohydrates and a protein source
(e.g., 200 mL of milk plus 2 Social Tea
biscuits) while waiting for the meal**

3. If the person is unconscious:
- Inject 1 mg of Glucagon SC or IM
  (dosage for adults and children weighing more than 20 kg (44 lbs).
- When the person has regained consciousness and is able to swallow, provide a substantial snack of 45 g of carbohydrates and a protein source (e.g., orange juice and a meat sandwich or cheese and crackers).

## CAUTION

1. For people with diabetes taking acarbose (Glucobay®) in combination with other medications that may cause hypoglycemia, the hypoglycemia should be corrected in one of the following ways:
   - o   3 tablets of Glucose BD® (1 tablet = 5 g of carbohydrates), or
   - o   4 tablets of Dex4® (1 tablet = 4 g of carbohydrates); or
   - o   5 tablets of Dextrosol® (1 tablet = 3 g of carbohydrates)
   - o   300 mL (1 1/4 cups) of milk, or
   - o   15 mL (3 tsp) of honey

2. For people with diabetes suffering from **kidney problems**, hypoglycemia should be corrected in one of the following ways:
   - o   3 tablets of Glucose BD® (1 tablet = 5 g of carbohydrates)
   - o   4 tablets of Dex4® (1 tablet = 4 g of carbohydrates); or
   - o   5 tablets of Dextrosol® (1 tablet = 3 g of carbohydrates)
   - o   3 packets of sugar dissolved in a little water

3. Hypoglycemia should never be dismissed as minor or unimportant. All appropriate measures should be taken to prevent it. When it occurs, it should be treated immediately.

# Self-monitoring:

## Blood Glucose and Glycosylated Hemoglobin (A1C)

### 1. What is self-monitoring?

Self-monitoring is a technique that people with diabetes use to **measure their own blood glucose levels**. Consequently, the approach usually also includes **adjusting** treatment according to the results obtained to bring and maintain blood glucose levels as close to normal as possible.

### 2. Why practice self-monitoring?

Self-monitoring allows people with diabetes to:

1) measure the impact of **nutrition, physical activity, stress and antidiabetic drugs** on blood glucose;
2) identify episodes of hypoglycemia and hyperglycemia and react quickly;
3) modify their behaviour with respect to nutrition, physical activity, antidiabetic drugs and stress, as required;
4) measure the impact of these changes on blood glucose;
5) feel confident, safe and independent in the management of their diabetes; and above all,
6) bring and maintain blood glucose levels as close to normal as possible.

### 3.  Why should people with diabetes try to maintain blood glucose levels as close to normal as possible?

People with diabetes should try to maintain their blood glucose levels as close as possible to normal to prevent complications associated with diabetes.

Two major studies (one American study on type 1 diabetes and one British study on type 2 diabetes) have shown that maintaining blood glucose levels as close to normal as possible significantly reduces the development and progression of microvascular complications due to diabetes:

- o   Retinopathy:     decrease of 21% to 76%
- o   Nephropathy:    decrease of 34% to 54%
- o   Neuropathy:     decrease of 40% to 60% or improvement in the existing neuropathy

### 4.  How is blood glucose measured from the fingertip?

A glucose meter is used to measure blood glucose in blood from the fingertip. The procedure involves two steps:

**Preparing the materials and checking the reagent strips**

1)  **Wash your hands** with soapy water and dry them thoroughly. This reduces the risk of infection and makes it easier to take the blood sample. Alcohol swabs are not recommended for home use because they can dry out the skin, which can lead to cracked fingertips.
2)  **Prepare the materials**: meter, test strip, holder, lancet, paper tissue.
3)  **Insert the lancet into the holder** and set it. A lancet must never be used more than once. It should not be thrown directly into the ordinary trashcan. Special containers are distributed at no charge in pharmacies and Community Health Centres. Once a container is full, it can be returned for safe disposal. Never use a lancet or a holder that another person has already used.
4)  Check the reagent strip container for the manufacturer's expiration date.
5)  If appropriate, write the date of first opening on the container to **keep track of the life expectancy of the strips.**
6)  **Take out a test strip.** If the strip comes from a vial, close it immediately.

**Blood analysis and recording of data**

1) Press the switch to start the device, if necessary.

2) Insert the test strip into the strip support on the device or automatically release a strip from the device.

3) Prick the **lateral extremity** of a finger (use a different finger each time you take a blood sample).

4) Produce a **large drop of blood** by applying pressure on the finger while pointing it downwards. Do not apply excessive pressure.

5) Place the **first drop of blood** on the reactive part of the strip or bring the reactive part of the strip into contact with the blood, depending on the device used.

6) Wait for the reading to be displayed.

7) Enter the result in the appropriate column of your glucose logbook.

## 5. Can other sites ("alternative sites") be used to measure blood glucose?

Blood glucose can be measured with blood drawn from other areas of the body ("alternate sites") such as the forearm, the arm, the palm, the abdomen or the thigh. Several glucose meters now offer this option.

Results from alternative sites are generally comparable to glucose readings taken from the fingertip before a meal. This method of measuring blood glucose is limited, however, and it is recommended that a blood glucose reading be taken from the fingertip at times when blood glucose can fluctuate rapidly. This can occur:

1) during an episode of hypoglycemia;

2) during physical activity;

3) up to two hours after a meal;

4) immediately after an insulin injection;

5) during an illness.

## 6. Which glucose meters are currently available, and what are their features?

The tables on pages 48 to 51 present a list of the latest generation of blood glucose meters on the market, along with some of their characteristics (list updated on May 1, 2008).

Blood glucose meters are frequently offered for free and many manufacturers will trade new meters for old ones at no cost. Continuous glucose monitors can cost as much as $2000.

Strips cost between $0.80 and $1.00 each. There are special offers on some strips. The price can also vary from one pharmacy to another.

### 7. What are the main causes of false glucose readings?

False readings occur when:
1) the glucose meter is dirty;
2) the glucose meter is calibrated incorrectly;
3) the user forgets to calibrate the meter, leaving out the calibration code for the current batch of reagent strips;
4) the strips have expired;
5) the strips have been exposed to humidity;
6) the strips have been exposed to extreme temperatures;
7) the drop of blood is too small;
8) the user's technique is faulty (e.g., the time of contact with the strip is too short);
9) the glucose meter is inaccurate.

### 8. How can the accuracy of glucose meter results be verified?

The accuracy of results taken from the glucose meter should be verified annually. The **fasting blood glucose** level from a laboratory blood test should be compared with the level the patient obtains from the blood glucose meter. Blood glucose should be tested **within five minutes after** the blood sample.

The result of the **fasting blood glucose** reading from a blood glucose meter should **vary by less than 20%** from the blood glucose reading taken in the laboratory. For glucose readings less than or equal to 4.2 mmol/L, the difference should be smaller.

## HOW CAN THE ACCURACY OF A GLUCOSE METER BE MEASURED?

### Fasting

1) Have a "fasting blood glucose" measured in the laboratory.
2) Take a glucose reading as usual, within the following five minutes.
3) Enter this information in the logbook and circle it.
4) Ask for the results of the blood test at the next visit to the doctor.
5) Calculate the accuracy of the meter (a difference of more or less 20%).

|  | Example | Your results |
|---|---|---|
| **Fasting blood glucose** (laboratory blood sample) | 10 mmol/L | ................ |
| **Blood glucose from fingertip** (taken within 5 minutes) | 9.2 mmol/L | ................ |
| Accuracy of the meter expressed as a percentage | | ................% |

### Formula for calculating the accuracy of meter

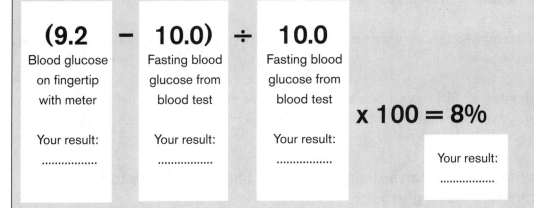

| **(9.2** | **−** | **10.0)** | **÷** | **10.0** |
|---|---|---|---|---|
| Blood glucose on fingertip with meter | | Fasting blood glucose from blood test | | Fasting blood glucose from blood test |

**x 100 = 8%**

Your result: ................

Your result: ................

Your result: ................

Your result: ................

A difference of 20% or less is considered acceptable.
Aim for a smaller difference for blood glucose levels below 4.2 mmol/L.

## 9. How often should blood glucose levels be measured?

Generally, people with **type 1** diabetes or those who are currently in a period of adjustment are advised to measure blood glucose **at least three times a day** at various intervals: **before each meal and before bedtime** (before snacking). Sometimes, the doctor responsible for treatment will advise a patient to measure blood glucose one or two hours after meals (generally timing it from the first mouthful) and even during the night.

People with **non-insulin dependent type 2** diabetes are generally advised to measure blood glucose **once a day,** alternating between measurements before meals and measurements before bedtime (before a snack). On some occasions they are instructed to measure blood glucose one or two hours after meals (generally timing it from the first mouthful), and in some cases, even during the night. People who are in a period of adjustment or insulin-requiring are advised to measure blood glucose several times a day.

It is also a good idea to measure blood glucose whenever unease or discomfort suggests the **possibility of hypoglycemia** or **hyperglycemia**. In the case of illness, blood glucose should be measured more often.

Blood glucose levels should be tested more often whenever **any change occurs**, whether the change is in diet, medication or stress levels.

When engaging in **physical activity,** blood glucose should be measured before, during and afterwards.

People with diabetes are advised to take a blood glucose reading before **driving a car** and every four hours during long drives in order to prevent hypoglycemia.

## 10. What information should be recorded in the logbook to help self-monitor blood glucose?

Blood glucose self-monitoring is easier when the following information is recorded in the logbook:

1) the result and date of **blood glucose** readings (in the column corresponding to the meal in question; for example, "Before lunch");

2) relevant comments, such as the explanation for the **hypoglycemia**, change in diet, physical activity, etc.;

3) the result of a **ketone bodies** reading from urine or blood, with the date and time (in the "Comments" column);

4) the name, dose and time of ingestion of **all prescribed antidiabetic drugs**; write down every change or omission in the "Comments" column;

5) the quantity of carbohydrates consumed in meals and snacks;

6) the area of the insulin injection, if applicable, the technique used, and so on (in the "Comments" column).

## 11. How should the information be recorded?

The information should be noted in the **self-monitoring logbook**. Each reading category should be entered in a clearly identified column:

1) in the first column, write down the results of blood glucose readings taken **before the morning meal** over the course of a single week;

2) in the second column, write down the results of blood glucose readings taken **after the morning meal** over the course of a single week;

3) in the next columns, enter the results of the **other blood glucose readings**, taken before and after the afternoon and evening meals, before bedtime (before a snack) and during the night;

4) **hypoglycemia** occurring outside the four usual periods of blood glucose readings should be noted in the following period (e.g., hypoglycemia occurring in the afternoon should be entered in the column corresponding to "Before the evening meal");

5) unmeasured hypoglycemia should be assigned a reading of **2 mmol/L**;

6) the **weekly average** of glucose readings should be entered at the foot of each column (do not include the results of hypoglycemic correction when calculating the average). See the example indicated by two asterisks (**) in the table on the next page;

7) when calculating averages, do not include readings associated with an exceptional, one-off, explainable situation; see the examples indicated by an asterisk (*) in the table on the next page;

8) enter any relevant remarks in the "Comments" column.

## Example of a self-monitoring logbook

| Week beginning Sunday: | 01 (day) | | | 05 (month) | | 2008 (year) | |
|---|---|---|---|---|---|---|---|
| Day of the week | Blood glucose measurements (mmol/L) | | | | | | Comments |
| | Breakfast | | Lunch | | Dinner | | Bedtime | |
| | Before | After | Before | After | Before | After | Before snack | |
| Sunday | 5.2 | | 12.1 | | | | | |
| Monday | 7.1 | | | | 8.1 | | | |
| Tuesday | 4.6 | | | | | | 4.1 | |
| Wednesday | 9.3 | | 10.4 | | | | | |
| Thursday | 5.5 | | | | 7.2 | | 6.7 | |
| Friday | 6.8 | | | | 3.5* | | 16.6** | *Exercise **Corrected hypoglycemia |
| Saturday | 3.9 | | 11.3 | | 18.1* | | | *Stress |
| Average | **6.1** | | **11.3** | | **7.7** | | **5.4** | |

The average is calculated by adding up all the numbers in the same column and dividing the total by the number of measurements in that column:

Example: Average blood glucose before lunch:
12.1 + 10.4 + 11.3 = 33.8 ÷ 3 = 11.3

## 12. Will the doctor prescribe other tests in addition to blood glucose readings to monitor blood glucose?

In addition to blood glucose readings, the doctor may prescribe blood tests to measure **glycosylated hemoglobin** or A1C and in some cases **fructosamine**. These two laboratory analyses show how well the diabetes has been managed.

1) Glycosylated hemoglobin or A1C

   **The glycosylated hemoglobin or AIC levels reflects how well blood glucose has been controlled over the last two to three months.**

   This type of hemoglobin results from the binding of blood glucose to the hemoglobin present in red blood cells. The higher the blood glucose, the higher the level of A1C, due to the binding of sugar molecules to hemoglobin.

   A blood test is used to measure the A1C value. It should be done two to four times a year, depending on how well the diabetes is managed. The A1C value is essential information, giving people an overall picture of their blood glucose management and making it possible to adjust treatment.

   A1C is complementary to the blood glucose meter readings. A1C does not indicate requiring blood glucose variations, hypoglycemia or hyperglycemia. It is recommended to target an A1C value of 7% (0.070) or less. When there is no hypoglycemia, a value of 6% (0.060) or less is recommended.

2) Fructosamine

   **Fructosamine levels reflect how well blood glucose has been controlled over the last two to three weeks.**

   Using fructosamine levels as a marker of the risk of complications of diabetes is a less well established practice. This kind of reading (which is carried out through a blood test) can nevertheless be useful in some cases, for example:

   o   short-term assessments of a change in treatment;
   o   assessment of blood glucose management when A1C levels are less reliable (e.g., in the presence of hemoglobin disease, severe anemia);
   o   follow-up on blood glucose levels during pregnancy.

   Normal fructosamine levels are generally considered to be between 200 and 290 µmol/L. Like A1C, fructosamine does not indicate blood glucose variations and is adjunctive to regular blood glucose measurements.

## LIST OF BLOOD GLUCOSE METERS (REVISED MAY 1, 2008)

| Blood glucose meter | Manufacturer | Range of results (mmol/L) | Range of temperature of strips (°C) | Length of test (sec.) |
|---|---|---|---|---|
| FreeStyle® Lite® (to come) | Abbott | 1.1 to 27.8 | 4 to 40 | 5 |
| FreeStyle® Mini® | Abbott | 1.1 to 27.8 | 5 to 40 | 7 |
| Precision Xtra® Blood glucose (G) Ketone bodies (K) | Abbott | G: 1.1 to 27.8 C: 0 to 6.0 | 15 to 40 | G: 5 C: 10 |
| iTest® | AgaMatrix Auto Control Medical | 1.1 to 33.3 | 10 to 40 | 4 |
| Ascensia®* Breeze 2® | Bayer | 0.6 to 33.3 | 10 to 40 | 5 |
| Ascensia® Contour®* | Bayer | 0.6 to 33.3 | 10 to 40 | 5 |
| OneTouch® UltraMini® (4 colours) | LifeScan | 1.1 to 33.3 | 6 to 44 | 5 |
| OneTouch® Ultra 2® | LifeScan | 1.1 to 33.3 | 6 to 44 | 5 |
| OneTouch® UltraSmart® | LifeScan | 1.1 to 33.3 | 6 to 44 | 5 |
| Guardian® ** REAL-Time | Medtronic MiniMed | 2.2 to 22.2 | sensors 2 to 27 | Initialization: 2 hrs 20 mins; calibration: 2-3/day with meter; results every 5 mins |
| Nova Max® | Nova Biomedical | 1.1 to 33.3 | 15 to 39 | 5 |
| Accu-Chek® Aviva | Roche Diagnostics | 0.6 to 33.3 | 4 to 44 | 5 |
| Accu-Chek® Compact Plus®*** | Roche Diagnostics | 0.6 to 33.3 | 10 to 40 | 5 |

\*   Speech synthesis is available at Pharmacie Danielle Desroches (905 Blvd. René-Lévesque E., tel: 514 288-8555 or 450 447-9280) for $495.
\*\*  Continuous monitor costing $2,000, plus $47.50 for a 72-hour sensor.
\*\*\* Accu-ChekMC Voicemate PlusMC speech synthesis to come.

| Blood glucose meter | Amount of blood required (µL) | Possibility of adding a second drop of blood | Cleaning required | Calibration of reactive strips | Lifespan of reactive strips |
|---|---|---|---|---|---|
| **FreeStyle® Lite®** (to come) | 0.3 | yes (within 60 seconds) | no | automatic | 18 months (after opening) |
| **FreeStyle® Mini®** | 0.3 | yes (within 60 seconds) | no | calibration code on every vial | date on vial |
| **Precision Xtra® Blood glucose (G) Ketone bodies (K)** | G: 0.6 C: 1.5 | yes (within 5 seconds) | no | calibration strip in every box | date on the packet |
| **iTest®** | 0.5 | no | no | calibration code on every vial | 3 months (after opening) |
| **Ascensia®\* Breeze 2®** | 1.0 | no | no | automatic | date on disc |
| **Ascensia® Contour®\*** | 0.6 | no | no | automatic | 6 months (after opening) |
| **OneTouch® UltraMini® (4 colours)** | 1.0 | no | no | calibration code on every vial | 3 months (after opening) |
| **OneTouch® Ultra 2®** | 1.0 | no | no | calibration code on every vial | 3 months (after opening) |
| **OneTouch® UltraSmart®** | 1.0 | no | no | calibration code on every vial | 3 months (after opening) |
| **Guardian® \*\* REAL-Time** | N/A | N/A | N/A | N/A | sensor lifespan: 72 hours ($47.50/sensor) |
| **Nova Max®** | 0.3 | no | Nova Biomedical | no coding necessary | 3 months (after opening) |
| **Accu-Chek® Aviva** | 0.6 | yes (within 5 seconds) | no | calibration chip in every box | date on vial |
| **Accu-Chek® Compact Plus®\*\*\*\*** | 1. 5 | yes (within 25 seconds) | yes | automatic | 3 months (after cartridge use) |

| Blood glucose meter | Reactive strips | Lifespan of control solution after opening | PC Programs/ Memory | Batteries and lifespan | Guarantee |
|---|---|---|---|---|---|
| **FreeStyle® Lite®** (to come) | in vial (sensitive to humidity) | 3 months | 400 | 1 lithium 3 V No. CR2032 500 tests | 5 years |
| **FreeStyle® Mini®** | in vial (sensitive to humidity) | 3 months | 250 | 2 lithium 3 V no CR2032 500 tests | 5 years |
| **Precision Xtra® Blood glucose (G) Ketone bodies (K)** | individually wrapped | 3 months | 450 | 1 lithium 3 V No. CR2032 1000 tests | 4 years |
| **iTest®** | in vial (sensitive to humidity) | 3 months | 300 | 2 lithium 3 V No. CR2032 1000 tests | 4 years |
| **Ascensia®* Breeze 2®** | 10-test disc | 6 months | 420 | 1 lithium 3 V No. CR2032 1000 tests | 5 years |
| **Ascensia® Contour®*** | in vial (sensitive to humidity) | 6 months | 480 | 2 lithium 3 V No. CR2032 1000 tests | 5 years |
| **OneTouch® UltraMini® (4 colours)** | in vial (sensitive to humidity) | 3 months | 500 | 1 lithium 3 V No. CR2032 1000 tests | 3 years |
| **OneTouch® Ultra 2®** | in vial (sensitive to humidity) | 3 months | 500 | 2 lithium 3 V No. CR2032 1000 tests | 3 years |
| **OneTouch® UltraSmart®** | in vial (sensitive to humidity) | 3 months | 3000 | 2 alkaline AAA, 1.5 V 540 tests | 3 years |
| **Guardian®** REAL-Time** | N/A | N/A | 288 readings/day; 21 days of information | 1 alkaline AAA, 1.5 V; 40 recharges of MiniLink 14 days | 1 year |
| **Nova Max®** | in vial (sensitive to humidity) | 3 months | 400 | 1 lithium, 3 V No. CR2450, 500 test | 3 years |
| **Accu-Chek® Aviva** | in vial (sensitive to humidity) | 3 months | 500 | 1 lithium, 3 V No. CR2032 less than 2000 tests | 5 years |
| **Accu-Chek® Compact Plus®***** | 17-strip cartridge | 3 months | 500 | 2 alkaline AAA, 1.5 V 1000 tests | 5 years |

| Blood glucose meter | Alternative sites | Lancing device | Lancet | Telephone assistance | Internet |
|---|---|---|---|---|---|
| **FreeStyle® Lite®** (to come) | yes | FreeStyle | FreeStyle 25 gauge | 1-888-519-6890 | www.abbott.com |
| **FreeStyle® Mini®** | yes | FreeStyle | FreeStyle 25 gauge | 1-888-519-6890 | www.abbott.com |
| **Precision Xtra® Blood glucose (G) Ketone bodies (K)** | yes | Freestyle | Abbott Thin Lancets 28 gauge | 1-888-519-6890 | www.abbott.com |
| **iTest®** | yes | iTest | iTest ultra-thin 33 gauge | 1-800-461-0991 | www.itestglucose.com |
| **Ascensia® * Breeze 2®** | yes | Microlet | Microlet  28 gauge | 1-800-268-7200 | www.ascensia.ca |
| **Ascensia® Contour® *** | yes | Microlet | Microlet  28 gauge | 1-800-268-7200 | www.ascensia.ca |
| **OneTouch® UltraMini®** (4 colours) | yes | OneTouch | OneTouch UltraSoft 28 gauge | 1-800-663-5521 | www.onetouch.ca |
| **OneTouch® Ultra 2®** | yes | OneTouch | OneTouch UltraSoft 28 gauge | 1-800-663-5521 | www.onetouch.ca |
| **OneTouch® UltraSmart®** | yes | OneTouch UltraSoft | OneTouch UltraSoft 28 gauge | 1-800-663-5521 | www.onetouch.ca |
| **Guardian® ** REAL-Time** | N/A | N/A | N/A | 1-866-444-4649 | www.guardianrealtime.ca |
| **Nova Max®** | yes | Nova | Nova automatic with alternate site testing cap 10 lancets | 1-800-260-1021 | www.novacares.ca |
| **Accu-Chek® Aviva** | yes | Accu-Chek Multiclix | Accu-Chek Multiclix 30 gauge (6-lancet cartridge) | 1-800-363-7949 | www.accu-chek.ca |
| **Accu-Chek® Compact Plus®****** | yes | Softclix Plus | Accu-Chek Softclix 28 gauge | 1-800-363-7949 | www.accu-chek.ca |

# Measuring Ketone Bodies

**1. What are ketone bodies?**

Ketone bodies are **by-products of the breakdown of body fat.**

**2. What does an increase of ketone bodies in the blood mean?**

An increase of ketone bodies in the blood indicates that a **lack of insulin** is causing a person with diabetes to use **fat** reserves stored in the body instead of **glucose**.

**Without insulin**, many cells in the body are unable to use glucose in the blood. When the body lacks insulin, it uses energy stored in the form of fat, and the breakdown of this fat leads to the production of **ketone bodies**. Ketone bodies are acids; their presence can lead to **diabetic ketoacidosis.**

Excess ketone bodies in the blood are eliminated through the urine. They may therefore be measured in either blood or urine.

**3. Why must people with diabetes check for excess ketone bodies in the blood or urine?**

People with diabetes—especially type 1—must check for excess ketone bodies in the blood or urine **because an excess indicates poor management of the disease** and a risk of diabetic ketoacidosis. Ketoacidosis can lead to coma. In some special cases, doctors recommend this type of monitoring for people with type 2 diabetes.

**4.** **When should people with diabetes check for excess ketone bodies in the blood or urine?**

People with diabetes should check for the presence of ketone bodies in the blood or urine when their **blood glucose is higher than 14 mmol/L or when a doctor recommends it.**

They should continue performing the test—in addition to measuring blood glucose four times a day or more often if necessary—until there are no excess **ketone bodies** in the **blood or urine and blood glucose is back to normal.**

They should also test for ketone bodies if they experience the following symptoms:
1) intense thirst;
2) abdominal pain;
3) excessive tiredness or drowsiness;
4) nausea and vomiting.

**5.** **What should a person with diabetes do if there are excess ketone bodies in the blood or urine?**

A person with diabetes who finds excess ketone bodies in the blood or urine should:
1) **drink 250 mL** of water every hour to hydrate and help eliminate ketone bodies through the urine;
2) **take extra doses of Humalog®, NovoRapid®, Humulin® R or Novolin® ge Toronto insulin, following the recommendations of the treating physician** (*see chapter 21 on hyperglycemic emergencies*);
3) call a doctor **immediately** or go to the emergency room if an excess of ketone bodies in the blood or urine persists despite treatment and if the following symptoms appear:
   o abdominal pain;
   o excessive tiredness or drowsiness;
   o nausea and vomiting.

**6.** **How is the presence of ketone bodies measured in urine?**

Ketone bodies in urine are measured with a reagent strip.

## Preparing the materials

1) Gather the materials: Ketostix® reagent strips, a clean, dry container, and a timer.
2) Check the manufacturer's expiry date indicated on the reagent strip container. Mark the container with the date it was first opened. It must be discarded **six months** after being opened.
   - o Ketostix® reagent strips must be stored at room temperature (between 18ºC and 25ºC).
3) Collect a **fresh** urine sample for analysis:
   - o empty the bladder completely and discard the urine;
   - o drink one or two glasses of water;
   - o urinate into a clean, dry container.
4) Take a reagent strip from the container and close the cover **immediately**.
   - o Compare the reagent strip with the colour chart on the container to ensure that the strip has not changed colour, which could give a false result.

## Testing the urine sample with the reagent strip

1) Dip the reactive part of the strip into the fresh urine sample and remove it right away.
2) Tap the excess fluid off the strip on the edge of the container and start the timer.

## Reading and entering the results

1) After **exactly 15 seconds**, place the reagent strip next to the colour chart on the strip container and compare the result under a bright light.

2) Enter the result in your glucose self-monitoring logbook.

| Negative | Trace | Small | Moderate | Large |
|----------|-------|-------|----------|-------|
| 0 | 0.5 mmol/L | 1.5 mmol/L | 4 mmol/L | 8 mmol/L to 16 mmol/L |

Reagent strips that simultaneously measure glucose and ketone bodies in the urine (e.g., Keto-Diastix®, Chemstrip® u G/K) are also available.

## 7. How is the level of ketone bodies measured from a fingertip blood sample?

Ketone bodies in the blood are measured with a ketone meter.

### Preparing the materials

1) Gather the materials: Precision Xtra® meter (to measure blood glucose and ketone bodies), reagent strips for measuring ketosis (ketone bodies), lancing device, lancet.
2) Check the expiry date on the reagent strip envelope.
3) Insert the ketone calibrator into the Precision Xtra® meter. The code on the screen must match the code on the strip.
4) Insert the ketone strip into the Precision Xtra® meter.

### Applying the blood sample to the reagent strip

1) Prick the fingertip with the lancing device.
2) Apply a drop of blood to the sensitive area of the strip.

### Reading and entering the result

1) Wait for the result to appear on the screen; it should appear within 10 seconds.
2) Write down the result in the self-monitoring logbook.

| Negative | Trace | Small | Moderate | Large |
|---|---|---|---|---|
| 0 | Less than 0.6 mmol/L | 0.6 mmol/L to 1.5 mmol/L | 1.5 mmol/L to 3 mmol/L | Over 3 mmol/L |

# Eating Well

1. **Why is it important for people with diabetes to eat well?**

   Eating well, along with exercising regularly and not smoking, is part of a wholesome routine to promote good health and control the disease more effectively.

   There are no "forbidden foods" and there is no "diabetic diet". Instead, the focus is on choosing foods wisely and managing serving/portion size. The diet of a person with diabetes should be satisfying, varied and balanced, not restrictive or punitive.

   A treatment regimen can consist solely of a dietary plan or include oral antidiabetic drugs or insulin as well. Either way, healthy eating is essential.

2. **Why is it particularly important for people with diabetes to eat well?**

   Eating well offers a number of advantages for a person with diabetes. A healthy diet:
   1) promotes better control of:
      - blood glucose;
      - weight;
      - blood pressure;
      - fat (lipid) levels in blood;
   2) satisfies the body's energy, vitamin and mineral requirements;
   3) promotes well-being.

3. **What does "eating well" mean for a person with diabetes?**

   Eating well means choosing **quality foods**, such as those mentioned in *Canada's Food Guide*:

1)  Eat at least one dark green and one orange vegetable every day; choose fresh vegetables or fruit over juice.
2)  Eat at least half of the recommended grain products in the form of whole grains;
3)  Drink skim, 1% or 2% milk or enriched soya beverages every day;
4)  Eat meat alternatives such as legumes and tofu often;
5)  Eat at least two portions of fish per week;
6)  Eat a small amount of good fats (such as olive oil or canola oil) every day;
7)  Drink water to quench your thirst.

Eating well also means choosing the **right quantity** for your energy needs. That means eating to satisfy your hunger…but no more.[1]

Some people have trouble recognizing and listening to the body's signals of hunger and satiety (fullness). Hunger can reveal many kinds of needs. It can be physiological, when the body needs energy in the form of nutrients (carbohydrates, proteins and fats) or vitamins and minerals. It can also be psychological, as a way of dealing with stress or negative thoughts or emotional states.

### 4. How can a person eat to satisfy hunger… but no more?

Eating to satisfy hunger but not going beyond that point requires moderation. This is the best way of avoiding the ravages associated with dieting or binging on food, both of which are bad for the health.[1]

### 5. Practically speaking, how is moderation achieved?

To achieve moderation, it is first necessary to become aware of your body and learn the difference between physiological hunger and psychological hunger. The former is the body's need for nourishment (a need for energy and certain nutrients), while the latter is a defence mechanism, a desire to eat as a way of dealing with uncontrollable emotions, either negative or positive. Being able to make the distinction between these two types of hunger is indispensable to eating the proper amount—that is, neither too much nor too little, but just enough.

1. G. Apfeldorfer, *Maigrir, c'est fou* (Éditions Odile Jacob, 2000), 301 pages.

Second, it is necessary to be able to recognize the feeling of being full, that turning point between the pleasure of eating and satiety, when the body has eaten enough to fulfil the body's needs.[2] This task requires constant effort, practice and perseverance.

## 6. How can I tell if I have eaten enough?

The following ten suggestions can help you know when you have eaten enough.[2]

1) **Feel your hunger:** try to eat nothing for four hours. This will help you rediscover the feeling of being hungry and re-establish a healthy relationship with food.

2) **Establish a routine:** have a similar breakfast every morning and eat meals at regular hours. This will help you feel hungry just before mealtime and then feel full after eating.

3) **Concentrate on the taste:** pay particular attention, taking small bites and chewing well, to savour the food.

4) **Slow down:** stretch out your meals to at least 20 minutes. This will help give the body's signals of hunger and satiety time to reach the brain. Putting your knife and fork down between each bite also helps slow down meals.

5) **Take a break in the middle of the meal:** this will give you a chance to assess whether you are still hungry or whether you have eaten enough. If eating has become less enjoyable, you have eaten enough;

6) **Avoid distractions:** just eat. Do not read the newspaper, watch television, or carry on an animated conversation. It may be helpful to take frequent breaks during the meal to talk or listen to ensure that you do only one thing at a time.

7) **Identify your cravings:** ask yourself whether your appetite is triggered by something besides a physiological need or a real hunger. If it is just a craving, take the time to figure out what emotions you are feeling at the time and write them down in a journal.

8) **Do not overeat now for the future:** wanting to stockpile "just in case" and the fear of "missing out" on food later are frequent consequences of dieting. Come back to the present, and ask yourself how hungry you are right now.

9) **Be your own judge:** stay tuned in to your own needs instead of eating to please someone else or not to give offence. This will ensure that you are the one who chooses how much you eat.

---

2. Collectif 2007, "Retrouver le plaisir de manger", *Psychologies*, Special issue.

10) **Practice moderation:** eating "just enough" can be done by eating more slowly to better savour the food, reducing portion size, consciously evaluating your hunger throughout the meal, and reducing the number of courses in one meal.

## 7. How can eating well help a person with diabetes manage blood glucose?

Of all the food groups, carbohydrates have the greatest influence on blood glucose levels. A person with diabetes will maintain better control over blood glucose if:

1)  meals are taken at regular hours, at the same time every day. This is particularly true for people with diabetes taking oral antidiabetic drugs that stimulate insulin secretion (for example, Diaβeta®) and those taking insulin. Large variations in blood glucose levels such as hyperglycemia or hypoglycemia can also be diminished;

2)  nutrients are spread out evenly over at least three meals, spaced four to six hours apart;

3)  carbohydrates are spread out evenly over three meals instead of being consumed once a day (such as in the evening meal);

4)  the amount of carbohydrates in meals (and, if necessary, between meals) is moderate and corresponds to the person's energy needs. Carbohydrates are essential, but too many can hamper proper blood glucose management;

5)  no meal is skipped;

6)  the carbohydrate content of each meal is consistent from one day to the next.

## 8. How can eating well help control weight?

Eating well can help some people lose weight when they **eat just enough to satisfy their hunger and choose foods containing fewer calories more often.**

For people who are overweight, losing between 5% and 10% of their weight may be enough to improve their control of blood glucose levels, blood pressure and fat levels in the blood.

## 9. How can eating well help control fat levels in blood?

Choosing **leaner foods** containing higher quality fats can help control fat levels in blood. High fat levels in the blood increase the risk of cardiovascular diseases.

### 10. How can eating well help manage blood pressure?

Choose a diet rich in:

- o fruits and vegetables;
- o skimmed or partly skimmed dairy products;
- o soluble dietary fibre, found in legumes, oatmeal and oat bran;
- o whole grains;
- o vegetable protein, low in saturated fats and cholesterol, as found in legumes and tofu.

This can help reduce blood pressure. These foods generally contain less salt than processed foods that are canned or preserved. Fresh fruits and vegetables also contain potassium, which helps lower blood pressure.

Alcohol should be consumed in moderation, following the Canadian low-risk drinking guidelines:

---

**HEALTHY ADULTS SHOULD LIMIT ALCOHOL CONSUMPTION
TO A MAXIMUM OF 2 DRINKS A DAY**

o Men: a maximum of 14 drinks a week

o Women: a maximum of 9 drinks a week

---

### 11. Can a person with diabetes still take pleasure in eating?

Some people, after being diagnosed with diabetes, might have trouble believing that eating will ever be a source of pleasure again. But getting the most out of eating means involving all of your senses, from meal planning, through preparation, to the final enjoyment of the food.

Taking the time to consult cookbooks, choosing the recipes and planning an imaginative meal are all ways of enhancing the pleasure of eating. Markets display an array of colourful and aromatic foods and can also present an opportunity to discuss flavours, aromas and recipes with other food lovers. Preparing meals alone or with others can be a simple task but still provide a chance to experiment with a variety of new flavours and sensations.

Attractive food presentation and an inviting table can also help maximize the pleasure of a delicious and healthy meal.

### 12. Does eating well mean avoiding cold cuts, French fries, chips and pastries?

These foods can be part of a healthy diet. While it is true that they are often high in fat, sugar and calories, excluding them from your diet altogether is an error, especially if you want to lose weight. It is said that excessive or complete deprivation of a certain food merely increases the desire for it and leads to overindulgence. It is therefore better to give yourself permission to enjoy a few chips once in a while, instead of developing an uncontrollable craving and eating an entire bag. Therefore, these foods play a small role in a balanced diet and can be eaten on occasion, simply for the pleasure they may give.[3]

### 13. What are some ways to develop better nutritional habits?

Here are some suggestions for improving your eating habits:
1) Set clear, measurable and realistic goals.
2) Go about it gradually, one modification at a time. Small changes can make a big difference.
3) Follow the meal plan created with the help of a dietician.
4) Be sure that you like the food you choose; being satisfied is the best way to prevent slips.
5) Replace food rewards with other treats. For example, buy a book or a CD or take a relaxing bath to pamper yourself.

### 14. What is a meal plan?

A meal plan is a personalized guide that is prepared by a dietician for a person with diabetes who wants to eat well. It encourages a varied diet of nutritious foods from all the different food groups, suggests quantities, and adheres to dietary recommendations for maintaining good health. It takes into consideration the drugs taken for the treatment of diabetes and other ailments associated with the disease.

---

3. Groupe Équilibre : www.equilibre.ca

The meal plan is built around the seven food groups:
- o   starches;
- o   fruits;
- o   vegetables;
- o   milk and alternatives;
- o   meats and alternatives;
- o   fats;
- o   other choices.

It suggests the **quantities or servings** appropriate to the individual's energy needs. It specifies the recommended carbohydrate content for each meal and snack, as well as the number of servings of meat and alternatives and fats.

The plan can be used as a template for your daily meals. It helps standardize the quantities and servings of food eaten from one day to the next, promoting better control of blood glucose levels while allowing room for a varied diet.

## 15. Are snacks necessary?

Snacking is not routinely necessary, but having snacks in your meal plan can help spread the carbohydrates out evenly over the course of a day, to better correspond with actual energy (or calorie) needs.

People who inject insulin are sometimes advised to have a snack containing carbohydrates at night, as close as possible to bedtime.

# How to Recognize Carbohydrates

**1.   Why is it necessary to know how to recognize carbohydrates?**

The amount of dietary carbohydrates consumed in a meal plays an important role in the increase of blood glucose after the meal. Keeping a watchful eye on the amount of carbohydrates consumed in meals and snacks can improve metabolic control.

**2.   Carbohydrates can raise blood glucose levels. Should they still be eaten?**

Even though they can raise blood glucose, foods containing carbohydrates are essential at every meal. Dietary carbohydrates should provide approximately half of a person's daily energy needs. For example, if a person needs 1800 calories per day, half (900 calories) should come from carbohydrates.

**3.   What are dietary carbohydrates?**

Digested dietary carbohydrates, which can be stored in the liver and muscles, are one of the body's main sources of fuel. Most of the carbohydrates we consume are from plants, which absorb energy from the sun and store it in the form of carbohydrates.

The main types of dietary carbohydrates are glucose, fructose, saccharose (sucrose), lactose, starch, dietary fibre and polyols (or sugar alcohols).

## 4. What information about carbohydrate content is listed on prepackaged food labels?

Prepackaged food labels list carbohydrate content in grams per portion specified. Carbohydrate content includes sugars, dietary fibre, starches, polyols (or sugar alcohols) and polydextrose.

- o The term "sugars" refers to glucose, fructose, saccharose (sucrose) and lactose. They may be naturally present or added to the product.
- o The term polyols (or sugar alcohols) refers to sugars such as maltitol, mannitol and sorbitol.

## 5. Which foods contain carbohydrates?

Essentially, there are four food groups that contain carbohydrates: **starchy foods, fruits, vegetables** and **milk**.

Starchy foods contain primarily starches, while fruit and vegetables contain fructose and milk contains lactose. Foods from these groups may also naturally contain glucose and sucrose.

## 6. How are meals planned for people with diabetes?

There are different meal-planning approaches. The most common are the following

1) The exchange system:

This system involves grouping foods according to their nutritional content (protein, carbohydrates and fats). All the foods within the same group have the same nutritional content, and single portions of food within the same group are known as exchanges or equivalents.

Foods within the same group are interchangeable, as long as the same number of exchanges per meal is consumed. Carbohydrate-containing foods from the starches, fruits, and milk and alternatives groups may also be interchanged to ensure a varied diet.

This system categorizes food into seven main groups:
- o Starches
- o Fruits

- ○ Vegetables
- ○ Milk and alternatives
- ○ Other choices
- ○ Meat and alternatives
- ○ Fats

An eighth group of "low calorie foods" has recently been added. There are no restrictions on the consumption of foods in this group, given their negligible effect on blood glucose and blood lipids.

Each exchange contains on average 15 g of carbohydrates or 3 teaspoons of sugar, except for vegetables, meat, and fats. One exchange of vegetables contains an average of 5 g of carbohydrates or 1 teaspoon of sugar. Most raw and cooked vegetables contain few carbohydrates and therefore have little effect on blood glucose. Vegetables with the highest carbohydrate content are included in the starches group, which do have an effect on blood glucose.

A few examples of exchanges:

| Foods | One serving corresponding to one exchange (15 g of carbohydrates or 3 teaspoons of sugar) |
|---|---|
| **Starches**<br>Bread<br>Cooked spaghetti<br>Lentils<br>Sweet peas | <br>1 slice (30 g serving)<br>75 mL (1/3 cup)<br>125 mL (1/2 cup)<br>250 mL (1 cup) |
| **Fruits**<br>Banana<br>Kiwi<br>Orange juice | <br>½ large (90 g serving)<br>2 small<br>125 mL (½ cup) |
| **Milk and alternatives**<br>Milk<br>Plain yogurt | <br>250 mL (1 cup)<br>175 mL (¾ cup) |

The exchange system is used mainly to plan meals for people with diabetes whose treatment includes diet, oral antidiabetic drugs or fixed-dose insulin.

This system is used by Diabetes Québec and a detailed explanation is provided in the brochure entitled *Meal Planning for People with Diabetes.*[1] It is also used by the American Diabetes Association (ADA). The system recommended by the Canadian Diabetes Association (CDA), which has recently been revised, closely resembles the one used by Diabetes Québec and the ADA. It is outlined in a new guide entitled *Beyond the Basics: Meal Planning for Healthy Eating, Diabetes Prevention and Management.*[2]

| AMOUNT OF CARBOHYDRATES IN ONE EXCHANGE | | |
|---|---|---|
| **Food groups** | **Systems** | |
| **DQ/CDA** | **DQ and ADA** | **CDA** |
| Starches/Grains and Starches | 15 g | 15 g |
| Fruits | 15 g | 15 g |
| Vegetables | 0 g to 5 g | – |
| Milk /Milk and Alternatives | 12 g to 15 g | 15 g |
| Other choices | 15 g | 15 g |
| Meat and Alternatives | 0 g | 0 g |
| Fats | 0 g | 0 g |
| Low calorie foods /Extras | < 5 g | < 5 g |

2) Basic carbohydrate counting
This method involves predetermining the grams of carbohydrates to be contained in each meal and snack.
Basic carbohydrate counting can be used by anyone with diabetes and is especially useful for people who have trouble using the food exchange system.
3) Advanced carbohydrate counting
Advanced carbohydrate counting involves counting the total number of carbohydrates from all meals as precisely as possible.

1. http://www.diabete.qc.ca/english/publications/pdf/meal_planning.pdf (updated version due in 2008).
2. http://www.diabetes.ca/section_about/btb2006.asp.

This method is particularly useful for people with diabetes who inject insulin according to a varied carbohydrate intake.

The amount of insulin for each meal is calculated using an insulin: carbohydrate ratio (that is, a number of units of insulin for every 10 g of carbohydrates). The insulin dose is thus proportionate to the amount of carbohydrates consumed.

The doctor first determines the insulin: carbohydrate ratio specific to a person. The ratio can also be done with the help of a dietary journal detailing the amount of carbohydrates consumed at every meal, the amount of insulin injected, and blood glucose readings. The ratio may differ from one meal to another over the course of the same day.

Advanced carbohydrate counting allows for a certain amount of flexibility, since it does not require planning the specific amount of carbohydrates for every meal and snack.

## 7. Can foods such as pastries, jams, and soft drinks be included in meals?

These foods fall under the "other choices" category in the guide *Meal Planning for People with Diabetes* and may be substituted for an equal quantity of carbohydrates in any other food.

**Foods containing fewer than 3 g of carbohydrates per serving** do not need to be counted in the meal's carbohydrate total, provided they are eaten one serving at a time.

For example:
The 2.5 g of carbohydrates contained in 10 ml or 2 teaspoons of light fruit jam are generally not added to the total breakfast carbohydrates.

**Foods containing more than 3 g of carbohydrate per serving** may be eaten as part of a meal and their carbohydrate content must be counted.

Pastries, pies, cookies, ice cream, chocolate, chips and crackers contain not only carbohydrates but also fats. These foods should be consumed only occasionally and in moderation because their high calorie content can cause weight gain

## 8. Where can information on the carbohydrate content of specific foods be found?

There are several ways to find out about the carbohydrate content of the foods we consume.

1) **Product labels:**

   Nutritional value is printed on food packaging.

2) **Food composition tables:**

   Health Canada publishes a useful table entitled "Nutrient Value of Some Common Foods" (2008). It is available in bookstores and on the Health Canada website.[3]

3) **Nutritional information provided by restaurants:**

   Some restaurants provide nutritional information about the food they serve. Be sure to ask.

4) **Cookbooks:**

   Many cookbooks list the nutritional value of their recipes.

5) **Food exchange lists:**

   A dietician can provide a list of food exchanges. The lists published by the Ministère de la Santé et des Services sociaux and Diabetes Québec (*Meal Planning for People with Diabetes*) and by the Canadian Diabetes Association (*Beyond the Basics: Meal Planning for Eating, Diabetes Prevention and Management*) are also available for consultation.

6) **Carbohydrate factors:**

   The carbohydrate factor is the amount of carbohydrates contained in 1 g of a given food.

   For example:

   > a 100 g pear with a carbohydrate factor of 0.12 contains 12 g total carbohydrates:
   > 100 g x 0.12 = 12 g of carbohydrates

   A table of carbohydrate factors can be found in the book "Pumping Insulin".[4]

3. http://www.hc-sc.gc.ca/fn-an/alt_formats/hpfb-dgpsa/pdf/nutrition/nvscf-vnqau_e.pdf.
4. Walsh John and Ruth Roberts, *Pumping Insulin*, 4th ed. (Torrey Pines Press, 2006).

**9. What amount of carbohydrates should be eaten daily?**

Total daily carbohydrate intake is determined by energy (or caloric) needs, which are evaluated according to a person's size, weight, sex, age and the amount of physical activity he or she engages in.

On average, carbohydrates should provide half of a person's caloric needs. The rest should be supplied by proteins, fats and alcohol.

To maintain adequate body function, a person should consume more than 130 g of carbohydrates a day. Generally, for an adolescent or an adult with diabetes, the amount should fall between 200 g and 300 g per day, or at least:

- o   6 exchanges of starches and
- o   3 exchanges of fruits and
- o   4 exchanges of vegetables and
- o   2 exchanges of milk and alternatives and
- o   6 exchanges of meat and alternatives and
- o   approximately 4 exchanges of fats and
- o   occasionally, 1 exchange of other choices

This corresponds to at least 60 g of carbohydrates per meal.

**10. Should the same quantity of carbohydrates be eaten every day?**

It depends on the individual's treatment regimen.

1)   **People with diabetes whose treatment consists solely of a dietary regimen or of a diet combined with a fixed medical treatment** (either oral antidiabetic drugs or insulin) should eat the same quantity of carbohydrates at every meal and schedule meals at regular times.

The total carbohydrate amount should be spread out over the course of the day. This will help avoid a spike in blood glucose after meals.

2)   **People who count carbohydrates and inject insulin according to the amount of carbohydrates ingested** may vary their carbohydrate consumption from one day to another. Eating balanced meals should remain a priority, however, because it is vital to good health and because overeating can lead to weight gain.

## 11. What is the glycemic index?

According to the CDA, the glycemic index is a scale ranking carbohydrate-rich foods by their tendency to raise blood glucose levels after consumption compared to a standard food (glucose or white bread).

Low glycemic index foods, such as dried beans, cause blood glucose to rise more gradually than high glycemic index foods, such as white bread or mashed potatoes. Some low glycemic index foods:

- o milled or stone ground whole grains,
- o oatmeal,
- o barley,
- o pasta,
- o legumes,
- o sweet potato.[5]

It has been found that taking the glycemic index of food into account when planning meals brings an additional benefit to carbohydrate counting. Low glycemic index foods are said to help control blood glucose levels after meals. Although studies are contradictory, it appears that the fibre in these foods may positively influence insulin sensitivity and even pancreatic function.

## 12. Why should fibre-rich foods be part of the diet of a person with diabetes?

Fibres are a form of carbohydrate. They resist digestion by human enzymes and are therefore not broken down in the small intestine. As a result, they arrive in the large intestine intact and do not raise blood glucose levels.

| Some sources of fibre |
| :---: |
| Fruits |
| Whole grains |
| Vegetables |
| Legumes |
| Nuts |
| Oat and wheat bran |

---

5. See http://www.diabetes.ca/files/Diabetes_GL_FINAL2_CPG03.pdf.

Eating a wide variety of fibre-rich foods is recommended, since they are also a good source of vitamins and minerals. Such foods should be introduced gradually to avoid unpleasant effects such as bloating and flatulence. It is also important to drink a sufficient amount of liquid to ensure that the fibres perform their function efficiently. The target amount of fibres for people with diabetes is the same as it is for the general population, namely, between 21 g and 38 g per day, depending on sex.

Moreover, fibres help:
1) **control blood glucose:** very large amounts of fibres (50 g/day) can help control blood glucose in some people with diabetes;
2) **avoid constipation:** fibres improve intestinal transit by increasing stool volume; fibres promote a healthy colon (large intestine);
3) **control blood cholesterol:** large amounts of fibres help lower blood cholesterol in some people with diabetes;
4) **control weight:** foods rich in fibre are low in calories but still leave you feeling full.

# Fats:
## Making the Right Choices

**1. Why should people with diabetes limit their fat consumption?**

People with diabetes have a serious risk of developing cardiovascular disease. If they also have elevated levels of triglycerides and bad cholesterol in their blood, the risk is even higher.

Limiting consumption of certain fats such as saturated and trans fats helps control blood lipids, also known as blood fats. The main types of blood lipids are:

- o   triglycerides;
- o   total cholesterol;
- o   HDL-cholesterol (good cholesterol);
- o   LDL-cholesterol (bad cholesterol).

Limiting fat consumption also helps control weight.

**2. Why does fat consumption lead to weight gain?**

One gram of carbohydrate or protein contains four calories, while one gram of fat contains nine calories, more than double.

- o   5 mL or 1 teaspoon of sugar (5 g of carbohydrates) contains 20 calories;
- o   5 mL or 1 teaspoon of oil (5 g of fat) contains about 45 calories.

### 3. If fats can be bad for the health, why is it necessary to eat them?

Fats are part of a balanced diet, just like carbohydrates and proteins. They are an excellent source of energy. They contain essential fatty acids, which help make up certain vitamins and hormones, and play a vital role in the body.

### 4. What is the recommended daily fat consumption for a healthy diet?

It is recommended that 30% to 35% of a person's daily calories should be ingested in the form of fats:

- o   less than 7% of calories from saturated or trans fats;
- o   higher intake of omega-3 from fish and vegetable sources;
- o   higher intake of monounsaturated and polyunsaturated fats.

### 5. Should people with diabetes count fats the way they count carbohydrates?

Not necessarily. In most cases, there are other ways (eating smaller portions of meat or choosing lower fat cheeses, for example) to reduce the amount of dietary fat to a satisfactory level. It should help to remember that people usually eat large quantities of fat on impulse because it adds flavour, making the food more appealing.

### 6. Which foods contain fats?

The following foods contain either visible or hidden fats:

| Visible fats | Hidden fats |
|---|---|
| Oils | Meats and cold cuts |
| Butter | Fatty fish (mackerel and herring, among others) |
| Margarine | Sauces (such as mayonnaise or béarnaise, white or cheese sauce) |
| Lard | Some types of prepared dishes |
| Vegetable fats | Nuts and seeds |
| Meats | Avocado |
| | Cookies, pastries, croissants, brioches |

## 7. Which fats are found naturally in foods?

The following types of fats occur naturally:
1) saturated fats, usually of animal origin;
2) cholesterol, always of animal origin;
3) unsaturated fats, primarily of vegetable origin (monounsaturated and polyunsaturated);
4) Trans fats, naturally present in small quantities in meats and dairy products.

No food contains only one type of fat. They are classified according to the predominant fat source.

For example:
Sunflower oil, very high in polyunsaturated fats, also contains small quantities of saturated and monounsaturated fats. It is classified as a source of polyunsaturated fats.

## 8. What are trans or hydrogenated fats?

These fats are produced by the food industry and do not occur naturally. They are made from oils that are processed to transform them from a liquid to a solid state. Examples include partially hydrogenated margarine, vegetable fats and fats used in bakery products.

Regular consumption of these fats increases the risk of cardiovascular disease because they are metabolized in the same way as saturated fats.

In June 2007, Health Canada adopted the recommendations of a working group that recommended reducing the trans fat content of foods. The food industry has two years to limit trans fat content to:
- 2% of the total amount of fat in oils and soft margarines;
- 5% of other foods, including prepared ingredients or ingredients sold in restaurants.

## 9. Why do we have to choose fats carefully?

Some people are predisposed to abnormally high fat levels in their blood. In such cases, different types of fats and the foods that contain them can have either beneficial or harmful effects.

Harmful effects:

|  | Triglycerides | Total Cholesterol | HDL Cholesterol | LDL Cholesterol |
|---|---|---|---|---|
| Cholesterol |  | ↑ |  | ↑ |
| Saturated fats |  | ↑ | ↓ | ↑ |
| Trans or hydrogenated fats |  | ↑ | ↓ | ↑ |

↑ increase    ↓ decrease

Beneficial effects:

|  | Triglycerides | Total Cholesterol | HDL Cholesterol | LDL Cholesterol |
|---|---|---|---|---|
| Monounsaturated fats | = | ↓ | ↑ OR = | ↓ |
| Polyunsaturated omega-3 fats | ↓ OR = | = | ↑ OR = | ↑ OR = |

↑ increase    ↓ decrease    = no change

Some types of fat are better for your heart and blood vessels than others. Foods containing **monounsaturated and polyunsaturated** fats should be preferred over anything containing saturated fats, trans or hydrogenated fats, or cholesterol.

## 10. Which foods contain which types of fat?

| SATURATED FATS | |
|---|---|
| **Animal origin*** | **Vegetable origin** |
| Butter | Coconut or copra oil |
| Cream, ice cream | Palm oil |
| Yogurt (8% m.f.) | Palm kernel oil |
| Cheeses | Coconut |
| Whole milk (3.25 % m.f.) | |
| Lard | |
| Eggs | |
| Tallow | |
| Meats | |
| Poultry and poultry skin | |

* These also contain cholesterol.

| UNSATURATED FATS | |
|---|---|
| **Monounsaturated** | **Polyunsaturated** |
| Almonds | Pumpkin seeds |
| Peanuts | Linseed |
| Avocado | Sunflower seeds |
| Sesame seeds | Borage oil |
| Peanut oil | Safflower oil |
| Canola oil | Pumpkin oil |
| Olive oil | Linseed oil |
| Hazelnut oil | Corn oil |
| Sesame oil | Walnut oil |
| Hazelnuts | Grapeseed oil |
| Cashew nuts | Soya oil |
| Brazil nuts | Sunflower oil |
| Olives | Evening primrose oil |
| Pecans | Walnuts |
| Pistachios | Pine nuts |
| | Fatty fish (e.g., salmon, mackerel) |

| UNSATURATED FATS<br>MONOUNSATURATED AND POLYUNSATURATED |
|---|
| Soft non-hydrogenated margarine (e.g. Becel®, Crystal®, Lactantia®, Nuvel®, Olivina®, etc.) |

| TRANS OR HYDROGENATED FATS (VEGETABLE ORIGIN) | |
|---|---|
| Hydrogenated vegetable oil | Soft margarine |
| Hard margarine | Vegetable oil shortening |
| Certain bakery products | Fast food |
| Snacks | |

## 11. How can the consumption of fats, and trans or hydrogenated fats in particular, be reduced?

It is useful to remember that:

1) all fats have comparable energy value: 5 mL or 1 teaspoon of oil, butter or margarine all contain 40 to 45 calories;

2) no oil is low-fat, even if it is called "light".

To eat less fat, do the following:

1) develop the habit of measuring fats with a teaspoon or tablespoon; one teaspoon equals 5 mL and one tablespoon equals 15 mL;*

2) choose leaner cuts of meat (10% or less of fat), poultry, fish, molluscs, and crustaceans on occasion; trim visible fat and remove skin before cooking;

3) eat reasonably sized servings of meat or alternatives, no bigger than the palm of your hand; a meat serving that size equals 90 g (3 oz) of meat;

4) eat fish more often, at least two or three times a week;

5) incorporate dishes with legumes (beans, etc.) into your meals;

6) eat less cheese or select leaner cheeses more often; leaner choices include unripened cheeses (for example, cottage, quark, goat's and cow's milk cheese). Cheese with over 20% fat content has two or three times more fat than meat;

7) drink partially skimmed or skimmed milk (1% m.f. or 2% m.f.) instead of whole milk (3.25% m.f.);

8) reduce daily consumption of fatty foods like butter and cream sauces, pastries, prepackaged muffins, croissants, brioches, cookies, and so on. Save these foods for special occasions only. Replace them with yogurt, mousses, skim or partially skim milk desserts, puddings, soy mousses, dry cookies, homemade muffins and dessert breads, etc.

## 12. Which cooking methods can lower fat content?

When cooking, use methods requiring the least amount of fat possible.

---

\* One tablespoon equals three teaspoons.

| Cooking method | Foods |
|---|---|
| Water | Boiled beef, boiled chicken |
| Steam | Vegetables, fish, pressure-cooked or steamed rice |
| Conventional oven or microwave | Poultry, roasts (beef, chicken, veal), fish, fruits, gratin with light béchamel |
| Double-boiler | Scrambled eggs |
| Braising | Mixed plate cooked in clay pot or pressure cooker |
| Grill | Cast-iron, oven or BBQ grill: meats, poultry, vegetables, higher-fat fish such as salmon |
| Frying | Non-stick frying pan for eggs, omelettes and sliced meats |
| Closed packet | Fish, lean meats, potatoes, fruits |
| Simmering or stewing | Stewing meats |
| Gros sel[2] | Fish, chicken |

## 13. Can some foods help lower blood fat levels?

Yes, it appears that some food components can lower blood fat. Vegetable phytosterols, omega-3 fatty acids and soluble fibre are the most well known.

1) **Vegetable phytosterols** (or sterols/stanols) have a beneficial effect on blood fat levels, primarily on total cholesterol and LDL or bad cholesterol. They are believed to prevent the absorption of cholesterol in the intestine, thereby reducing the amount of bad cholesterol in the blood. The recommended daily consumption is 2 to 3 grams of vegetable sterols, which are found primarily in vegetable oils, nuts, seeds, and whole grains, but only in very small quantities. Because huge quantities of these foods would have to be consumed in order to have an effect, sterols/stanols are marketed as supplements and added to certain foods (not sold in Canada).

2) **Omega-3 fatty acids** help protect against cardiovascular disease. Among other things, they help reduce blood triglyceride and cholesterol.

---

2. Heat the gros sel (coarse sea salt) in the oven between two aluminum plates for approximately 30 minutes at 500°F (260°C). Remove from the oven and place the chicken or fish in the salt. Allow to cook 30 minutes at 350°F (175°C).

They are found in:

o    foods of both vegetable origin, such as canola oil, linseed oil, and linseed (alphalinolenic or ALN acid);

o    foods of animal origin, such as fish and fish oil (DHA and EPA).

The most significant effects on cardiac health have been observed with omega-3 of fish origin.

The protective effects of omega-3 fatty acids from fish have led to recommendations for the general population and people with diabetes in particular to eat fish two or three times a week. As for omega-3 fatty acids of vegetable origin, the recommended daily intake is the following: 1 g of ALN for women and 1.6 g for men.

The following chart presents a few examples of food sources of omega-3 fatty acids:

| Foods | Total amount (g) | ALN | EPA | DHA |
|---|---|---|---|---|
| Natrel® omega-3 milk beverage, 1% or 2% m.f. (250 mL or 1 cup) | 0.30 | 0.30 | 0.00 | 0.00 |
| Naturegg® Break-Free Omega 3 liquid eggs (50 mL) | 0.32 | 0.03 | 0.15 | 0.14 |
| Naturegg® Omega 3 shell eggs* (50 g or 1 unit) | 0.40 | 0.31 | 0.01 | 0.08 |
| Becel Omega3plus® margarine (10 g or 2 tsp) | 0.60 | 0.55 | 0.05 | |
| Soya oil (15 mL or 3 tsp) | 0.94 | 0.94 | 0.00 | 0.00 |
| Canola oil (15 mL or 3 tsp) | 1.32 | 1.32 | 0.00 | 0.00 |
| Linseed oil (15 mL or 3 tsp.) | 7.74 | 7.74 | 0.00 | 0.00 |
| Chopped walnuts (60 mL or 30 g) | 2.69 | 2.69 | 0.00 | 0.00 |
| Ground linseed (10 mL or 2 tsp) | 1.09 | 1.09 | 0.00 | 0.00 |
| Salba** (30 mL or 2 tbsp) | 2.45 | 2.45 | 0.00 | 0.00 |

| Foods | Total amount (g) | ALN | EPA | DHA |
|---|---|---|---|---|
| Cooked wild or farmed rainbow trout (75 g or 2 ½ oz) | 0.93 | 0.06 | 0.25 | 0.62 |
| Baked or broiled blue mackerel (75 g or 2 ½ oz) | 0.99 | 0.09 | 0.38 | 0.52 |
| Baked or grilled fresh red tuna (75 g or 2 ½ oz) | 1.13 | 0.00 | 0.27 | 0.86 |
| Canned white tuna, in water (75 g or 2 ½ oz) | 0.70 | 0.05 | 0.18 | 0.47 |
| Atlantic sardines, in oil, drained, with bones (75 g or 2 ½ oz) | 1.11 | 0.37 | 0.36 | 0.38 |
| Baked or broiled Atlantic herring (75 g or 2 ½ oz) | 1.61 | 0.10 | 0.68 | 0.83 |
| Atlantic herring, smoked and salted (75 g or 2 ½ oz) | 1.72 | 0.11 | 0.73 | 0.88 |
| Canned pink salmon, drained, with bones, salted (75 g or 2 ½ oz) | 0.84 | 0.05 | 0.27 | 0.52 |
| Canned keta salmon, drained, with bones, salted (75 g or 2 ½ oz) | 0.93 | 0.04 | 0.36 | 0.53 |
| Canned sockeye salmon, drained, with bones, salted (75 g or 2 ½ oz) | 1.46 | 0.07 | 0.55 | 0.84 |
| Cooked Atlantic salmon (75 g or 2 ½ oz) | 1.70 | 0.09 | 0.52 | 1.09 |
| Quinnat salmon, smoked (75 g or 2 ½ oz) | 0.34 | 0.00 | 0.14 | 0.20 |

3) **Soluble fibres** also have a beneficial effect on bad cholesterol. The recommended daily intake is 10 g to 25 g. Soluble fibres are often part of a low-saturated fat and cholesterol diet, in combination with drug therapy.

---

\* Eggs from hens raised on linseed feed
\*\* Grain high in omega-3 fatty acids and antioxidants

The following foods provide 3 g of soluble fibres per serving:

| Food | Amount |
|------|--------|
| All-Bran Buds® | 75 mL (⅓ cup) |
| Psyllium husks or powder | 5 mL (1 tsp) |
| Metamucil® | 15 mL (1 tbsp) |
| Cooked oat bran or porridge | 250 mL (1 cup) |
| Red kidney beans | 125 mL (½ cup) |
| Ground linseed | 75 mL (⅓ cup) |
| Roasted soy seeds | 75 mL (⅓ cup) |
| Canned artichoke hearts | 2 |

## 14. Are there other ways to lower blood fat levels?

The following factors can help control fat levels in blood:

| | Triglycerides | Total cholesterol | HDL Cholesterol | LDL Cholesterol |
|------|------|------|------|------|
| Increasing physical activity | ↓ | ↓ | ↑ OR = | ↓ |
| Losing weight | ↓ | | | |
| Quitting smoking* | ↓ | ↓ | ↑ | ↓ |

↓ decreases  ↑ increases  = no change

---

* The effects of smoking on blood fats that have been observed may be linked to other factors associated with quitting smoking.

# How to Read Food Labels

1. **What information is listed on prepackaged food labels?**

   The following nutritional information is found on prepackaged food labels:

   1) the Nutrition Facts table;
   2) the list of ingredients;
   3) the product's nutritional and health claims.

   Health Canada regulates food labelling in Canada through the *Food and Drugs Act*. This labelling statute was updated and its final version published on January 1, 2003. Since December 2007, nutritional labelling has been mandatory on all prepackaged foods. The Canadian Food Inspection Agency (CFIA) is charged with protecting the public against fraud or misrepresentation*.

2. **What information is listed in the Nutrition Facts table?**

   The Nutrition Facts table on prepackaged food labels provides information about a specified quantity of the food. This information includes:

   1) the caloric value of the food in the specified serving;
   2) the content of 13 listed nutrients in the specified serving;
   3) the percentage of the recommended Daily Value (% DV) represented by that serving.

---

\* See the following web sites on food labelling in Canada:
http://www.hc-sc.gc.ca/fn-an/label ctiquet/nutrition/index_e.html
http://www.hc-sc.gc.ca/fn-an/label-etiquet/index_e.html

| Nutrition Facts per 125 mL (87 g) | | |
|---|---|---|
| **Amount** | | **% Daily Value** |
| **Calories** 80 | | |
| **Fat** 0,5 g | | **1** % |
| Saturated Fat 0 g | | |
| + trans Fat 0 g | | |
| **Cholesterol** 0 mg | | |
| **Sodium** 0 mg | | **0** % |
| **Carbohydrate** 18 g | | **6** % |
| Fibre 2 g | | **8** % |
| Sugars 2 g | | |
| **Protein** 3 g | | |
| Vitamin A | 2 % | Vitamin C 10 % |
| Calcium | 0 % | Iron 2 % |

**3. What information is in the list of ingredients?**

The list includes all the food's ingredients presented in decreasing order of weight; in other words, the ingredients present in the greatest amount are listed first.

**4. What is important to know about the manufacturer's nutritional claims?**

The new nutrient labelling regulation permits two types of nutritional claims:

1) **nutrient content claims**: these are statements or expressions describing the nutritional elements of a food;

2) **health claims**: these include any representation affirming, suggesting or implying a relationship between a food or an ingredient in the food and a health effect.

Nutrient content and health claims are useful for people with diabetes as they enable them to make better-informed nutritional choices.

## 5.   What type of nutrient content claims appears on labels?

The following chart presents several examples of nutrient content claims on food product labels, along with their meanings.

| Claims | Meaning per specified serving |
|---|---|
| **Calories** | |
| "Calorie reduced" | At least 25% fewer calories than the food to which it is compared |
| "Low calorie" | No more than 40 calories |
| "Calories free" | Less than 5 calories |
| **Fats** | |
| "Fat free" | Less than 0.5 g of fat |
| "Low fat" | No more than 3 g of fat |
| "Low saturated fat" | No more than 2 g of saturated fat and trans fat in total, and no more than 15% of total calories derived from saturated fat and trans fat |
| "No trans fatty acids" | Less than 0.2 g of trans fatty acids and "low in saturated fats" |
| **Cholesterol** | |
| "Cholesterol free" | Less than 2 mg of cholesterol and low in saturated fat |
| **Carbohydrate and sugar** | |
| "Sugar free" | Less than 0.5 g of sugar |
| "Reduced sugar" | At least 25% less sugar than the regular version than the food to which it is compared |
| "No sugar added" | No added sugar such as saccharose, fructose, glucose, molasses, fruit juice, honey, syrup, etc. |
| **Fibre** | |
| "Source of fibre" | 2 g or more of fibre |
| "Good source of fibre" | 4 g or more of fibre |
| "Very good source of fibre" | 6 g or more of fibre |
| **Calcium** | |
| "Good source of calcium" | At least 165 mg of calcium |

If a manufacturer wants to use the term "light" to describe a product, the label must indicate precisely what in fact makes the product "light". If the term refers to nutritive value, it is authorized only for food products with a reduced amount of **calories** or **fats**.

## 6. What kinds of health claims are authorized?

For the first time in Canada, manufacturers may include claims regarding diet on a food product. Only claims based on scientifically demonstrated links between the food product and a reduced risk of chronic disease are authorized. Such links include the following:

- o   A low-sodium and high-potassium diet may reduce the risk of high blood pressure;
- o   A healthy diet with adequate calcium and vitamin D may reduce the risk of osteoporosis;
- o   A diet low in saturated and trans fats may reduce the risk of cardiovascular disease;
- o   A diet rich in fruits and vegetables may reduce the risk of certain types of cancer.

An example of a health claim:
*"A healthy diet including a variety of fruits and vegetables may help reduce the risk of certain types of cancer."*

It is also permitted to make claims regarding cavities for candy, gum or breath fresheners, since they contain only minute quantities of carbohydrates that promote tooth decay.

## 7. How is the law applied?

The Canadian Food Inspection Agency (CFIA)* is in charge of implementing inspections to determine whether nutritional information is in compliance with the regulations enacted by the government in 2003.

---

*   www.inspection.gc.ca/english/toce/shtml

### 8. What is a sugar substitute?

A sugar substitute is a substance that replaces table sugar (saccharose or sucrose) as a food sweetener. Some add calories or carbohydrates and are therefore known as **nutritive** sweeteners; others do not and are called **non-nutritive**. Any calories or carbohydrates added by nutritive sweeteners can affect blood glucose levels to varying degrees and must be calculated in the carbohydrate count or meal plan. Non-nutritive sweeteners have no calories and little effect on blood glucose.

### 9. What types of nutritive sugar substitutes are found in prepackaged foods?

The following chart presents the various nutritive sugar substitutes that raise blood glucose, along with a few of their properties.

| Nutritive sugar substitute | Some properties |
|---|---|
| Fructose | • Possible effect on blood glucose, triglycerides, cholesterol and weight;<br>• Consumption of more than 60 g per day is not recommended for people with diabetes;<br>• Risk of gastro-intestinal symptoms |
| Sorbitol<br>Mannitol<br>Xylitol<br>Isomalt<br>Maltitol<br>Erythritol<br>Hydrogenated starch hydrolysate | • Provides fewer calories than sugars because they are only partly absorbed<br>• Glycemic response is weaker than sugars<br>• Do not cause cavities<br>• Risk of gastro-intestinal symptoms due to varying degrees of laxative effect |
| Lactitol | • Not absorbed; provides calories<br>• No glycemic effect<br>• Risk of gastro-intestinal symptoms due to varying degrees of laxative effect |

In the above table, the sugar substitutes ending with "-ol" and hydrogenated starch hydrolysate are also known collectively as "polyols" or "sugar alcohols". They come from plants such as fruits or berries, but they can also be synthetically manufactured.

Compared to table sugar (sucrose), sugar alcohols provide fewer calories and carbohydrates and do not raise blood glucose as much because they are digested more slowly or only partially absorbed by the intestine. Foods that contain nutritive sugar substitutes include gum, candy, chocolate, jam, ice cream, syrup, nutrition bars, and cough drops.

Polydextrose is also a sugar alcohol. This food additive is used primarily to add texture to prepackaged foods. Unlike other sugar alcohols, it does not have a sweet taste. Very little is absorbed, it provides very few calories, and it does not increase blood glucose.

## 10. What non-nutritive sugar substitutes are authorized in Canada and are found in some prepackaged foods?

The following chart presents the various non-nutritive sugar substitutes that do not increase blood glucose and their properties.

| Non-nutritive sugar substitutes | Commercial names and/or foods that contain them | Sources | ADI* mg/kg/ day | Maximum daily consumption** (mg) |
|---|---|---|---|---|
| Acesulfame-potassium (K) | Not authorized for purchase | • Prepackaged foods or drinks | 15 | 750 |
| Aspartame | Equal®<br>NutraSweet®<br>Sweet'N'Low®<br>Private brands | • Packets, tablets or powders<br>• Prepackaged foods or drinks | 40 | 2000 |
| Cyclamates | Sucaryl®<br>SugarTwin®<br>Sweet'N'Low®<br>Private brands | • Packets, tablets, powder or liquid<br>• Unauthorized in prepackaged food or drink | 11*** | 550 |
| Saccharine | Hermesetas® | • Packets, tablets<br>• Unauthorized in prepackaged foods or drinks | 5*** | 250 |
| Sucralose | Splenda® | • Packets or powder<br>• Prepackaged foods or drinks | 9 | 450 |
| Neotame | | • Prepackaged foods or drinks | 2 | 100 |
| Thaumatine | Talin®**** | • Prepackaged foods | unspecified | – |

\*  ADI = Acceptable Daily Intake.
\*\*  For a 50-kg (110 lb) adult
\*\*\*  Not recommended during pregnancy or while breastfeeding
\*\*\*\*Not available in retail

Recently, the Natural Health Products Directorate (NHPD) provisionally authorized the use of Stevia and its extracts such as stevioside as a medicinal ingredient and sweetening agent in natural health products. The daily intake for extracts such as stevioside was set at 1 mg/kg/day up to 70 mg and a maximum of 280 mg/day for an adult taking powdered Stevia leaves. Stevia is available in packet, powder or liquid form. Stevia is not recommended by Health Canada for children, pregnant or nursing women, or people with hypotension (low blood pressure).

### 11. How are sugar alcohols listed in the Nutrition Facts chart on prepackaged foods?

They are listed under total carbohydrates and are often referred to by their specific names or as sugar alcohols.

### 12. How are carbohydrates that can affect blood glucose measured in products containing sugar alcohols?

Here is an excerpt from a Nutrition Facts table providing information on the carbohydrate content:

| Carbohydrates | 19 g |
|---|---|
| Sugars | 3 g |
| Sorbitol | 16 g |

Despite the notable differences between them, one rule applies to nearly all sugar alcohols. Because only half of them is digested or absorbed, their carbohydrate content must be divided by two and subtracted from the total carbohydrate count.

In the above example, the body will not absorb 8 g of sorbitol. From the total carbohydrate count (19 g), only 11 g of carbohydrates will have any effect on blood glucose:

16 g of sorbitol ÷ 2 = 8 g of carbohydrates not absorbed

19 g total carbohydrates – 8 g of unabsorbed sorbitol = 11 g of carbohydrates

Because of their physiological properties, lactitol and polydextrose are not absorbed at all and their carbohydrate content should be subtracted in total from the carbohydrate count of the food.

# Preparing meals

**1. How should people with diabetes go about preparing their meals?**

Example: Spaghetti with meat sauce.

**Step 1**

- o    Refer to the **meal plan**.
- o    In the sample menu, find the recommended number of servings of each food group for the appropriate meal.

Example:

| Sample menu | |
|---|---|
| **Lunch** | |
| Starches | 3 servings |
| Fruits | 1 serving |
| Vegetables | 2 servings |
| Milk | 1 serving |
| Meat and alternatives | 3 servings |
| Fats | 1 serving |

**Step 2**

- o    Assign the meal chosen to the appropriate food group.

Spaghetti with tomato meat sauce:
  - spaghetti = starches
  - tomato and meat sauce = meats and alternatives, vegetables.

### Step 3

o   Find the serving size for each type of food.

| Starch group 1 serving = 15 g of carbohydrates | |
| --- | --- |
| **Food:** | **1 serving:** |
| Spaghetti (cooked) | 75 mL ($^1/_3$ cup) |

| Meat and meat substitutes | |
| --- | --- |
| **Food:** | **1 serving:** |
| Lean ground beef | 30 g (1 ounce) |

### Step 4

o   Figure out how many servings you will eat.
    Example:

| 75 mL ($^1/_3$ cup) of spaghetti | = | 1 serving |
| --- | --- | --- |
| Therefore: | | |
| 250 mL (1 cup) | = | 3 servings |
| Tomato and meat sauce containing 90 g (3 ounces) | = | 3 servings of meat and alternatives, 1 serving of vegetables |

**In this case, the meal contains all the recommended servings of starches and meat and alternatives, as well as one serving of vegetables. The menu should then be completed with the other food groups (one serving each of milk, vegetables, fruit, and fat).**

## 2.   How is the nutritional value of a recipe calculated?

To figure out the nutritional value of a recipe, you need the following information:
1)   the number of servings* or units produced by the recipe;
2)   the nutritional value, in grams (g), of carbohydrates, proteins and fats provided by one serving or unit of the recipe.

*   One serving as defined in the recipe does not necessarily correspond to one serving of a food group (for example, one muffin equals one recipe serving, but it also equals two servings of 15 g of carbohydrates, or 30 g per muffin).

Example:

| Prune muffins | |
|---|---|
| Ingredients: | flour, prunes, sugar, oil, eggs, baking soda |
| Servings or units: | 18 muffins |
| Nutritional value per muffin: | 28 g carbohydrate and 5 g fat |

**3.  How is the nutritional value of a recipe adapted to a meal plan?**

If the meal plan is divided into 15 g servings of carbohydrates, the number of 15 g servings in the food to be eaten has to be determined. Let us take as an example one prune muffin, from the above recipe.

28 g ÷ 15 g = 1.9 = 2 servings of 15 g

Knowing the meal plan well will help you classify the food according to the correct food groups.

In this example, the prune muffin counts as one fruit serving containing 15 g of carbohydrates and one starch serving containing 15 g of carbohydrates.

The prune muffin also contains 5 g of fat. Since foods from the starch and fruit groups are not sources of fat, there is therefore one serving of fat in this muffin. This must be accounted for in the daily food record.

Fit the muffin into the number of servings in the appropriate meal in your sample menu.

Example:

| Sample menu | |
|---|---|
| **Dinner** | |
| Starches | 3 servings |
| Fruits | 1 serving |
| Vegetables | 2 servings |
| Milk | 1 serving |
| Meat and alternatives | 3 servings |
| Fats | 1 serving |

**In this example, one muffin counts as one serving of fruit, one serving of starch, and one serving of fat.** Complete the meal with one serving of milk, two additional servings of starch, three servings of meat and alternatives, and two servings of vegetables.

If the meal plan is divided into fixed amounts of carbohydrates per meal, keep track of the carbohydrate content of the muffins you eat. Complete the menu to reach the recommended carbohydrate content.

4.  **What if the serving yield and nutritional value of a recipe are unknown? Is it still possible to figure out the carbohydrate content?**
    Yes. If you do not know the nutritional value of a recipe, it can be calculated from the list of recipe ingredients, using a food composition table. For carbohydrate content, divide the total value by the number of servings (or units) in the recipe.

# Special Situations

## Eating in Restaurants

### 1. Can people with diabetes eat out in restaurants?

Yes. Occasional restaurant dining is one of life's pleasures, and there is no need to eliminate it because of diabetes. People with diabetes have to find ways to enjoy the experience while following the meal plan.

It is still possible to manage blood glucose levels, even if you eat out everyday (for lunch, for example). It is a question of being careful about food choices and amounts. However, remember that the fat content of restaurant food is on average 20% to 25% higher than food prepared at home, and often the meals are not served well balanced. Restaurant food is also generally higher in sodium (salt). These factors must be taken into account.

### 2. How should people with diabetes choose a meal from a restaurant menu?

There are several strategies to help people with diabetes choose meals in restaurants.
1) Know your meal plan.
2) Find out about the ingredients of the dishes on the menu.
3) Choose carbohydrates first. Go for a simple dish such as grilled meat rather than a mixed au gratin dish. This will make it easier to adapt your choice to the food groups in your meal plan.
4) Pay particular attention to amounts.
5) Order food prepared with a minimum of fat, such as grilled skewered meats or poached fish.
6) Do not eat chicken skin.

7) Ask for sauces and salad dressing on the side whenever possible.

8) Share your French fries, cake or pizza with a friend.

9) Order half-servings or servings from the children's menu.

10) Order two starters rather than a starter and a main course.

To learn how to estimate serving sizes at a glance, practice measuring and weighing food. Some people find that trial and error is the best way to learn to estimate the carbohydrate content of restaurant food. Serving sizes can also be estimated by comparing them to hand size. For more information, speak to a dietician.

# Delayed Meals

## 1. How are blood glucose levels affected if a meal is delayed?

A delayed meal can lead to hypoglycemia if the person with diabetes injects insulin or takes medications that stimulate the pancreas to produce more insulin (for example, glyburide, gliclazide, repaglinide).

1) **If the meal is delayed by approximately one hour**:
Have a snack providing 15 g of carbohydrates at the scheduled mealtime and subtract this amount from the usual carbohydrate content of the meal.

2) **If the meal is delayed two to three hours:**
Have the equivalent of one or two servings of starches (15 g to 30 g of carbohydrates) with a small amount of protein. Then subtract these servings from the eventual meal or, if it is the evening meal, switch the evening snack with the delayed meal.

In all of these cases, take oral antidiabetic medications or insulin with the delayed meal.

# Alcohol

### 1. Can people with diabetes drink alcohol?

People with diabetes can drink alcohol if their diabetes is well controlled. It should always be remembered, however, that excessive alcohol consumption can affect blood glucose levels and can lead to increases in:

1) blood pressure;
2) triglycerides;
3) weight.

### 2. What effect does alcohol have on blood glucose?

There are two types of alcoholic drinks:

1) **alcoholic drinks containing sugar;** these include beer, aperitif wines, and sweet wines. They can raise blood glucose;
2) **alcoholic drinks that do not contain sugar;** these include dry wines and distilled alcohol such as gin, rye, rum, whisky, vodka, cognac, armagnac, and so on. They do not raise blood glucose if they are consumed in small quantities.

Drinking alcohol on an empty stomach can cause hypoglycemia in people with diabetes, particularly those who inject insulin or take medications to stimulate the pancreas to produce insulin (for example, glyburide, gliclazide, repaglinide).

All types of alcohol can trigger **late hypoglycemia.** If alcohol is consumed with the evening meal, it can produce nocturnal hypoglycemia.

To avoid this risk:

1) have a snack before bed;
2) check blood glucose during the night, if recommended.

### 3. What factors should be considered when drinking alcohol?

1) Alcohol has a **high calorie content.** Regular consumption can hinder weight loss or even cause weight gain, because the calories in the alcohol are added to the calories in the meal plan.
2) Alcohol **does not belong to a food group in your meal plan.** Excessive drinking can

be harmful to your health, especially if highly nutritive foods are left out of the regular food plan.

3) Excessive drinking can increase **levels of triglycerides** (a type of blood fat) and **blood pressure**.

## 4. What are the main recommendations regarding alcohol consumption?

1) Drink alcohol only if your diabetes is well controlled.
2) Drink alcohol with food, never on an empty stomach.
3) Drink in moderation:
   o women should have no more than one drink a day (a maximum of nine a week);
   o men should have no more than two drinks a day (a maximum of fourteen a week).
4) Drink slowly.
5) Avoid drinking alcohol before, during or after physical activity.

| **One drink corresponds to:** |
| :---: |
| 1 ½ oz (45 mL) of distilled alcohol |
| 5 oz (150 mL) of dry red or white wine |
| 2 oz (60 mL) of dry sherry |
| 12 oz (340 mL) of beer |

**Remember:**
   o Just one drink can cause hypoglycemia.
   o Just one drink is enough to make your breath smell like alcohol.
   o Because the symptoms of hypoglycemia and drunkenness are very similar, people around you may confuse the two and delay appropriate treatment. Wear a bracelet or pendant that identifies you as diabetic.

## 5. What are the calorie and carbohydrate contents of alcoholic drinks?

The following chart presents the calorie and carbohydrate contents of some alcoholic drinks.

| Alcoholic drinks | Amount | Energy (calories) | Carbohydrates (grams) |
|---|---|---|---|
| Regular beer | 340 mL (12 oz) | 150 | 13 |
| Light beer | 340 mL (12 oz) | 95 | 4 |
| Beer with 0,5 % alcohol | 340 mL (12 oz) | 60 to 85 | 12 to 18 |
| Low-carbohydrate beer | 340 mL (12 oz) | 90 | 2.5 |
| Wine coolers | 340 mL (12 oz) | 170 | 22 |
| Vodka Ice®, Tornade® | 340 mL (12 oz) | 260 | 50 |
| Sweet sherry | 60 mL (2 oz) | 79 | 4 |
| Sweet vermouth | 60 mL (2 oz) | 96 | 10 |
| Scotch | 45 mL (1 ½ oz) | 98 | 0 |
| Rhum | 45 mL (1 ½ oz) | 98 | 0 |
| Dry white wine | 150 mL (5 oz) | 106 | 1 |
| Dry red wine | 150 mL (5 oz) | 106 | 2 |
| Champagne | 150 mL (5 oz) | 120 | 2.5 |
| Porto | 60 mL (2 oz) | 91 | 7 |
| Crème de menthe | 45 mL (1 ½ oz) | 143 | 21 |
| Coffee liqueur | 45 mL (1 ½ oz) | 159 | 17 |
| Cognac | 45 mL (1 ½ oz) | 112 | 0 |

## 6.  What are some alternatives to alcoholic drinks?

Alcoholic drinks can be replaced with the following:

- o  low-sodium carbonated water;
- o  diet soft drinks;
- o  tomato juice with lemon or Tabasco sauce;
- o  water with lemon and ice.

# Minor Illnesses

### 1.	What effects do minor illnesses have on diabetes?

Minor illnesses such as a cold, the flu or gastroenteritis are sources of stress on the body and can destabilize and increase blood sugar levels. This occurs for two reasons:

- o	An increase in the secretion of certain hormones causes glucose stored in the liver to enter the bloodstream;
- o	These same hormones increase resistance to insulin and prevent glucose from entering the cells.

These two reactions can lead to hyperglycemia.

### 2.	What precautions should be taken in the case of a minor illness?

If a person with diabetes has a cold or the flu but is not ill enough to warrant a visit to the doctor, he or she should follow these five rules:

1)	**Continue taking oral antidiabetic medications or insulin.**

Insulin needs can increase during an illness. Doctors can provide a sliding scale based on blood glucose readings to adjust insulin dosage for patients on insulin injection treatment. The following is an example:

Add one unit of rapid-acting insulin (Humalog® or NovoRapid®) or short-acting insulin (Humulin® R or Novolin® ge Toronto) for every mmol/L higher than 14 mmol/L before each meal and at bedtime, and during the night if required.

2)	**Check blood glucose levels at least four times a day or every two hours if they are high.**

3)	**Check for ketone bodies in urine or blood when blood glucose is higher than 14 mmol/L.**

4)	**Drink a lot of water to avoid dehydration.**

5)	**Consume the recommended amount of carbohydrates in easily digested foods.**

### 3.	Should the same precautions be taken for gastroenteritis?

Gastroenteritis generally causes diarrhea and vomiting that can in some cases lead to dehydration and a loss of electrolytes (such as sodium and potassium) because sufferers are unable to eat or drink.

**Important!!!**
See your doctor or go to the emergency room if any of the following situations occur:
1)  your blood glucose is higher than 20 mmol/L;
2)  urine or blood tests show moderate or large levels of ketone bodies;
3)  you are vomiting and cannot retain liquids;
4)  you have a fever with a temperature higher than 38.5°C (101.3°F) for more than 48 hours.

A three-phase approach will avoid dehydration and reduce diarrhea and vomiting:

**Phase 1: Liquid food for the first 24 hours**
Consume only liquids. In particular, drink water, bouillon or consommé at any time. Every hour, drink liquids containing about 15 g of carbohydrates. If you have trouble tolerating large amounts, try drinking 15 mL or 1 tablespoon every 15 minutes instead.

Commercially available oral rehydrating solutions such as Gastrolyte® and Pedialyte® are helpful, or try a homemade preparation: mix 250 mL (1 cup) of orange juice, the same amount of water, and 2 mL (½ tsp) of salt. One cup (250 mL) provides 15 g of carbohydrates.

Gradually replace these drinks with juice, flavoured gelatine, regular non-caffeinated flat soft drinks and nutritional supplements (such as Glucerna®, Resource Diabetic® or Boost Diabetic®, for example).

**Phase 2: Low-residue foods (gentle on the large intestine)**
Add solid foods gradually, increasing consumption by portions of 15 g of carbohydrates, until you reach the recommended carbohydrate content of the meal plan. For example:
- o  fruits: 1 small raw apple (grated), ½ a ripe banana, 125 mL (½ cup) unsweetened orange juice, etc.;
- o  starches: 2 rusks, 8 soda crackers, 4 melba toasts, 1 slice of toast, 75 mL (⅓ cup) of plain pasta or rice, etc.;
- o  vegetables: carrots, beets, asparagus, string or wax beans, etc.;
- o  meats: lean meats such as white chicken or turkey, fish cooked without fat, mild cheese, etc.

**Phase 3: Eat normally**

Gradually resume your normal diet according to the meal plan, but continue to limit your intake of certain items:

- o foods that produce intestinal gas such as corn, legumes (chickpeas, red beans, and so on), cabbage, onions, garlic and raw vegetables;
- o foods that are irritants, including anything fried or spiced, as well as chocolate, coffee, and cola.

# Planning a Trip

### 1. How should a person with diabetes plan a trip?

When preparing for a trip, people with diabetes should take the following precautions.

1) Make sure your diabetes is **well controlled**.
2) Get a **doctor's letter** stating that you have diabetes and describing your treatment, particularly if you require insulin injections.
3) Carry a **piece of identification** or bracelet indicating that you have diabetes.
4) Find out what coverage is provided by **insurance companies** for pre-existing diseases incurring medical expenses abroad. Also find out whether your travel costs to get home in case of medical emergency are covered.
5) Find out about the **habits and customs** of the country you are visiting.
6) **Alert the transportation company** that you have diabetes.
7) Find out about the required vaccines or other treatments (for example, malaria prevention) from a **travellers' clinic** or your doctor.
8) Prepare a **medication kit** with treatments for diarrhea, vomiting and travel sickness. Include antibiotics if your doctor advises.
9) Bring at least two pairs of **comfortable shoes**.
10) **If possible, do not travel alone.**

### 2. Should any precautions be taken when travelling with equipment and medication for the treatment of diabetes?

Everything that is required to treat diabetes should be kept in a carry-on bag (not in stored luggage). The items should include the following:

1) All medications with the identifying pharmacy label.
2) Twice the normal amount of insulin required, in case some vials break or insulin is not available abroad. It should be noted that in some countries, insulin is packaged and sold in a different concentration (40 units/mL). When injecting, make sure the syringe corresponds to the concentration of insulin used.
3) An insulation kit to protect insulin.
4) Extra syringes, even if you use a pen-injector.
5) A self-monitoring kit (meter, test strips, etc.).
6) Emergency food provisions in case of hypoglycemia or a delayed meal (for example, dried or fresh fruits, juice, nuts, packets of peanut butter or cheese and crackers).

## 3. Is there any special advice for diabetic travellers?

When travelling, people with diabetes should heed the following recommendations:
1) Follow your regular meal and snack schedule as closely as possible.
2) Because your habits or routine could change, continue to check your blood glucose levels regularly to make sure the diabetes is still well controlled.
3) Always carry food provisions in case of hypoglycemia or a delayed meal (for example, dried or fresh fruits, juice, nuts, packets of peanut butter or cheese and crackers).
4) Check your feet daily to check for cuts or contusions;

## 4. How should people following the "split-mixed" insulin regimen adapt their insulin doses for time differences of more than three hours?

The "split-mixed" insulin regimen is a combination of intermediate-acting (Humulin® N or Novolin® ge NPH) and rapid-acting (Humalog® or NovoRapid ®) or short-acting insulin (Humulin® R or Novolin® ge Toronto), injected before the morning and evening meals.

Take for example a trip from Montreal to Paris with a six-hour time difference. Suppose you normally take the following insulin doses:

- ○ Novolin® ge NPH 16 units and NovoRapid® (NR) 8 units before breakfast;
- ○ Novolin® ge NPH 6 units and NovoRapid® (NR) 6 units before dinner.

**Montreal to Paris:**
The departure day will be six hours shorter, so **reduce the NPH dose by 50% before dinner. Eat only half of your dinner before leaving and the other half during the flight. Take 50% of the NR dose before dinner in Montreal and 50% before the evening in-flight meal.**

| Meals | Blood glucose | Insulin | Meals |
|---|---|---|---|
| Montreal: breakfast | Yes | NPH 16 units<br>NR 8 units | normal |
| Montreal: lunch | Yes | – | normal |
| Montreal: dinner | Yes | NPH 3 units<br>NR 3 units | 50% |
| In-flight: evening meal | Yes | NR 3 units | 50% |
| In-flight: breakfast | Yes | NPH 16 units<br>NR 8 units | normal |

**Paris-Montreal.**
The return day will be six hours longer, so **have the evening meal during the flight** with the regular amount of NR insulin. Also, **have an additional evening meal** containing 50% of a regular evening meal's carbohydrates, **preceded by a dose of NR equal to 50% of the usual pre-dinner dose.** The NPH dose should be delayed until the second evening meal.

| Meals | Blood glucose | Insulin | Meals |
|---|---|---|---|
| Paris: breakfast | Yes | NPH 16 units<br>NR 8 units | normal |
| Paris: lunch | Yes | – | normal |
| In-flight: dinner | Yes | NR 6 units | normal |
| Montreal: evening meal | Yes | NPH 6 units<br>NR 3 units | 50% |

**5. How should people following the "multiple daily injections (MDI)" insulin regimen with fixed carbohydrates adapt their insulin doses for time differences of more than three hours?**

The "MDI" insulin regimen with fixed carbohydrates consists of one injection of rapid-acting (Humalog® or NovoRapid®) or short-acting (Humulin® R or Novolin® ge Toronto) insulin before each meal and one injection of intermediate acting (Humulin® N or Novolin® ge NPH) or long-acting (Levemir® or Lantus®) insulin at bedtime.

The time difference between Montreal and Paris is six hours. Suppose you normally take:

- NovoRapid® (NR) 8 units before breakfast;
- NovoRapid® (NR) 8 units before lunch;
- NovoRapid® (NR) 8 units before dinner;
- Novolin® ge NPH 8 units before bedtime.

**Montreal-Paris.**

The departure day will be six hours shorter, so **move the NPH dose up before the dinner and take only 50% of it.** Have half the dinner meal before leaving and the other half during the in-flight evening meal. **Take 50% of the NR dose before dinner in Montreal and 50% before the in-flight evening meal.**

| Meals | Blood glucose | Insulin | Meals |
|---|---|---|---|
| Montreal: breakfast | Yes | NR 8 units | normal |
| Montreal: lunch | Yes | NR 8 units | normal |
| Montreal: dinner | Yes | NPH 4 units NR 4 units | 50% |
| In-flight: evening meal | Yes | NR 4 units | 50% |
| In-flight: breakfast | Yes | NR 8 units | normal |

**Paris-Montreal:**

The return day will be six hours longer, so eat the in-flight dinner with the regular amount of NR insulin. You should also eat **an additional evening meal** containing 50% of the usual evening meal carbohydrates, **preceded by 50% of the usual pre-dinner NR dose.** In addition, delay the NPH dose until bedtime.

| Meals | Blood glucose | Insulin | Meals |
|---|---|---|---|
| Paris: breakfast | Yes | NR 8 units | normal |
| Paris: lunch | Yes | NR 8 units | normal |
| In-flight: dinner | Yes | NR 8 units | normal |
| Montreal: evening meal | Yes | NR 4 units | 50% |
| Montreal: bedtime snack | Yes | NPH 8 units | snack |

## 6. How should people following the "multiple daily injection (MDI)" insulin regimen with variable carbohydrate adapt their insulin doses for time differences of more than three hours?

The "MDI" insulin regimen with variable carbohydrates consists of one injection of rapid-acting (Humalog® or NovoRapid®) or short-acting (Humulin® R or Novolin® ge Toronto) insulin before each meal and one injection of intermediate acting (Humulin® N or Novolin® ge NPH) or long acting (Levemir® or Lantus®) insulin at bedtime.

The time difference between Montreal and Paris is six hours. Suppose you normally take:

- o Humalog® (Hg) 1.2 units/10 g of carbohydrates before breakfast;
- o Humalog® (Hg) 1.0 unit/10 g of carbohydrates before lunch;
- o Humalog® (Hg) 1.0 unit/10 g of carbohydrates before the evening meal;
- o Lantus® 12 units at bedtime.

Because long acting insulin (Lantus®) has an extended duration, it is not necessary to change the dose.

**Montreal-Paris.**

The departure day will be six hours shorter, so **move the Lantus® dose up before departure.** Although it is possible for people on the "MDI" insulin regimen with variable carbohydrates to wait and eat dinner on the plane, a **light meal before departure is recommended,** along with Hg insulin according to the amount of carbohydrates consumed. An in-flight evening meal is also possible, again with

Hg insulin according to the amount of carbohydrates consumed. **The next morning during the flight, Hg insulin should be taken before breakfast as usual.**

| Meals | Blood glucose | Insulin | Meals |
|---|---|---|---|
| Montreal: breakfast | Yes | Hg 1.2 units /10 g of carbohydrates | normal |
| Montreal: lunch | Yes | Hg 1.0 unit /10 g of carbohydrates | normal |
| Montreal: dinner | Yes | Lantus® 12 units; Hg 1.0 unit /10 g of carbohydrates | 50% |
| In-flight: evening meal | Yes | Hg 1.0 unit /10 g of carbohydrates | normal or 50% |
| In-flight: breakfast | Yes | Hg 1.2 units /10 g of carbohydrates | normal |

**Paris-Montreal.**

The return day will be six hours longer, so **eat the dinner during the flight with the same dose of Hg insulin, and eat an additional evening meal**, along with the usual pre-dinner dose of Hg. **Take Lantus® at bedtime as usual.**

| Meals | Blood glucose | Insulin | Meals |
|---|---|---|---|
| Paris: breakfast | Yes | Hg 1.2 units /10 g of carbohydrates | normal |
| Paris: lunch | Yes | Hg 1.0 unit /10 g of carbohydrates | normal |
| In-flight: dinner | Yes | Hg 1.0 unit /10 g of carbohydrates | normal |
| Montreal: evening meal | Yes | Hg 1.0 unit /10 g of carbohydrates | normal or 50% |
| Montreal: bedtime snack | Yes | Lantus® 12 units | snack |

7. **How should people following the "premixed" insulin regimen adapt their insulin doses for time differences of more than three hours?**

The "premixed" insulin regimen consists of one injection of a mix of rapid-acting or short-acting insulin and intermediate acting insulin (Humulin® 30/70, Novolin® ge 30/70, 50/50, 40/60, Humalog® Mix 25, etc.) before breakfast and dinner.

The time difference between Montreal and Paris is six hours. Suppose you normally take the following doses of Humulin® (H) 30/70:
- o    20 units before breakfast;
- o    10 units before dinner.

**Montreal-Paris.**
The departure day will be six hours shorter, so **have half the dinner meal before leaving and the other half during the in-flight evening meal.** Also, take **half the insulin dose for the dinner meal before leaving and the other half before the in-flight evening meal.**

| Meals | Blood glucose | Insulin | Meals |
|---|---|---|---|
| Montreal: breakfast | Yes | H 30/70 20 units | normal |
| Montreal: lunch | Yes | – | normal |
| Montreal: dinner | Yes | H 30/70 5 units | 50% |
| In-flight: evening meal | Yes | H 30/70 5 units | 50% |
| In-flight: breakfast | Yes | H 30/70 20 units | normal |

**Paris-Montreal.**
The return day will be six hours longer, so **have an additional evening meal** (50% of the usual carbohydrate content) **preceded by a dose of insulin equivalent to 50% of the usual pre-dinner dose.**

| Meals | Blood glucose | Insulin | Meals |
|---|---|---|---|
| Paris: breakfast | Yes | H 30/70  20 units | normal |
| Paris: lunch | Yes | --- | normal |
| In-flight: dinner | Yes | H 30/70  10 units | normal |
| Montreal: evening meal | Yes | H 30/70  5 units | 50% |
| Montreal: bedtime snack | Yes | – | snack |

# Oral Antidiabetic Drugs

1.  **What are oral antidiabetic drugs?**
    Oral antidiabetic drugs are medications taken **orally to lower blood glucose levels.**

2.  **When should oral antidiabetic drugs be used to treat diabetes?**
    Oral antidiabetic drugs are used to treat type 2 diabetes **if diet, exercise and weight loss programs are not sufficient to normalize blood glucose levels.** They can be taken alone or in combination.

> WARNING! Oral antidiabetic drugs are complementary treatments. They **do not replace** diet, exercise and weight loss programs.

### 3. How many classes of oral antidiabetic drugs are there?

There are seven classes of oral antidiabetic drugs:

| Class | Drug |
|---|---|
| Sulfonylureas* | Chlorpropamide (e.g., Apo®- Chlorpropamide)<br>Gliclazide (e.g., Diamicron®)<br>Glimepiride (Amaryl®)<br>Glyburide (e.g., Diaβeta®, Euglucon®)<br>Tolbutamide (e.g., Apo®-Tolbutamide) |
| Amino acid derivatives*<br>Meglitinides* | Nateglinide (Starlix®)<br>Repaglinide (GlucoNorm®) |
| Biguanides | Metformin (e.g., Glucophage®) |
| Thiazolidinediones | Pioglitazone (Actos®)<br>Rosiglitazone (Avandia®) |
| Alpha-glucosidase inhibitors | Acarbose (Glucobay®) |
| Dipeptidyl peptidase-4 (DPP-4) inhibitors | Sitagliptin (Januvia®) |

\* Insulin secretagogues

### 4. What are the characteristics of sulfonylureas (e.g., Diaβeta®, Diamicron®, Amaryl®)?

1) **Mechanism of action:** Sulfonylureas **stimulate the pancreas to produce more insulin** (they are known as insulin secretagogues). They are therefore ineffective if the insulin-producing cells of the pancreas no longer function.

2) **Adverse effects: Hypoglycemia** is the adverse effect most commonly attributed to sulfonylureas. It can occur at any time of day or night; dosage should therefore be adjusted accordingly. To minimize the risk of hypoglycemia, meals and snacks should be eaten on a regular schedule as set out in the meal plan. Sulfonylureas should not be taken at bedtime.

3) **When to take them:** Sulfonylureas should be taken **before meals, but never more than 30 minutes beforehand.** Sulfonylureas that are taken once a day, such as modified release gliclazide (Diamicron® MR) and glimepiride (Amaryl®), should be taken with breakfast.

5. **What are the characteristics of nateglinide (Starlix®) and repaglinide (GlucoNorm®)?**

   1) **Mechanism of action:** Like sulfonylureas, nateglinide and repaglinide **stimulate the pancreas to produce more insulin** (they are insulin secretagogues). They are therefore ineffective if the insulin-producing cells of the pancreas no longer function. They are faster and shorter acting than sulfonylureas.

   2) **Adverse effects: Hypoglycemia** is the adverse effect most commonly attributed to nateglinide and repaglinide. Dosage should be adjusted accordingly. To minimize the risk of hypoglycemia, meals and snacks should be eaten according to a regular schedule as set out in the meal plan. Nateglinide and repaglinide should not be taken at bedtime.

   3) **When to take them:** They should be taken as close as possible to the beginning of a meal (0 to 15 minutes), but never more than 30 minutes beforehand.

6. **What are the characteristics of metformin (for example, Glucophage®)?**

   1) **Mechanism of action:** The primary action of metformin is to **reduce the production of glucose by the liver.** It also lowers insulin resistance or, in other words, renders insulin more efficient.

   2) **Adverse effects: Intestinal problems**, especially diarrhea, are the side effects most commonly attributed to metformin. Some patients also note a slight metallic aftertaste. When taken on its own, metformin is very rarely associated with hypoglycemia.

   3) **When to take it:** Take metformin at mealtime in order to minimize adverse intestinal effects.

7. **What are the characteristics of pioglitazone (Actos®) and rosiglitazone (Avandia®)?**

   1) **Mechanism of action:** Pioglitazone and rosiglitazone **lower insulin resistance** or, in other words, increase the effectiveness of insulin. This results in an increase in the use of glucose by muscle tissue in particular and by adipose (fatty) tissue.

   2) **Adverse effects: Edema (swelling due to water retention) and weight gain** are possible adverse effects. These drugs must be used with caution or avoided by

people with cardiovascular disease. When taken on their own, pioglitazone and rosiglitazone are generally not associated with hypoglycemia.

3) **When to take them:** These drugs should always be taken at the same time of day, usually in the morning. They do not have to be taken with meals.

## 8.  What are the characteristics of acarbose (Glucobay®)?

1) **Mechanism of action:** Acarbose **slows the absorption of carbohydrates ingested at meals.** It also helps control rising blood glucose levels **after meals.**

2) **Adverse effects:** The adverse effects most commonly attributed to acarbose are **intestinal problems, particularly bloating and flatulence (gas).** When taken on its own, acarbose is not associated with hypoglycemia.

3) **When to take it:** To ensure effectiveness, acarbose should be taken with the first mouthful of a meal.

## 9.  What are the characteristics of sitagliptin (Januvia®)?

1) **Mechanism of action:** Sitagliptin **intensifies the effect of certain intestinal hormones** (such as GLP-1) involved in the control of blood sugar. It causes an increase in insulin secretion and decrease in the secretion of glucagon (a hyperglycemic hormone), but only if blood sugar is high.

2) **Adverse effects:** DPP-4 inhibitors such as sitagliptin are generally well tolerated. When taken alone, sitagliptin is very rarely associated with hypoglycemia.

3) **When to take it:** This drug should always be taken at the same time of the day, usually in the morning. It is not necessary to take it with food.

## 10.  What should be done if a dose is missed?

1) If you notice the omission quickly, take the dose immediately. If not, skip the missed dose and wait for the next scheduled one.

2) **Never double the dose.**

3) It is not a good idea to take sulfonylureas, nateglinide or repaglinide at bedtime, as they can cause a risk of nocturnal hypoglycemia.

4) Acarbose is effective only if it is taken **with a meal.** If forgotten at mealtime, there is no point in taking it afterwards.

### 11. Why are antidiabetic drugs taken together?

Any given class of antidiabetic drugs acts according to a particular mechanism. Secretagogues, for example, stimulate the release of insulin via the pancreas, while biguanides decrease the production of glucose by the liver. In many cases, combining agents with different modes of action is a way to increase the effectiveness of treatment.

### 12. Do oral antidiabetic drugs interact with other medications?

All drugs can potentially interact with other agents. The responsibility for anticipating and preventing such interactions falls on pharmacists and doctors, but the patient also has a role to play.

People taking medication should keep an up-to-date list of their prescriptions, ideally one provided by their pharmacist. They are strongly advised to **bring their medication containers** when seeing the doctor, who will use them to guide any decisions about treatment. It is also a good idea for people with diabetes to use the same pharmacist at all times; in such a case, the pharmacist will be better able to detect potential problems and advise appropriately (regarding duplicate prescriptions, adverse effects or interactions, for example).

### 13. Are oral antidiabetic drugs lifelong treatments?

At this point, diabetes is a disease that can be controlled but not cured. Generally speaking, therefore, oral antidiabetic drugs are long-term treatments. The doctor will regularly adjust treatment, either increasing or decreasing dosages. The goal of such treatment is to **normalize** blood glucose levels without causing adverse effects such as hypoglycemia.

## MOST COMMON ORAL ANTIDIABETIC DRUGS

| Drug | Glyburide | Gliclazide | Modified release Gliclazide | Glimepiride |
|---|---|---|---|---|
| Class | Sulfonylureas (insulin secretagogues) | Sulfonylureas (insulin secretagogues) | Sulfonylureas (insulin secretagogues) | Sulfonylureas (insulin secretagogues) |
| Brand name (non-exhaustive list) | Diaßeta Euglucon Apo-Glyburide Gen-Glybe Novo-Glyburide | Diamicron Gen-Gliclazide Novo-Gliclazide | DiamicronMR | Amaryl |
| Form marketed | 2.5 mg and 5 mg tablets (divisible into two) | 80 mg tablets (divisible into four) | 30 mg tablets (non-divisible) | 1 mg, 2 mg and 4 mg tablets (divisible into two) |
| Daily dosage | 1.25 mg to 20 mg | 40 mg to 320 mg | 30 mg to 120 mg | 1 mg to 8 mg |
| Number of daily doses | 1 to 3 | 1 to 3 | 1 | 1 |
| When to take it | 0 to 30 mins. before meals | 0 to 30 mins. before meals | With breakfast | With breakfast |
| Most common adverse effects | Hypoglycemia | Hypoglycemia | Hypoglycemia | Hypoglycemia |
| Risk of hypoglycemia | Yes | Yes | Yes | Yes |

| Repaglinide | Nateglinide | Acarbose | Metformin | Extended release metformin | Pioglitazone |
|---|---|---|---|---|---|
| Meglitinides (insulin secretagogues) | Amino acid derivative (insulin secretagogue) | Alpha-glucosidase inhibitor | Biguanides | Biguanides | Thiazolidinediones |
| GlucoNorm | Starlix | Glucobay | Glucophage Apo-Metformin Gen-Metformin Novo-Metformin | Glumetza | Actos |
| 0.5 mg, 1 mg and 2 mg tablets (non-divisible) | 60 mg, 120 mg and 180 mg tablets (non-divisible) | 50 mg and 100 mg tablets (divisible into two) | 500 mg tablets (divisible into two) and 850 mg tablets (non-divisible) | 500 mg and 1000 mg tablets | 15 mg, 30 mg and 45 mg tablets (non-divisible) |
| 1 mg to 16 mg | 180 mg to 540 mg | 50 mg to 300 mg | 250 mg to 2500 mg | 500 mg to 2000 mg | 15 mg to 45 mg |
| 2 to 4 (according to the number of meals) | 3 | 1 to 3 | 1 to 4 | 1 | 1 |
| 0 to 15 mins. before meals | 0 to 15 mins. before meals | With the first bite of a meal | With meals | With dinner | With or without food |
| Hypoglycemia | Hypoglycemia | Bloating, flatulence, diarrhea | Diarrhea/metallic taste | Diarrhea | Edema/weight gain |
| Yes | Yes | No | No | No | No |

| Drug | Rosiglitazone | Rosiglitazone and metformin | Rosiglitazone and glimepiride | Sitagliptin |
|---|---|---|---|---|
| Class | Thiazolidinediones | Thiazolidinediones and biguanides | Thiazolidinediones and sulfonylureas | Dipeptidyl peptidase-4 inhibitor |
| Brand name (non-exhaustive list) | Avandia | Avandamet | Avandaryl | Januvia |
| Form marketed | 2 mg, 4 mg and 8 mg tablets (non-divisible) | 1 mg/500 mg, 2 mg/500 mg 4 mg/500 mg 2 mg/1000 mg 4 mg/1000 mg tablets (rosiglitazone/metformine) (non-divisible) | 4 mg/1 mg 4 mg/2 mg 4 mg/4 mg tablets (rosiglitazone/ glimepiride) | 100 mg tablets (non-divisible) |
| Daily dosage | 4 mg to 8 mg | 2 mg/1000 mg to 8 mg/2000 mg | 4 mg/1 mg to 4 mg/4 mg | 100 mg |
| Number of daily doses | 1 to 2 | 2 | 1 | 1 |
| When to take it | With or without food | With meals | With breakfast | With or without food |
| Most common adverse effects | Edema/weight gain | Edema/weight gain/diarrhea/metallic taste | Edema, weight gain, hypoglycemia | Well tolerated |
| Risk of hypoglycemia | No | No | Yes | No |

## MECHANISM OF ACTION OF ORAL ANTIDIABETIC DRUGS

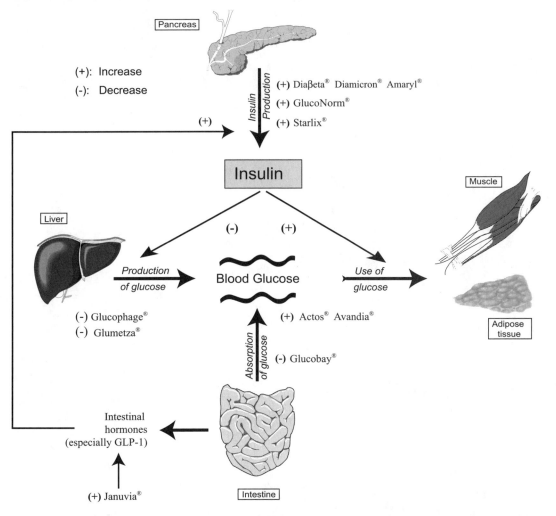

(+): Increase

(-): Decrease

(+) Diaβeta® Diamicron® Amaryl®

(+) GlucoNorm®

(+) Starlix®

---

o Diaβeta®, Diamicron®, Amaryl®, GlucoNorm® and Starlix® stimulate the pancreas to produce more insulin (insulin secretagogues).

o Glucophage® (metformin) decreases the production of glucose by the liver.

o Actos® and Avandia® augments the action of insulin, which in turn increases the use of glucose by the muscle tissue in particular, and by adipose (fatty) tissue.

o Glucobay® delays the absorption of dietary carbohydrates.

o Januvia® (sitagliptin) enhances the action of certain intestinal hormones (such as GLP-1) that increase the secretion of insulin by the pancreas when blood glucose is high.

# Over-the-counter Drugs

### 1.   What are over-the-counter drugs?

Over-the-counter drugs include all medications sold without prescription. Some may be obtained only after consulting a pharmacist, although most can be purchased on the spot.

### 2.   When and how should over-the-counter drugs be used?

Over-the-counter drugs allow people to self-medicate for **mild health problems**. They should only be used for **short periods of time** to ensure that they are not masking the symptoms of a more serious condition. All directions and warnings printed on the product's packaging should be followed closely.

### 3.   Are over-the-counter drugs free of side effects?

No drug is completely free of side effects. Certain over-the-counter drugs can cause adverse effects in some cases. Some drugs should be avoided or used with caution by people with certain illnesses. There is also a risk of interactions between over-the-counter and prescription drugs.

### 4.   How can I be sure that the over-the-counter drugs I choose are safe?

It is strongly recommended that you speak with your pharmacist before selecting an over-the-counter drug. Your pharmacist can recommend the most suitable product for your condition, taking into account your symptoms, health problems, and any other drugs you are taking, possibly even suggesting non-pharmacological alternatives. The pharmacist will recommend that you see your doctor if he or she believes that your condition requires it. Always have your prescriptions filled by the same pharmacist; this will ensure that your file is always up-to-date and that the pharmacist has all the information necessary to properly advise you.

## 5. Which over-the-counter drugs should be avoided or used with caution by people with diabetes?

The following drugs should be used with caution:

1) oral decongestants (for the treatment of nasal congestion);
2) medications containing sugar;
3) keratolytic preparations (for the treatment of corns, calluses and warts);
4) high doses of acetylsalicylic acid or ASA (e.g., Aspirin®).

## 6. Why should oral decongestants be used with caution?

Oral decongestants (e.g., Sudafed®) are medications in syrup, tablet or powder form that reduce nasal congestion. Most oral decongestants contain what is known as a "sympathomimetic" ingredient (e.g., pseudoephedrine) that can have a **hyperglycemic** effect, especially if recommended doses are exceeded. These types of products are frequently overconsumed. Cold medications often contain a mixture of ingredients (to relieve coughs, fight fevers, etc.), including a sympathomimetic decongestant. It is not uncommon for people to take two different products when treating a cold or the flu, thereby unwittingly doubling the dosage of the decongestant.

This type of oral decongestant is also not recommended for people with vascular problems, high blood pressure, hyperthyroidism or cardiac diseases such as angina.

Recommended alternative treatments include drinking plenty of water, keeping the room humidified and using a saline nasal vaporizer. If the condition persists, a nasal decongestant vaporizer may be used, but for no longer than 72 hours (to avoid rebound congestion).

**7.  Why should drugs containing sugar be used cautiously?**

People with diabetes need to know which drugs contain sugar so that they do not unwittingly hamper their control of their blood glucose levels. Sugar is found not only in syrups, but also in powders, chewable tablets, lozenges, etc. People with diabetes must avoid any drug that contains more than **20 calories** (5 g of carbohydrates) **per dose or provides more than 80 calories** (20 g of carbohydrates) **per day**. If these drugs are taken on occasion, they should be included in the overall carbohydrate tally of the meal plan. If the sugar content of a product is not printed on the packaging, the pharmacist can provide this information.

There are a number of "sucrose-free" or "sugar-free" preparations. They usually contain sugar substitutes and can be used by people with diabetes at the recommended dose, as long as the active ingredient is not contraindicated for another reason.

**8.  Why should keratolytic preparations (for the treatment of corns, calluses and warts) be used with caution?**

Adhesive plasters, pads, ointments or gels containing products such as salicylic or tannic acid are often used to treat corns, calluses and warts. These acids are highly irritating. See a doctor, a podiatrist or a nurse specializing in foot care before using these products.

**9.  Why should high doses of acetylsalicylic acid be used with caution?**

High doses of acetylsalicylic acid (e.g., Aspirin®, ASA, Anacin®, Entrophen®, etc.) can cause **hypoglycemia** if the daily dose exceeds 4,000 mg, the equivalent of more than 12 tablets of 325 mg per day or more than 8 tablets of 500 mg each.

Acetaminophen (e.g., Tylenol®, Atasol®, etc.) does not contain acetylsalicylic acid and is a safe alternative for the treatment of fever and pain.

**10.  Is there a simple way at the pharmacy to find out which over-the-counter drugs should be used with caution or avoided?**

In Quebec, the Ordre des pharmaciens du Québec has developed a program called the "Code médicament" ("Drug Caution Code"). It consists of six letters, each letter corresponding to a specific warning. These code letters usually appear on the price sticker or the particular shelf where the medication is placed.

**Code letter "E"** specifically concerns people with diabetes. Products bearing an "**E**" are **not recommended**. There are three types:
1)  oral decongestants;
2)  drugs with a sugar content in the recommended dose that equals 20 calories or more **per dose** or 80 calories or more **per day**;
3)  keratolytic preparations (for the treatment of corns, calluses and warts).

In Quebec, a personalized "code médicament" card from your pharmacist will indicate the code letters that apply to you.

Elsewhere, ask your pharmacist whether there is a similar program in your area.

## 11. Can "natural health products" be used by people with diabetes?

There are a number of so-called "natural health products" on the market; it is important, however, to know that "natural" does not necessarily mean "harmless". In fact, some natural health products can have adverse effects, interact with prescribed drugs or be contraindicated for various illnesses.

In addition, the quality of natural health products on the market can vary widely, and it is not always possible to know exactly what they contain. An eight-digit natural product number (NPN) identifies products that are authorized for sale in Canada.

People with diabetes who choose to use a natural health product should ask a pharmacist to confirm whether the product is suitable. Doctors should also be informed of the products their patients use.

## 12. Can natural health products affect blood glucose levels?

Some natural health products can raise blood glucose levels, while others can lower them. For example, glucosamine, a supplement used for osteoarthritis, can increase glucose levels. Animal studies have also shown that it increases insulin resistance, although the effect of glucosamine on humans appears to be minimal. Nevertheless, because data is limited, people who decide to take glucosamine are advised to measure blood glucose levels regularly to observe the effects. Products that can lower blood glucose include fenugrec, vanadium, bitter melon (Momordica charantia), Gymnema sylvestre, chromium, American ginseng, and ivy gourd (*Coccinia grandis*).

It is generally advisable to consult a pharmacist or doctor before taking a natural health product to make sure it is both safe and effective. People with diabetes who decide to take a potentially hyperglycemic or hypoglycemic product should take care to observe its effect on their blood glucose levels.

According to currently available information and research, there are no natural products that can be recommended to replace oral antidiabetic drugs or insulin.

# Insulins

### 1. What is the role of insulin?

Insulin is a hormone that plays an important role in controlling blood glucose. It acts as a kind of "manager", keeping blood glucose levels down by allowing the glucose in the blood to enter the cells of the body and lowering the production of glucose by the liver.

### 2. When is insulin an appropriate treatment for diabetes?

Insulin is routinely used to treat **type 1 diabetes** because in this form of the disease, the pancreas does not produce insulin. It can also be used for **type 2 diabetes** if diet, exercise, weight loss and oral antidiabetic drugs are not enough to control blood glucose.

### 3. How are insulins produced?

Insulins are primarily manufactured in laboratories through biogenetic techniques using genetically programmed bacteria or yeast.

There are two categories of insulin:
1) **Human insulin:** This type is identical to the insulin produced by the pancreas. All insulins called Humulin® or Novolin® belong to this category.
2) **Analogue insulin:** This type is similar to the insulin produced by the pancreas, although its structure has been slightly modified in order to give it new properties. Some examples of this type include Humalog®, NovoRapid,® NovoMix,® Lantus® and Levemir®.

Some types of insulin are of animal origin (purified pork insulin), but they are rarely used. They are mentioned here for informational purposes only.

## 4. What are the different types of insulin?

Insulins are classified according to their action time:

- o **onset of action:** the time insulin takes to start working;
- o **peak of action:** the time during which the insulin is at maximum effectiveness;
- o **duration of action:** the duration of the insulin's effectiveness in the body.

There are six types of insulin:

1) rapid-acting;
2) short-acting;
3) intermediate-acting;
4) long-acting;
5) **premixed insulin** made of a mixture of rapid-acting and intermediate-acting insulins;
6) **premixed insulin** made of a mixture of short-acting and intermediate-acting insulins.

## 5. What are the action times of the different types of insulin?

| Type of insulin | Onset of action | Peak of action | Duration of action |
|---|---|---|---|
| **Rapid-acting** | | | |
| Humalog® (lispro)<br>NovoRapid® (aspart) | 0 to 15 minutes<br>0 to 10 minutes | 1 to 2 hours<br>1 to 3 hours | 3 to 4 hours<br>3 to 5 hours |
| **Short-acting** | | | |
| Humulin® R (Regular)<br>Novolin® ge Toronto | 30 minutes | 2 to 4 hours | 6 to 8 hours |
| **Intermediate-acting** | | | |
| Humulin® N<br>Novolin® ge NPH | 1 to 2 hours | 6 to 12 hours | 18 to 24 hours |
| **Long-acting** | | | |
| Lantus® (glargine)<br>Levemir® (detemir) | 1 hour<br>1 to 3 hours | Insignificant<br>Insignificant | 24 hours<br>20 to 24 hours |
| **Premixed rapid-acting and intermediate-acting** | | | |
| Humalog® Mix 25*<br>Humalog® Mix 50* | 0 to 15 minutes | 1 to 2 hours<br>and<br>6 to 12 hours | 18 to 24 hours |
| NovoMix® 30** | 10 to 20 minutes | 1 to 4 hours | up to 24 hours |
| **Premixed short-acting and intermediate-acting**\*\*\* | | | |
| Humulin® 30/70<br>Novolin® ge 30/70<br>Novolin® ge 40/60<br>Novolin® ge 50/50 | 30 minutes | 2 to 4 hours<br>and 6 to<br>12 hours | 18 to 24 hours |

\*   Humalog® Mix 25 is a mixture of 25% lispro insulin (rapid-acting insulin) and 75% lispro protamine insulin (intermediate-acting insulin).

Humalog® Mix 50 is a mixture of 50% each of these two types of insulin.

\*\*  NovoMix® 30 is a mixture of 30% aspart insulin (rapid-acting insulin) and 70% aspart protamine insulin (intermediate-acting insulin)

\*\*\*The first number corresponds to the percentage of short-acting insulin and the second to the percentage of intermediate-acting NPH insulin.

Note: The values indicated in the table may vary from one individual to another.

## TIME-ACTION PROFILE OF THE DIFFERENT TYPES OF INSULIN

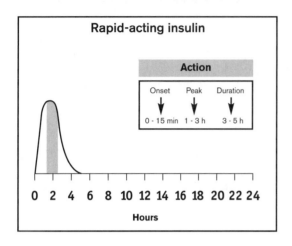

### Rapid-acting insulin

| Action | | |
| --- | --- | --- |
| Onset | Peak | Duration |
| 0 - 15 min | 1 - 3 h | 3 - 5 h |

Hours

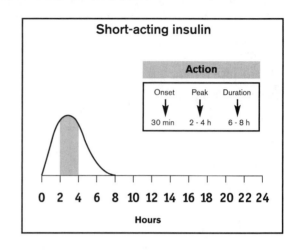

### Short-acting insulin

| Action | | |
| --- | --- | --- |
| Onset | Peak | Duration |
| 30 min | 2 - 4 h | 6 - 8 h |

Hours

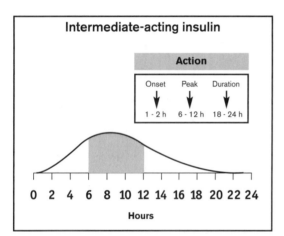

### Intermediate-acting insulin

| Action | | |
| --- | --- | --- |
| Onset | Peak | Duration |
| 1 - 2 h | 6 - 12 h | 18 - 24 h |

Hours

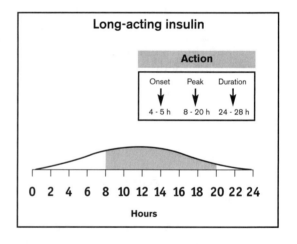

### Long-acting insulin

| Action | | |
| --- | --- | --- |
| Onset | Peak | Duration |
| 4 - 5 h | 8 - 20 h | 24 - 28 h |

Hours

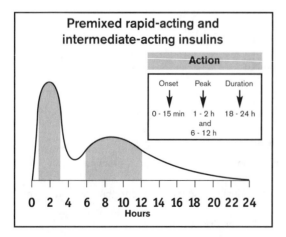

### Premixed rapid-acting and intermediate-acting insulins

| Action | | |
| --- | --- | --- |
| Onset | Peak | Duration |
| 0 - 15 min | 1 - 2 h and 6 - 12 h | 18 - 24 h |

Hours

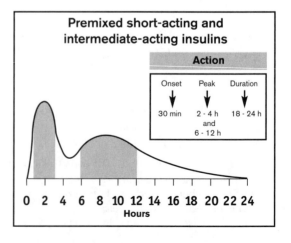

### Premixed short-acting and intermediate-acting insulins

| Action | | |
| --- | --- | --- |
| Onset | Peak | Duration |
| 30 min | 2 - 4 h and 6 - 12 h | 18 - 24 h |

Hours

**6. How many insulin injections are required daily?**

In general, insulin therapy requires from one to four injections daily. The number and timing of injections as well as the types of insulin vary from one person to another, and treatment is adapted to his or her lifestyle. The goal is to maintain blood glucose levels as close as possible to normal.

**7. What are the most frequently prescribed insulin regimens?**

There are several insulin regimens. Here are four of the most frequently prescribed:

1) The "**split-mixed**" regimen consists of injecting intermediate-acting and rapid or short-acting insulin before breakfast and dinner. The injection of intermediate-acting insulin before the evening meal is sometimes administered at bedtime to control glucose levels overnight and to help prevent nocturnal hypoglycemia.

2) The "**basal-prandial**" regimen consists of injecting rapid-acting or short-acting insulin before each meal and intermediate-acting or long-acting basal insulin at bedtime (also called and MDI regimen i.e. multiple daily injections). Although basal insulin is usually administered in one injection, it can also be given as two (occasionally more) injections throughout the day.

The rapid-acting or short-acting insulin dose may be fixed (fixed carbohydrate diet) or may correspond to the amount of carbohydrates consumed in the meal (variable carbohydrate diet). In a variable carbohydrate diet, the dose is defined as a ratio, as in 1 unit: 10 g of carbohydrates (1 unit of insulin for every 10 g of carbohydrates consumed).

3) The "**premixed**" regimen involves injecting a mixed dose of rapid-acting or short-acting insulin and intermediate-acting insulin before breakfast and dinner.

4) The "**combined**" regimen involves injecting intermediate-acting or long-acting

**8. What is intensive insulin therapy?**

Intensive insulin therapy consists of multiple insulin injections (for example, the "basal-prandial" regimen) or the use of an insulin pump, combined with monitoring blood glucose measurements and self-adjusted insulin doses. This therapy tries to imitate the normal release of insulin from the pancreas. The goal is to maintain blood glucose levels as close as possible to normal.

## 9. How much insulin is required to control blood glucose?

Insulin doses are initially determined by the doctor and vary according to blood glucose readings. The doses are measured in **units**. Some people inject fixed doses and others calculate their doses according to the carbohydrate content of meals. Whatever the regimen, doses should be regularly modified according to factors such as diet, exercise and illness.

## 10. How should insulin injections be timed in relation to meals and bedtime?

**Meals:**

o **Rapid-acting insulin** should be injected **just before meals** (or in the case of Humalog®, no more than 15 minutes before and NovoRapid®, no more than 10 minutes before), whether or not the insulin is premixed.

o **Short-acting insulin** should be injected **15 to 30 minutes before** meals, whether or not it is premixed.

This allows the peak action of the insulin to coincide with the peak absorption of the carbohydrates consumed.

**Bedtime:**

o **Intermediate-acting or long-acting insulin** is generally injected at approximately **10 p.m.** The injection time should be as regular as possible.

In the case of intermediate-acting insulin, the peak action coincides with breakfast.

## OPTIMAL INSULIN INJECTION TIMES

| Insulin | Optimal Injection Time |
|---|---|
| Humalog®<br>NovoRapid®<br>Humalog® Mix<br>NovoMix® | • Immediately before meals (at the most, 10 minutes beforehand for Novo and 15 minutes beforehand for Humalog).<br><br>• May be administered immediately after meals (e.g., in the case of variable appetite and unpredictable dietary intake). |
| Humulin® R<br>Novolin® ge Toronto<br>Humulin® 30/70<br>Novolin® ge 30/70, 40/60, 50/50 | • 15 to 30 minutes before meals. |
| Humulin® N<br>Novolin® ge NPH | • If taken at bedtime, always at the same time, usually around 10 p.m.<br><br>• If at breakfast and supper, at the same time as rapid or short-acting insulin |
| Lantus®<br>Levemir® | • Always at the same time, usually at bedtime, around 10 p.m.<br><br>• If twice a day, in the morning and at bedtime or with supper |

## 11. What is the most common adverse effect of insulin treatment?

**Hypoglycemia** is the most common adverse effect seen in people taking insulin. The risk of hypoglycemia is much higher when insulin action is at its peak. Being well-informed about insulin and the rules governing dosage adjustment can lower the risk.

## 12. How can insulin be used to effectively control diabetes?

To control diabetes with insulin injections, it is important to:

1) closely follow your **meal plan;**
2) **check blood glucose levels regularly;**
3) **be well-informed about the insulin you use;** and
4) **self-adjust** your insulin doses after receiving the necessary training from your diabetes health care team.

## 13. What time of day should a person with diabetes who is taking insulin check blood glucose?

A person with diabetes on insulin treatment should measure blood glucose before meals and at bedtime (before a snack). It is also helpful to occasionally measure blood glucose after meals (one or two hours after the first mouthful) or during the night (around 2 a.m.) to check for nocturnal hypoglycemia. If the person is sick, blood glucose measurements should be taken more often. It should also be measured every time the person feels discomfort that could indicate hypoglycemia or hyperglycemia.

## MAIN INSULIN REGIMENS

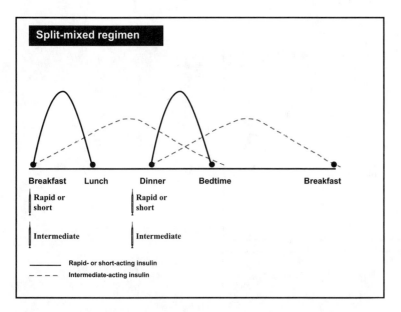

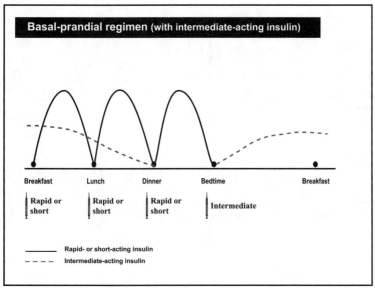

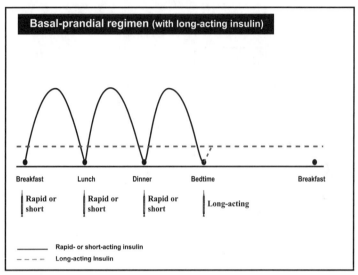

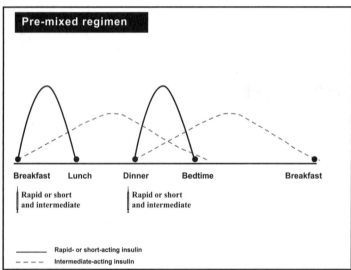

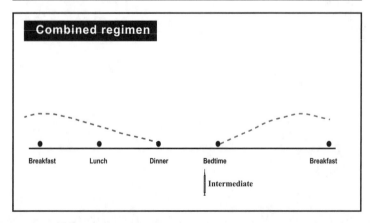

# Preparation and Injection of Insulin

### 1. What devices are used to inject insulin?

Two types of devices are available for insulin injection

1) **The syringe**: This device consists of a cylinder and a plunger equipped with a fine needle. Syringes have different capacities: 100 units, 50 units or 30 units. The finer the needle, the greater the gauge (for instance, a 30-gauge needle is finer than a 29-gauge needle). In addition, the finer the needle, the shorter it is (8 mm as opposed to 12.7 mm). Syringes also come with different scale graduations (½ unit, 1 unit and 2 units).

2) **The pen-injector**: This device is slightly larger than a pen and consists of three parts: the cap, which covers the pen, the cartridge-holder, which contains the insulin cartridge, and the pen body, which contains the plunger. A dosage ring allows you to select the desired dose.

### 2. What is involved in preparing and injecting a specific type of insulin with a syringe?

There are three steps involved in preparing and injecting a specific type of insulin with a syringe.

**Preparing the materials**
1) **Wash your hands** with soap and water and dry them well.
2) Lay out the **materials**: syringe, insulin vial, alcohol swab, cotton ball.
   - o   Use a new syringe for each injection.
   - o   Use a vial of insulin stored at room temperature.

3) Check the label of the vial to make sure you have the right **type of insulin.**

4) Check the **expiry dates** on the label: the date printed by the manufacturer and the date recorded after the vial was opened (*see the table in chapter 17 on page 154 listing the temperatures and maximum storage times recommended by insulin manufacturers*).

   o Do not prepare syringes in advance if the insulin used is Lantus®, which becomes foggy, or Levemir®, because of a lack of information regarding its stability.

**Drawing up the insulin**

1) If the **contents are opaque**, roll the vial between your hands and turn it upside down to mix the suspension well (**do not shake**). Replace the vial and place it on the table.

2) Disinfect the cap of the vial with the alcohol swab.

3) **Pull back the plunger** of the syringe to draw up an amount of air equal to the amount of insulin to be injected.

4) **Insert the needle** in the rubber cap of the insulin vial.

5) **Inject the air** into the vial.

6) **Turn the vial and syringe** upside down.

7) **Pull the plunger back slowly** to draw up the number of insulin units to be injected.

   o Make sure there are no air bubbles in the syringe; bubbles may cause a smaller amount of insulin to be injected.

   o Push and pull the plunger until any air bubbles disappear.

   o Check the syringe to make sure no insulin has been lost; if there has, repeat this step.

**Injecting the insulin and recording the data**

1) **Choose the injection area.**

   o Avoid injecting insulin into a limb or part of the body used for any physical activity (for example, a thigh if you intend to take a walk, an arm if you intend to play tennis, etc.).

2) **Choose the injection site** in the area, paying attention to the condition of the skin.

   o Avoid any crease, bump, growth, bruise, blotch or painful spot.

3) **Wash the skin** with soapy water, rinse and let dry.

   o Make sure the injection site is clean. The use of alcohol at home is optional.

4) **Pinch the skin between the thumb and forefinger and keep it pinched** until the end of the injection.

5) Hold the syringe like a pencil and **pierce the skin**.
   o The insulin should be injected into subcutaneous tissue (tissue beneath the skin).
6) **Inject all the insulin**, pushing the plunger all the way.
   o **Do not pull the plunger back:** raising the plunger to check whether the injection is at the right spot can damage the skin.
   o **Leave the needle in place** for about **5 seconds**.
7) **Withdraw the needle** and carefully press the cotton ball to the injection site.
8) **Record the number of insulin units** injected as well as the type of insulin in the appropriate column of the self-monitoring logbook.

## 3. What precautions should be taken when mixing two types of insulin in the same syringe?

When mixing clear and opaque insulin in the same syringe, certain precautions are necessary:

1) It is important to avoid contaminating a vial of one insulin with another insulin. The order of drawing up the insulins may vary from one diabetes clinic to another. Some clinics recommend drawing up clear rapid-acting insulin Humalog® or NovoRapid®) or short-acting insulin (Humulin® R or Novolin® ge Toronto) before opaque insulin (Humulin® N or Novolin® ge NPH). **Other clinics advise drawing up opaque insulin before clear insulin so that any contamination of the clear by the opaque can be easily detected.**

2) If one insulin is contaminated by another, the contaminated vial must be discarded because there is a risk that its time of action (start, peak, duration) has been modified. Insulin contaminated by another insulin can hinder the control of blood glucose.

3) It is important to always draw up the insulins in the same order; this will help avoid errors.

4) It is generally recommended to avoid mixing insulins from different manufacturers in the same syringe.

5) **Lantus® (glargine) and Levemir® (detemir) insulins must never be mixed with another insulin.**

**4. What is involved in preparing and injecting two types of insulin with the same syringe?**

There are three steps involved in preparing and injecting two types of insulin with the same syringe.

**Preparing the materials for injection**

1) **Wash your hands** with soap and water and dry them well.
2) Lay out the **materials**: syringe, insulin vials, alcohol swab, cotton ball.
   o   Use a new syringe for each injection.
   o   Use vials of insulin stored at room temperature.
3) Check the labels of the vials to make sure you have the right **types of insulin**.
4) Check the **expiry dates** on the labels: the date printed by the manufacturer and the date recorded after the vials were opened (*see the table in chapter 17 on page 154, listing the temperature and maximum storage times recommended by insulin manufacturers*).
   o   Do not prepare the syringes in advance if the insulin used is Lantus®, which becomes foggy, or Levemir®, because of a lack of information regarding its stability.

**Drawing up the insulins**

**The order of drawing up the insulins may vary from one diabetes clinic to another.**

1) **Roll the vial of opaque insulin** between your hands and turn it upside down to mix the suspension well (**do not shake**). Replace the vial and place it on the table.
2) **Disinfect the caps** of the vials of opaque insulin and clear insulin with an alcohol swab.
3) **Inject air into the vial of clear insulin.**
   o   Pull back the plunger of the syringe to draw in an amount of air equal to the amount of clear insulin to be injected. Insert the needle in the rubber cap of the clear insulin vial. Inject the air into the vial. Do not touch the insulin or draw any up. Withdraw the needle from the vial.
4) **Inject the air into the vial of opaque insulin.**
   o   Pull back the plunger of the syringe to draw in air equal to the amount of opaque insulin to be injected. Insert the needle in the rubber cap of the opaque insulin vial. Inject the air into the vial. Leave the needle in the vial.
5) **Draw up the required dose of opaque insulin.**
   o   Turn the opaque insulin vial and the needle upside down. Pull the plunger

back slowly to draw up the number of units of opaque insulin to be injected. Withdraw the needle from the vial.

- o Make sure there are no air bubbles in the syringe; bubbles may cause a smaller amount of insulin to be injected.
- o Push and pull the plunger until the bubbles disappear.
- o Check the syringe to make sure no insulin has been lost; if there has, repeat this step.

6) **Draw up the required dose of clear insulin.**

- o Turn the clear insulin vial upside down. Insert the needle in the rubber cap of the clear insulin vial. Do not introduce any opaque insulin into the clear insulin vial. Pull the plunger back slowly to draw up the number of units of clear insulin to be injected. Withdraw the needle from the vial.

  **If you have drawn up too much clear insulin:**
  - **discard** the insulin drawn up, but save the syringe;
  - **start** the process again, from the beginning.

  **If the vial of clear insulin is contaminated by opaque insulin:**
  - **discard** the vial of clear insulin;
  - **start** the process again from the beginning with a new vial.

### Injecting the insulins and recording the data

1) **Choose the injection area.**
   - o Avoid injecting insulin into a limb or part of the body used for any physical activity (for example, a thigh if you intend to take a walk, an arm if you intend to play tennis, etc.).
2) **Choose the injection site** in the area, paying attention to the condition of the skin.
   - o Avoid any crease, bump, growth, bruise, blotch or painful spot.
3) **Wash the skin** with soapy water, rinse and let dry.
   - o Make sure the injection site is clean. The use of alcohol at home is optional.
4) **Pinch the skin between the thumb and forefinger and keep it pinched** until the end of the injection.
5) Hold the syringe like a pencil and **pierce the skin**.
   - o The insulin should be injected into subcutaneous tissue (tissue beneath the skin).
6) **Inject all of the insulin**, pushing the plunger all the way.
   - o **Do not pull the plunger back**: raising the plunger to check whether the injection is at the right spot can damage the skin.
   - o Leave the needle in place for about **5 seconds**.

7) **Withdraw the needle** and carefully press the cotton ball to the injection site.
8) **Record the number of insulin units** injected as well as the type of insulin in the appropriate column of the self-monitoring logbook.

## 5. What different types of pen-injectors are currently available?

There are several models of pen injectors available (list revised as of May 1, 2008):

| Pen-injectors | Manufacturers | Cartridges | Graduation | Dosage dial |
|---|---|---|---|---|
| Huma Pen® Luxura HD | Eli Lilly Canada Inc. | 3 mL | 0.5 units at a time | 0.5 to 30 units |
| HumaPen® Luxura | Eli Lilly Canada Inc. | 3 mL | 1 unit at a time | 1 to 60 units |
| Humulin® N Pen (disposable) | Eli Lilly Canada Inc. | 3 mL | 1 unit at a time | 1 to 60 units |
| Humalog® Pen (disposable) | Eli Lilly Canada Inc. | 3 mL | 1 unit at a time | 1 to 60 units |
| Humalog® Mix 25 Pen (disposable) | Eli Lilly Canada Inc. | 3 mL | 1 unit at a time | 1 to 60 units |
| Novolin-Pen® Junior | Novo Nordisk Canada Inc. | 3 mL | 0.5 units at a time | 0.5 to 35 units |
| Novolin-Pen® 4 | Novo Nordisk Canada Inc. | 3 mL | 1 unit at a time | 1 to 60 units |
| Autopen® 24 (green) | sanofi aventis Canada Inc. | 3 mL | 1 unit at a time | 1 to 21 units |
| Autopen® 24 (blue) | sanofi aventis Canada Inc. | 3 mL | 2 units at a time | 2 to 42 units |
| Lantus® SoloSTAR (disposable) | sanofi aventis Canada Inc. | 3 mL | 1 unit at a time | 1 to 80 units |

• Check the product monograph for the type of insulin and the type of needle that can be used with the pen-injector selected.
• If using two types of insulin which have not been premixed, you may use two pen-injectors.

### 6.  How do you prepare for insulin injection with a pen-injector?

The preparation and injection of insulin with a pen-injector involves three steps.

**Preparing the materials**
1) **Wash your hands** with soap and water and dry them well.
2) Lay out the **materials**: pen-injector, insulin cartridge, needle, alcohol swab.
   - Use a new needle for each injection.
   - Use an insulin cartridge stored at room temperature.
3) Check the **type of insulin and the quantity of insulin** remaining in the cartridge.
4) Check the expiry dates on the label: the ones printed by the manufacturer and the ones recorded after the cartridges were opened (*see the table in chapter 17 on page 154, listing the temperatures and maximum storage time recommended by insulin manufacturers*).
   - Do not refrigerate the pen-injector; cold temperatures can damage it or cause air bubbles to form in the cartridge.
   - Do not share a pen-injector with anyone else.

**Selecting a dose of insulin**
1) **Bring opaque insulin to a uniform appearance.** Roll the pen between your palms about ten times to loosen the insulin from the sides, then turn the pen-injector over the same number of times. There is a glass marble inside the opaque insulin cartridge that slides from one end to the other to mix the insulin. Do not shake the pen vigorously, as this could harm the insulin and reduce its effectiveness.
2) **Screw the needle onto the pen and fill up the empty space in the needle** by selecting one unit of insulin at a time until a drop of insulin appears at the tip of the needle when pointed upwards.
3) **Select the insulin dose** by turning the dosage ring to the desired number of units.

**Injecting the insulin and recording the data**
1) **Choose the injection area.**
   - Avoid injecting insulin into a limb or part of the body used for any physical activity (for example, a thigh if you intend to take a walk, an arm if you intend to play tennis, etc.).
2) **Choose the injection site** in the area, paying attention to the condition of the skin.
   - Avoid any crease, bump, growth, bruise, blotch or painful spot.
3) **Disinfect the skin** with an alcohol swab and let it dry.
   - Make sure the injection site is clean. The use of alcohol at home is optional.

4) **Pinch the skin between the thumb and forefinger and keep it pinched** until the end of the injection with **needles measuring 8 mm to 12 mm.**

5) It is generally recommended not to pinch the skin when using **shorter needles (5 mm).**

6) Hold the pen injector like a pencil and **pierce the skin.**
   - o The insulin should be injected into subcutaneous tissue (tissue beneath the skin).

7) **Inject all of the insulin,** pushing the plunger down all the way.
   - o Leave the needle in place for about 15 seconds.

8) **Withdraw the needle** and carefully press the cotton ball to the injection
   - o **Remove** the needle from the pen-injector when the injection is complete. Discard the needle.

9) **Record the number of insulin units** injected as well as the type of insulin in the appropriate column of the self-monitoring logbook.

## 7. What are the recommended insulin injection techniques?

Insulin should be injected into subcutaneous tissue (the tissue beneath the skin).

1) The proper techniques for injecting insulin are a **subject of controversy.**

2) To ensure a personalized insulin injection technique, it should be chosen with the help of a **health professional.** Several factors have to be taken into account, including age (child or adult) and weight (thin or obese). The length of the needle, the need to pinch the skin, and the angle of injection can vary from person to person.
   - o **Most people can reach subcutaneous tissue by injecting at a 90° angle.** However, **thin people or children** may need to pinch the skin, use short needles or inject at a 45° angle to avoid injecting into muscle tissue, especially in the thigh.
   - o **Blood** at the injection site can indicate that a muscle has been penetrated. If this occurs, injections should be done at a 45° angle or with short needles (5 mm and 6 mm).
   - o A **white area** appearing when the needle is withdrawn can indicate that the insulin has not been injected deeply enough.
   - o When the technique requires injection into a **cutaneous fold,** pinch the skin between the thumb and forefinger and keep it pinched until the injection is finished.

    o    Blood glucose levels must be checked more carefully if a **change is made from a long needle to a short needle**. Insulin absorption must remain at the same level.

3) There have not yet been any studies concerning the maximum subcutaneous insulin dose that can be administered at one site. Several factors have to be taken into account, such as the volume of insulin injected at once, the method of injection, the speed of insulin absorption and pain at the injection site.

    o    **In some cases it is recommended that the dose be distributed between two injection sites to make absorption easier.**

    o    One of the factors affecting the speed of subcutaneous insulin is the volume injected. The greater the volume of insulin, the more slowly it is absorbed, and the longer it will take before noticeable absorption begins.

    o    Studies have shown that in most cases, pain at the injection site increases when the volume injected is greater than 50 units.

## 8. What should be done with used prefilled disposable pen injectors, syringes, needles and lancets?

A system for the disposal of used prefilled disposable pen injectors, syringes, needles and lancets has been implemented to ensure that these items are not left in inappropriate places and cause accidents.

Ideally, special containers that may be obtained for free in pharmacies and in Community Health Centres should be used for disposal. Once filled, the container may be brought to one of four places for disposal: a pharmacy, a Community Health Centre, a diabetes clinic or a participating community organization. If no special containers are available, the used material may be placed in a safely sealed plastic container for disposal.

# Insulin Injection: Injection Site Rotation

1.  **What part of the body is the best place to inject insulin?**
    Insulin can be injected in different regions of the body. There are eight standard **"injection areas"**:

|                   |               |                                                                            |
| ----------------- | ------------- | -------------------------------------------------------------------------- |
| **Areas 1 and 2** | **Abdomen:**  | right and left sides, except for 2.5 cm (1 inch) around the belly button   |
| **Areas 3 and 4** | **Arms:**     | antero-external surface                                                     |
| **Areas 5 and 6** | **Thighs:**   | antero-external surface                                                     |
| **Areas 7 and 8** | **Buttocks:** | fleshy upper parts                                                         |

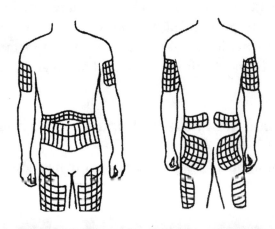

Unless it is possible to fold the skin (create a cutaneous fold), injecting into the distended abdomen of a pregnant woman can damage the skin and is not recommended.

**2. How many injection sites are there in each area?**

There are a number of places within each **injection area**, known as "**injection sites**", where insulin can be injected. The entire surface of each area can be used, as long as the same injection site **is not used more than once a month**.

**3. What distance should there be between injection sites within the same area?**

Within the same area, each **injection site** must be at least 1 cm (1/2 inch) from the site of the previous injection:

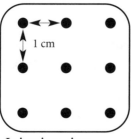

Injection sites

**4. Why should a new site be used for each injection?**

Injection sites should be rotated **for each insulin injection** to prevent **lipodystrophy** (bumps and cracks from repeated injections at the same site). Not only are these subcutaneous deformations unattractive, more importantly, they hamper the absorption of insulin and the proper control of blood glucose.

**5. Does the injection area have an impact on the absorption of the insulin injected?**

Yes. The speed of absorption of any one type of insulin varies according to the injection area used.

Insulin is absorbed most quickly in the abdomen, followed by the arms, thighs and buttocks, in that order.

> **Speed of absorption: abdomen > arms > thighs > buttocks**
>
> > = greater than

## 6. What other factors influence the speed of insulin absorption?

Intense exercise increases the rate of absorption if the insulin is injected into the part of the body being exercised.

- o   For example, insulin injected into your thigh is absorbed more quickly if you take a walk or play tennis afterwards.

Other factors such as heat (sun, bath, etc.), the depth of the injection, or massage near the site can affect the speed of absorption.

## 7. How can the amount of insulin absorbed be maintained at a stable level despite injection site rotation?

To ensure that the amount of insulin absorbed varies as little as possible, the following steps should be taken:

1) Inject rapid-acting and short-acting insulin into the **abdomen**, either alone or mixed with intermediate-acting insulin. Change the injection site each time.
2) For greater convenience, regularly inject rapid-acting or short-acting insulin into the **arm** before lunch. This will ensure that the peak effect of the midday injection will be more or less the same every day, allowing dosages for this time of day to be adjusted accordingly.
3) To ensure that absorption is as slow as possible, inject intermediate-acting or long-acting insulin that is not mixed with rapid-acting or short-acting insulin into the **thigh or buttocks**.
4) If several injections are administered at different times of the day, the same injection area should be used at the same time every day.
5) A particular area (taking into account speed of absorption) should be used for a given insulin (taking into account time of action) according to the time of injection (taking into account activity level).

6) Lantus® (glargine) and Levemir® (determir) insulins are long-acting and can meet basal insulin needs with one daily injection. Sometimes two injections are necessary. These insulins are usually injected in areas of slow absorption, such as the thigh. The speed of absorption of Lantus, however, is the same regardless of the area of injection.

In summary:

| TYPE OF INSULIN | SUGGESTED AREAS OF INSULIN INJECTION | | |
|---|---|---|---|
| | Abdomen | Arm | Thighs and buttocks |
| Rapid-acting or short-acting, alone | Preferable | Before lunch, for greatest convenience | – |
| Rapid-acting or short-acting mixed with intermediate-acting | Preferable | – | – |
| Intermediate-acting, alone | – | – | Preferable |
| Long-acting, alone | – | – | Preferable |

# Storage of Insulin

### 1. Why should precautions be taken when storing insulin?

Insulin is fragile. To ensure that they do not lose their effectiveness, insulin solutions should be stored according to the manufacturers' recommendations. Using improperly stored insulin can impair blood glucose control.

### 2. What precautions should be taken when storing insulin?

1) Insulin that is **currently in use** can be stored for up to **one month at room temperature**. Injecting cold insulin can cause pain at the injection site.

2) **Reserve supplies** of insulin should be kept in the **refrigerator**. If stored this way, the insulin will remain usable until the expiry date indicated by the manufacturer.

3) Insulin should never be exposed to direct sunlight or heat. Although the product will not necessarily change in appearance, if it is exposed to excessive heat it must be discarded.

4) Insulin should never be frozen. Although the product will not necessarily change in appearance, if it freezes it must also be discarded.

5) A pen injector must not be stored in the refrigerator; this could damage it or create air bubbles in the cartridge.

6) Spare insulin syringes that have been prepared in advance should be kept in the refrigerator in an upright or slightly slanted position, with the needle (and its cap) pointing upwards. This will prevent insulin particles from clogging the needle.

7) The date the insulin was opened should be written in the space provided for this purpose on the container.

8) There should always be a reserve of insulin stored in the refrigerator for an emergency, such as breakage.

### 3. What are some specific recommendations for storing insulin?

The following table shows the temperatures and storage times recommended by insulin manufacturers, listed by the format and brands they sell.

| Format | Brand | Recommended temperature | Maximum storage length |
|---|---|---|---|
| Unopened vial or cartridge | Humulin® Humalog® | 2 °C-8 °C | Expiry date on container |
| | Novolin® NovoRapid® NovoMix® | 2 °C -10 °C | Expiry date on container |
| | Lantus® Levemir® | 2 °C -8 °C | Expiry date on container |
| Opened vial | Humulin® | 18 °C -25 °C (max. 25 °C) | 1 month |
| | Humalog® | 18 °C -25 °C (max. 30 °C) | 1 month |
| | Novolin® | 18 °C -25 °C (max. 25 °C) | 1 month |
| | NovoRapid® | 18 °C -25 °C (max. 37 °C) | 1 month |
| | NovoMix® | 18 °C -25 °C (max. 30 °C) | 1 month |
| | Lantus® | 15 °C-30 °C (max. 30 °C) | 1 month |
| Opened cartridge | Humulin® | 18 °C -25 °C (max. 25 °C) | 1 month |
| | Humalog® | 18 °C -25 °C (max. 30 °C) | 1 month |
| | Novolin® NovoRapid® | 18 °C -25 °C (max. 37 °C) | 1 month |
| | Lantus® | 15 °C -30 °C (max. 30 °C) | 1 month |
| | Levemir® | 18 °C -25 °C (max. 30 °C) | 42 days |

| Format | Brand | Recommended temperature | Maximum storage length |
|---|---|---|---|
| Unopened preloaded disposable pen injector | Humulin® N Pen<br>Lantus®<br>SoloSTAR | 2°C - 8°C | Expiry date on container |
| | Humalog® Pen<br>Humalog® Mix 25 Pen | 2°C - 10°C | Expiry date on container |
| Opened preloaded disposable pen injector | Humulin® N Pen | 18°C - 25°C<br>(max. 25°C) | 1 month |
| | Humalog® Pen | 18°C - 25°C<br>(max. 30°C) | 1 month |
| | Humalog® Mix 25 | 18°C - 25°C<br>(max. 30°C) | 1 month |
| | Lantus® SoloSTAR | 15°C - 30°C<br>(max. 30°C) | 1 month |
| Syringe, prepared in advance* | Humulin®<br>Humalog® | 2°C - 8°C | 3 weeks |
| | Novolin®<br>NovoRapid® | 2°C - 10°C | Use as quickly as possible |

\* It is not recommended to prepare syringes in advance when using Lantus® because it becomes foggy or Levemir® because of a lack of data regarding its stability.

## 4. What should insulin look like?

Insulin comes either in a clear solution that resembles water or in a cloudy suspension that is milky in appearance.

| Clear Insulin | | Cloudy Insulin | |
|---|---|---|---|
| Rapid: | Humalog®<br>NovoRapid® | Intermediate: | Humulin® N<br>Novolin® ge NPH |
| Short: | Humulin® R<br>Novolin® ge Toronto | Premixed: | Humulin® 30/70<br>Humalog® Mix 25<br>Humalog® Mix 50<br>Novolin® ge 30/70<br>Novolin® ge 40/60<br>Novolin® ge 50/50<br>NovoMix® 30 |
| Long: | Lantus®<br>Levemir® | | |

## 5. When should clear insulin be discarded?

**Clear** insulin should be discarded if:

  o   it looks cloudy;
  o   it is thick;
  o   the solution contains solid particles;
  o   it has been exposed to extreme temperatures (heat or cold);
  o   the recommended expiry date has passed.

## 6. What precautions should be taken with cloudy insulin?

Cloudy insulin is a suspension that needs to be **mixed well** before being used.

A whitish deposit at the bottom of the vial or in the cartridge is normal, but it must be remixed into the suspension. The vial should be rolled between the palms and turned upside down, or the cartridge should be turned over in the pen injector several times. **Do not shake.**

Improperly mixed cloudy insulin can hamper the precision of measured insulin doses.

7.  **When should cloudy insulin be discarded?**

Cloudy insulin should be discarded if:

- o    a deposit remains at the bottom of the vial or in the cartridge;
- o    there are specks floating in the insulin;
- o    particles are stuck to the sides of the vial or cartridge, making the containers look frosty;
- o    it has been exposed to extreme temperatures (heat or cold);
- o    the expiry date has passed.

# Insulin Dose Adjustment

### 1.  Why do insulin doses need to be adjusted?

The goal of insulin dose adjustment is to improve the control of blood glucose levels. Ideally, a person with diabetes self-adjusts doses after receiving the appropriate information from his or her health care team.

### 2.  What blood glucose levels should be targeted when adjusting insulin doses?

Most people with diabetes should aim for **target blood glucose levels** between 4 mmol/L and 7 mmol/L before meals and between 5 mmol/L and 10 mmol/L one or two hours after meals. In cases where there is no risk, however, they are advised to aim for **normal blood glucose levels**, that is, between 4 mmol/L and 6 mmol/L before meals and between 5 mmol/L and 8 mmol/L one or two hours after meals.

### 3.  What are the rules governing insulin dose adjustment?

The following rules are a guide to making safe decisions about insulin dose adjustment. The basic principles are the following:

- o   insulin lowers blood glucose levels;
- o   current blood glucose reflects what happened before.

Before any insulin dose adjustment, time must be taken to analyze blood glucose levels by taking the average of the last three readings for each period of the day (morning, noon, evening and bedtime), going back a maximum of seven days. Only levels recorded since the last adjustment should be considered.

The six suggested rules for adjusting insulin doses are the following:

1) The calculation of the average should not take into account any measurement below 4 mmol/L or above 7 mmol/L that is associated with a **situation that is isolated, exceptional or explainable.**

2) Never adjust insulin doses based on only **one blood glucose test.** Generally speaking, adjusting an insulin dose to correct blood glucose at one given moment is not recommended.

3) Always adjust **only one insulin dose** at a time, at one time of day.

4) Correct **hypoglycemia** first, starting with the first of the day, then the second, etc.
   - **Hypoglycemia** can be identified by the following:
     - the average is below 4 mmol/L for a given period of the day;
     - even if the average for a given time of day is greater than or equal to 4 mmol/L, the last two readings or three non-consecutive readings over the last seven days have revealed hypoglycemia.
   - A value of 2 mmol/L is assigned to any hypoglycemia that has not been measured.
   - A hypoglycemic reading taken outside the four usual blood glucose measuring periods should be recorded for the following period (for example, a hypoglycemic reading measured in the morning should be recorded in the "before lunch" column).

5) Next, correct **hyperglycemia**, that is, when average blood glucose at a given time of day is higher than 7 mmol/L. Begin with the first episode of the day, then the next, and so on.
   - Watch out for **rebound hyperglycemia**. Rebound hyperglycemia is a blood glucose reading **above** 7 mmol/L that follows hypoglycemia. This type of hyperglycemia should not be considered when calculating the average. Nocturnal hypoglycemia can cause rebound hyperglycemia upon waking. When in doubt, take a blood glucose reading around 2 a.m. and if necessary correct the hypoglycemia instead of waiting to correct the hyperglycemia.

6) It is recommended to wait at least two days after an adjustment before making any new modifications. The only exception is when there are two consecutive nocturnal or morning hypoglycemic readings, in which case the rule must be disregarded and the dose of insulin that caused it must be decreased.

## 4. What are the most frequently prescribed insulin regimens?

There are a number of different insulin regimens. The four most commonly prescribed are the following.

1) The **split-mixed regimen** involves injecting one intermediate-acting insulin (e.g. Humulin® N or Novolin® ge NPH) and one rapid-acting (Humalog® or NovoRapid®) or short-acting insulin (Humulin® R or Novolin® ge Toronto) before breakfast and dinner. Sometimes, the injection of intermediate-acting insulin before dinner should be delayed until bedtime to avoid nocturnal hypoglycemia.

2) The **basal-prandial regimen** consists of injecting one rapid-acting (Humalog® or NovoRapid®) or short-acting insulin (Humulin® R or Novolin® ge Toronto) before each meal and one intermediate-acting (for example, Humulin® N or Novolin® ge NPH) or long-acting insulin (Lantus® or Levemir®) at bedtime. Although basal insulin is usually administered in one injection, it can also be administered in more than one injection during the course of the day. The dose of rapid-acting or short-acting insulin can be fixed (fixed carbohydrate regimen) or measured according to the amount of carbohydrates consumed in a meal (variable carbohydrate regimen). In the variable carbohydrate regimen the dose is determined according to a ratio, such as 1 unit: 10 g of carbohydrates, that is, 1 unit of insulin per 10 g of carbohydrates consumed.

3) The **premixed regimen** involves injecting one premixed insulin (for example, Humulin® 30/70, Novolin® ge 50/50, Humalog® Mix 25, NovoMix®30, etc.) before breakfast and dinner.

4) The **combined regimen** involves injecting one intermediate-acting insulin (Humulin® N or Novolin® ge NPH) or long-acting insulin (Lantus® and Levemir®) at bedtime, in addition to oral antidiabetic drugs during the day.

## 5. In the split-mixed regimen, which insulins affect blood glucose levels during the day?

| Insulin | affects | blood glucose levels measured |
|---|---|---|
| Intermediate-acting before dinner | ⟶ | before breakfast |
| Rapid-acting or short-acting before breakfast | ⟶ | before lunch |
| Intermediate-acting before breakfast | ⟶ | before dinner |
| Rapid-acting or short-acting before dinner | ⟶ | at bedtime (before the snack) |

Blood glucose levels at any given moment reflect the action of the previous insulin injection.

## 6. How should insulin doses be adjusted in the split-mixed regimen?

In general, when **hypoglycemia (average blood glucose below 4 mmol/L)** occurs before meals and at bedtime (as defined in the adjustment rules), the insulin dose should be **decreased** by two units at a time. If the **total daily dose** of insulin is less than or equal to 20 units, the dose that caused it should be reduced by one unit at a time.

In general, when **hyperglycemia (average blood glucose above 7 mmol/L)** occurs before meals and at bedtime (as defined in the adjustment rules), the insulin dose should be **increased** by two units at a time. If the **total daily dose** of insulin is less than or equal to 20 units, the dose that caused it should be increased by one unit at a time.

It is recommended to wait at least two days after any insulin dose adjustment before making any new changes. In the event of hypoglycemia or hyperglycemia, the insulin dose that caused it must be adjusted within one week.

7.  **In the basal-prandial regimen, which insulins affect blood glucose levels at different times of day?**

| Insulin | affects | blood glucose levels measured |
|---|---|---|
| Intermediate- or long-acting at bedtime | ⟶ | before breakfast |
| Rapid acting or short acting before breakfast | ⟶ | before lunch |
| Rapid-acting or short-acting before lunch | ⟶ | before dinner |
| Rapid-acting or short-acting before dinner | ⟶ | at bedtime (before the snack) |

> Blood glucose levels at any given moment reflect the action of the previous insulin injection.

8.  **How should insulin doses be adjusted in the basal-prandial with fixed carbohydrate regimen?**

    In general, when **hypoglycemia (average blood glucose below 4 mmol/L)** occurs before meals and at bedtime (as defined by the adjustment rules), the insulin dose should be **decreased** by two units at a time. If the **total daily dose** of insulin is less than or equal to 20 units, however, the dose that caused it should be reduced by one unit at a time.

    In general, when **hyperglycemia (average blood glucose above 7 mmol/L)** occurs before meals and at bedtime (as defined by the adjustment rules), the insulin dose should be **increased** by two units at a time. If the **total daily dose** of insulin is less than or equal to 20 units, however, the dose that caused it should be increased by one unit at a time.

It is recommended to wait at least two days after an insulin dose adjustment before making any new changes. The only exception is when two consecutive episodes of hypoglycemia occur during the same period, in which case the rule must be disregarded and the dose of insulin that caused it must be decreased. In the event of hypoglycemia or hyperglycemia, the insulin dose that caused it must be adjusted within one week.

9. **How should insulin doses be adjusted in the basal-prandial with variable carbohydrate regimen?**

When **hypoglycemia (average blood glucose below 4 mmol/L)**, as defined by the rules of adjustment, occurs:

1) during the night or before breakfast, the dose of intermediate-acting (for example, Humulin® N or Novolin® ge NPH) or long-acting insulin (Lantus® or Levemir®) must be decreased by two units at a time. If the daily dose of intermediate-acting or long-acting insulin is less than or equal to 10 units, however, the dose should be decreased by only one unit at a time;

2) before lunch, dinner or bedtime, the dose of insulin that caused it (Humalog®, NovoRapid®, Humulin® R or Novolin® ge Toronto) must be **decreased** by 0.2 units/10 g of carbohydrates. If the dose of insulin is less than or equal to 0.5 units/10 g of carbohydrates, however, the dose should be decreased by only 0.1 unit/10 g of carbohydrates at a time.

If **hyperglycemia (average blood glucose above 7 mmol/L)**, as defined by the rules of adjustment, occurs:

1) during the night or before breakfast, the dose of intermediate acting (for example, Humulin® N or Novolin® ge NPH) or long acting insulin (Lantus® or Levemir®) should be increased by two units at a time. If the daily dose of intermediate acting or long acting insulin is less than or equal to 10 units, however, the dose should be increased by only one unit at a time;

2) before lunch, dinner or bedtime, the dose of insulin that caused it (Humalog®, NovoRapid®, Humulin® R or Novolin® ge Toronto) must be increased by 0.2 units/10 g of carbohydrates. If the dose of insulin is less than or equal to 0.5 units/10 g of carbohydrates, the dose should be increased by only 0.1 unit/10 g of carbohydrates at a time.

It is recommended to wait at least two days after an insulin dose adjustment before making any new changes. The only exception is when two consecutive episodes of hypoglycemia occur during the same period, in which case the rule must be disregarded and the dose of insulin that caused it must be decreased. In the event of hypoglycemia or hyperglycemia, the insulin dose that caused it must be adjusted within one week.

### 10. In the premixed regimen, which insulins affect blood glucose levels at different times of day?

| Premixed insulin | affects | blood glucose levels measured |
|---|---|---|
| Rapid-acting or short-acting and intermediate-acting insulin before breakfast | ⟶ | before lunch and before dinner |
| Rapid-acting or short-acting and intermediate-acting insulin before dinner | ⟶ | at bedtime (before the snack) and before breakfast |

Blood glucose levels at any given moment reflect the action of the previous insulin injection.

### 11. How should insulin doses be adjusted in the premixed regimen?

In general, when **hypoglycemia (average blood glucose below 4 mmol/L)** as defined by the adjustment rules occurs before meals and at bedtime, the mixed insulin dose that caused it should be **decreased** by two units at a time. If the **total daily dose** of insulin is less than or equal to 20 units, however, the dose should be reduced by only one unit at a time.

In general, when **hyperglycemia (average blood glucose above 7 mmol/L)** as defined by the adjustment rules occurs, the mixed insulin dose that caused it should be **increased** by two units at a time. If the **total daily dose** of insulin is less than or equal to 20 units, the dose should be increased by only one unit at a time.

It should be recalled that premixed insulins are responsible for two periods of the day at a time. Consequently, if there is a difference between blood glucose at bedtime and in the morning (for example, elevated at bedtime and low in the morning) or between blood glucose before lunch and before dinner, **a doctor should be consulted, as this could mean that the mixture has to be changed.**

It is recommended to wait at least two days after an insulin dose adjustment before making any new changes. In the event of hypoglycemia or hyperglycemia, the insulin dose that caused it must be adjusted within one week

## 12. In the combined regimen, which blood glucose reading is affected by insulin administered at bedtime?

In the combined regimen, **morning blood glucose** is affected by intermediate acting or long acting insulin administered at bedtime.

## 13. How should insulin doses be adjusted in the combined regimen?

In general, when morning **hypoglycemia (average blood glucose below 4 mmol/L)** as defined by the adjustment rules occurs, the bedtime insulin dose should be **decreased** by two units at a time. If the total daily dose of insulin is less than or equal to 10 units, however, the dose should be reduced by only one unit.

In general, when morning **hyperglycemia (average blood glucose above 7 mmol/L)** as defined by the adjustment rules occurs, the bedtime insulin dose must be **increased** by two units at a time. If the total daily dose of insulin is less than or equal to 10 units, however, the dose should be increased by one unit.

It is recommended to wait at least two days after an insulin dose adjustment before making any new changes. In the event of hypoglycemia or hyperglycemia, the insulin dose that caused it must be adjusted within one week.

### Practical Examples

It is important to understand the rules of adjustment described in this chapter before attempting any insulin dose adjustment. The following practical examples can be useful:

### Example 1
Treatment: Split-mixed regimen:

| | |
|---|---|
| Humulin® R | 12 units at breakfast and 10 units at dinner |
| Humulin® N | 20 units at breakfast and 14 units at dinner |
| Total daily dose of insulin = 56 units | |

**Self-monitoring logbook:**

| | Blood Glucose | | | |
|---|---|---|---|---|
| **Date** | **Before breakfast (mmol/L)** | **Before lunch (mmol/L)** | **Before dinner (mmol/L)** | **At bedtime (mmol/L)** |
| 16/05 | 6.4 | 7.7 | 6.5 | 5.7 |
| 17/05 | 7.1 | 9.3 | 7.0 | 5.4 |
| 18/05 | 5.9 | 7.5 | 6.2 | 6.0 |
| Average | 6.5 | 8.2 | 6.6 | 5.7 |

### Analysis:
In this example, blood glucose levels before lunch are above 7 mmol/L (hyperglycemia). The appropriate adjustment is to increase the morning dose of short-acting insulin by two units.

### Example 2
Treatment: basal-prandial with fixed carbohydrate regimen:

| | |
|---|---|
| NovoRapid® | 8 units at breakfast, 6 units at lunch, 6 units at dinner |
| Novolin® ge NPH | 16 units at bedtime |
| Total daily dose of insulin = 36 units | |

**Self-monitoring logbook:**

| Date | Blood Glucose | | | |
| --- | --- | --- | --- | --- |
| | Before breakfast (mmol/L) | Before lunch (mmol/L) | Before dinner (mmol/L) | At bedtime (mmol/L) |
| 03/01 | 12.0 | 9.0 | 8.0 | 6.5 |
| 04/01 | 13.0 | 8.7 | 7.2 | 5.8 |
| 05/01 | 11.7 | 8.9 | 7.8 | 5.6 |
| Average | 12.2 | 8,.9 | 7.7 | 6.0 |

**Analysis:**

In this example, hyperglycemia occurs before breakfast, lunch and dinner. The first hyperglycemia of the day, the one occurring before breakfast, should be corrected first. To do so, the NPH insulin taken at bedtime should be **increased** by 2 units to 18 units. It is still a good idea to **check blood glucose** at 2 a.m., however, to ensure there is no nocturnal hypoglycemia that could cause rebound hyperglycemia in the morning. If nocturnal hypoglycemia does occur, the bedtime dose of NPH insulin should be **decreased** by 2 units.

**Example 3**

Treatment: basal-prandial with variable carbohydrate regimen:

| Humalog® | 1.2 units/10 g of carbohydrates at breakfast |
| --- | --- |
| | 1.0 unit/10 g of carbohydrates at lunch |
| | 0.8 units/10 g of carbohydrates at dinner |
| Lantus® | 12 units at bedtime |

Self-monitoring logbook:

| Date | Blood Glucose | | | |
|---|---|---|---|---|
| | **Before breakfast (mmol/L)** | **Before lunch (mmol/L)** | **Before dinner (mmol/L)** | **At bedtime (mmol/L)** |
| 13/04 | 5.4 | 6.4 | 4.4 | 5.8 |
| 14/04 | 5.9 | 6.0 | 3.6 | 5.0 |
| 15/04 | 5.3 | 5.6 | 2.8 | 5.2 |
| Average | 5.5 | 6.0 | 3.6 | 5.3 |

**Analysis:**

In this example, two episodes of **hypoglycemia** are detected in the last two blood glucose readings taken before dinner. The appropriate adjustment is to **decrease** the insulin dose before lunch by 0.2 units/10 g of carbohydrates, or in other words, from 1.0 unit/10 g to 0.8 units/10 g of carbohydrates.

# The Insulin Pump:
## Another Treatment Option

### 1.  What is an insulin pump?

An insulin pump is a device consisting of:

1)  a reservoir or cartridge containing insulin;
2)  an electric motor to inject insulin from the reservoir;
3)  a catheter (cannula) attached to the insulin reservoir and equipped with a small needle that is inserted beneath the skin of the abdomen, where the insulin is injected.

An insulin pump administers insulin subcutaneously on a continual basis, 24 hours a day; this is called the **basal rate**. The basal rate fills all insulin needs regardless of meals (basal dose). The pump can be programmed to provide different basal rates to meet insulin needs that vary according to the time of day. Before meals, an extra dose is injected via the pump to meet insulin needs associated with meals; this is called the **bolus dose**. The continual release of insulin along with the pre-meal bolus imitates the normal function of the pancreas.

Generally, insulin pumps use rapid-acting insulin such as Humalog® or NovoRapid®.

The insulin pump is not an artificial pancreas. It does only what it is programmed to do.

### 2.  What are the indications for using an insulin pump?

Current indications for using an insulin pump tend to be restrictive because the equipment is expensive. The following indications are usually recognized:

1) serious hypoglycemia (requiring the help of a third person) on more than one occasion (two or more over the last twelve months);
2) great blood glucose lability (instability) requiring repeated medical attention (two or more hospitalizations over the last twelve months);
3) inadequate control of blood glucose (glycosylated hemoglobin ≥ 8%) despite an attempt at intensive insulinotherapy;
4) accelerated progression of complications (retinopathy and/or neuropathy) with sub-optimal control of blood glucose (glycosylated hemoglobin > 7%).

The insulin pump can also be an option in the following situations:
1) pregnancy;
2) a request from a diabetic person who wants to intensify treatment;
3) a person with a very irregular schedule or very active lifestyle.

### 3. How much does insulin pump treatment cost?

An insulin pump costs approximately $6,500, and the materials required (needles, catheters, insulin, etc.) can cost between $2,000 and $4,000 a year.

### 4. Is insulin pump treatment covered by medical insurance?

No. Provincial medical insurance does not cover the purchase cost of an insulin pump or the materials required. Some private insurance companies, however, will cover up to 80% of the costs if the justification for this type of treatment is accepted. Other companies will contribute a maximum, non-renewable amount.

### 5. What should I do if I think I could benefit from insulin pump treatment?

First, discuss it with your endocrinologist. If insulin pump treatment is appropriate, you must:
1) check with your insurance company to see whether it covers insulin pump treatment costs;
2) get the following from your doctor:
    o   a prescription for an insulin pump;
    o   a letter justifying the indication for insulin pump treatment, to be submitted to your insurance company.

## 6. What procedures should be followed when using an insulin pump?

Using an insulin pump requires instruction from a qualified health care team.

An endocrinologist prescribes and adjusts insulin doses. The instructions received should include:
1) how the pump functions;
2) how to install the catheter and how to choose the injection area;
3) how to calculate carbohydrates;

The endocrinologist will provide information about the procedures to follow and the people to contact.

## 7. How is insulin pump dosage determined?

Generally, rapid-acting insulin (Humalog® or NovoRapid®) is used. To determine the **basal dose**, begin with 50% of the total insulin dose for the day according to prior treatment (for example, total dose for 24 hours = 40 units, so 40 ÷ 2 = 20 units for the basal dose). When determining the daily distribution of the basal dose, the two following two points must be considered: 1) generally speaking, people are most sensitive to insulin between midnight and 4 a.m. and are therefore the most vulnerable to hypoglycemia during these hours; 2) people are generally most resistant to insulin between 4 a.m. to 8 a.m and therefore more insulin is required during this period. The midnight basal rate should therefore be decreased by 25% and the 4 a.m. rate increased by 25-50%.

For example, if the amount of insulin is 20 units per 24 hours, the basal rate is 0.8 units/hour (20 units ÷ 24 hours = 0.8 units/hour). However, when the information above is taken into account, the basal rate can be decreased by 25% between midnight and 4 a.m. (to 0.6 units/hour) and increased by 50% between 4 a.m. and 8 a.m. (to 1.2 units/hour).

To determine the **pre-meal bolus insulin dose**, begin with 1.0 unit per 10 g of carbohydrates for each meal, then adjust the dose as needed. For example, a meal containing 60g of carbohydrates requires a dose of 6 units: (60 g ÷ 10 g) x 1.0 unit = 6 units.

## 8. Are there always different basal rates for different times of day?

Not necessarily. However, there are five distinct periods in a day and it is possible for basal requirements to vary with each one

**Period 1:** 12 a.m. (midnight) – 4 a.m. People are most vulnerable to hypoglycemia during these hours and it may be necessary to deliver less insulin.

**Period 2:** 4 a.m. – 8 a.m. People are more insulin-resistant during this period and may need more insulin

**Period 3:** 8 a.m. – 12 p.m. (noon). This is a more active period of the day and may require a lower basal rate.

**Period 4:** 12 p.m. (noon) – 6 p.m. This is a more active period of the day and may require a lower basal rate.

**Period 5:** 6 p.m. – 12 a.m. (midnight). This less active period may require a higher basal rate.

## 9. Which blood glucose readings are used to adjust the basal rate?

It is important to identify the blood glucose readings during the day that reflect the basal rate for each period. These readings can be used as a basis for making adjustments.

| Period | | Basal blood glucose |
|---|---|---|
| Midnight to 4 a.m. | ⟶ | 2 a.m. |
| 4 to 8 a.m. | ⟶ | before breakfast (around 7-8 a.m.) |
| 8 a.m. to 12 noon | ⟶ | before lunch (around 11 a.m.-noon) |
| 12 noon to 6 p.m. | ⟶ | before dinner (around 4-6 p.m.) |
| 6 p.m. to midnight | ⟶ | bedtime (around 11 p.m.-midnight) |

## 10. Which blood glucose readings are used to adjust the pre-meal bolus dose?

The bolus for each meal is adjusted according to the postprandial blood glucose reading (1 or 2 hours after the meal).

| Meal | Postprandial blood glucose (1 or 2 hours after a meal) |
|------|--------------------------------------------------------|
| Breakfast ⟶ | after breakfast |
| Lunch ⟶ | after lunch |
| Dinner ⟶ | after dinner |

## 11. What are the target blood glucose levels?

**Basal blood glucose:**

Most people are advised to target a blood glucose level between 4 mmol/L and 7 mmol/L before meals and at bedtime (before the snack). If there is no risk, however, normal blood glucose should be targeted, that is, between 4 mmol/L and 6 mmol/L before meals and bedtime (before the snack).

**Postprandial blood glucose:**

The recommended postprandial blood glucose level is higher than the pre-meal blood glucose. Most people should aim for a postprandial target blood glucose level between 5 mmol/L and 10 mmol/L (1 or 2 hours after the meal). If there is no risk, however, normal blood glucose should be targeted, that is, between 5 mmol/L and 8 mmol/L 1 or 2 hours after meals.

## 12. What are the insulin adjustment rules?

Before insulin doses are adjusted, blood glucose levels should be analyzed by calculating the average of the last two or three readings for each period of the day (before meals, after meals and at bedtime), going back no further than seven days. Only readings done since the last adjustment should be taken into account.

There are six insulin adjustment rules:

1) In the calculation of the average, do not take into account any measurements lower than 4 mmol/L or higher than 7 mmol/L that are associated with an **isolated, exceptional and explainable** situation.

2) Never adjust insulin doses on the basis of only **one blood glucose reading**. Adjusting insulin dosage to correct blood glucose at any one given moment is generally discouraged.

3) Adjust **only one insulin dose** at a time (basal or bolus) and for one time of day only.

4) Correct **hypoglycemia** first, starting with the first of the day.
   - **Basal hypoglycemia** occurs when:
     - the basal blood glucose average for a given period of the day is below 4 mmol/L;
     - the last two readings or two of three non-consecutive hypoglycemic readings taken over the last seven days for the same time of day reveal hypoglycemia, even if the average is equal to or greater than 4 mmol/L.
   - **Postprandial hypoglycemia** occurs when:
     - average postprandial blood glucose levels after a meal are lower than average blood glucose levels before the same meal;
     - the last two postprandial readings or two of three non-consecutive readings over the last seven days for the same meal reveal blood glucose levels lower than before the meal, even if average postprandial blood glucose levels are higher than average blood glucose levels before the meal.
   - Assign a value of 2 mmol/L to any hypoglycemia that has not been measured.
   - Hypoglycemia that occurs outside the usual blood glucose measuring periods should be recorded under the following period (for example, hypoglycemia occurring at 11 a.m. is entered in the "before lunch" column).

5) Next, correct **hyperglycemia**, which occurs when the basal blood glucose level for the same time of day is greater than 7 mmol/L or the postprandial blood glucose level is greater than 10 mmol/L. Begin with the first of the day, followed by the second, and so on.
   - **Watch out for rebound hyperglycemia.** Rebound hyperglycemia is a basal blood glucose level above 7 mmol/L that follows hypoglycemia. This type of hyperglycemia should not be considered when calculating the average.

6) Wait at least two days after adjusting a dose before making any other changes.

## 13. How should insulin doses be adjusted?

The basal rate is determined according to blood glucose measured at 2 a.m., before meals and at bedtime. The bolus rate is determined according to blood glucose measured 1 or 2 hours after meals. These values are then used to adjust insulin doses as follows:

**Basal:**
- If hypoglycemic → decrease the corresponding basal rate by 0.1 unit/hour to 0.2 units/hour.
- If hyperglycemic → increase the corresponding basal rate by 0.1 unit/hour to 0.2 units/hour.

**Bolus:**
- If hypoglycemic → decrease the bolus by 0.1 unit to 0.2 units/ 10 g of carbohydrates.
- If hyperglycemic → increase the bolus by 0.1 unit to 0.2 unit/10 g of carbohydrates.

## 14. What types of insulin pumps are available in Canada?

The following table presents a list of the latest generation of insulin pumps currently on market, along with a few of their features (list revised as of May 1, 2008, adapted from a document entitled "Comparaison des pompes à insuline" from the Quebec University Hospital).

| MODEL | Accu-Chek® Spirit | Animas® 2020 | Cozmo® | Paradigm® • 522 • 722 |
|---|---|---|---|---|
| **Manufacturer or distributor** | Disetronic Medical Systems Inc. | Johnson & Johnson | Auto Control Médical | Medtronic |
| **Weight of pump (in grams)** | 79 | 88 | 90 | 100 108 |
| **Size (cm)** | 8.1 x 5.6 x 2.1 | 7.62 x 5.08 x 2.18 | 8.8 x 5 x 1.9 | 8.6 x 5 x 1.8 9.6 x 5 x 1.8 |
| **Colour** | blue | blue, silver, black, pink and green | blue, black, purple | transparent, smoke, blue, purple |
| **Reservoir** | 315 units | 200 units | 300 units | 176 units 300 units |
| **Connection** | Luer lock | Luer lock | Luer lock | Luer lock Paradigm |
| **Suggested batteries** | AA alkaline or rechargeable (1 battery) | AA alkaline or lithium (1 battery) | AAA alkaline (1 battery) | AAA alkaline (1 battery) |
| **Battery lifespan** | alkaline (1 month); rechargeable (1 week) | lithium (5-7 weeks) alkaline (2-3 weeks) | 1 month | 4-6 weeks |
| **Watertightness** | 60 mins at 2.5 metres | 24 hrs at 3.6 metres | 3 mins at 3.6 metres or 30 mins at 2.4 metres | 30 mins at 1 metre |
| **Base delivery** | 0.1 to 25 units/hr | 0.025 to 25 units/hr | 0.05 to 35 units/hr | 0.05 to 35 units/hr |
| **Basal release** | Every 3 mins | Every 3 mins | Every 3 mins | Total dose administered over 60 minutes in increments or stages of 0.05 |
| **Temporary basal rate** | 0% to 250% 15 mins – 24 hrs | 0% to 200% 30 mins – 24 hrs | 0% to 250% 30 mins – 72 hrs | 0% to 200% 30 mins – 24 hrs |
| **Bolus calculator** | On a Palm PDA | yes | yes | yes (touch screen) |

| MODEL | Accu-Chek® Spirit | Animas® 2020 | Cozmo® | Paradigm® • 522 • 722 |
|---|---|---|---|---|
| **Bolus** | 0.1 to 25 units (in increments or stages of 0.1, 0.2, 0.5, 1 and 2) | 0.05 to 35 units (increments or stages of 0.05) | 0.05 to 75 units (increments or stages of 0.05 – 0.1 – 0.5 – 1 – 2 and 5) | 0.1 to 25 units (increments or stages of 0.1) |
| **Length of bolus for 1 unit** | 5 secs | 1 or 4 secs | adjustable 1-5 mins | 40 secs |
| **Memory** | 30 events per categories (bolus, alerts, daily totals, temporary basal rate) | 500 bolus, 120 daily totals | 4,000 events | 90 days (through software) 24 bolus on pump |
| **downloading software** | yes Accu-check Smart Pix | yes Ezmanager | yes Cozmanager | yes Carelink Pro software (for professionals) or Carelink Personnal (for patients) or Web site at www.carelink.minimed.com |
| **Blood glucose meter** | Aviva or Compact Plus | One Touch model | Cozmonitor Freestyle IR (communicates results in the pump via infrared) | Contour® Link (communicates results in the pump via radio frequency) |
| **Specific features** | Bolus calculator on a Palm PDA; 12 languages; reversible screen; tactile buttons; emergency pump | Colour screen Personalized food list with carbohydrates option | Blood glucose meter that attaches to the pump | Continual REAL Time blood glucose system on pump screen Alarms for hypo/hyperglycemia |

| MODEL | Accu-Chek® Spirit | Animas® 2020 | Cozmo® | Paradigm® • 522 • 722 |
|---|---|---|---|---|
| **Technical support** | 1-866-703-3476 | 1-866-406-4844 | 1-800-630-0864 | 1-800-284-4416 |
| **Price** | $6,395 for pump, Palm PDA and emergency pump | $6,895 | $6,500 | $6,800 (Minilink Transmitter $700) |
| **Internet address** | www.disetro nic-ca.com www. accuchek.ca | www.animas. ca | www.autocon trol.com | www.minimed.ca www.medtro nic.com |

\* Prices may vary. Additional material can cost between $2,000 and $4,000 a year.

## 15. When should the injection site be changed?

1) Immediately:
   o if you feel pain or discomfort;
   o if two corrective bolus doses fail to reduce an elevated blood glucose (blocked catheter);
   o if ketone bodies are present in the blood or urine, for no apparent reason;
   o if you see blood in the catheter.

2) Every 24 to 48 hours:
   o if you use a steel needle set;
   o if you are pregnant.
3) Every 48 to 72 hours:
   o if you use a flexible cannula set.

It is generally recommended that the **perfusion device (that is, the reservoir, tubing and catheter) be replaced every 48 to 72 hours**. The suggested frequency of replacement varies according to the pump, brand of insulin and type of catheter used.

# Physical activity

### 1. What is physical activity?

Physical activity is defined as any bodily movement produced by the muscles and requiring an expenditure of energy.

### 2. Why is regular exercise so important?

Regular exercise is beneficial for everyone, whether or not they have diabetes. There are certain risks associated with inactivity.

Regular physical activity leads to the following benefits:
1) better health, improved physical fitness, increased self-esteem;
2) better posture and balance;
3) strengthening of the muscles and bones;
4) energy recovery;
5) weight control;
6) lower blood lipid levels;
7) relaxation and stress control;
8) increased autonomy in later years;

The risks associated with inactivity are the following:
1) early death;
2) heart disease;
3) obesity;
4) high blood pressure;
5) diabetes;
6) osteoporosis;
7) stroke;
8) depression;
9) colon cancer.

3. **What are the benefits of a regular exercise program for people with glucose intolerance (pre-diabetic state) or people with diabetes?**

People with glucose intolerance and people with diabetes derive the same benefits from exercise as people with normal glucose tolerance. However, people who are glucose intolerant and engage in moderate regular physical activity decrease their risk of developing diabetes. People with type 2 diabetes who engage in regular physical activity decrease their resistance to insulin and are better able to control their diabetes.

Regular exercise is as beneficial for people with type 1 diabetes as it is for people who do not have diabetes. It is vital, however, for people with diabetes to control their illness and adjust insulin doses and diet according to their physical activity.

4. **How should a successful exercise program be approached?**

1) First, choose a sport or activity that you like. Dancing, mild gymnastics, swimming, working out, and speed-walking are all examples of simple and pleasant physical activities. The important thing is to choose something that appeals to you. This will increase the likelihood that you will do it on a daily basis.

2) Include the activity in your daily schedule. The more physical activity a person engages in every day, the greater his or her sense of well-being. Daily life offers a number of opportunities for exercise:

   o   walking or biking to work;

   o   taking the stairs instead of the elevator;

   o   doing manual tasks such as sweeping, cleaning windows, gardening, etc.

According to recent recommendations, all adults between 18 and 65 years old should have at least **150 minutes of moderate physical activity per week, or 30 minutes, five times a week.**

5. **What is considered a good physical fitness program to help control diabetes?**

1) The exercises selected require **moderately intense levels of effort**.

2) The person exercises most days of the week, **at least five days a week.**

3) The person exercises an average of **at least 30 minutes a day**. The physical activity can be performed for shorter periods of at least 10 minutes per session.

The most accessible exercise is **speed-walking**. Walking quickly, but at a pace that allows conversation without breathlessness, is considered to be an activity of moderate intensity.

The energy expended by engaging in regular physical activity helps people maintain a healthy weight.

6. **What are some low, moderate, and elevated intensity exercises?**
   The following chart ranks examples of physical activities according to the length and intensity of effort they generally require.

| | |
|---|---|
| Washing and waxing a car (45-60 mins) | **Less intense**<br>**Longer** |
| Washing floors and windows (45-60 mins) | |
| Gardening (30-45 mins) | |
| Moving around in a wheelchair (30-40 mins) | ↑ |
| Walking 3 km in 35 minutes (12 mins/km) | |
| Dancing (fast, for 30 mins) | |
| Walking with a baby (2.5 km in 30 mins) | |
| Raking leaves (30 mins) | |
| Walking 3.5 km in 30 minutes (8½ mins/km) | |
| Aqua-fitness (30 mins) | |
| Swimming (20 mins) | |
| Biking 6.5 km in 15 minutes | |
| Running 2.5 km in 15 minutes (6 mins/km) | ↓ |
| Shoveling snow or climbing stairs (15 mins) | **More intense**<br>**Shorter** |

## 7. How can the exercise be pleasurable, effective and safe? How can I ensure that I progress at my own speed?

It is strongly recommended that people beginning an exercise program start out slowly and increase their pace little by little. Knowing how to measure out your physical effort is therefore critical and a good way to assess your abilities and progress. There are a number of ways to set your own pace.

1) **The degree of breathlessness:** Find the level where your breathing is deeper than when at rest but you are still able to have a conversation.

2) **Pulse or heart rate (HR):** Exercise is considered moderate when your pulse falls between 50% and 70% of your maximum heart rate. If an exact measurement of your maximum heart rate is not available, it can be estimated by subtracting your age from 220 beats per minute. To determine the moderate zone, this result should be multiplied by 50% or 70%.

For example, if a person is 45 years old:

(220 - 45) x 50% = 87.5

(220 - 45) x 70% = 122.5

Moderate exercise means a heart rate between 88 and 123 beats per minute. This estimate does not, however, take into account drugs that can affect heart rate.

The following table can help you determine whether the intensity is appropriate:

| Time needed depends on effort | | | | |
|---|---|---|---|---|
| Very Light Effort | Light Effort<br>*60 minutes* | Moderate Effort<br>*30-60 minutes* | Vigorous Effort<br>*20-30 minutes* | Maximum Effort |
| • Strolling<br>• Dusting | • Light walking<br>• Volleyball<br>• Easy gardening<br>• Stretching | • Brisk walking<br>• Biking<br>• Raking leaves<br>• Swimming<br>• Dancing<br>• Water aerobics | • Aerobics<br>• Jogging<br>• Hockey<br>• Basketball<br>• Fast Swimming<br>• Fast aerobics | • Sprinting<br>• Racing |
| | How does it feel? How warm am I? What is my breathing like? | | | |
| • No change from rest state<br>• Normal breathing | • Starting to feel warm<br>• Slight increase in breathing rate | • Warmer<br>• Greater increase in breathing rate | • Quite warm<br>• More out of breath | • Very hot/perspiring heavily<br>• Completely out of breath |
| | Range needed to stay healthy | | | |

Handbook for *Canada's Physical Activity Guide to Healthy Active Living*. Ottawa, Ontario, K1A 0S9. Tel.: 1-888-334-9769; Website: http://www.phac-aspc.gc.ca/pau-uap/paguide/index.html

3) **The Borg Perceived Effort Scale:** This scale, which measures an individual's subjective perception of his or her effort, is easy to use. It is an excellent way to assess the intensity of physical activity undertaken by people who are taking drugs that affect their heart rate. An intensity of 12-13 corresponds to a moderate level of effort (see illustration below). Although the measurement is subjective, an estimate of perceived effort can provide a fairly reliable assessment of the person's actual heart rate during the physical activity.

The Borg scale should be referred to while the physical effort is taking place. The scale ranges from 6 to 20, with 6 signifying "no effort at all" and 20 signifying "exhaustion" or "maximal effort". Choose the number the best corresponds to your perception of your effort. It will give a good idea of the intensity of your physical activity and will guide you either to accelerate or slow down your movements to achieve the intensity you want. An accurate estimate depends on your being as honest as possible in your evaluation of your exertion.

| BORG SCALE | |
|---|---|
| **Perceived effort** | |
| | 6 |
| Extremely light (7.5) | 7 |
| | 8 |
| Very light | 9 |
| | 10 |
| Light | 11 |
| | 12 |
| Somewhat hard | 13 |
| | 14 |
| Hard | 15 |
| | 16 |
| Very hard | 17 |
| | 18 |
| Extremely strenuous | 19 |
| | 20 |

8. **When is exercise dangerous for people with diabetes?**

Exercise can be risky and contraindicated when a person's diabetes is poorly controlled and blood glucose is:

1) lower than 4 mmol/L;
2) above 14.0 mmol/L and there are ketone bodies in the urine or blood;
3) above 17.0 mmol/L, whether or not there are ketone bodies in the urine or blood.

In some cases, people with diabetes can engage in regular physical activity, although they must always make careful choices regarding the type of activity they engage in.

For example:

1) **if the person with diabetes has a heart problem**, he or she should only undertake an exercise program under medical supervision;
2) **if the person with diabetes has eye problems with a risk of hemorrhage**, he or she should take up physical activities such as swimming, walking and riding a stationary bike instead of anaerobic activities such as weightlifting or activities that can involve blows or jolts, such as boxing, racket sports (tennis, badminton) and jogging;
3) **if the diabetic person has serious neuropathy with complete loss of sensation in the feet**, he or she should take up activities such as swimming, biking, rowing, arm exercises or exercises performed while seated.

Generally speaking, walking for short periods remains one of the least risky activities, even in such special cases.

9. **What potential risks does exercise present for a person with diabetes who is taking oral antidiabetic medications or insulin?**

People with diabetes being treated with insulin or drugs that stimulate the pancreas to produce more insulin (e.g. glyburide, gliclazide, repaglinide) run a higher risk of **hypoglycemia**, especially if the activity is unplanned, prolonged, and of moderate intensity.

It should be remembered that:

1) moderate exercise sustained for several hours can cause delayed hypoglycemia as long as 12 to 16 hours after the activity. For example, cross-country skiing, house-cleaning or even several hours of shopping can all provoke delayed hypoglycemia;

2) the more regular the activity (schedule, duration and intensity), the lower the risk of hypoglycemia.

## 10. What precautions should be taken when planning to exercise?

1) Blood glucose should be measured **before** any physical activity, regardless of the treatment regimen.
2) The condition of the feet should be checked **before and after** any exercise.
3) Alcohol should not be consumed **before, during or after** exercise.
4) People with diabetes should always wear a diabetic ID bracelet or pendant.
5) People with diabetes should also have quickly metabolized carbohydrate sources on hand.
6) People taking insulin are advised to use an injection site in an area that will be the least involved in the exercise, such as the abdomen.

## 11. What can people with diabetes who are taking insulin do to prevent hypoglycemia when exercising?

**People with diabetes who are taking rapid or short acting insulin** before meals should know how to adapt their treatment to prevent hypoglycemia when exercising.

1) When the activity is **planned and takes place 1 to 2 hours after a meal**, the insulin dose before the meal should be reduced, according to the type of exercise, its duration, its intensity, the training involved and above all, the person's **experience**.

The following table provides an example of how to decrease the insulin dose before the meal:

| Intensity of effort | Percentage (%) reduction in the rapid or short acting insulin dose, according to duration of exercise | |
|---|---|---|
| | 30 minutes | 60 minutes |
| Low | 25% | 50% |
| Moderate | 50% | 75% |
| Elevated | 75% | 100% |

Let us take, for example, a man with diabetes who injects 10 units of insulin before a meal. He plans on taking an hour-long walk at moderate intensity immediately after the meal. He can reduce the insulin dose by 75% and inject 2.5 (or 3) units before the meal.

75% x 10 units = 7.5 units

10 units – 7.5 units = 2.5 (or 3) units.

2)  When the activity is **unplanned and takes place immediately before or after a meal,** or when the activity is **planned but takes place more than two hours after a meal:**

   o   **for blood glucose below 5.0 mmol/L**, have a carbohydrate snack (15 g to 30 g) at the beginning of the activity, and approximately every 30 to 45 minutes afterward, while the activity lasts;

   o   **for blood glucose above 5.0 mmol/L**, have a snack of about 15 g of carbohydrates every 30 to 45 minutes while the activity lasts.

Blood glucose should always be measured immediately **after exercising** to adjust the amounts of insulin and carbohydrates required.

In all cases, the need for insulin can decrease after exercise. This sometimes requires reducing the insulin dose for the next meal or at bedtime.

## 12. What can people with diabetes do to prevent hypoglycemia when exercising if they are taking oral antidiabetic drugs that stimulate the secretion of insulin?

For people with diabetes who are taking **drugs that stimulate the pancreas to produce insulin (for example, glyburide, gliclazide, repaglinide)**, the only way to lower the risk of hypoglycemia is to consume more carbohydrates while exercising. Anyone who regularly experiences hypoglycemia after exercising, however, is strongly advised to contact his or her doctor.

The recommendations are:

   o   **for blood glucose below 5.0 mmol/L**, have a carbohydrate snack (15 g to 30 g) at the beginning of the activity and then approximately every 30 to 45 minutes afterwards, while the activity lasts.

o **for blood glucose above 5.0 mmol/L,** additional carbohydrates are only necessary if the hypoglycemia occurs during the exercise. It is essential to check the blood glucose levels before eating, in order to avoid overeating. If more carbohydrates are needed, have a snack of about 15 g of carbohydrates every 30 to 45 minutes during the activity can provide what is necessary.

The following chart* can serve as a guide for adding carbohydrates during exercise. Additional carbohydrates are especially useful during unplanned exercise and almost always necessary during exercise that lasts a long time or is quite intense, resulting in a significant expenditure of energy.

| Type of exercise | Blood glucose (mmol/L) | Additional carbohydrates |
|---|---|---|
| Short duration (< 30 min) at light intensity | < 5.0<br>> 5.0 | 10 g to 15 g<br>not necessary |
| Moderate duration (30 to 60 min) at moderate intensity | < 5.0<br>5.0 - 9.9<br>10.0 - 13.9 | 30 g to 45 g<br>15 g every 30 to 45 min of exercise<br>not necessary |
| Long duration (> 60 min) at elevated intensity | < 5.0<br>5.0 - 9.9<br>> 9.9 | 45 g<br>30 g to 45 g<br>15 g per hour |

*Adapted from Hayes C. *J Am Diet Assoc 97* (suppl 2): S167-S171

## 13. What precautions are appropriate for people with diabetes who take insulin or oral antidiabetic drugs that stimulate the secretion of insulin?

People with diabetes treated with insulin or oral antidiabetic drugs that stimulate the secretion of insulin must do the following:

1) always measure blood glucose before, during and after a session of exercise, and more often than normal in the 24 hours following prolonged physical activity;
2) always carry foods containing carbohydrates to correct hypoglycemia.

## 14. Should exercise be done in one long session or several shorter ones?

A 30-minute session of exercise has a hypoglycemic effect, which is often desired, but it also requires adjusting insulin doses or eating more carbohydrates. The same amount of exercise performed in three ten-minute sessions has little hypoglycemic effect and requires little or no insulin adjustment or additional carbohydrates, but it still provides the sought-after benefits.

| Risk of hypoglycemia from physical activity according to antidiabetic medication* | |
| --- | --- |
| **Class of medication** | **Risk of hypoglycemia** |
| Biguanides (e.g., metformin) | No |
| Alpha-glucosidase inhibitors (e.g., acarbose) | No |
| DPP-4 inhibitors (e.g., sitagliptin) | No |
| Thiazolidinedione (e.g., pioglitazone) | No |
| Sulfonylureas (p. ex., glyburide) | Yes |
| Non-sulfonylurea secretagogues (e.g., repaglinide) | Yes |
| Insulin | Yes |

* People taking drugs associated with a risk of hypoglycemia must speak with their doctor about dose adjustment or whether to ingest carbohydrates when exercising.

# Hyperglycemic Emergencies:

## Diabetic Acidosis and the

## Hyperosmolar State

**1.   What are the two hyperglycemic emergencies that can affect a person with diabetes?**

The two hyperglycemic emergencies that can affect a person with diabetes are:

- o    diabetic acidosis;
- o    the hyperosmolar state.

These two conditions are caused by a lack of insulin. Diabetic acidosis is more common in people with type 1 diabetes. Hyperosmolar states occur primarily in people with type 2 diabetes, usually when they are older. It is possible, however, for both conditions to occur simultaneously in people with either type 1 or type 2 diabetes.

**2.   What is diabetic acidosis?**

Diabetic acidosis is caused by a lack of insulin. It is characterized by hyperglycemia and an accumulation of ketone bodies in the blood. The ketone bodies, which are acids, are produced by the breakdown of fats. They make the blood acidic, which can cause **excessive fatigue, abdominal pains, nausea and vomiting**. Diabetic acidosis also gives the breath a fruity odour and causes intense thirst as well as deep and rapid breathing; in some cases, it provokes disorientation and confusion. It can also sometimes result in a **coma**, which can be fatal if not treated.

Diabetic acidosis occurs primarily in people with type 1 diabetes, although it can also occur in people with type 2 diabetes when there are other aggravating factors such as infection, myocardial infarction (heart attack), pancreatitis or stroke.

### 3. What causes diabetic acidosis?

Diabetic acidosis is always caused by a **shortage of insulin** in the blood. When there is insufficient insulin, glucose cannot enter certain cells of the body and accumulates in the blood at extremely high levels. The body is then forced to draw on its reserves of fat for energy. The **breakdown of fats** causes the liver to produce ketone bodies. The ketone bodies, which are acids, then accumulate in the blood and spill over into the urine.

This complication of diabetes can occur if **insulin injections are skipped or doses miscalculated.**

Diabetic acidosis is sometimes caused by an **increased need for insulin** (this can happen, for example, when a person gets an infection or is under exceptional stress).

### 4. How is diabetic acidosis detected?

Diabetic acidosis is detected by the **presence of ketone bodies** in the urine or blood; these are accompanied by elevated blood glucose levels, often higher than **20 mmol/L.**

### 5. How can diabetic acidosis be avoided?

Diabetic acidosis can be avoided in most cases by taking the following precautions:
1) **Check blood glucose levels regularly.** If necessary, check for ketone bodies in the urine using Ketostix® test strips or determine the level of ketone bodies in a blood sample from the fingertip, using the Precision Xtra® meter. Take these readings **more frequently** when ill, under exceptional stress, and especially if glucose readings are **higher than 14 mmol/L.**
2) Follow a **dietician-recommended meal plan.**
3) **Take insulin** as prescribed.

4)  **Follow the advice and instructions** of the doctor and dietician concerning the nutrients that should be ingested in both solid and liquid form and the **insulin** doses that should be injected when an illness makes it difficult or impossible to follow a normal diet.

5)  **Call the doctor or go to the emergency room if any one of the following five situations occurs:**
    o   **blood glucose is higher than 20 mmol/L;**
    o   the **ketosis level reading (ketone bodies) in the urine is moderate (4 mmol/L) or large (8 mmol/L –16 mmol/L);**
    o   **the ketosis level reading from the fingertip is above 3 mmol/L;**
    o   **you are vomiting continually and cannot retain liquids;**
    o   the **following conditions persist** despite treatment: excessive fatigue, weakness, dizziness, abdominal pains, nausea and vomiting, fruity breath odour, intense thirst, fast and heavy breathing.

## 6.  What is a hyperosmolar state?

A hyperosmolar state usually occurs in people with type 2 diabetes who develop an **increased resistance to insulin**. Insulin resistance prevents **glucose** from entering the cells properly, leading to its **accumulation in the blood.**

If kidney function is slightly impaired, it is more difficult to eliminate excess sugar in the blood through the urine. Sugar can therefore accumulate in the blood until it reaches very high levels (**above 30 mmol/L**), especially if not enough fluids are ingested. The small amount of insulin present in the blood at this point is usually sufficient to prevent the breakdown of fats, however, and diabetic acidosis generally does not develop.

In a hyperosmolar state, blood glucose levels rise and the person feels extremely tired and thirsty (although some elderly people feel no thirst). Frequent and profuse urination also occurs, leading to dehydration. This can be followed by a drop in blood pressure and in some cases disorientation, which can lead to coma and, if left untreated, even death.

**7.   What causes a hyperosmolar state?**

In all cases, a hyperosmolar state is caused by a **shortage of insulin** in the blood. Because there is not a complete absence of insulin, however, ketone bodies do not form and diabetic acidosis does not develop.

This complication of diabetes can occur if antidiabetic drugs (insulin or pills) are **skipped**.

A hyperosmolar state is sometimes caused by an **increased need for insulin** (for example, in the case of illness, infection or exceptional stress, or when the subject is using certain medications such as cortisone).

Most of the time, a hyperosmolar state occurs in people who **do not feel thirst** or who are unable to hydrate themselves, which is sometimes the case for elderly people or individuals who have lost autonomy.

**8.   How is a hyperosmolar state detected?**

The symptoms of a hyperosmolar state are generally **intense thirst, frequent and increased urination over several days**, and in particular, **blood glucose levels over 30 mmol/L**. There is usually no accumulation of ketone bodies in the blood or urine.

**9.   How can a hyperosmolar state be avoided?**

The following tips can generally help a person avoid a hyperosmolar state.

1)   **Stay hydrated**; drink 250 mL of water every hour if blood glucose levels are high or if high glucose levels cause an increased amount and frequency of urination.
2)   **Measure blood glucose levels regularly** during illness or in times of exceptional stress.
3)   **Follow the meal plan** recommended by the dietician.
4)   Take antidiabetic **drugs** (pills or insulin) as prescribed.
5)   **Follow the recommendations** of the doctor and dietician concerning the appropriate **nutrients** to consume in solid and liquid form and the **antidiabetic drug dosages** (pills or insulin) to be taken when illness makes it impossible to follow a normal diet.

| Suggested approach to the detection and treatment of diabetic acidosis and/or hyperosmolar states | | | |
|---|---|---|---|
| **Blood glucose (mmol/L)** | **Ketosis level reading (mmol/3) in urine or blood** | **Symptoms** | **Suggested action** |
| 13 - 14 | None, or trace Urine: 0.5 Blood: less than 0.6 | Frequent urination Intense thirst | • Drink 250 ml of water every hour • Measure blood glucose levels every 6 hours |
| 14 - 20 | small Urine: 1.5 Blood: 0.6 to 1.5 | Frequent urination Intense thirst | • Drink 250 ml of water every hour • Measure blood glucose every 4 hours • Adjust insuline doses according to the **rules of adjustment** • Contact your doctor |
| 14 - 20 | Moderate Urine: 4 Blood: 1.5 to 3 | Frequent urination Intense thirst Nausea Vomiting Abdominal pain (Diarrhea) | • Measure blood glucose and ketone bodies every 4 hours • **Immediately** adjust the insulin dose to follow the **sick day recommendations** (see boxed insert, next page) • Contact the doctor or go to the emergency room if there is no improvement |
| More than 20 | Moderate to large Urine: 8 to 13 Blood: more than 3 | Nausea Vomiting Abdominal pain (Diarrhea) Fruity breath | • Go to the hospital* |
| More than 30 | None or small Urine: 0 to 1.5 Blood: 0 to 0.6 | Frequent urination Intense thirst Extreme weakness | • Go to the hospital** |

\*   Diabetic acidosis
\*\* Hyperosmolar state

## SLIDING SCALE FOR ADJUSTING INSULIN DOSES ON SICK DAYS

For example, in addition to units calculated for meals, one unit of rapid- or short-acting insulin may be added for each mmol/L above a blood glucose level of 14 mmol/L before each meal, at bedtime or if necessary, at night.

Example : **Lunch:**   Carbohydrate content of meal = 60 g
Ratio = 1.0 unit/10 g of carbohydrates
Blood glucose = 23 mmol/L
Ketone bodies = moderate
      If measured in the urine: 4 mmol/L
      If measured in the blood: 1.5 to 3 mmol/L

**Inject:**
1) **Meal:**

$$\frac{1.0 \ unit \ x \ 60 \ g}{10 \ g} = 6 \ units$$

2) **Adjustment of insulin doses for sick days:**
23 mmol/L – 14 mmol/L = 9 units for dosage adjustment

3) **total amount to inject:**
6 units for the meal + 9 units for dosage adjustment = 15 units

## SUMMARY

**Appropriate action is determined on the basis of:**

1)   blood sugar levels;
2)   the presence or absence of ketone bodies in the blood or urine;
3)   the presence of signs and symptoms.

# Chronic Complications

1. **What are the long-term complications of diabetes?**

   After several years, if blood glucose levels are not well managed, complications can develop and affect:
   1) the **eyes (diabetic retinopathy)**;
   2) the **kidneys (diabetic nephropathy)**;
   3) the **nervous system (diabetic neuropathy)**;
   4) the **heart** and **blood vessels (cardiac or peripheral atherosclerosis)**.

2. **How does diabetes affect the eyes?**

   Over time, hyperglycemia can cause **changes to the small vessels in the back of the eye** that can compromise blood circulation and cause hemorrhage: this is called **diabetic retinopathy**. If diabetes and retinopathy are not adequately treated, they can lead to blindness. Diabetic retinopathy is the leading cause of blindness in the 20 to 64 year old age group.

3. **How do I know if my eyes have been affected by diabetes?**

   If your eyes are affected, you may see **spiderwebs** or **spots** in your field of vision. Consult an ophthalmologist (a doctor who specializes in eye diseases) or an optometrist, who will examine the eyes by dilating the pupil to take a look at the retina. Examinations with special digital cameras that take photos of the back of the eye can also detect abnormalities. If any are found, an examination by an ophthalmologist is necessary to confirm the diagnosis. Temporary changes in vision (blurriness) can result from blood glucose variations. **Hyperglycemia and hypoglycemia can cause blurry vision**, which is corrected when blood glucose is normalized.

## 4. When should I have my eyes examined?

It is fairly common for damage to the retina, a light sensitive layer at the back of the eye, to occur without causing any vision problems. It is therefore very **important to consult an ophthalmologist or optometrist regularly.**

People with type 1 diabetes should consult an ophthalmologist or optometrist five years after the initial diagnosis and once a year afterwards. People with type 2 diabetes should consult an ophthalmologist or optometrist at the time of diagnosis and every one to two years afterwards. In the case of both type 1 and type 2 diabetes, however, it might be necessary to visit an ophthalmologist more often if the eyes show any signs of damage progression.

## 5. How can I protect my eyes?

The eyes can be protected by:
1) keeping **blood glucose levels** as close to normal as possible;
2) consulting an **ophthalmologist** or **optometrist** regularly;
3) controlling your **blood pressure**;
4) **quitting smoking**, if applicable.

## 6. What are the possible long-term of diabetes on the kidneys?

In the long term, hyperglycemia can cause changes in the **small blood vessels of the kidneys**, compromising their blood filtration and purification functions: this is called **diabetic nephropathy**. If diabetes is not properly controlled, this condition can develop into complete loss of renal function. In such a case, dialysis (artificial kidney) or a kidney transplant is necessary. Diabetes is the main cause of dialysis in the Western world.

## 7. How do I know if my kidneys have been affected by diabetes?

The effect of diabetes on the kidneys can only be detected through a laboratory analysis to detect **microalbuminuria** (small amounts of albumin in the urine). This test requires only a urine sample. In some cases, the doctor will ask for urine samples from a 24 hour period to better assess the severity of the nephropathy. A rise in blood pressure can also signal the onset of damage to the kidneys.

### 8.   How can I protect my kidneys?

The kidneys can be protected by:
1)  keeping **blood glucose levels** as close to normal as possible;
2)  checking for **albumin** in the urine once a year;
3)  checking **blood pressure** regularly and treating high blood pressure aggressively;
4)  **quitting smoking**, if applicable;
5)  taking drugs to slow the progression of the nephropathy. These drugs are also used to control blood pressure and heart failure. The doctor may suggest them if indicated.

### 9.   What are the possible long-term effects of diabetes on the nerves?

In the long term, hyperglycemia can **damage the nerves**, particularly in the extremities but also in such organs as the intestines, stomach, bladder, heart and genitals. This is known as **diabetic neuropathy**.

### 10.  How do I know if the nerves in my extremities have been affected by diabetes?

In most cases, nerve damage manifests as a **decrease in sensitivity of the extremities to pain, heat and cold**. Another sign is a tingling or burning sensation. The diagnosis can be confirmed by your doctor or by a special test called electromyography (EMG). This type of complication is also known as "peripheral diabetic neuropathy" and affects the lower limbs more often than the upper limbs.

### 11.  What is the biggest danger when nerves in the extremities are affected?

The biggest danger of a loss of sensation, particularly in the feet, is **unwilling self-injury** (from ill-fitting shoes, hot water, a needle, etc.). After such an injury, infection can occur and, if circulation is compromised, can lead to gangrene and amputation.

12. **How do I know if the nerves in my intestines have been affected by diabetes?**

When the nerves in the intestines are affected by diabetes, stool evacuation can be compromised: this is called **constipation**. In an advanced state, when stools stagnate in the colon, normal intestinal bacteria can multiply, liquefying the stool and triggering sudden, intense diarrhea several times a day, especially at night: this is called **diabetic diarrhea.**

The first line of treatment for constipation is diet. Fibre consumption should be increased gradually and plenty of water consumed. Fibre supplements in capsules or powder form (e.g. Metamucil®) can help make the stool firmer and help with evacuation. If fibre and water are not effective, there are drugs available to treat constipation.

Constipation can be treated with drugs that cause the intestines to contract (for example, domperidone or metoclopramide). Laxatives, such as docusate sodium or sennosides, are also an option.

Diabetic diarrhea can also be treated with antibiotics such as tetracycline or erythromycin. Sometimes, anti-diarrheal agents such as loperamide or diphenoxylate must be added.

13. **How do I know if the nerves of my stomach have been affected by diabetes?**

When the nerves of the stomach are affected, the stomach empties more slowly: this is **diabetic gastroparesis.** This usually manifests as a feeling of bloating and/or regurgitation after a meal. Food absorption becomes irregular, which can explain poor control of blood glucose (hyperglycemia and hypoglycemia). The diagnosis can be confirmed by a nuclear medicine test called gastric emptying.

Gastroparesis can be treated with small and frequent meals and, if necessary, drugs such as domperidone or metoclopramide that cause the stomach to contract. In very serious cases, a gastric pacemaker can sometimes improve the symptoms.

14. **How do I know if the nerves of my bladder have been affected by diabetes?**

When the nerves of the bladder are affected by diabetes, it is more difficult to sense when the bladder is full. Furthermore, the bladder does not empty completely during urination: this is called **neurogenic bladder**. It can result in overflow loss of urine and, if urine stagnates in the bladder, there is a risk of urinary tract infection that can extend to the kidneys.

Neurogenic bladder can be diagnosed with an echography of the bladder after urination, which will reveal any urine retention.

To avoid overflow loss of urine, it is advised to urinate regularly, while exerting pressure on the bladder. In the case of significant urine retention, drugs that cause the bladder to contract such as betanechol can be used.

Nerve damage to the bladder can also manifest as hyperactive bladder, which has the following symptoms:
- increased frequency of urination;
- urgency of urination;
- urinary incontinence.

This condition results from damage to the nerves, causing them to send a signal to the bladder to contract at inappropriate times. Drugs such as oxybutinine (Ditropan®, Oxytrol®) can help control these symptoms.

15. **How do I know if the nerves of my heart have been affected by diabetes?**

Most of the time, when the nerves of the heart are affected, the condition is asymptomatic. In some cases, an accelerated heartbeat (tachycardia) and/or arrhythmia are noticeable. The diagnosis can be confirmed by electrocardiogram (ECG).

There is no specific treatment. If the accelerated heartbeat persists, beta-blockers such as metoprolol, atenolol, etc. can be prescribed.

### 16. How does a man know if the nerves in his genitals have been affected by diabetes?

When the nerves in the genitals are affected, men with diabetes have difficulty achieving and maintaining erection, making sexual relations difficult or impossible; this is known as **erectile dysfunction**.

This can be treated with certain oral medications such as Viagra®, Cialis® and Levitra®. Sometimes, more aggressive treatments are necessary, such as prostaglandin, either introduced into the urethra (urinary duct) in the form of suppositories (for example, Muse®) or injected into the base of the penis (for example, Caverject®).

### 17. How can nerve problems and their complications be prevented?

Nerve problems and their complications can be prevented by:
1) keeping **blood glucose levels** as close to normal as possible;
2) taking measures to avoid **trauma** and **burns** to the feet;
3) **inspecting the feet** daily;
4) consulting a **doctor** in the event of even the slightest lesion;
5) reporting any **digestive problems**;
6) reporting any **bladder problems**;
7) reporting any **erectile dysfunction**;
8) reporting any a**ccelerated or irregular heartbeat**;
9) seeking aggressive treatment for **high blood pressure**.

### 18. How can diabetes affect the heart and blood vessels?

Diabetes can affect the heart and blood vessels by accelerating the process of **arteriosclerosis**. This is a thickening and hardening of the arteries, which can block circulation in certain parts of the body, such as the heart, lower limbs, and even the brain. Damage to the blood vessels in the heart is the main cause of morbidity and death in people with diabetes.

**19. What are the possible dangers of damage to the heart and blood vessels?**

The dangers of arteriosclerosis depend on the part of the body affected:

1) if the heart is affected, **myocardial infarction** can result;
2) if the brain is affected, a **stroke can result, possibly causing paralysis or speech impairment**;
3) if the lower limbs are affected, **pain when walking** and **intermittent claudication can result.**

**20. How do I know if my heart and blood vessels have been affected by diabetes?**

Certain signs reveal arteriosclerosis and circulation problems:

1) **slow healing** of wounds;
2) **chest pain** and/or **difficulty breathing** during physical exertion;
3) **pain in the calves** when walking (intermittent claudication).

In some cases, however, arteriosclerosis is asymptomatic, particularly in its early stages, and can be diagnosed only by medical examination or by means of special tests such as an electrocardiogram at rest or during exertion, cardiac scintigraphy (MIBI), abdominal X-ray (to identify vessel calcification), or a Doppler test (to examine the condition of blood vessels using ultrasound) of vessels in the neck or the lower limbs.

**21. How can I prevent damage to my heart and blood vessels due to my diabetes?**

Reduce the risk of damage to the heart and blood vessels by:

1) keeping **blood glucose levels** as close to normal as possible;
2) checking **blood pressure** regularly and treating high blood pressure aggressively;
3) avoiding **saturated fats** (especially of animal origin) as much as possible;
4) having **blood lipid levels** checked regularly and treating any anomalies aggressively;
5) **quitting smoking**, if applicable;
6) **exercising**;
7) taking an **aspirin a day** (unless contraindicated).

## 22. What is high blood pressure?

In the general population, blood pressure is considered high if it is greater than or equal to 140/90. In people with diabetes, however, the criteria are more rigorous and blood pressure is considered high if it is greater than or equal to 130/80.

## 23. Why should people with diabetes treat high blood pressure aggressively?

High blood pressure significantly increases the complications of diabetes that affect the eyes, nerves, kidneys, heart and blood vessels.

It has been clearly shown that treating high blood pressure in people with diabetes significantly decreases the development and progression of complications associated with the disease.

## 24. What is considered a blood lipid anomaly in a person with diabetes?

A person with diabetes is said to have a blood lipid anomaly if:
1) bad cholesterol (LDL cholesterol) is greater than or equal to 2 mmol/L;
2) good cholesterol (HDL cholesterol) is less than 1.0 mmol/L;
3) triglycerides are greater than or equal to 1.5 mmol/L; or
4) the ratio between total cholesterol and HDL cholesterol is greater than or equal to 4.0.

## 25. Why should all blood lipid anomalies be treated aggressively?

Blood lipid anomalies should be treated aggressively because they represent major risk factors for arteriosclerosis and therefore for diseases of the heart and blood vessels. Because people with diabetes have an elevated risk of developing diseases of the heart and blood vessels, these anomalies must be treated with added vigilance.

# Foot Care and General Hygiene

### 1. Why is diabetic foot a public health issue?

Foot complications due to diabetes are a major public health issue because they are the primary cause of non-trauma-related amputations. In the long term, poorly controlled diabetes is associated with peripheral neuropathy, especially of the feet. Loss of sensitivity to touch, pain, heat and cold are some of the symptoms. This loss of sensitivity makes people with diabetes vulnerable to injuries that go unnoticed. A lesion can become infected and if there are circulatory problems, gangrene can develop, possibly requiring amputation. However, if people with diabetes take good care of their feet, 80% of these amputations can be prevented. Hence the importance of learning about proper foot care.

### 2. What problems can lead to diabetic foot complications in people with diabetes?

The feet of people with diabetes are more fragile than those of people who do not have the disease. In the long term, hyperglycemia can cause the following foot problems:

1) **nerve damage** resulting in loss of sensitivity to touch, pain, heat and cold;
2) **a tendency for the skin to get thinner and drier**, to become more easily irritated and to develop calluses (hyperkeratosis) at pressure points;
3) a tendency for **arteries to thicken and harden**, thereby reducing circulation in the feet;

4) **a susceptibility to infection** because the body is less able to defend itself against microbes when blood glucose levels are high.

## 3. How should the feet be examined?

The responsibility for foot care should be shared between the person with diabetes and his or her healthcare team. If you have diabetes, do the following to prevent complications:

1) examine your feet closely every day after a bath or shower;
2) sit down and, under a good light source, examine both feet from every angle (top, bottom and between the toes);
3) use a mirror to examine the soles of the feet if you lack the flexibility to see them otherwise;
4) ask another person for help if your vision is impaired or if you cannot reach your feet with your hands;
5) follow up the self-exam with a thorough professional examination every time you visit a doctor, podiatrist or nurse specializing in foot care.

## 4. What should I look for?

Look carefully for:

1) **lesions between the toes** caused by fungi that thrive in humid conditions (athlete's foot);
2) **calluses:** heavily callused skin (often located under the foot) can make the skin fragile and vulnerable to infection, thus providing a good place for microbes to multiply;
3) **corns:**
   o  on the toes, produced by friction with shoes;
   o  between the toes, known as "soft corns" (or "kissing corns"), caused by the toes being compressed together;
4) **cracks:** crevices in callused skin (often on or around the heel) are particularly well-suited for microbial growth. Excess callused skin can always be traced to a specific cause:
   o  poor foot posture (position, compression); see your doctor as soon as possible;

o    the use of instruments that can harm the feet: razor blades, knives, graters or corn-removal preparations;

o    foreign bodies in the shoes or seams that can injure the feet; check by running your hand along the inside of your shoes.

### 5.    What are the first signs of foot problems?

The feet should be examined for the following problems:

1) changes in skin colour, unusual redness;
2) unusually high skin temperature;
3) swollen feet or ankles;
4) pain in the legs or feet;
5) ingrown toenails;
6) toenail fungi;
7) open sores that heal slowly;
8) calluses that bleed or appear to be infected;
9) dry and fissured skin, especially around the heel;
10) scratches;
11) bunions;
12) warts;
13) loss of sensation in the feet.

### 6.    How can a person with diabetes reduce the risk of foot problems?

To limit the risk of developing foot problems:

1) keep blood glucose as close to normal as possible;
2) quit smoking, if applicable;
3) lose weight, if necessary;
4) reduce alcohol consumption, if applicable;
5) get regular exercise;
6) see a doctor, podiatrist, or nurse specialized in foot care, or any other specialist, as needed.

## 7. What are the top-ten foot care suggestions for people with diabetes?

1) **Examine your feet every day** and ask for help from family and friends if needed:
   - examine the feet closely all over, looking for lesions, cuts or any malformation;
   - regularly check the sensitivity level of the feet (following the doctor's recommendations):
     - run a cotton ball lightly over and under the foot to detect any areas lacking sensation;
     - put a dry pea in your shoe and walk a few steps to see whether you can detect the foreign body; remove the pea immediately to avoid injuring yourself.

2) **Do not walk barefoot**, not even in the house, and especially not on a beach or in any public area:
   - put on slippers when you get out of bed;
   - during the day, wear comfortable shoes.

3) **Wash your feet every day:**
   - check the water temperature with your wrist, elbow or a thermometer; the water should be lukewarm (below 37°C);
   - wash your feet with mild soap (for example, unscented Dove®, Aveeno®, Cetaphil®, Neutrogena®, Keri®, etc.);
   - avoid soaking your feet for longer than 10 minutes to avoid maceration and softening of the skin;
   - dry your feet carefully, especially between and under the toes; humidity encourages the development of fungi such as athlete's foot.

4) **Be sure the skin is completely dry:**
   - apply a thin layer of neutral (unscented) moisturizing cream (for example, Nivea®, Lubriderm®, Vaseline Intensive Care® lotion, Glycerodermine®, etc.), except between the toes;
   - once or twice a week after a bath or shower, use a moistened pumice stone to rub areas where hyperkeratosis (thickening of the skin) has developed. Avoid rubbing back and forth, and use long, continuous movements instead. Never use a metal grater, which can cause injury.

5) **Avoid cutting your toenails too short:**
   - nails should be cut straight across, a little beyond the tips of the toes, and the corners filed after a bath or shower. This will prevent the development of ingrown toenails and wounds;

o   nails should be filed with an emery board instead of being cut; this will help avoid injury;

o   handle round-ended scissors and nail clippers with care. Anyone lacking in dexterity or suffering from impaired or reduced vision should avoid using them altogether;

o   never tear your toenails.

6) **Never self-treat for calluses, corns or blisters:**

o   avoid so-called "bathroom surgery": never use pointy scissors, sharp clippers, razor blades, lancets, scalpels, or metal files to remove a corn;

o   never use over-the-counter solutions or plasters with a salicylic acid base; they can cause skin necrosis;

o   see a professional specializing in foot care, taking care to tell him or her that you have diabetes.

7) **Change socks every day:**

o   wear clean socks (or stockings); wash them every day;

o   wear socks that fit; be sure they are loose and long enough and do not squeeze the toes; avoid wearing tight socks that leave marks on the calves and cut off circulation;

o   avoid thick stitching; if the socks have seams, wear them inside out;

o   avoid shoes with holes or patches that create points of friction;

o   wear socks that keep the feet dry, made from a blend of cotton and synthetic fibres (acrylic, orlon, polypropylene, Coolmax, etc.); people who sweat profusely should avoid socks that contain nylon.

8) **Choose your shoes carefully:**

o   always wear socks with shoes;

o   choose shoes fastened with laces, buckles or velcro; they should be made from supple leather or canvas and roomy enough to let the toes move;

o   choose non-skid soles;

o   buy shoes in the late afternoon; when feet are swollen, it is easier to choose shoes that fit correctly;

o   break in new shoes gradually by wearing them only a half-hour a day at first;

o   carefully inspect the inside of your shoes before wearing them; run your hand inside to find any foreign bodies or seams that could injure your feet;

o   avoid pointy shoes and shoes with high heels (over 3 cm).

9) **Watch out for burns or frostbite:**

o   wear socks, even in bed, if your feet are cold; avoid hot-water bottles, electric blankets or hot water;

    o    use sunscreen with at least 15 SPF (sun protection factor) to lower the risk of sunburns;

    o    never use powerful products or irritants (for example, Parisienne® or other bleaches);

    o    make sure the skin is covered, especially in cold and dry winter weather.

10) **Immediately contact your foot care specialist** (doctor, podiatrist or nurse) if you notice discoloration, loss of sensation or a lesion.

Everyone with diabetes should have a foot examination at least twice a year. People at higher risk should have more frequent exams.

## 8. Which moisturizing creams should a person with diabetes use for foot care?

For skin that has a tendency to dry out, use a moisturizer daily. Unscented products without coloring are preferable. Avoid applying cream between the toes, which will soften the skin excessively. Apply a thin layer after a bath or shower.

There are three main kinds of moisturizing products:

1) **hydrating products with humectants**, which soften the skin and diminish fine lines (e.g., Nivea®, Glycerodermine®, Glaxal Base®, Aquatain®, Complex-15®, etc.);

2) **anti-dehydration products**, which reduce the evaporation of moisture by creating a film on the skin (e.g., Moisturel®, Lubriderm® (Lotion), Cetaphil®, Aveeno® (Lotion), Keri® (Lotion), Vaseline Intensive Care® (Lotion), Neutrogena®, Aquaphor®, Prevex®, Barrier Creme®, Akildia®, Curel®, Eucrin®, Elta®, etc.);

3) **hydrating products with keratolytic and exfoliating properties**, which help remove dead skin cells. These products should be **used with care and be applied only on the stratum corneum, or top layer, of the skin**. Urea may cause a burning or tingling sensation on dry or cracked skin (e.g., Uremol-10®, Uremol-20®, Dermal Therapy® at 10%, 15%, 20% or 25% urea, Lacticare® Lotion, Lac-Hydrin® Lotion, Urisec®, etc.).

9. **Which antiseptic products should a person with diabetes use for sores or lesions on the feet?**

Wash the sore with water and mild soap, then rinse and dry it well.

1) Disinfect the skin with an antiseptic (according to a doctor's recommendations):
   - 70% alcohol swab;
   - Proviodine swab;
   - 0.05% chlorhexidine gluconate (e.g., Hibidil®, Baxedin®).

2) **If there is inflammation**, apply a compress soaked in physiological saline solution three or four times a day. Watch for signs of infection over the next 24 to 48 hours. Avoid using adhesive tape directly on the skin. If redness worsens or if there is pus, see a doctor immediately.

3) **If your doctor recommends foot baths**, use one of the following products in one litre of lukewarm boiled water for no more than 10 minutes:
   - 15 ml (1 tbsp.) of Proviodine®;
   - 15 ml (1 tbsp.) of Hibitane® 4% (chlorhexidine gluconate 4%);
   - 30 ml (2 tbsp.) of Hibitane® 2% (chlorhexidine gluconate 2%).

Wash your feet again in running water and dry them well, especially between the toes. See a doctor if the sore does not heal.

It is important to discover the cause of the problem so that it is does not recur.

10. **How can circulation in the feet be improved?**

There are a number of simple, readily available methods that can improve circulation and maintain or improve the flexibility of the feet.
   - Do not smoke.
   - Do not cross your legs when sitting.
   - Keep moving – do not remain standing or sitting in one place for too long.
   - Walk as much as you can, within your limits and abilities.
   - When seated, rest your legs on a footstool whenever possible.
   - Do foot exercises regularly – repeat each one 20 times:
     - put a towel on the floor and try to pick it up with your toes;
     - stand on the tips of your toes, then lower your body weight down onto your heels; use a support if necessary (be careful not to fall);
     - flex your ankle, pointing your feet up and down;

- rotate your feet, first in one direction, then the other;
- rock in an armchair, pushing with your toes.

## 11. What is diabetic neuropathic pain?

The term "diabetic neuropathy" refers to nerve disease associated with diabetes. Neuropathic pain occurs when damage to the nerves causes pain.

## 12. What are the symptoms of diabetic neuropathic pain?

Some people with diabetes suffering from neuropathic pain use many different terms to describe it. Neuropathic pain may be accompanied by:

- burning sensations;
- numbness;
- stinging;
- tingling;
- a feeling of electric shock;
- sensitivity to touch or cold;
- formication;
- a feeling of being crushed;
- deep, shooting pains;
- a feeling of walking on cotton batten.

## 13. How is diabetic neuropathic pain treated?

People with diabetes can lower the risk of developing neuropathic complications by properly managing their blood sugar levels. In some cases, proper control of diabetes, physical exercise, meal plans and relaxation exercises combined with drug treatment can help reduce pain. The doctor may prescribe medications such as amitriptyline, gabapentine (Neurontin®) or pregabaline (Lyrica®).

## 14. What is a diabetic foot ulcer?

A diabetic foot ulcer is a foot sore or wound resulting from neuropathy; it develops on pressure points on the bottom of the foot, due to calluses or other foot deformations. In many cases people with diabetes continue to walk around despite such foot injuries because they lack sensitivity in their feet, unwittingly making them worse. In some cases, a sore develops in the middle of a callus, which can worsen and become infected, especially if blood glucose is poorly controlled. If the ulcer does not receive adequate treatment, it can become gangrenous and amputation may be necessary.

If you have any questions about the nature of a sore on your foot, see your doctor as quickly as possible. Foot ulcers will heal with the appropriate treatment.

### 15. Why is dental hygiene particularly important for people with diabetes?

People with diabetes should manage their dental health with as much care as their skin or feet for two major reasons:

1) Poorly controlled diabetes causes a high risk of cavities, gum sores or infection.
2) Any infection can raise blood glucose levels and hamper the control of diabetes.

### 16. What are the main types of oral lesions?

1) **Cavities**

   Cavities destroy teeth. The main cause of cavities is dental plaque, a whitish deposit that sticks to the enamel. The formation of dental plaque is encouraged by sweet foods, failure to brush the teeth and gums, and alcohol, which reduces acidity levels in the mouth.

2) **Gingivitis**

   Gingivitis is caused by the deposit of bacteria that create plaque between the teeth and gums. The gum becomes bright red, inflamed and swollen, and tends to bleed if touched.

3) **Periodontitis**

   Periodontitis develops if gingivitis remains untreated. The germs along the roots of the affected teeth multiply, and the inflammation spreads to areas deep within the gums and the bone supporting the teeth. The teeth become loose and may even fall out painlessly.

## 17. What kind of dental hygiene measures should people with diabetes practice?

The main preventive dental hygiene measures are:

1) maintain blood glucose levels as close to normal as possible;
2) brush your teeth carefully after every meal;
3) use dental floss every day;
4) see a dentist twice a year or more often if necessary;
5) see a denturologist once every five years to adjust dental prostheses, if necessary;
6) consume alcohol in moderation, so as not to reduce acidity in the mouth;
7) do not smoke.

People with diabetes should always inform the health professionals they consult that they have diabetes. In the event of an intervention, antibiotics may be prescribed to prevent infection.

# Living with Diabetes

1.  **What does it mean to live with diabetes?**

    Diabetes is increasingly widespread. Many people, however, find that **it is not easy to live with diabetes**.

    People who have been diagnosed with diabetes face a series of challenges that will be there for the rest of their lives. These challenges include the following:
    1)  **Realizing that diabetes is a chronic illness** that cannot be cured.
    2)  **Admitting that it is a serious illness**, even if the symptoms are barely noticeable and not painful.
    3)  **Accepting the necessity of establishing a daily routine** (meals, sleeping, exercise, etc.), especially if insulin treatment is necessary.
    4)  **Self-motivating to change certain habits,** since medication alone is not enough to treat diabetes.
    5)  **Taking personal responsibility** for treatment.

    The challenges of living with diabetes are considerable, but surmountable.

2.  **Is there anything to help a person who has just been diagnosed with diabetes?**

    Advances in knowledge about diabetes in terms of both medical science and the psychosocial sphere are cause for optimism. People with diabetes should remember the following:
    1)  diabetes **can be controlled effectively**;
    2)  good control of blood glucose **significantly decreases the risks of developing serious complications** over the long term;
    3)  there are information and training resources (such as diabetes teaching units) that allows people with diabetes to acquire the necessary skills to **adapt diabetes treatment to daily life and individual needs**;

4) diabetes can be an **opportunity to learn** how to improve diet, exercise regularly, manage stress more effectively, and generally learn how to live better.

Most people with diabetes are able to live long, active, healthy and satisfying lives.

## 3. How do people with diabetes accept their illness?

A diagnosis of diabetes delivers an emotional shock, whether or not the person is aware of it. The shock is provoked by the need to face up to the reality that the disease will inevitably entail some losses.

Whether or not the person wants to, he or she will begin a grieving process, which will eventually, at the person's own speed, lead to a state of acceptance of the illness and its treatment.

A better understanding of the disease can make the grieving process a little easier. Acceptance comes through knowledge; it is therefore important to learn about the disease.

## 4. What is a grieving process?

Grieving is a process of maturation that everyone goes through when they deal with a loss. In the case of diabetes, the process involves grieving the loss of health, along with other equally important losses, such as the loss of liberty, spontaneity, and former habits. It can even involve grieving the loss of self-esteem or a feeling of invulnerability.

The grieving process evolves in a number of stages that correspond to different emotions that vary in intensity and duration. These emotions, which are entirely normal, help the person with diabetes reach a new state of emotional equilibrium and greater acceptance.

## 5. What are the stages of grief?

The following chart presents the five stages of grief. They may appear in a different order, according to the individual.

| Stage | Description | Characteristic statements |
|---|---|---|
| *1) Denial or negation* | Ignoring the unbearable aspects of the illness or treatment.<br>Acting as though there is no illness or as though it is not serious. | "I can't be diabetic, I don't feel sick." |
| *2) Anger or revolt* | Seeing the illness as an injustice.<br>Being angry at everyone.<br>Blaming others.<br>Seeing only the negative aspects of treatment. | "Diabetes is the worst disease possible, and it's preventing me from living my life." |
| *3) Negociating or bargaining* | Taking on certain aspects of the disease, but leaving out whatever is displeasing. Acceptance remains very conditional. | "I take pills to lower my blood sugar, so I don't have to worry about what I eat." |
| *4) Depressive feelings or reflection* | Realizing that denying the illness is useless.<br>Exaggerated perception of limitations.<br>Possible feelings of powerless or retreating into dependency. | "Is this kind of life worth living?" |
| *5) Acceptance* | Realistic perception of the illness and its treatment.<br>Deciding to take concrete and positive action. | "I'd rather not have diabetes, but since I don't have a choice, I'm going to do my best." |

## 6. How can the grieving process be influenced and acceptance encouraged?

Being open to actively learning about the process will make the stages of grief more clearly recognizable and make it possible to identify the related emotions. Above all, it will help the person with diabetes get in touch with himself or herself through these emotions. This is a journey of self-discovery.

The next step involves learning to transform negative feelings, whether guilt, anger or fear, into positive ones. It is normal to have negative feelings or emotions, and they are not bad in themselves. They are simply unpleasant.

Being aware of negative feelings can help motivate the will to change. They are often the expression of psychological pain related to specific problems. The best way to ease this pain is to find solutions to the problems that cause them.

These steps can influence the grieving process and thereby the process of acceptance, which ultimately makes it possible to adapt to the disease and its treatment.

## 7. Are some emotional problems more common in people with diabetes?

Yes. We know that depression and anxiety affect a good number of people in the general population, but studies suggest that **depression** and **anxiety disorders** are more common in people with a chronic physical illness such as diabetes.

It is estimated that depression affects people with diabetes up to three times more than those in the general population (20% compared to 5% to 10%). Similarly, anxiety disorders are up to six times more common (30% compared to 5%).

Accurate diagnosis of these two psychological problems is therefore important, since they can significantly influence the control of blood glucose. The more depressed or anxious a person feels, the harder it is to control the diabetes.

## 8. How is depression recognized?

It is first necessary to distinguish between depressive feelings, which are normal emotions that play a part in the grieving process, and depression, which is an illness. Someone whose mood is depressed will not necessarily be diagnosed with depression.

Depression **becomes an illness** when the symptoms listed below last several weeks and begin to **affect work and social life**:
1) feeling depressed, sad, hopeless, discouraged, "at the end of my rope" most of the day, almost every day;
2) loss of interest or pleasure in almost all activities;
3) loss of or significant increase in appetite or weight;
4) insomnia or a need to sleep more than usual;
5) agitation (for example, difficulty sitting still) or the slowing down of psychomotor

functions (for example, slowed speech, monotone voice, long delay before answering questions, slower bodily movements);

6)  lack of energy, tiredness;
7)  feelings of loss of dignity, self-blame, excessive or inappropriate guilt;
8)  difficulty concentrating, thinking or making a decision;
9)  recurring thoughts of death, suicidal impulses, death wishes or actual suicide attempts.

## 9.  What should you do if you think you are suffering from depression?

If you have experienced some or many of these symptoms for at least two weeks, inform your doctor to determine whether the symptoms are due to diabetes, other physical problems (for example, hypothyroidism) or depression. The doctor can then prescribe the appropriate treatment or refer you to a mental health specialist, as needed.

Although depressive feelings are often a normal part of the grieving process after a diagnosis of diabetes, a doctor should be consulted if these feelings intensify and last for several weeks.

Depression is one of the most easily treated mental health problems, especially if diagnosed promptly. Most people who suffer from depression are treated with antidepressant medications and/or psychotherapy, and the combination of these two therapeutic approaches has been recognized as the most effective treatment. The support of family, friends and outreach groups is also important.

## 10.  How are anxiety disorders recognized?

Anxiety disorders are mental health problems in which anxiety is the predominant disturbance. In people with diabetes, anxiety disorders such as phobias (for example, a fear of needles or of low blood glucose) and especially **generalized anxiety** are the most frequent.

A diagnosis of a generalized anxiety disorder is possible if the following symptoms are present:

1)  anxiety and excessive worry most of the time, for at least six months, with respect to different events or activities;
2)  difficulty controlling this type of worry;

3)  intense distress;

4)  agitation or feeling on edge;

5)  easily fatigued;

6)  difficulty concentrating or memory lapses;

7)  irritability;

8)  muscle tension;

9)  disturbed sleep.

## 11. What should you do if you think you are suffering from an anxiety disorder?

If you show signs of generalized anxiety or a phobia, speak to your doctor, who will evaluate your situation and recommend the appropriate treatment or refer you to a mental health professional, as needed.

Anxiety disorders can be treated with drugs and/or psychotherapy. Relaxation techniques are common therapeutic tools to treat these conditions.

## 12. Where can you find help if you suffer from depression?

Speak to your doctor. In some cases, if indicated, drug treatment can begin right away. Your doctor can also refer you to a mental health professional, that is, a psychiatrist or psychologist who works in the public healthcare system. You can find these professionals at a hospital's department of psychiatry or psychology, or through the mental health services offered by some Community Health Centres.

Psychiatrists and psychologists in private practice are also available for consultation. Their contact information is available through their respective professional associations.

## 13. Is it true that people with diabetes go through personality changes and become angrier or more aggressive?

No. **Anger is not a typical personality trait of people with diabetes**. There of course may be people with diabetes who are short-tempered, but this has nothing to do with the fact that they have the disease.

However, **sudden character changes** or irritable or angry **mood swings** could be a sign that a person with diabetes is **in a hypoglycemic state**. These signs will disappear once the hypoglycemia has been corrected.

Mood swings can also occur **when a person with diabetes becomes very tired** because of elevated or fluctuating blood glucose. These mood swings usually stop relatively quickly when blood glucose is better controlled and the person recovers energy.

Irritability can also **signify a failure to accept the illness**. In such cases, the people have become "embittered by their illness". This phenomenon is not specific to diabetes and can be experienced by anyone with a chronic disease who has been unable to accept the condition.

It is therefore important for people who are near a diabetic person to be able to distinguish the different reasons for any mood swings. This will make it easier to understand and help.

---

**Remember:**

o Your personality shapes how you react to your diabetes.

o You cannot totally control the emotions you feel or even the way you manage them, but you are responsible for your behaviour.

o You cannot control the time it takes to go through the grieving process, but you are responsible for learning about it, observing your reactions, and influencing the process if possible.

o Your diabetes is not your fault, but managing it is your responsibility.

# Managing Daily Stress

1.  **Why should people with diabetes be concerned about daily stress?**

    Stress can increase blood glucose levels in some people with diabetes. Stress acts directly on blood glucose by encouraging the secretion of hormones such as adrenalin, which release glucose reserves from the liver into the bloodstream and decrease the effectiveness of insulin by increasing resistance to it in the cells. Stress can also act indirectly by causing people to neglect their self-care.

2.  **Does stress cause diabetes?**

    No, it does not. In someone who is genetically predisposed, however, stress can be one of the factors that trigger the disease.

3.  **What is stress?**

    Stress is what you feel when you think that you are unable to effectively deal with a situation that you perceive as threatening.

    The following four characteristics create a stressful situation: the feeling of a lack of control over the situation, its unpredictability, its newness, and the feeling of a threatened ego. The brain detects a stressful situation and responds to the stress only if at least one of these four characteristics is present.

    Stress is largely the result of an individual's perception of an event, and not simply the event itself.

Stress is a part of life. No one can go through life without encountering stress. Essentially, it is a coping mechanism that has enabled humanity to survive. Everyone has a different tolerance to stress and, depending on a number of factors, it can be experienced as either good or bad.

### 4.   What is "good stress"?

A person's capacity to deal with a threatening situation effectively is what determines whether or not that person perceives stress as good or bad. It can be a positive force in a person's life. For example, resolving a very difficult problem and falling in love are events that potentially cause good stress because they increase the pleasure and satisfaction that can be taken from life. On the other hand, if these situations are perceived by the person as beyond his or her ability to deal with them, the stress will probably be experienced more intensely and perceived as bad.

### 5.   What are the sources of stress?

Stressors fall into three broad categories:

1) **physical stressors:**
   o   illness and its consequences;
   o   fatigue;
   o   pain.
2) **psychological stressors:**
   o   emotions;
   o   attitudes;
   o   behaviour.
3) **social stressors:**
   o   interpersonal and professional relationships;
   o   death of a loved one;
   o   major life changes (marriage, moving, retirement).

It should be noted that stress can be triggered by happy events (marriage, birth of a child, promotion) as well as difficult ones.

### 6.   What affects a person's response to stress?

Several factors affect a person's response to stress, including:

1) **personal factors**: personality, genetics, past experiences, attitudes;
2) **emotions**: guilt, anxiety, sadness, fear, etc.;
3) **personal resources**: coping strategies, social support, information.

### 7.   How are the symptoms of stress recognized?

There are many possible indicators of stress:

1) **physical symptoms:**
   o   increased heartbeat;
   o   rise in blood pressure;
   o   increased muscle tension;
   o   faster breathing;
   o   chronic fatigue;
   o   headache, backache;
   o   tightness in the chest;
   o   digestive problems;
   o   tics, twitching.

2) **psychological symptoms:**
   o   aggressiveness;
   o   depression;
   o   crying jags or an inability to cry;
   o   feeling empty, dissatisfied;
   o   ambivalence;
   o   decreased ability to concentrate or pay attention;
   o   decreased motivation;
   o   loss of self-esteem;
   o   nightmares.

3) **behavioural symptoms:**
   o   irritability;
   o   angry outbursts;
   o   very critical attitude;
   o   forgetfulness, indecision;
   o   loss of productivity;

o   increased consumption of some foods or substances (tobacco, alcohol, medications) or loss of appetite;

o   sexual problems.

Although humans are equipped to deal adequately with occasional stress, persistent, intense and frequent stress can overtax our bodies and cause undesirable physical states. Stress is a part of human life and cannot be eliminated. It is possible, however, to learn how to manage and minimize its negative effects.

## 8.  How should you respond to stress?

1)  **Recognize your stress level**: First, know how to recognize the symptoms and sources of stress. Awareness of your own stress level is a starting point.

2)  **Recognize good stress and bad stress**: Understand what makes stress positive or negative for you.

3)  **Develop strategies to cope with stress**: Research on coping strategies has shown that the people who are best adapted have strategies focused on solving problems instead of on their emotional response only.

## 9.  What is a problem-solving approach?

It is a logical process, whereby a stressful situation is analyzed and different solutions are explored. The steps are:

1)  **First step: Define the problem**. Define the problem in simple, clear and concrete terms.

2)  **Second step: Seek out solutions**. Imagine as many solutions as possible, without being overly self-critical.

3)  **Third step: Evaluate every possible solution**. Look at the advantages and disadvantages of each solution. Organize them according to the ease or difficulty of application and your intention of putting them into action immediately.

4)  **Fourth step: Prepare a plan of action**. Decide which of the solutions you will keep as your goal. Prepare a plan of action that defines the concrete steps that need to be made.

**10. What daily coping strategies can help manage stress related to emotions?**

- o Learn how to express negative emotions appropriately, both to yourself and to others.
- o Avoid belittling yourself or over-dramatizing; try to perceive the real situation accurately.
- o Rely on some positive self-affirmations to control any emotions that are paralyzing (for example, "I can do it", "I've made it through worse than this", "Everything's okay, this is a step in the right direction").
- o Practice relaxation techniques to reduce the symptoms of stress.

**11. What daily coping strategies can help manage stress related to behaviour?**

- o Express your needs, while respecting the needs of others.
- o Avoid passively submitting to events and living like a victim of circumstance.
- o Learn to say no when you truly cannot or do not want to say yes.
- o Do not allow problems to accumulate.
- o Temporarily remove yourself from stressful situations.

**12. What daily coping strategies can help manage stress related to lifestyle?**

- o Plan out a balanced program that includes regular exercise, creative and relaxing activities.
- o Seek out activities that you find fulfilling and pleasurable.
- o Organize your time and establish realistic deadlines.
- o Maintain some distance between your professional life and your personal life.
- o Do not seek to deal with your stress by consuming alcohol or food to excess or by using drugs.

### 13. What attitudes and behaviours can help people with diabetes manage stress related to their illness?

1) **Manage the illness well:**
   - check blood glucose regularly;
   - eat well;
   - exercise;
   - take medications as prescribed;
   - learn about diabetes.

2) **Deal with external stressors:**
   - practice time management (plan, define priorities);
   - change environments, if necessary;
   - engage in satisfying activities;
   - use relaxation techniques;
   - put things in motion as soon as possible;
   - make changes gradually; avoid "all-or-nothing" reactions.

3) **Deal with psychological stressors:**
   - control irrational thoughts (for example, perfectionism);
   - question your beliefs (for example, "What I don't know can't hurt me, so I think about diabetes as little as possible");
   - open yourself up to other ways of seeing (for example, instead of seeing life in black and white, open yourself up to shades of grey);
   - build a social support network (family, friends, outreach groups) and let them know that you appreciate their support (avoid making members of your family responsible for your treatment);
   - speak with a person you trust, sharing your emotions; confiding in someone is an effective way to feel better and combat any feelings of isolation that are be caused by the illness;
   - consult a specialist if your own resources seem inadequate. A psychologist is a specialist in human behaviour, and can help you identify the sources of your stress and your reactions, and change your attitudes and behaviour to better manage stress.

### 14. What is relaxation?

Relaxation is an important tool in stress management. Stress provokes a number of reactions, stimulating several physiological functions (cardiovascular, respiratory, muscular). Relaxation, on the other hand, produces the opposite effect with respect to these functions, re-establishing physiological and psychological equilibrium. Relaxation is more than just "rest"; its effect is deeper.

### 15. Are there any easy relaxation exercises?

There are a number of easy techniques. The most common are:
1) active relaxation, which involves alternating tension and release;
2) passive relaxation, which involves gradually relaxing each part of the body as each one is named inwardly.

The important thing is to stop, get away from external stimuli (noise, light, activity), sit down, close your eyes and breathe deeply, finding your own rhythm. After a few minutes, your breathing will slow down. Then conduct an inventory of every part of your body, starting at the feet and moving up to the head. You will begin to feel more relaxed, with sensations of warmth, heaviness and calm overtaking you. With practice, five minutes will be enough to attain this relaxation state anywhere, even in public places. It is just a matter of practice; it's easy, accessible to anyone and, above all, very effective.

### 16. Are there any tools that promote relaxation?

There is a wide variety of CDs that provide information on relaxation techniques. Experiment and explore to discover your preferences.

Here are some suggestions for beginners:
- *Progressive Relaxation and Breathing.* 1987. Oakland, CA: New Harbinger Publications Inc. Jacobson's complete Deep Muscle Technique, shorthand relaxation of muscle groups, deep breathing, etc.
- *Applied Relaxation Training.* 1991. Oakland, CA: New Harbinger Publications Inc. How to relax all your muscles except those you actually need for a given activity, to reduce stress while driving, working at a desk or walking.

There are also a number of books on relaxation techniques and stress management. Browse through a bookstore to find something that is appealing to you. The following is one recommendation to get you started:

- o  Martha Davis *et al.*, *Relaxation and Stress Reduction Workbook*, 5th ed. Oakland, CA: New Harbinger Publications, 2001.

### 17.  Should you talk about your disease with your family and friends?

It is important to realize that your family and friends will share your feelings of shock, especially when you are first diagnosed. It is important to speak with them. They are worried about you and need information to help you properly. Communication is always the best choice. Your role involves instructing your family and friends, providing them with general information about diabetes, your lifestyle regimen and any possible complications. This will ensure that you get the appropriate aid and support. Expressing your needs and expectations is the first step toward mutual understanding and a way to ensure your safety.

### 18.  What reactions should you expect from your family and friends?

In most cases, family and friends want to help, but they do not always do so in the right way. You may sometimes get the impression that they all want to tell you what you should and should not do, or that they minimize the seriousness of the illness and lure you away from what you should be doing. It is important to inform your loved ones and let them know what you need and expect. You are an autonomous person and it is normal for you to want to exert as much control over your life as possible.

### 19.  Should you talk about your condition at work?

It is important to find allies who can help you in an emergency. You are responsible for creating a climate of safety around yourself. Your stress level will depend greatly on how successful you are at doing this.

# The Motivation to Change

### 1. What is motivation?

Motivation is the action of conscious and unconscious forces that determine behaviour.

For example, smoking is behaviour that is determined and conditioned by a number of forces, including advertising, fashion, relaxation, or emotional conflict.

Analyzing the reasons we come up with for continuing or changing behaviour can help us become aware of these forces.

### 2. Why is motivation important in the treatment of diabetes?

First and foremost, motivation is an important issue in the treatment of diabetes because the disease requires people to care for themselves (self-care) and control their own blood glucose levels (self-monitoring).

Self-care and self-monitoring only work if people change their lifestyle and choose to eat better, exercise and manage their stress.

The requirements of the treatment of diabetes demand a great deal of personal motivation to adopt and maintain healthy behaviour.

3. **What are the main factors behind the motivation to change?**

There are three main factors:

1) **The will to change**

In large part, the will to change is determined by personal beliefs about health, diabetes, and the treatment of the disease.

The collection of opinions known as "health beliefs" has been shown to positively influence a person to adopt healthy behaviours (for example, the belief that the proposed treatment regimen is effective).

On the other hand, there are also erroneous beliefs, which are very personal perceptions of the disease and its treatment that can negatively affect the will to change.

2) **The steps toward change**

Any transformation is accomplished step by step, each one defined by the feeling of being more or less ready to take action. For each step toward change, there are recommendations about how to continue progressing.

3) **Confidence in the capacity to change**

A person's confidence in his or her capacity to change can be reinforced by learning skills that make change easier to envisage.

Two such skills are the manner of setting goals and familiarity with the plan or strategy for change.

4. **How do the health beliefs of people with diabetes reinforce the will to change?**

Health beliefs are a collection of beliefs that a person holds about diabetes and treatment. They can play a positive role in reinforcing the will to change behaviour.

The more closely health beliefs are adhered to, the stronger the will to adopt behaviours that promote good health (eating better, checking blood glucose regularly, etc.). To assess the sincerity of your will to change, do the following exercise. Ask yourself how much you really believe:

1) that you really do have diabetes;
2) that the disease can have serious consequences;
3) that following the advice of your healthcare providers will benefit your health;
4) that the benefits of treatment balance out the limitations it imposes;
5) that you feel capable of putting the advice of caregivers into action.

5. **Can erroneous beliefs about the illness and its treatment be obstacles to the will to change?**

   Of course. Erroneous beliefs, forged from false information, rumours, family stories and cultural perceptions, are a negative influence. They are often used as justifications to avoid taking proper care of oneself, to administer inadequate treatment, or to abandon a poorly understood treatment.

---

**Most common erroneous beliefs among people with diabetes**

o If I take pills to treat diabetes, I can eat whatever I want.

o My diabetes is minor or my sugar levels are just a little bit high; I therefore don't need treatment.

o I have to eliminate all sugars from my diet.

o Taking drugs to treat diabetes creates an addiction because the drugs are "chemicals". They should be taken as little as possible.

o If I inject insulin, I will become a "junkie".

o I got diabetes because I ate too much sugar.

o Diabetes treated with insulin is much worse than diabetes treated with oral antidiabetic medications.

o My diabetes is cured because my glucose level has returned to normal.

o Since I don't have any obvious symptoms, I must not have the disease.

o If I ignore the problems, they will disappear.

o No matter what I do, I'm still going to end up with complications and dying.

---

6. **What can be done to reinforce the positive effects of health beliefs and reduce the negative effects of erroneous beliefs?**

   1) Review your health beliefs regularly.
   2) Question your personal convictions about diabetes and treatment regularly.
   3) Seek out information:
      o read up on diabetes;
      o speak to your doctor;
      o follow a training course at a diabetes teaching center;
      o exchange information with other people with diabetes.

### 7. What are the steps to changing behaviour?

The following chart presents the steps that must be taken when changing behaviour. Being familiar with these steps can help you to identify what you need to do to get from one stage to the next.

| Step | Description | Action |
|---|---|---|
| **Pre-contemplation** | You have no intention of changing your behaviour. | 1) Remain open.<br>2) Seek out information that can make you more aware of the importance of the changes you have to make. |
| **Contemplation** | You have started to think about making changes over the next six months. | 1) Determine the obstacles to change.<br>2) Assess the advantages and disadvantages of change.<br>3) Ask the people around you for help. |
| **Preparation** | You have decided to make a change over the coming month. | 1) Draw up a plan, setting clear goals.<br>2) It can be useful to set up a verbal agreement with your doctor or diabetes health care professional. Also speak to your spouse or significant other. |
| **Action** | You have made a change. You have maintained it for fewer than six months. | Seek support, especially during periods when you feel more vulnerable, such as during vacations or periods of high stress. |
| **Maintenance** | You have made a change. You have maintained it for six months. | Reward yourself if you have achieved your goal (for example, treat yourself to a massage or set aside some money for a night out). |

### 8. How can you set achievable goals?

The following is a list of elements to take into account to increase the likelihood of reaching your goals. Goals should be:

1) **specific:**

   The plan must be clear. For example, instead of saying "I will eat more regularly", it is better to specifically say "I will eat three meals a day, five out of every seven days".

2) **measurable:**
   It is easier to assess your progress when your goals can be checked or measured.

3) **self-directed:**
   You must participate in establishing the goals. They are yours, after all.

4) **realistic:**
   Plan your progress in small steps. Success breeds success.

5) **limited in time:**
   Decide on a starting date, a time limit and how often you will keep track of your progress.

6) **assessed in terms of the expected support:**
   Determine whether you need the support of your family, friends or caregivers to reach your goal.

## 9.   What strategies can motivate you to exercise more?

1) **Exercise with a goal in mind:**
   Walk the dog or ride a bicycle to work, for example.

2) **Start off moderately:**
   It is better to walk only ten minutes a day than not at all.

3) **Remind yourself of the benefits of the exercise:**
   Exercise has been shown to be an excellent way to combat stress and depression and to protect from heart disease. It also helps control blood glucose levels in people with diabetes.

4) **Make exercise a regular part of your life:**
   Program your exercise regimen the way you program your work schedule or your social activities.

5) **Be flexible:**
   Do exercises that are accessible; when planning your activities, take into account your schedule, budget and abilities.

6) **Make it enjoyable:**
   Vary your physical activities to learn which ones you enjoy the most.

7) **Exercise with other people:**
   Find partners to walk, play tennis or go bird-watching with.

## 10. What strategies can motivate you to eat better?

Following the meal plan is probably the most difficult part of diabetes treatment. Here are a number of suggestions to help you succeed[1].

1) Develop a clear and realistic meal plan with your dietician.

2) Exert control over your environment to make it easier. For example, do not buy cookies if you know you cannot resist them.

3) Keep things in perspective if you seem to fall short of your expectations. For example, use glycosylated hemogoblin instead of just the week's blood glucose levels to assess the impact of weight loss on the control of your diabetes.

4) Beware of being too strict and depriving yourself; this can provoke an urge to abandon all your efforts.

5) Focus on the new habits you need to develop instead of the old ones you need to leave behind.

6) If your day-to-day life seems boring to you and eating has become your only pleasant and stimulating activity, you have to put some serious thought into reorganizing things. There are many options, such as volunteering or picking up a hobby.

7) Develop self-affirmation skills, especially if you are someone who finds it difficult to say "no".

---

1. Taken from *Diabetes Burnout* by W. Polonsky. Alexandria VA; American Diabetes Association, 1999.

# Sex and Family Planning

1. **Can diabetes affect the sex lives of people with diabetes?**

   Diabetes can cause problems affecting sexuality in both men and women. In women, these problems are less obvious and do not directly impede the sex act. It is worth noting, however, that there has been less research into the problems experienced by women and they are therefore less understood. As for men, on the other hand, chronic elevated blood glucose can cause difficulty in achieving and maintaining an erection and therefore the inability to have satisfactory sexual relations: this is known as **erectile dysfunction.**

2. **Do all men with diabetes suffer from erectile dysfunction?**

   **No.** Not all men with diabetes necessarily develop erectile dysfunction.

3. **How does diabetes cause erectile dysfunction in men?**

   In the long term, hyperglycemia can cause two problems:
   1) nerve damage;
   2) thickening and hardening of the arteries, which can hamper circulation.

   These two problems, either separately or in combination, can lead to the partial or complete inability to achieve erection (erectile dysfunction).

   Poorly controlled diabetes and an illness affecting general health can also cause erectile dysfunction. In such a case, correcting hyperglycemia generally enables a return of normal sexual function.

### 4. When men with diabetes have erectile dysfunction, is it always caused by the disease?

**No**. Erectile dysfunction in men with diabetes is often due to causes that have nothing to do with the disease. Possible causes include:

1) medications;
2) hormonal problems;
3) psychological problems.

### 5. How can men with diabetes prevent erectile dysfunction?

The risk of erectile dysfunction can be reduced by:

1) keeping blood glucose levels as close to normal as possible;
2) following the meal plan's recommendations on fats;
3) quitting smoking, if applicable;
4) maintaining control of high blood pressure and any blood lipid abnormalities;
5) stopping or decreasing alcohol consumption, if applicable.

### 6. How is erectile dysfunction assessed?

The following tests are performed to assess erectile dysfunction:

1) Doppler test to measure penile blood flow;
2) electromyography (EMG) of the penis to measure neurological conductivity;
3) measurement of hormone levels;
4) evaluation of nocturnal erections; the occurrence of nocturnal erections suggests the problem has a psychological origin;
5) psychological evaluation if these tests are negative.

### 7. Can erectile dysfunction be treated in men with diabetes?

**Yes**. The key is to identify the problem in order to find the appropriate treatment:

1) better control of blood glucose can help in some cases;
2) any hormonal problems should be corrected;
3) any drugs that disturb sexual function should be eliminated, if possible;
4) in some cases, drugs can be used to induce erection and eventually make full sexual relations possible:
   ○ medications taken orally, such as Viagra®, Cialis® or Levitra®;

      o      insertion of prostaglandin suppositories (Muse®) into the urethra;

      o      injection of prostaglandin at the base of the penis (Caverject®);

5)   in the case of severe organic erectile dysfunction, a penile prosthetic device can be used;

6)   sex therapy is often useful; it can either help the person adapt to his sexual difficulties or resolve any psychological conflicts that are at the root of the sexual problem.

## 8. Are there any risks associated with pregnancy in women with diabetes?

**Yes.** Pregnancy can cause certain risks for women with diabetes, especially if blood glucose is poorly controlled. There are three types of risk:

1)   **risks to the mother:**

      o      aggravation of the complications of diabetes;

      o      urinary infections;

      o      acidosis in women with type 1 diabetes;

      o      severe hypoglycemia.

**2)  risks to the baby:**

      o      spontaneous miscarriage;

      o      malformation;

      o      death in utero;

      o      premature birth;

      o      hypoglycemia at birth.

3)   **risks to both mother and baby:**

      o      toxemia of pregnancy, characterized by high blood pressure, protein in the urine and edema of the lower limbs;

      o      macrosomia (excessive birth weight of more then 4 kg at full term).

The risk of complications is significantly reduced if blood glucose is properly controlled both before and during pregnancy.

## 9. How can women with diabetes prevent complications associated with pregnancy?

Complications can generally be avoided. It is essential for a woman with diabetes to **consult her doctor** before deciding to become pregnant. It is very important to:

1) assess and treat any complications that could worsen during pregnancy, especially if they involve the eyes;
2) control blood glucose, prior to conception, as much as possible to reduce the risk of congenital malformation.

A woman with diabetes should consider becoming pregnant only once these issues have been addressed.

## 10. Are there risks of complications during pregnancy in women with diabetes?

**Yes**. Some of the complications related to diabetes carry high risks for pregnant women, especially if blood glucose is poorly controlled:
1) progression of retinopathy;
2) progression of kidney damage with severe loss of renal function;
3) severe high blood pressure;
4) heart failure if there is prior heart damage.

If these complications develop, it may be necessary to consider a **therapeutic termination of the pregnancy.**

## 11. What are the risks of a child developing diabetes if one of the parents has the disease?

If one of the parents has **type 1 diabetes**, the long-term risk of the child developing diabetes is **5%**. The risk is higher if the father has diabetes.

If one of the parents has **type 2 diabetes**, the long-term risk of the baby developing diabetes is **25%**.

## 12. What contraceptive methods are available to women with diabetes?

There are no contraceptive methods specifically designed for women with diabetes. Some methods do carry greater risks for these women, however.

There are two types of contraceptives:

1) **hormonal contraceptives:**
   o **combined birth control pills,** which contain two hormones, estrogen and progestin. They are effective, but they carry certain risks for blood glucose levels and blood vessels. There is also a skin patch and a vaginal ring that releases a combination of estrogen and progestin;
   o **low-dose progestin pills,** which contain a small amount of progestin. They are effective and have little impact on blood glucose, but their long-term effect on blood vessels is unknown;
   o intramuscular injections of progestin or intra-uterine devices (IUDs) with progestin. They are effective and have no impact on blood glucose or on blood vessels;

2) **mechanical contraception:**
   o intra-uterine devices (IUDs) are effective and present no risk of infection, provided blood glucose levels are properly controlled;
   o localized methods such as condoms, diaphragms and spermicide can be used by women with diabetes without risk.

The choice of method should be guided by the woman's age, how long she has had diabetes, how well it is managed, whether there are complications, whether she smokes, how many times she has been pregnant before, the effectiveness of the contraceptive, and above all, the preferences of the woman and her partner.

### 13. Can a woman with diabetes use emergency oral contraception (the "morning-after pill")?

Emergency oral contraception, which is used after unprotected sexual intercourse, is not contraindicated for women with diabetes. On the other hand, it is not recommended for regular use. It involves taking an oral contraceptive in one of the following ways:

1) a 100 µg dose of ethinylestradiol (an estrogen) combined with 500 µg of levonorgestrel (a progestin) as soon as possible after intercourse, and a second dose 12 hours later (for example, two doses of two Ovral® tablets); or

2) one dose of 750 µg of levonorgestrel (Plan B®) as soon as possible after intercourse and a second dose 12 hours later.

Emergency oral contraception should be prescribed by a doctor or, in Quebec, by a doctor or pharmacist.

## 14. What sterilization methods are available to women with diabetes and their partners?

Sterilization is an option that is worth considering when women with the disease have been pregnant a number of times, especially if they have experienced complications related to diabetes. The options are:

1) tubal ligation, for the woman;
2) vasectomy, for the man.

## 15. Can a menopausal woman with diabetes take hormones?

Menopausal women with diabetes can take estrogen, either with or without progestin. It has recently been demonstrated, however, that combined hormonal therapy (estrogen and progestin) in menopausal women is associated with a minimal but significant risk of breast cancer, thrombophlebitis (blood clots), strokes and heart disease. Menopausal women should therefore only take hormones (estrogen and progestin) if menopausal symptoms are difficult (for example, hot flashes) and only for a maximum of four years. Afterwards, medication should be discontinued if the symptoms are gone.

When deciding whether to take estrogen, the following high-risk situations should be taken into account:

1) prior thrombophlebitis;
2) prior cerebrovascular problems, especially in women who smoke;
3) a history of breast cancer.

# Community Resources

**This book was written by the multidisciplinary team of the diabetes day unit of the CHUM Hôtel-Dieu Hospital.**

The CHUM Hôtel-Dieu diabetes day unit opened its doors in March 1995 in response to a need for education, research and development in the area of diabetes.

Every week, the diabetes day unit welcomes about a dozen people and their families for a four-day training session. Individual and group encounters give people an opportunity to learn more about every aspect of diabetes. This type of knowledge can help people with diabetes become more independent with respect to their illness.

A multidisciplinary team of endocrinologists, nurses, dieticians, and psychologists offers the following training programs to people with diabetes:
- four-day course (regular program);
- one-day intensive course;
- one-day refresher every six months (after initial training);
- two hours a month for amblyopic or blind people;
- four hours a month for people with cystic fibrosis.

Everything is offered free of charge, and every person with diabetes receives a copy of the book *Understand Your Diabetes and Live a Healthy Life.*

Recommendations are sent to the treating physician.

All interested parties can contact:
> **Diabetes Day Unit**
> CHUM Hôtel-Dieu
> 3840 Saint-Urbain Street
> Montreal, Quebec H2W 1T8
> Tel.: 514 890-8000, extension 14658

There are a number of other diabetes teaching centres accessible through the health network. The Diabetes Québec magazine *Plein Soleil* and the Diabetes Québec website contain a list of these centres. The local branches of the Canadian Diabetes Association, present in all provinces except Quebec, are also a valuable source of information.

# Physical Activity

1.  ## What exercise services and facilities are available to people with diabetes?

> **Amicale des diabétiques des hôpitaux Notre-Dame et Maisonneuve-Rosemont**
> (aquafitness, gentle conditioning, group walking)
> 2065 Alexandre-de-Sève Street
> 9th floor, suite Z-9903-4
> Montreal, Quebec  H2L 2W5
> Tel.: 514 890-8000, extension 25358
> E-mail: amicale.diabetique.chum@ssss.gouv.qc.ca

> **Centre ÉPIC**
> 5055 Saint-Zotique Street East
> Montreal, Quebec  H1T 1N6
> Tel.: 514 374-1480
> Fax: 514 374-2445
> Website: www.icm-mhi.org

**Clinique de kinésiologie**
CEPSUM–Université de Montréal
2100 Édouard-Montpetit Blvd., suite 205
C. P. 6128, Succ. Centre-ville
Montreal, Quebec  H3C 3J7
Tel.: 514 343-6150
Fax: 514 343-2188
E-mail: cliniquekin@kinesio.umontreal.ca
Website: www.kinesio.umontreal.ca
www.cepsum.umontreal.ca

**Centre de santé et de services sociaux Jeanne-Mance**
Health motivation education centre
1051 Saint-Hubert Street
Montreal, Quebec  H2L 3Y5
Tel.: 514 521-7663, extension 6559
Website: www.santemontreal.qc.ca/csss/jeannemance

**Fédération québécoise de la marche**
*Marche-Randonnée* magazine
4545 Pierre-de-Coubertin Avenue
C.P. 1000, succ. M
Montreal, Quebec  H1V 3R7
Tel.: 514 252-3157  or toll-free 1 866 252-2065
Fax : 514 252-5137
Website: www.fqmarche.qc.ca

**Outdoor recreational activity groups (for people who are more active)**
www.actionpassion.com
www.aventuremonde.com
www.azimutaventure.com/
www.bougex.com
www.horizonroc.com/
www.aventuriers.qc.ca
www.cycloconcept.ca
www.cyclonature.org

246 Understand Your Diabetes and Live a Healthy Life

www.detournature.com
www.karavaniers.com
www.groupeoxygene.qc.ca
www.pulsations.ca
www.passionaventure.com

**Kino-Québec**
www.kino-quebec.qc.ca
www.actimetre.qc.ca (adult physical activity assessment software and recommendations)

# Socioeconomic support

## 2. What kind of socioeconomic support is available?

○ **Access to welfare**
People with diabetes who are eligible for welfare receive an additional $20 per month. They must communicate with the agent responsible for their file for further information.
  • Solidarité sociale, Bureau des renseignements et plaintes
    Tel. toll-free: 1 888 643-4721

○ **Family allowance**
An extra $167 per month is added to the family allowance for parents with a dependent child who has diabetes. The request for the supplement must be filled out and signed by the pediatrician.
  • Régie des rentes du Québec
    Tel.: 514 864-3873 or 1 800 667-9625 (benefits for handicapped children)

○ **Régie des rentes du Québec**
Tel.: 514 864-3873 or 1 800 667-9625 (benefits for han dicapped children)

○ **Tax credit**
People with chronic diseases requiring daily care may be entitled to a federal tax credit.

o **Loans and Bursaries**

Full-time CEGEP or university students with diabetes are reimbursed for the cost of their medication.

Students must make a loan and bursary request at the financial aid office of their school and follow the steps set out in the program.

The cost of medications is reimbursed by the Ministère de l'Éducation, according to the *Act respecting financial assistance for education expenses*. Tel.: 418 643-3750 or toll-free 1 877 643-3750

# Insurance

## 3. What factors should people with diabetes consider when taking out insurance?

**Important facts**

- Insurance taken out before the diagnosis of diabetes remains in force under the same terms.
- When a new application for insurance is made, people with diabetes must undergo a medical assessment to determine their new level of risk. Each person with diabetes is considered as a separate case.
- In the case of mortgage life insurance, the benefit is usually not available if the diabetes is pre-existing or if the disease is diagnosed before the renewal of the policy.

**Group insurance**

- Like all other employees, people with diabetes benefit from compulsory coverage. People with diabetes may take out optional coverage with no additional premium if the request is made before the imposed deadline. Beyond the deadline, coverage is usually refused.
- When a person leaves a particular employment, group insurance policies can often be converted into individual insurance.

**Individual life insurance**
- People with diabetes should consult with several insurance companies before signing a contract. Every insurer has its own method of evaluation.
- There are many possible types of insurance for people with diabetes:
  - additional premiums that vary widely, possibly increasing from one year to the next; the premium depends on each individual's risk assessment
  - "health option" flat rate, where the admissibility and maintenance of the protection depends on criteria related to how well the diabetes is controlled.

# Associations

## 4. What associations provide support to people with diabetes?

**Canadian Diabetes Association**
1400-522 University Avenue
Toronto, Ontario  M5G 2R5
Tel.: 1 800 226-8464
Website: www.diabetes.ca
Magazine : *Diabetes Dialogue*

**American Diabetes Association**
1701 North Beauregard Street
Alexandria, VA 22311
United States of America
Tel.: 1 800 342-2383
Website: www.diabetes.org
Magazine: *Diabetes Forecast*

**Diabetes Québec**
8550 Pie-IX Blvd., suite 300
Montreal, Quebec  H1Z 4G2
Tel.: 514 259-3422 or 1 800 361-3504
E-mail: info@diabete.qc.ca
Website: www.diabete.qc.ca
Magazine: *Plein soleil*

# Blind or Amblyopic

5.  **What services are offered to people with diabetes who are blind or amblyopic?**

**Philips Lifeline**
Remote surveillance (two-way vocal communicator)
774 Décarie Blvd., suite 100
Saint-Laurent, Quebec H4L 3L5
Tel.: 514 735-2101 or 1 877 423-9700
Website: www.lifeline.ca

**Montreal Association for the Blind**
7000 Sherbrooke Street West
Montreal, Quebec  H4B 1R3
Tel.: 514 489-8201
Fax: 514 489-3477
Website: www.mab.ca

**Institut de réadaptation en déficience physique du Québec**
525 Wilfrid-Hamel Blvd., Wing J
Quebec City, Quebec G1M 2S8
Tel.: 418 529-9141
Fax: 418 529-3699
Website: www.irdpq.qc.ca

**Canadian National Institute for the Blind**
215 Guy Street, suite 750
Montreal, Quebec  H3H 2R9
Tel: 514 934-4622 or 1 800 465-4622
Fax: 514-934-2131
Website: www.inca.ca

**Institut Nazareth et Louis-Braille**
1111 Saint-Charles Street West
Longueuil, Quebec  J4K 5G4
Tel.: 450 463-1710 or 1 800 361-7063
Fax: 450 463-0243
Website: www.inlb.qc.ca

**Specialized equipment for amblyopic or visually impaired people**
- Braille blood glucose notebook
  CHUM Hôtel-Dieu diabetes day unit
  Tel.: 514 890-8000, extension 14658
- CD for people who are visually impaired
  - Diabetes Québec
    *Plein soleil* magazine
    Tel.: 514 259-3422 or 1 800 361-3504
  - CHUM Hôtel-Dieu diabetes day unit
    1) *Understand Your Diabetes and Live a Healthy Life*
    2) Recipes with calculated carbohydrates for the visually impaired: *Recettes faciles pour diabétiques et semi-voyants 2006* Distributed by the Service québécois du livre adapté
       Tel.: 514 873-4454 or 1 866 410-0844
- Blood glucose metres
  - **Bayer Ascensia® Contour** ® with speech synthesis distributed by Pharmacie Danielle Desroches
    Tel.: 514 288-8555 or 450 447-9280
  - **Accu-Chek® Compact Plus®** from Roche Diagnostics
    A reader emitting beeps; upcoming model with speech synthesis
    Tel.: 1 800 363-7949

- Syringe support for the blind
  Institut de réadaptation en déficience physique du Québec
  Tel.: 418 529-9141

### Regroupement des aveugles et amblyopes du Montréal métropolitain

5215 Berri Street, suite 200
Montreal, Quebec  H2J 2S4
Tel.: 514 277-4401
Fax: 514 277-8961
Website: www.raamm.org

### Service québécois du livre adapté

475 de Maisonneuve Blvd. East
Montreal, Quebec  H2L 5C4
514 873-4454 or 1 866 410-0844
Website: www.banq.qc.ca/portal/dt/sqla/sqla.htm

# Diabetes Québec

### 6.   What services are offered by Diabetes Québec?

**Diabète Québec**
8550 Pie-IX Blvd., suite 300
Montreal (Quebec) H1Z 4G2
Tel.: 514 259-3422 or toll-free 1 800 361-3504
Website: www.diabete.qc.ca
Email: info@diabete.qc.ca

Diabetes Québec is a non-profit association bringing people with diabetes and health professionals together. Its mission is education, sensitization, and prevention. There are four general aspects to the work done by this organization: training, encouraging research, defending the rights of people with diabetes, and ensuring that services are provided. Some of its services are free, while others are offered at a nominal price.

- o The *Plein soleil* magazine, which features useful information about diabetes;
- o lectures;
- o educational materials (books, brochures, and the videocassette entitled "Foot Care for Diabetics");
- o training tailored to specific groups of people with diabetes and health professionals;
- o an information phone line:
  InfoDiabetes
  Tel.: 514 259-3422, extension 233 or toll-free 1 800 361-3504
  E-mail: infodiabete@diabete.qc.ca

# Grieving

## 7. What bereavement services are available to people with diabetes?

**Services commémoratifs Mont-Royal**
(sharing and discussion groups on bereavement)
1297 Chemin de la Forêt
Outremont, Quebec H2V 2P9
Tel.: 514 279-7358
Fax: 514 279-0049
Website: www.mountroyalcem.com

**Vie nouvelle** (information about the grieving process and discussion groups)
CHUM Hôtel-Dieu
3840 Saint-Urbain Street
Montreal, Quebec H2W 1T8
Tel.: 514 890-8000, extension 15000

# Children

## 8. What services are offered to children with diabetes?

**Camp pour enfants diabétiques de l'est du Québec**
11 Crémazie Street East
Quebec City, Quebec G1R 1Y1
Tel.: 418 523-6159
E-mail: info@cedeq.org
Website: www.cedeq.org

**Juvenile Diabetes Research Foundation**
2155 Guy Street, suite 1120
Montreal, Quebec  H3H 2R9
Tel.: 514 744-5537 or 1 877 634-2238
Fax: 514 744-0516
E-mail: montreal@jdrf.ca
Website: www.jdrf.ca

**The Diabetic Children's Foundation and Camp Carowanis**
785 Plymouth Street, suite 210
Mont-Royal, Quebec H4P 1B3
Tel.: 514731-9683 or 514 731-9683 or 1 800 731-9683
Fax: 514 731-2683
E-mail: carowanis@diabete-enfants.ca
Website: www.diabetes-children.ca

# Medical Identification

### 9. Where can I get a medical bracelet or pendant?

Jewellery stores

**Canadian Medic-Alert Foundation**
2005, Sheppard Avenue East, suite 800
Toronto, Ontario M2J 5B4
Tel.: 416 696-0267 or 1 800 668-6381
Website: www.medicalert.ca

**Pharmacies**

# Feet

### 10. What foot care services are available?

**Association des infirmières et infirmiers en soins de pieds du Québec**
3850 Jean-Talon Street West, Suite 122
Montreal, Quebec H3R 2G8
Tel.: 514 344-7212 or toll-free 1 800 771-9664
Fax: 514 344-0766
E-mail: info@aiispq.qc.ca

**Clinique d'évaluation et de traitement podologique pour patients atteints de diabète (pied diabétique)**
CHUM Hôtel-Dieu
3840 Saint-Urbain Street
Montreal, Quebec H2W 1T8
Tel.: 514 890-8151 (make an appointment at Centre des rendez-vous)

**Ordre des podiatres du Québec**
300 Saint-Sacrement Street, Suite 102
Montreal, Quebec H2Y 1X4
Tel.: 514 288-0019
Website: www.ordredespodiatres.qc.ca

# Driver's Licence

## 11. What factors should people with diabetes consider when getting a driver's licence?

### Important facts

- Diabetes can cause problems that affect visual sharpness and field of vision. Obviously, vision plays a fundamental role in driving an automobile.
- Driving is a **privilege**, not **a right to be taken for granted** or bestowed without reservation.
- The SAAQ (Société de l'assurance automobile du Québec) establishes the rules governing the acquisition and holding of this privilege. These rules revolve around a person's ability to **drive safely**, as regards himself or herself and all others. The state of the driver's health is taken into account.

### Medical assessment

- A medical assessment form is sent out to people with diabetes at varying intervals.
- The report must be filled out by the treating doctor and/or optometrist within the time frame specified (three months).

> The SAAQ medical assessment takes into account how well the diabetes is controlled.

The SAAQ bases its decision on this medical opinion. It places more weight on functional limitations than on the diagnosis.

### Hypoglycemia and driving

- Hypoglycemia can compromise the ability of a person with diabetes to drive safely. It occurs most often in people with diabetes who are treated with insulin and less frequently in those who take medications to stimulate the production of insulin (sulfonylureas, meglitinides).
- Necessary preventive measures include the following:
  - always have rapidly absorbed sugars nearby;
  - avoid driving for long periods without a break;
  - never skip meals or snacks;
  - carry an emergency food supply in case a meal is delayed.

## Legal obligations

The law provides the following:

- Holders of a **driver's licence are under a legal obligation** to inform the SAAQ of any disease or change that is, in particular, related to their physical and mental health when they first apply for their permit and within 30 days of the change in their health. Knowingly providing false or misleading information is an offence and can lead to the suspension of the person's driver's licence and a fine.

- Holders of a driver's licence are under a legal obligation to respond to a request for a medical report within the specified time.

> Any person providing false or misleading information is guilty of an offence and may be subject to prosecution. A false declaration renders the driver fully responsible, which could have serious repercussions in the case of an accident.

For more information, contact the Service de l'évaluation médicale at the SAAQ:

> Service de l'évaluation médicale, SAAQ
> P.O. 19500,
> Quebec City, Quebec G1K 8J5
> Tel.: 418 643-5506 or toll-free 1 800 561-2858
> Website: www.saaq.qc.ca

# Professionals

### 12. What nutritional resources are available to people with diabetes?

Dieticians

- **Association des diététistes au Québec**
  Tel.: 514 954-0047
  Fax: 514 932-8108
  Website: www.adaqnet.org

- **Ordre professionnel des diététistes du Québec**
  2155 Guy Street, Suite 1220
  Montreal, Quebec  H3H 2R9
  Tel.: 514 393-3733 or toll-free 1 888- 393-8528
  Website: www.opdq.org

Books about diabetes and nutrition
- Isabelle Galibois, *Le diabète de type 1 et ses défis alimentaires quotidiens* (Quebec City: Les Presses de l'Université Laval, 2005).

Cookbooks with carbohydrate counts
- Anne Lindsay, *Smart Cooking: Quick and Tasty Recipes for Healthy Living* (Canadian Cancer Society, 1997).

- *Anne Lindsay's Light Kitchen* (Wiley, 1991)

- Anne Lindsay, in collaboration with Denise Beatty of the Canadian Medical Association, *Anne Lindsay's New Light Kitchen* (Random House Canada, 1998).

- Manon Poissant, Céline Raymond & Josée Rouette, *La nouvelle cuisine santé* (Éditions Stanké, 1998).

- Karen Graham, *Meals for Good Health* (Canadian Diabetes Association, 2005).

- Manon Robitaille & Daniel Lavoie, *Le dessert se fait léger* (Éditions Diabète Québec, 2007).

- N. Delisle, M. Forget & S. Larouche, *Les sucres et pourquoi pas* (Métro Richelieu et Diabète Québec, 2001).

- N. Delisle, M. Forget & S. Larouche, *Les sucres... Question d'équilibre* (Éditions Profil-Santé, 2007).

- Helen Bishop, et al., *Eat Well, Live Well: The Canadian Dietetic Association's Guide to Healthy Eating.*, (Macmillan of Canada, 1990).

- Katherine E. Younker, *The Best Diabetes Cookbook* (published in cooperation with the Canadian Diabetes Association, R. Rose, 2005.)

- *Qu'est-ce qu'on mange?* Vol. 4. (Cercle des fermières du Québec, 1997)

- Various authors, *Simplement délicieux*, Éditions du Trécarré, 2007.

**Web sites on diabetes and nutrition**
- Recipe analyzer
  - Dieticians of Canada:
    Website: http://www.dietitians.ca/public/content/eat_well_live_well/english/recipeanalyzer/recipeanalyzer.asp

- Carbohydrate calculator (advanced method):
  www.diabete.qc.ca
  (for download)

- L'Épicerie television show on Radio-Canada
  www.radio-canada.ca/actualite/v2/lepicerie/

- Extenso, Centre de référence sur la nutrition humaine (information on human nutrition)
  www.extenso.org

- Fédération des producteurs maraîchers du Québec
  www.legumesduquebec.com

- Canada's Food Guide
  http://www.hc-sc.gc.ca/fn-an/food-guide-aliment/index-eng.php

- Passeport santé

- SOS cuisine
  www.soscuisine.com

- Nutritional value of foods
  - CalorieKing
    www.calorieking.com
  - Canadian Nutrient File
    http://www.hc-sc.gc.ca/fn-an/nutrition/fiche-nutri-data/cnf_
    downloads-telechargement_fcen-eng.php
  - Nutritional values of some common foods
    www.hc-sc.gc.ca/fn-an/alt_formats/hpfb-dgpsa/pdf/nutrition/nvscf-
    vnqau_f.pdf

### Websites featuring recipes with carbohydrate counts
  - Canadian Diabetes Association
    www.diabetes.ca/recipes/recipesIndex.asp
  - American Diabetes Association
    vgs.diabetes.org/recipe/index.jsp
  - Diabetes Québec
    www.diabete.qc.ca/html/alimentation/recette/recette.html

# Nursing Services

### 13. What nursing care resources are available to people with diabetes?

**Nurses**

**Ordre des infirmières et infirmiers du Québec**

4200 Dorchester Blvd. West

Westmount, Quebec H3Z 1V4

Tel.: 514 935-2501 or toll-free 1 800 363-6048

Fax: 514 935-1799

E-mail: inf@oiiq.org

Website: www.oiiq.org

**Info-Santé**

CLSC (Quebec community health centres) telephone help line, available 24 hours a day to provide answers to health questions. Since April 2008, this service can be reached by dialing **811**.

All **CLSCs** are open from 8 a.m. to 4 p.m.

# Medical services

### 14. How can you get medical assistance?

Collège des médecins du Québec

2170 René-Lévesque Blvd. West

Montreal, Quebec  H3H 2T8

Tel.: 514 933-4441 or toll-free 1 888 633-3246

Fax: 514 933-3112

Website: www.cmq.org

**DOCTORS**

My family doctor: _____   Tel._____

My endocrinologist_____   Tel._____

Endocrinologist on call
at my hospital:_____   Tel._____

# Pharmacists Services

## 15. How can you get help from a pharmacist?

**Ordre des pharmaciens du Québec**
266 Notre-Dame Street West, suite 301
Montreal, Quebec H2Y 1T6
Tel.: 514 284-9588 or toll-free 1 800 363-0324
Website: www.opq.org

**Any pharmacy**

**Régime public d'assurance-médicaments (Quebec)**
· Contact the Régime de l'assurance maladie du Québec
  Tel.: 1 888 435-79999
  Website: www.ramq.gouv.qc.ca

**PHARMACISTS**

My pharmacist: _____   Tel._____

My pharmacy: _____   Tel._____

# Psychological Services

## 16. What psychological services are available to people with diabetes?

### Psychologists

- **Ordre des psychologues du Québec**
  1100 Beaumont Avenue, suite 510
  Mont-Royal, Quebec H3P 3H5
  Tel.: 514 738-1881 or toll-free 1 800 363-2644
  Website: www.ordrepsy.qc.ca

### Anxiety and mood disorders

- **Hôpital Louis-Hippolyte LaFontaine**
  7401 Hochelaga Street
  Montreal, Quebec H1N 3M5
  Note: Ask for the Evaluation-Liaison Module
  (medical reference necessary)
  Tel.: 514 251-4000, extension 2495
  Fax: 514 251-7527
  Website: www.hlhl.qc.ca

- **Anxiety disorder clinic/ Depressive disorder clinic**
  Douglas Mental Health University Institute
  6875 Lasalle Blvd.
  Montreal, Quebec H4N 1R3
  Note: Ask for the Evaluation-Liaison Module
  (medical reference necessary)
  Tel.: 514 888-4469
  Website: www.douglas.qc.ca

### Services for addiction, alcohol abuse, drug abuse, and problem gambling

- **Centre Dollard-Cormier**
  950 de Louvain Street East
  Montreal, Quebec H2M 2E8
  Tel.: 514 385-1232
  Website: ww.centredollarcormier.qc.ca

# Sex therapy services

**17.  What resources are available regarding sexual concerns related to diabetes?**

> Sex therapists
> *   **Association des sexologues du Québec**
>     7400 Boul Saint Laurent, office 404
>     Montreal, Quebec H2R 2Y1
>     Tel.: 514 270-9289
>     Website: www.associationdessexologues.com
>
> *   **Sexual Dysfunction Unit at the CHUM Hôpital St-Luc**
>     Édouard-Asselin Building, 5th floor
>     264 René-Lévesque Blvd. East
>     Montreal, Quebec H2X 1P1
>     Tel.: 514 890-8351

# Websites

**18.  What are some useful websites on diabetes?**

> o   Canadian Food Inspection Agency (information on food labelling and advertising)
>     Tel.: 450 928-4300 or toll-free 1 800 442-2342
>     www.cfia-acia.agr.ca
>
> o   American Diabetes Association
>     www.diabetes.org
>
> o   American Dietetic Association
>     www.webdietitians.org
>
> o   Canadian Diabetes Association
>     www.diabetes.ca

o  Association de langue française pour l'étude du diabète et des maladies métaboliques
www.alfediam.org

o  CDC Diabetes Public Health Resource
www.cdc.gov/diabetes

o  CH Baie-des-Chaleurs
www.chbc.qc.ca/lediabete/default.htm

o  Children with Diabetes
www.childrenwithdiabetes.com/index_cwd.htm

o  Diabetes Québec
www.diabete.qc.ca

o  Diabetes Insight
www.diabetic.org.uk

o  Diabetes.com Health Library
www.diabetes.com/tools/health_library/index.html

o  European Association for the Study of Diabetes
www.easd.org

o  International Diabetes Federation
www.idf.org

o  Joslin Diabetes Center
www.joslin.harvard.edu

o  Juvenile Diabetes Research Foundation Canada
www.jdfc.ca

o  Diabetes in Canada
www.phac-aspc.gc.ca/publicat/dic-dac2/english/05contents_e.html

- o   Le diabète au jour le jour
  www.ciminfo.org/diabete/index.html

- o   Dieticians of Canada
  www.dietitians.ca

- o   Medline plus: diabetes
  www.nlm.nih.gov/medlineplus/diabetes.html

- o   National Diabetes Education Program
  www.ndep.nih.gov

- o   National Institute of Diabetes & Digestive & Kidney Diseases
  www.niddk.nih.gov/health/diabetes/diabetes.htm

- o   National Institutes of Health
  www.niddk.nih.gov

- o   Programme d'enseignement diabète
  www.hopitallaval.qc.ca

# Smoking

### 19. What services are offered to people with diabetes who want to quit smoking?

**Centre d'abandon du tabagisme**

Free assistance and personalized support is available everywhere in Quebec.

- Speak to a specialist on the telephone on the J'Arrete line:
  1-866-jarrete or 1 866 527-7383.

- Resources to help you keep your resolve are available online at www.jarrette.qc.ca.

- Meet with a professional at a Centre d'abandon du tabagisme (centre for quitting smoking) nearest you for personalized services to help you quit.

- For the address of the Centre d'abandon du tabagisme nearest you, call 1 866-jarrete or 1 866 527-7383.

- At the CHUM: to make an appointment, call 514 890-8226; for information only, call 514 890-8000, extension 15983.

# Work

### 20. What workplace concerns should people with diabetes keep in mind?

**People with diabetes should tell people at their workplace about their disease.**

- The *Charter of Rights and Freedoms* protects people with diabetes against any and all discrimination.
- People with diabetes should be as candid as possible with their employer and a few select colleagues, keeping in mind workplace context (for example, it is a good idea to inform people of what to do in the event of serious hypoglycemia).

**Some jobs or professions should be avoided.**

- People with diabetes are discouraged from taking certain jobs:
  - for example, airplane pilot, fireman, emergency vehicle driver, high-voltage lineworkers, etc.
- Certain jobs can be difficult for people with diabetes:
  - for example, garbage collector (increased risk of infection), cook (difficult to follow the meal plan), jeweller (requires good eyesight), etc.

**Workplace behaviour**

- Employers or colleagues may change the way they interact with a co-worker who has diabetes when they first learn of the disease. This is a temporary and foreseeable stage of the adaptation process.
- Like everyone else, people with diabetes have the fundamental right to be full members of society. Work is one of the most important tools to help achieve personal growth and self-realization.
- The International Association of Machinists—Center for Administering Rehabilitation and Employment Services (AIM CARES) can help you. This association offers a free specialized job search service.

> 750 Marcel-Laurin Blvd., suite 450
> Saint-Laurent, Quebec H4M 2M4
> Tel.: 514 744-2944 or 514 744-2613
> E-mail: emploi@aimcroitqc.org
> Website: www.aimcroitqc.org

---

### YOUR STRONG POINTS

People with diabetes who are looking for a job can actually take advantage of the constraints their illness imposes when they are looking for a job. People with diabetes have had to acquire a number of positive qualities including discipline, consistency, perseverance, dedication to a healthy lifestyle, and so on.

# Travel

## 21. What services are offered to people with diabetes who want to travel?

**Travel Health Clinics in Canada**
Public Health Agency of Canada
Web\site: http://www.phac-aspc.gc.ca/index-eng.php

**Regional Quebec office**
Suite 218, Complexe Guy-Favreau
200 René-Lévesque Blvd. West, East Tower
Montreal, Quebec H2Z 1X4
Tel.: 514 283-2306
Fax: 514 283-6739

**Clinique Santé-Voyage Saint-Luc (Saint-Luc Travel Health Clinic)**
1001 Saint-Denis Street, 6th floor
Montreal, Québec H2X 3H9
Tel.: 514 890-8332
Fax: 514 412-7362
E-mail: info@santevoyagesaint-luc.com
Website: www.santevoyagesaint-luc.com

# Research:
## What the Future Holds

There have been steady advances in research into diabetes over recent years. This chapter will outline the main questions that have been answered, as well as those that are still receiving the attention of researchers.

**1.   What is the cause of type 1 or "juvenile" diabetes?**
Alterations in the pancreatic beta cells, caused by environmental factors such as a viral infection, can lead to loss of recognition of one's own cells. Mistaking them for foreign cells, the body produces antibodies to destroy them. The capacity to create antibodies against its own cells has a genetic component and these antibodies can be detected approximately five years before the development of the disease.

**2.   Are there ways to prevent diabetes?**
A number of different methods have been attempted to prevent the appearance of the disease in people at high risk.
   1)   treatments attempting to block the production of antibodies as soon as they appear and treatments using insulin injections or orally administered doses failed to prevent type 1 diabetes;
   2)   an international nutritional study currently underway is trying to determine whether early introduction of solid foods or cow's milk to young children at risk could influence the risk of development of type 1 diabetes later on;
   3)   there is currently research underway into the genes involved in the development and progression of diabetes, whether type 1 or type 2. Teams from Montreal have made

a number of discoveries in this area. Gene KIAA0350, which codes for a protein that binds molecules containing sugar, has been associated with type 1 diabetes. Several genes (including TCF7L2) that are involved in the development and the function of pancreatic beta cells and in metabolic mechanisms have variants that create a predisposition to type 2 diabetes in approximately 70% of cases.

## 3. What is the cause of type 2 diabetes?

There are two major factors involved in the development of the type 2 diabetes: insulin resistance (meaning that a great deal more insulin is required to maintain normal blood glucose levels) and a decrease in the capacity of pancreatic cells to produce the insulin. In most cases, insulin resistance precedes the development of diabetes by several years. As long as the pancreatic cells can compensate by producing more insulin, blood glucose levels remain normal. It is only once the pancreatic cells are no longer able to compensate and insulin production decreases that blood glucose levels increase. At first, blood glucose levels rise, especially after meals. This is known as impaired glucose tolerance, and it characterizes the pre-diabetic stage. If insulin production decreases further, blood glucose levels rise even higher after meals and eventually even before meals. This is diabetes proper.

## 4. What factors contribute to insulin resistance?

Susceptibility to insulin resistance and a lowered capacity for insulin production are in part hereditary. Excess weight and a lack of physical activity contribute to insulin resistance and an increased risk of developing diabetes. Research has shown that efforts to reduce insulin resistance in people who are glucose intolerant have significantly reduced the risk of developing diabetes.

## 5. What types of interventions have positive effects on the prevention of type 2 diabetes?

The ideal is to intervene as early as possible. This is quite a challenge, however, because in some cases, an increased risk for diabetes can begin before birth if the fetus is exposed to unfavourable conditions inside the uterus. Gestational diabetes in the mother and low birth weight are possible risk factors for the development of diabetes as an adult.

Some interventions have been shown to be effective in preventing type 2 diabetes:
1)  improved nutrition and greater physical activity (lifestyle modifications);
2)  metformin and thiazolidinediones (drugs that decrease insulin resistance and glucose production by the liver);
3)  acarbose (drug that slows down carbohydrate absorption);
4)  orlistat (drug used to control weight gain);
5)  possibly inhibitors of the renin-angiotensin system (drugs used for the treatment of high blood pressure, heart failure, and diabetic nephropathy). This class of medication requires further research because benefits were not observed in all the studies;
6)  bariatric surgery, or weight-loss surgery, which involves reducing the size of the stomach or inducing malabsorption.

## 6.  What factors are responsible for the development of the complications of diabetes?

In the 1990s, two major studies definitively confirmed that the microvascular complications of diabetes (retinopathy, nephropathy, neuropathy) are primarily related to high blood glucose over several years. The first study, an American-Canadian trial (DCCT) published in 1993, followed 1440 patients with type 1 diabetes. The second, a British trial (UKPDS) published in 1998, followed 4209 patients with type 2 diabetes. Both studies found that diabetes, whether type 1 or type 2, must be aggressively treated and that the complications of diabetes can be prevented by keeping target blood glucose levels as close to normal as possible.

A number of more recent studies have confirmed the importance of optimal blood glucose control to avoid complications, particularly microvascular complications (retinopathy, nephropathy, neuropathy). The STENO-2 study demonstrated that intensive treatment of multiples factors including blood glucose, blood pressure, and cholesterol not only reduced microvascular complications (retinopathy, nephropathy, neuropathy), but also lowered mortality rates and cut the number of cardiovascular events (infarcts, stroke). The study also confirmed the importance of controlling all the risk factors.

Long-term follow-up in the DCCT and STENO-2 studies has shown that the benefits of treatment continue for several years after the intensive treatment.

### 7. Is it possible to prevent the appearance of complications?

The prevention of complications presents one of the great challenges of research into diabetes. Thanks to our better understanding of the physiopathological mechanisms responsible for the complications of diabetes, there are a few studies now evaluating drugs that may be able to prevent the complications of diabetes, regardless of blood glucose control.

We have already mentioned the major role that high blood glucose levels play in the development of the complications of diabetes. A number of studies have shown that high blood sugar is associated with an overproduction of an enzyme called kinase C, and that this enzyme is involved in the development of the complications. The pharmaceutical industry has developed a kinase C protein inhibitor and demonstrated that this drug can prevent complications in animals with diabetes.

Studies of the effects of kinase C inhibitors on diabetic retinopathy and neuropathy in humans are currently underway. Such drugs could eventually make it possible to prevent complications even when optimal control of blood glucose is difficult. Researchers are also beginning to study drugs inhibiting growth factors that play a role in the development of retinopathy (pegaptanib, ranibizumab and bevacizumab).

### 8. Is it easy to control diabetes?

DCCT and UKPDS studies have shown that it is difficult to reach normal blood glucose levels. In Canada, the DICE study looked at patients followed by front-line doctors and revealed that close to 50% of people with type 2 diabetes did not attain their recommended treatment targets. Making this task easier depends not only on using the medications that already exist, but also looking for new treatments.

### 9. How is it possible to prevent a gradual deterioration of glycemic control over time?

Interventions to preserve the function of the pancreatic beta cells and a residual secretion of insulin are also important topics of research at the moment. In animals, thiazolidinedione and incretin drugs have been shown to have a positive effect on the beta cells by decreasing cell death and increasing cell proliferation.

## 10. What is new in the treatment of diabetes?

A number of antidiabetic drugs and new techniques are currently being studied or will soon be available in Canada. The following are worth noting:

1) drugs that slow gastric emptying, giving time to the pancreas to react, such as pramlintide (Symlin®);

2) drugs that slow gastric emptying simulate the secretion of insulin by the pancreas (in response to elevated blood sugar) and decrease the production of glucagon (a hormone that blocks the effect of insulin and increases blood sugar). Such drugs include GLP-1 analogs (incretin drugs) such as exenatide (Byetta®) and liraglutide. These drugs are administered subcutaneously, although a form that will be delivered intranasally is currently in development. These drugs also have a positive side effect, as they induce weight loss;

3) new rapid-acting insulin analogues, such as glulisine;

4) new ways of administering insulin; Oralin®, for example, is delivered orally and absorbed through the mucous membranes of the mouth;

5) cannabinoid system inhibitors, such as rimonabant. This drug is also used to treat obesity;

6) inhibitors of glucose transport in the kidney that increase the elimination of glucose through the urine, such as sergliflozin and dapagliflozin;

7) new technical procedures to connect an insulin pump to a continuous blood glucose monitor, to create a kind of artificial pancreas.

## 11. What are the challenges of transplants?

○ **Pancreas transplants** have been successfully executed in various Canadian hospitals, including the CHUM Notre-Dame Hospital. The two major obstacles to pancreas transplants are the shortage of donors and the side effects of anti-rejection drugs.

○ More recently, there has been progress made in the transplants of **islets of Langerhans**, which involve the injection insulin-making pancreatic cells. An innovative group of researchers from Edmonton, Alberta have improved the technique of isolating the islets of Langerhans and used new combinations of anti-rejection drugs (without cortisone). These transplants are performed under local anesthesia on ambulatory patients. A catheter is inserted into the portal vein entering the liver and the islets are injected with a syringe, after which the patient goes home. One of the difficulties encountered is the fact that the isolation technique enables the recovery of only 20% of the islets. Therefore, two and sometimes three donor pancreases are required to obtain a sufficient amount of islets of Langerhans for the transplant. In addition, the destruction of the islets over time means that the cure offered by this technique is temporary. The problem of donor shortage is therefore all the more acute. Improved techniques for isolating the islets, however, should provide a partial solution to this problem.

o   New avenues are also being explored with the goal of finding insulin-producing and secreting cells for transplant. **Genetic engineering** now enables us to take cells from the intestine or liver and genetically program them to produce insulin. These specialized cells respond to changes in blood glucose: an increase in blood glucose increases the production and secretion of the hormone, and a decrease in blood glucose decreases the production and secretion of the hormone. If these cells are genetically reprogrammed to produce insulin, they are stimulated by hyperglycemia and inhibited by a lowering of blood glucose. Researchers have demonstrated that this is effective in mice and can cure diabetes in animals—even without anti-rejection drugs. There remains a lot of work to do before this technique can be used on human, of course, but it is all within the realm of the possible!

o   Over the past few years, there has been a great deal of discussion about embryonic stem cells and stem cells from adult human bone marrow. These stem cells have the innate capacity to become any type of mature cell, including insulin-producing pancreatic cells. Experiments in this area have only just begun, but they have been very encouraging.

## 12.  What benefits can diabetes research bring?

It is clear that diabetes represents an immense challenge due to the rapidly increasing frequency of the disease, caused primarily by the aging of the population and the ever-rising number of people who are overweight. Research, however, has brought us new pharmacological and technological advances that can not only control blood glucose but , maybe one day, actually cure the disease and its complications.

Research into diabetes, which involves participation of a number of Canadian researchers, is being carried out all over the world and continues to bring a great deal of hope to people with diabetes.

# Diabetes Follow-up Tools

## 1. How is diabetes "managed"?

Managing diabetes presents a number of challenges. Medical follow-ups, blood glucose self-monitoring, diet, exercise and medication are all important aspects of treatment that people with diabetes have to keep in mind at all times.

It can all seem overwhelming. Diabetes requires people to reconsider their entire lifestyle and make a long-term commitment to managing the condition. Therefore, the easiest way to improve treatment is to take things one step at a time instead of trying to change every habit at once. People should set clear and realistic goals, **congratulate themselves for each goal successfully achieved, and learn from any difficulties they encounter.**

## 2. Are there any tools to help with diabetes follow-up?

People with diabetes have several tools available to help them follow up on their disease. A self-monitoring logbook is obviously essential. Another useful tool is a "journal of personal goals", which should list the goals of the person with diabetes as they relate to five important aspects of the follow-up: medical follow-up, care, diet, medication and well-being. People are advised to select any number of these objectives and rank them in order of priority (for example, from 1 to 5).

It is a good idea to consult this journal from time to time. Checking it periodically can help keep track of progress, understand why some goals are more difficult to reach, determine the means to reach them, or set new objectives. (*See the Model journal on pages 279 to 281.*)

## 3. Is there a tool to help manage diet?

A meal plan drawn up with the aid of a dietician is an essential tool for people with diabetes.

## 4. Which tests and targets help achieve optimal control of diabetes?

Medical follow-up of a person with diabetes includes various tests, including tests for blood glucose, glycosylated hemoglobin (A1C), lipid profile and blood pressure. Remember that glycosylated hemoglobin is used to determine how the blood sugar has been controlled over the last three months.

Target values for the various tests or measurements are presented in the "Targets for optimal control" chart on page 282.

## 5. How are the test results used?

Test results enable a doctor to choose the appropriate treatment for a person with diabetes, to assess its effectiveness, and to make the necessary adjustments. The "Test follow-up journal" (*see page 283*) can be used to keep track of relevant information, including test results. These results enable a person with diabetes to follow the treatment as it evolves and discuss it with the doctor. They can even be used as a motivational tool.

## JOURNAL OF PERSONAL GOALS

What follows is a list of goals relevant to a person with diabetes. Choose the ones that are most important to you (a maximum of 5) and number them according to their priority. Revise the objectives you have chosen periodically.

| DATES | | | | | |
|---|---|---|---|---|---|
| **MEDICAL FOLLOW-UP** | | | | | |
| See the doctor at least twice a year | | | | | |
| Inquire about the results of tests and examinations | | | | | |
| Check blood pressure regularly | | | | | |
| Check microalbuminuria once a year | | | | | |
| See the opthalmologist regularly, as recommended | | | | | |
| **CARE AND RECOMMENDATIONS** | | | | | |
| Enter blood glucose levels in my self-monitoring logbook and analyze them as advised | | | | | |
| In case of illness, check blood glucose levels more often | | | | | |
| Compare readings from the glucose meter with a blood test at least once a year | | | | | |
| Keep carbohydrates within reach at all times (at least two portions of 15 g each) | | | | | |
| Examine my feet every day | | | | | |
| Do not smoke | | | | | |
| Do physical activity regularly (everyday if possible) | | | | | |
| Wear a diabetic ID bracelet or pendant | | | | | |

| **DATES** | | | | | |
|---|---|---|---|---|---|
| Inform driving authorities (in Quebec, the Société d'assurance automobile du Québec (SAAQ)) | | | | | |
| **DIET** | | | | | |
| Eat the recommended amount of carbohydrates at each meal | | | | | |
| Eat balanced meals (carbohydrates, proteins, fats) | | | | | |
| Choose fibre-rich foods | | | | | |
| Have evening snacks, as recommended | | | | | |
| Keep regular mealtimes | | | | | |
| Measure food portions from time to time | | | | | |
| Keep a regular food journal | | | | | |
| Eat only fats that are recommended | | | | | |
| Drink alcohol only with food | | | | | |
| **MEDICATION** | | | | | |
| Take medications as prescribed by the doctor | | | | | |
| Know the names of my antidiabetic drugs | | | | | |
| Enter all the antidiabetic drugs I take and any changes of dosage in the self-monitoring logbook | | | | | |
| Keep a complete and up-to-date list of all drugs (names, doses) and bring it to all medical appointments | | | | | |
| Follow the insulin adjustment rules | | | | | |
| Know the best times to take the drugs | | | | | |

| DATES | | | | | |
|---|---|---|---|---|---|
| Know how to manage skipped doses of antidiabetic drugs | | | | | |
| Make sure that any antidiabetic drugs or natural health products do not worsen my condition | | | | | |
| **WELL-BEING** | | | | | |
| Identify stress factors with the most effect | | | | | |
| Improve my reaction to stress | | | | | |
| Set aside at least 10 minutes a day for relaxation | | | | | |
| Speak to my support network about my diabetes | | | | | |
| Manage my time in a way that meets my needs | | | | | |
| **MY PERSONAL GOALS** | | | | | |
| | | | | | |
| | | | | | |
| | | | | | |
| | | | | | |
| | | | | | |

Signature: _____

## TARGETS FOR OPTIMAL CONTROL

| Glucose | |
|---|---|
| Glycosylated hemoglobin (A1C) | ≤ 0.070 (≤ 0.060 if possible) |
| Fasting or pre-meal blood glucose | 4 mmol/L – 7 mmol/L<br>(4 mmol/L – 6 mmol/L if possible) |
| Blood glucose 1 to 2 hours after meals | 5 mmol/L – 10 mmol/L<br>(5 mmol/L – 8 mmol/L if possible) |
| **Lipid Profile** | |
| LDL Cholesterol | ≤ 2.0 mmol/L |
| Total cholesterol / HDL Cholesterol | < 4 |
| Triglycerides | < 1.5 mmol/L |
| **Kidneys** | |
| Albumin/creatinine ratio | M: < 2.0 mg/mmol; W: < 2.8 mg/mmol |
| Microalbuminuria | < 20 µg/min or < 30 mg/day |
| **Others** | |
| Blood pressure | ≤ 130/80 mm Hg |
| Normal weight | < 65 years old: BMI* 18.5 – 24.9<br>≥ years old: BMI 18.6 – 29.9 |
| Waist | M: < 102 cm; W: < 88 cm |

* BMI: body mass index (weight in kg/height in m²)

Name: _____

## TEST FOLLOW-UP JOURNAL

| Date | | | | | | | |
|---|---|---|---|---|---|---|---|
| Weight (kg) | | | | | | | |
| Height (m) | | | | | | | |
| BMI (kg/m²) | | | | | | | |
| Waist circumference (cm) | | | | | | | |
| Blood pressure (≤ 130/80 mm Hg) | | | | | | | |
| Blood glucose (blood test) Before meal: 4 mmol/L – 7 mmol/L (4 mmol/L – 6 mmol/L if possible) | | | | | | | |
| After meal: 5 mmol/L – 10 mmol/L (5 mmol/L – 8 mmol/L if possible) | | | | | | | |
| Glycosylated hemoglobin (A1C) (≤ 0.070 or ≤ 0.060 if possible) | | | | | | | |
| Triglycerides (< 1.5 mmol/L) | | | | | | | |
| LDL Cholesterol (≤ 2.0 mmol/L) | | | | | | | |
| HDL Cholesterol M ≥ 1.0 mmol/L W ≥ 1.3 mmol/L | | | | | | | |
| Total cholesterol / HDL Cholesterol (< 4) | | | | | | | |
| Albumin: creatinin ratio M < 2.0 mg/mmol W < 2.8 mg/mmol) | | | | | | | |
| Microalbuminuria (< 20 µg/min ou < 30 mg/day) | | | | | | | |
| Creatinine clearance (>1.5 mL/s) | | | | | | | |

# Annexe

## BLOOD GLUCOSE CONVERSION CHART

| mmol/L* | mg/dL** | mmol/L | mg/dL |
|---------|---------|--------|-------|
| 1.4 | 25 | 11.2 | 202 |
| 1.6 | 29 | 11.6 | 209 |
| 1.8 | 32 | 12.0 | 216 |
| 2.0 | 36 | 12.4 | 223 |
| 2.4 | 43 | 12.8 | 230 |
| 2.8 | 50 | 13.2 | 238 |
| 3.2 | 58 | 13.6 | 245 |
| 3.6 | 65 | 14.0 | 252 |
| 4.0 | 72 | 14.4 | 259 |
| 4.4 | 79 | 14.8 | 266 |
| 4.8 | 86 | 15.2 | 274 |
| 5.2 | 94 | 15.6 | 281 |
| 5.6 | 101 | 16.0 | 288 |
| 6.0 | 108 | 16.4 | 295 |
| 6.4 | 115 | 16.8 | 302 |
| 6.8 | 122 | 17.2 | 309 |
| 7.0 | 126 | 17.6 | 317 |
| 7.2 | 130 | 18.0 | 324 |
| 7.6 | 137 | 18.5 | 333 |
| 8.0 | 144 | 19.0 | 342 |
| 8.4 | 151 | 19.5 | 351 |
| 8.8 | 158 | 20.0 | 360 |
| 9.2 | 166 | 20.5 | 369 |
| 9.6 | 173 | 21.0 | 378 |
| 10.0 | 180 | 21.5 | 387 |
| 10.4 | 187 | 22.0 | 396 |
| 10.8 | 194 | 22.5 | 405 |

Target values before meals and at bedtime (shaded region: 4.0/72 to 7.0/126)

\* mmol/L x 18 = mg/dL

\*\* mg/dL ÷ 18 = mmol/L